A Concise Encyclopaedia of Psychiatry

A Concise Encyclopaedia of Psychiatry

Edited by

Denis Leigh MD BSc FRCP
The Maudsley Hospital, London

C. M. B. Pare MD FRCP DPM
St Bartholomew's Hospital, London

John Marks MA MD MRCP FRCPath
Downing College, Cambridge

MTP

The *Concise Encyclopaedia of Psychiatry* is based upon a series of publications originally sponsored and issued under the Roche Continuing Medical Education Campaign. (The contributors to the original series are listed at the end of the book.) The Publishers would like to thank Roche Products Ltd for their kind permission to reproduce the material from this series, which has now been revised and up-dated by the editors.

Published by
MTP Press Ltd
St Leonard's House
Lancaster, England

ISBN 0 85200144-4

Printed in Great Britain by R. & R. Clark, Ltd, Edinburgh

Subject Classification

To assist readers, general accounts of the basic principles of key topics are included, viz.

For the central nervous system active drugs there are descriptions of the properties of groups (in the main text) and individual insertions according to the generic names (in an Appendix). The most widely internationally used trade names (indicated R) are given after the generic names but trade names are not accorded separate insertions. In any such compendium a selection has to be made of groups of drugs that are included. We have included drugs with psychotropic action (neuroleptics, tranquillizers and antidepressants); sedatives and hypnotics; narcotic analgesics and drugs with abuse liability. Non-narcotic analgesics and antiepileptics have been excluded.

Preface

Psychiatry is a discipline that crosses many frontiers, involving a knowledge of the anatomy, physiology and biochemistry of the nervous system, of general medicine, of sociology, of psychology, of the law and of all those subjects which comprise the behavioural sciences. Moreover, in the field of psychiatry the explosion of knowledge has led to an increase in specialization in sub-disciplines.

To all those interested in psychiatry this diversity causes real problems. They may have to consult a wide variety of sources before finding the answer to what may be in fact a relatively simple question.

This encyclopaedia aims at providing straightforward answers to the many questions that may arise. The editors wish to stress that this is not intended to be an advanced treatise on the minutiae of the subject. There will be entries with the contents of which some experts may disagree; others which may seem to err on the side of simplicity or of dogmatism. For whatever imperfections there may be, the editors take full responsibility. They hope that no major topics have been omitted and that the coverage is sufficiently comprehensive as to provide the reader, whether he be directly involved in psychiatry or not, with a useful and practical guide to the subject.

Abortion

The law relating to abortion differs from one country to another. In some countries to induce any abortion is illegal, while in others abortions are freely permitted. A typical compromise position defining therapetic grounds for abortion is that a pregnancy may be terminated if two registered medical practitioners are of the opinion that (a) continuance of the pregnancy would endanger the life of the pregnant woman or constitute a serious threat to the physical or mental health of that woman or any existing children of her family or (b) that there was a substantial risk that the child, if born, would suffer from a serious mental or physical handicap. Differing views exist on whether one of the doctors should be a psychiatrist. The indications for abortion on psychiatric grounds are as wide or as narrow as the prejudices of the psychiatrist concerned. Schizophrenia, paranoid psychoses, affective psychoses, severe psychopathy or gross immaturity; all these diagnostic categories may constitute adequate grounds for termination.

The more difficult and common problem is the woman whose distress is a direct reaction to the pregnancy, commonly the young single girl and the elderly multipara. In the young girl the psychiatrist has to assess her ability to cope with the pregnancy, with or without support from her family, and the effect of continuation of the pregnancy on her future mental health. In the elderly married multipara the problem is not so much the pregnancy as her ability to bear the burden of another child. Mild symptoms of tension or depression increasing in severity and duration as the family increases, and adverse social and marital conditions are all factors which may together justify termination of pregnancy and sterilization.

Methods of termination have changed considerably in recent years: (a) up to twelve weeks vacuum curettage is the optimal method; (b) from twelve to sixteen weeks the alternatives are hysterotomy or hysterectomy; (c) after sixteen weeks the options are hysterectomy or extraction of amniotic fluid through the abdominal wall and its replacement with 20% saline; the last method, though efficacious, carries the risk of introducing hypertonic saline into the mother's circulation.

Follow-up studies have shown that termination of pregnancy rarely results in psychiatric symptoms of more than temporary duration, provided that the woman really wants the operation. On the other hand refusal of termination may result in long-term mental ill-health involving hospitalization. A considerable proportion of mothers who continue the pregnancy and remain medically well still regret that termination was not carried out and show evidence of rejecting the child. Scandinavian studies suggest that children of pregnancies for which termination was requested show a much higher incidence of delinquency and other psychiatric disturbances than do controls.

Eugenic grounds for abortion apply (a) if the mother has already given birth to a mongol or phenylketonuric child, or (b) the mother has been infected with rubella in the first three months of pregnancy, or (c) the mother carries or is suspected of carrying a dominant pathogenic gene, e.g. Huntington's chorea.

Habitual abortion has been related to the woman's unconscious rejection of pregnancy, or of the unborn foetus. It is more likely to be due to somatic factors – anatomical disorder or endocrine imbalance.

Abreaction
(Synonym: Catharsis)

This is the process of bringing to consciousness material which has been made unconscious, usually by the mental mechanism of repression (q.v.). Abreaction includes not only the intellectual aspect of recollection of forgotten memories and experiences, but also their reliving and re-enacting with appropriate emotional expression and discharge. The method used to achieve the end result of abreaction is termed catharsis.

Catharsis, from the Greek, meaning to purge, describes the process, and was a term first introduced by Breuer to describe the emotional discharge occurring during a course of hypnotic treatment. The cathartic method was used in the first case treated by Breuer and Freud. Firstly, the revival of forgotten memories without the expression and discharge of

the appropriate affect is not likely to be therapeutically beneficial.
Secondly, attempts to obtain abreaction are in general more successful if a special traumatic event has been recent and severe. Catharsis has been used with success in many subjects of 'shell-shock' in war time. Hypnosis (q.v.) may be used, during which the subject is given suggestions to relive the traumatic event. The success of this technique depends on the experience of the therapist and the full co-operation of the subject. The use of intravenous short-acting barbiturates in subhypnotic doses, which may be combined with methedrine, is more reliable. Catharsis by ether inhalation in subanaesthetic doses is still held by many to be the most successful in the production of an excitatory abreaction. Abreaction by hallucinogenic drugs, e.g. LSD is now less frequently used.

Abstinence syndrome
(withdrawal symptoms)

This term is applied to the syndrome which occurs in a drug-dependent person when the drug is withheld. Such syndromes have specific clinical features related to states of physical dependence such as occur in opiate type dependence and severe varieties of barbiturate (q.v.) and alcohol (q.v.) dependence. Psychic symptoms relating to psychological dependence occur in all varieties of drug dependence and generally are characterized by subjective distress and craving. Treatment includes either continuation of the drug or replacement by an acceptable substitute and the use of tranquillizers. SEE ALSO Addiction and Withdrawal symptoms.

Abulia

Abulia is the absence of will power. It is usually seen in the less pronounced form – hypobulia. There is an inability to reach and act on decisions. It is a common complaint in depressive illness and has to be differentiated from the indecisiveness which may be observed in the obsessional patient.

Acalculia

Calculation is a complex process involving memory, attention, concentration and the capacity to abstract and think in symbolic terms. Number manipulation is impaired in general disturbances of brain function, e.g. delirium, senile dementia. A specific inability to calculate may be associated with finger agnosia, right-left disorientation, and dysgraphia. This is known as Gerstmann's syndrome (q.v.).

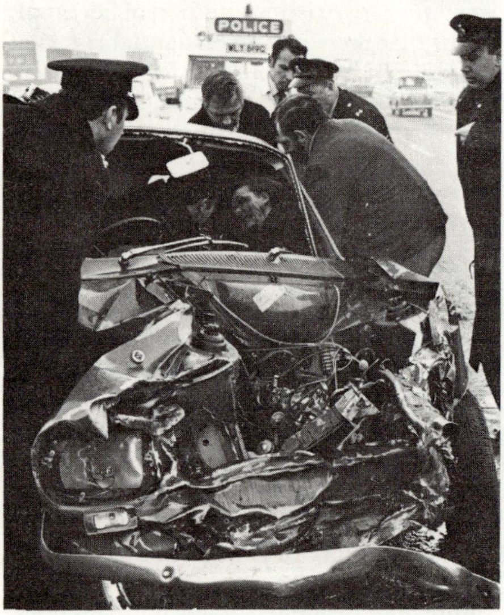

Accident proneness

The majority of accidents (work and motor) affect only a small percentage of the labour force and this same group tends to be involved in multiple accidents. While the emotional state of the individual at the time is important and many vehicle accidents are thought to result from the driver being in a mood of angry frustration, yet the personality is probably the important predisposing factor. The typical accident-prone subject is young, male, impulsive, concentrating on short-term goals and satisfactions. He likes danger, dislikes planning, is a guilty rebel who is perhaps unconsciously provoking accidents to express rebellion and atone for guilt. Fatigue, hunger and anoxia are physiological factors tending to impair judgement and motor co-ordination. In women accidents tend to occur in the pre-menstrual phase, probably correlated with the tension and irritability experienced at this time. Management in industry consists in identifying predisposed subjects and appropriately altering the job requirements.

Acetylcholine

Acetylcholine (ACh) is the chemical transmitter of the parasympathetic nervous system, of sympathetic ganglia and the neuro-muscular junction. It is also widely distributed in the brain where there is good evidence that it is the transmitter of the reticular activating (arousal) system, in the basal ganglia, in the cerebral cortex and is probably concerned in pain sensibility. It appears to act in all sites as an excitatory transmitter.

There are two different modes of action (involving different receptors) – muscarinic (blocked by atropine) and nicotinic (blocked by curare). Interference with the brain ACh system (atropine, hallucinogenic glycol esters) leads to a psychotic state which is different from the state produced by LSD with features of delirium (q.v.), with disorientation (q.v.) and clouding of consciousness (q.v.).

Much less is known of the relevance of brain acetylcholine to psychiatry than in the case of the monoamines (q.v.). However, the addictive action of nicotine suggests that nicotinic receptors are important in the brain. Many psychotropic drugs (e.g. the tricyclic anti-depressants) have atropine-like properties, which lead to annoying side effects, such as blurred vision and a dry mouth. Abnormal balance between the opposing actions of dopamine and acetylcholine in the basal ganglia probably account for the clinical manifestations of Parkinson's (q.v.) and Huntington's chorea (q.v.). ACh is inactivated at the synapse by hydrolysis by the enzyme – acetylcholine esterase. Blockers of this enzyme – e.g. the nerve gas DFP – also cause a delirious psychosis.
SEE ALSO Synapse – transmission in.
For brief account of importance SEE Biochemical and neurophysiological background to mental disease.

Acetylcholinesterase

The enzyme which inactivates acetylcholine in the synaptic cleft.
SEE ALSO Acetylcholine, and for a general description SEE ALSO Biochemical and neurophysiological background to mental disease.

Acridan derivatives

One of the groups of tricyclic antidepressant compounds. The only representative of the group in current clinical use is dimethacrine (q.v.).

Acrocephaly

A skeletal deformity caused by a dominant gene in which there is an abnormally high or pointed head. This is usually associated with mental defect. Also known as oxycephaly, hypsicephaly, turricephaly, steeplehead, and towerhead.

Acromegaly

Excessive secretion of growth hormone, usually due to a tumour of the acidophil cells of the anterior pituitary. Amenorrhoea and loss of libido are very common symptoms and many patients are mildly or moderately depressed. The psychological changes can be regarded as a reaction to a troublesome chronic disease, but in some patients affective disturbance occurs early in the illness.

Acrophobia

Fear of heights. The request for psychiatric treatment for this fear is sometimes occasioned by social changes, such as removal to a high block of flats rather than by increased fear. Visual perceptual factors influence the intensity of fear; it is usually harder to walk downstairs towards a receding spatial edge than upstairs.
SEE ALSO Phobia.

Acting out

Acting out is a term often applied to the unreasonable use of the motor aspects of emotion, although technically it is the evocation of inappropriate behaviour patterns during the course of psychotherapy. Acting out in the transference involves the projection of the patient's attitudes toward his therapist on to other persons in his environment; instead of expressing hostility to the therapist, the patient might, for example, act out towards his wife or his boss.

Action potential

The electrical charge which is associated with the transmission of impulses along a nerve fibre. It depends upon ionic interchanges across the membrane on the surface of the nerve.
SEE ALSO Nerve fibre transmission.

Acute confusional state

(Synonyms: Acute brain syndrome; acute delirium)

Literally a state of disorder. In psychiatry it is limited to the syndrome secondary to clouding of consciousness from organic disorders of the brain. It is characterized by impairment of comprehension, orientation and memory and these intellectual defects are associated with emotional instability.
The patient's impaired comprehension of incoming perceptions leads to disorientation in time and place, his memory for events during his illness is profoundly impaired and these with his impaired comprehension of events going on around him may lead to illusions and delusional misinterpretations. These symptoms are associated with marked affective changes, usually of fear but sometimes of depression or even euphoria. Characteristically there are marked fluctuations in the mental state, symptoms usually being worse in the evening when tiredness and failing daylight decrease the impact of incoming perceptions. In contrast the patient may be temporarily improved by vigorously arousing his attention. Restlessness and insomnia are prominent, making management difficult and leading to exhaustion.
In distinguishing these states from dementia the acute onset and the fluctuations in the mental state are the most important features. When lucid the patient's intellect may be found to be intact and his memory, except for the period of his illness, good. The EEG shows prominent bilaterally synchronous slow wave activity. The prognosis depends on the underlying condition of which febrile illness, cardiac failure and intoxication with alcohol or drugs are the commonest.
In acute psychoses, the patient's perplexity and inattention may simulate an acute confusional state. Sudden removal of visual cues, as in the 'patch delirium' of ophthalmic patients or after transfer to unfamiliar surroundings, may precipitate confusion but in such cases an underlying arteriosclerotic or senile dementia should be suspected.
Treatment should be directed to the underlying disorder. Restlessness may be controlled with phenothiazine drugs such as chlorpromazine. In delirium tremens the benzodiazepines or chlormethiazole are preferred.
SEE ALSO Clouding of consciousness, Delirium.

Adaptation disorders

Pre-school behaviour problems in the areas of feeding, sleeping and response to frustration are also termed 'management problems'. Although, because there is an absence of physical aetiology, they are often regarded as of rather minor importance, there is nothing trivial in symptoms which can produce quite severe parental depression or lay the foundations for long-standing difficulties in parent-child relationships.
Even before children are born, their parents have expectations about how they will behave derived from memories of their own childhood, their observations of their friends' children, and other sources. Parents are often unprepared for the individuality their children may show; yet in the process of mutual parent-child adaptation that occurs between birth and school entry the temperament of the child may be as important a factor as the personality of the parent. Most important of

all is the capacity of the parents to be sensitive to the child's needs and feelings, and flexible in their handling. Flexibility does not mean permissiveness. Indeed, an important aspect of flexible child rearing involves awareness of situations where children require firm control. Nor does flexibility mean the parents should sacrifice the convenience of their own lives to that of their children. It does involve ability to recognize when a child's biological make-up does not allow him to fit easily into the routine his parents require and to alter the situation accordingly.

Obesity is a more common symptom in western society than malnutrition, yet mothers are more frequently concerned about under than overfeeding. In the absence of physical illness, mothers can be reassured that young children differ in their need for food considerably. Persistence of the problem calls for understanding why the mother remains dissatisfied although her child is feeding adequately.

Children vary too in the amount of sleep they require. If they wake up in the middle of the night they may cry and demand attention until they get back to sleep. Parents, deprived of their own sleep, may become irritable with the child who may then develop insecurity, aggravating his sleep difficulty. There is no magic answer to this problem. Some children can be 'broken' of the habit of waking if they are left to cry it out, but parents may not wish to do this, especially if the child is frightened. Hypnotics, such as chloral and phenergan, often help to break into the vicious circle of insomnia and irritability, but if used habitually the child may develop tolerance to them. Reassurance to the parents that the child will come to no harm whatsoever through lack of sleep may be helpful in reducing anxiety. Recurrent waking in the night associated with nightmares and excessive nocturnal fear may be associated with a more generalized emotional disorder requiring further investigation.

Undue whining, temper-tantrums, and breath-holding are reactions to frustration which need to be understood in terms of the emotional climate of the home, and the amount of attention the child is deriving from his negative behaviour. In advising about treatment it is important to remember that the child may be receiving a good deal of reward from the mother in the amount of attention she gives to him when he is 'naughty'. It is better for her to ignore him when difficult but reward his good behaviour with her undivided attention.

Addiction

There is no general agreement about the meaning of the word 'addiction'. Medical men stress its physical aspects, sociologists its social aspects and lawyers its legal aspects. Nevertheless the term is so widely used that it is unlikely to be discarded. Because of the difficulties of definition, there is a growing tendency to use the word dependence which has been defined by the World Health Organisation in a way that qualifies each type of dependence by the generic name of the drug involved. These types will be described but their usefulness is often limited by the fact that the majority of drug users employ a multiplicity of drugs to satisfy their personal needs. Basic World Health Organisation definitions include:

Drug: any substance that when taken into the living organism may modify one or more of its functions.

Drug abuse: persistent or sporadic excessive drug use inconsistent with or unrelated to acceptable medical practice.

Drug dependence: a state, psychic and sometimes also physical, resulting from the interaction between a living organism and a drug, characterized by behavioural and other responses that always include a compulsion to take the drug on a continuous or periodic basis in order to experience its psychic effects and sometimes to avoid the discomfort of its absence. Tolerance may or may not be present. A person may be dependent on more than one drug.

Clearly the term 'drug' as defined by the World Health Organisation covers a wide range of substances, but in the field of drug abuse and dependence the drugs involved are those which share the common characteristic of producing a change, usually pleasurable, in the mental state of the taker. These drugs fall into three classes. First, drugs which have a depressant effect on consciousness, these include narcotic analgesics (e.g. opiates and opiate-like drugs) and the hypnosedative drugs (e.g.

barbiturates (q.v.) and non-barbiturate sedatives). Secondly, drugs whose action is primarily stimulant (e.g. amphetamines (q.v.), amphetamine-like drugs and cocaine (q.v.). Thirdly, drugs whose effect is hallucinogenic (q.v.) (e.g. LSD, psilocybin and mescalin). Cannabis (q.v.) is often included in this group, though strictly speaking cannabis produces its own pattern of dependence and abuse.

The World Health Organisation definition of dependence, though succinct, requires elaboration. A distinction is made between *physical and psychological dependence*, and though the distinction may appear to be arbitrary, it has practical uses. Physical dependence is best understood as being the end result of presumably neurobiochemical change, no doubt transient, possibly prolonged, which creates in the taker a real physical need to continue taking the drug to avoid physically determined abstinence symptoms. Abstinence syndromes are often heavily overlaid with psychologically determined symptoms, but the consensus of opinion favours certain abstinence symptoms with a physical basis, e.g. many opiate withdrawal symptoms and barbiturate withdrawal confusion and convulsions are physically determined. Psychological dependence covers not only subjective pleasure from a drug but also the emotional drives that lead the taker to persist. Also psychological dependence includes the relief of feelings of distress within the taker, e.g. feelings of anxiety, depression or general discontent. Added to this, psychological dependence extends into those extreme degrees of personal involvement in drug use that frequently occur. Such a situation is found when a drug user radically alters his life-style in such a way that his life may come to revolve around drug taking. He spends all his time in the company of drug users who reinforce his dependence and bring about important social changes in him. He adopts a shared value system based on drug use and comes to regard himself as alienated from society not only because of society's apparent rejection of him, but because he comes to overvalue the state of being totally identified with drug use. Thus drug use provides him with a life style and a career, albeit deviant, and a career that is hard to alter.

The drug user may become a member of a subculture of drug users whose behaviour has important consequences for its members and society at large, particularly when they offend against the norms of society. A heightened sense of alienation from society tends to be self-perpetuating and to lead to the rejection of the customary goals, such as earning a living. Special modes of dress and speech may become badges of the subculture – far removed from the drug effects but important consequences. Though they are social consequences they are part of the overall picture of psychological dependence, since membership of such a subculture may meet psychological needs related to drug use.

Tolerance is the action, specific for some drugs, in which it is necessary for the taker to increase dosage in order to achieve the desired effect.

Descriptions of the actions of cannabis and opium go back as far as 2000 BC, but in Britain the history of drug misuse relates to the past two centuries. The abuse of alcohol in the eighteenth and nineteenth centuries is well documented. It showed a decline from the mid nineteenth century following the Temperance Campaign. These reforms were based on social necessity, since alcoholism had become grotesque in its extent, constituting a public and national disgrace.

Drug abuse, of opium and tincture of

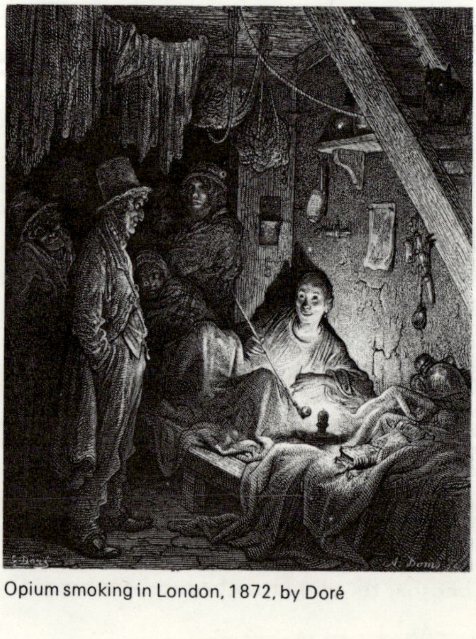

Opium smoking in London, 1872, by Doré

opium (laudanum), dates in England from 1700 when the virtues of opium were described by Dr John Jones. After this, oral opiate preparations became so common in England that by the mid nineteenth century there were very few people who had not taken them. This was particularly true for the poor and thousands of deaths were caused by the use of opiates for ailing children. Many notable literary and public figures were opiate takers.

The invention of the hypodermic needle and syringe provided a more potent method of administration. Morphinism became a fashionable upper class disorder in the nineteenth century. But control of opiate use was achieved by laws, so that by the beginning of the twentieth century – indeed until after World War II – the number of known opiate addicts in the United Kingdom was rarely more than 500. Eighty-five per cent of these were therapeutic addicts using morphine, were middle aged and scattered all over the country, 10% were doctors and nurses and only 5% were non-therapeutic addicts – a special group of deviant people who kept their drug use to themselves.

A dramatic change has occurred in the United Kingdom since the 1950's with the unexpected emergence of a youthful population of non-therapeutic heroin users. It is this change that caused public concern and re-examination of 'the British System' – the system by which any doctor could prescribe narcotics for an addict if he felt that cure of his addiction was impossible. The Brain Committee related the spread of heroin addiction to overprescribing and recommended, amongst other things, the limiting of the prescribing of heroin to specially licensed doctors in the United Kingdom. Different rules apply in other countries. Spread of dependence, however, cannot entirely be explained in terms of 'epidemic spread'. Evidence to date suggests that drug users are likely to show psychiatric and social pathology before drug use.

Drug dependence is a complex disorder related not only to the conditions of modern urban life, but to the further complexities of psychological disturbance. Supposed drug effects need to be regarded cautiously for they are related not only to known pharmacological action, but also to the mood of the taker and his expectations.

PATTERNS OF DRUG DEPENDENCE

1. *Drugs with depressant action*

(a) Narcotic analgesics: Morphine type. The type of dependence produced by these drugs is categorized by the World Health Organisation as *drug dependence, morphine type*. Some drugs included are morphine, diamorphine, methadone, pethidine and all analgesic drugs that are opiate derivatives and synthetic opiate-like drugs.

This type of dependence is characterized by severe physical and psychological dependence and tolerance. This means the user may crave the drug, though this is not inevitable. A characteristic abstinence syndrome occurs when the drug is stopped The symptoms include restlessness, rubbing the face and body, irritability, apprehension, yawning, salivation, nausea, vomiting, abdominal cramps, joint pains, running eyes and nose, diarrhoea, and, in later stages, elevated blood pressure, raised blood sugar and spontaneous ejaculation or orgasm. The dependency-producing potential of these drugs is high – probably the highest of all. The pleasure caused by opiates does not persist and as tolerance increases euphoria decreases. So that the ultimate reason for continuing is the avoidance of withdrawal distress. Initial subjective pleasure and later abstinence distress produce a strong drive to continue. Morphine-like drugs render people passive and inert with the social consequence of failure to function adequately as a social being. Though the hazards of these drugs *per se* are not spectacular (apart from death from overdose), there are very real hazards from unsterile self-injection including abscesses, thrombophlebitis, septicaemia, jaundice, pneumonia, endocarditis and, rarely, tetanus and malaria. Also there are the major social hazards of drug use as a way of life, associated with the criminality and inertia. An impressive catalogue.

(b) Barbiturate type. Properly speaking, alcohol is included here since dependence on alcohol and barbiturates are very similar. Under barbiturate type dependence are included dependence on non-barbiturates, sedatives, hypnotics and tranquillizers. This type of dependence when mild is mainly psychological – probably most commonly seen in the person who has been taking doses of say 300 mg of a barbiturate nightly for years and who cannot stop. If a dose of 700 mg of barbiturate per 24 hours is exceeded for a period of over six weeks, the taker is likely to become physically dependent. This leads to chronic intoxication (ataxia, dysarthria and nystagmus). Mild symptoms of physical dependence include nausea, dizziness, orthostatic hypotension and trembling. The major hazard of physical dependence is the appearance of barbiturate withdrawal fits. These can be fatal if vomit is inhaled. Also states of confusion and delirium may occur.

2. *Stimulant drugs*

(a) Cocaine type. Psychological dependence is often severe. There is no physical dependence and true tolerance does not occur. The subjective stimulant effect is often highly valued and large quantities may be taken. Psychotic excitement with hallucinosis and paranoid content can occur.
(b) Amphetamine type. May be caused by all amphetamines and amphetamine-like drugs. It is characterized usually by fairly severe psychological dependence and the slow development of tolerance. There is no physical dependence. Excitement, hilarity, restless irritability and repetitive overactivity are often found, as are outbursts of aggression and depressed mood when the drug is stopped. A serious hazard is the amphetamine psychoses which is schizophrenic in form and characterized by paranoid content, loosely held fleeting delusions and hallucinations. The euphoria of amphetamine taking is short lived as tolerance grows and higher doses are needed. Self-criticism may be impaired by amphetamines thus leading to antisocial acts.

3. *Hallucinogenic drugs*

The most commonly used hallucinogen is lysergic acid diethylamiamide (LSD) (q.v.). Other commonly used preparations include psilocybin (q.v.), mescalin (q.v.), dimethyl tryptamine (DMT) (q.v.) and Ditran.
Dependence on hallucinogens is entirely psychological, physical dependence does not occur. Psychological dependence often leads to radical alteration of life style. Tolerance to LSD and psilocybin occurs but develops only slowly with mescalin. Hallucinogenic activity is stressed but in fact is not the main action of this group. Emotional changes are far more marked and include feelings of ecstasy, anxiety, terror, nameless dread, even depression. These are often followed by perceptual changes including not only true hallucinations, but also distorted perceptions in the visual, auditory and tactile spheres. A feeling of cosmic revelation is often described, of a sense of awareness of metaphysical union with the universe etc. – these effects are often found and highly valued by the user. It is likely that a consequence of such experiences is that the user overvalues the effects, sometimes with disastrous social consequences to himself and family. Adverse reactions to hallucinogens are well described, particularly following LSD. These include periods of intense psychotic excitement – often schizophrenic in form – also depressed mood, prolonged anxiety reactions and persistent feelings of unreality (depersonalization).

4. *Cannabis dependence* (q.v.)

No physical dependence occurs, there is no tolerance, but severe degrees of psychological dependence may be found. In these latter there is a strong drive to continue taking the drug. There is no unequivocal evidence of permanent damage following long-term cannabis usage, but states of chronic cannabis intoxication are associated with deteriorated social behaviour, apathy, indolence and inertia. The heavy user becomes preoccupied with cannabis effects to the exclusion of all else. Short-lived psychotic states with paranoid content have been described though there is disagreement as to whether or not they are cannabis related or released by cannabis. The effects of cannabis in mild concentration are those of hilarity, jocularity, a carefree attitude and flippancy. On these grounds some regard it as a harmless intoxicant. But this ignores the real states of psychological dependence that can occur. There is no pharmacological reason linking cannabis to progression to other drugs, but social links may be present by association.

There is much evidence linking drug dependence with pre-existing severe personality disorders. Also many American studies link drug dependence with social pathology – social and material deprivation blocked opportunity and membership of low status racial minority groups. This combination of social and personal pathology provides fertile soil for development of dependence. In the United Kingdom recent research shows a high incidence of personality disorders in opiate users but no clear pattern of social pathology is noted. It is found in all social classes and a wide range of family backgrounds, though the presence of parental alcoholism, psychiatric disorders, delinquency and separation is noted in a minority. A minority of drug users appear to develop their dependence against a background of pre-existing anxiety or depression relieved by the drug. Men outnumber women in the ratio 5:1. The links of drug dependence with criminality, though demonstrable, are not easily defined.

The diagnosis of drug dependence is based on history and examination. Supportive evidence of drug dependence includes the finding of injection marks, needle tracks, thrombophlebitis, abscesses, ulcers from self-injection and sometimes abstinence symptoms.

Final proof that the drug is being taken is achieved by thin layer or gas chromatographic examination of the urine. Urine should be collected whenever the patient is seen.

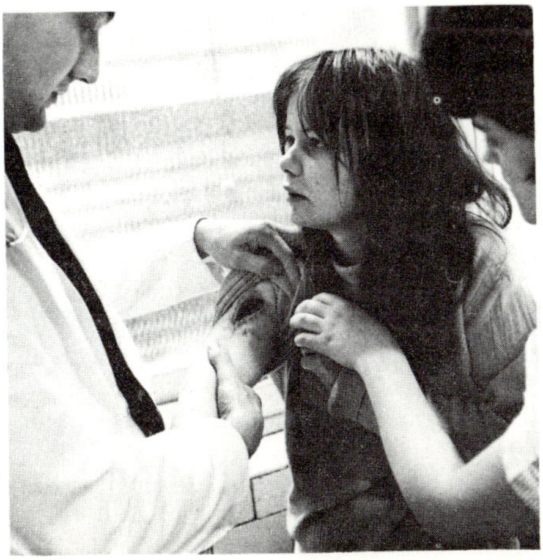

Consequences of non-sterile injection

The ultimate goal of treatment is total abstention from drugs based on total social and psychological rehabilitation. This is so often a near impossibility to achieve that many regard total abstention as a primary treatment goal as unrealistic whilst acknowledging it as an ultimate goal. Relapse rates are very high in the first six months (90%), but follow-up studies in the United States of America suggest that heroin users may show a remission rate of up to 30% at five years.

With this in mind initial treatment is often directed at the medical and psychiatric complications of drug dependence. Long-term support is then aimed at gradual re-education to more stable habits of living, and ultimately to total abstention. The most difficult task is to get the user to realize the real dangers of drug dependence and to accept a drug-free life as worthwhile. Withdrawal from drugs and abstinence syndromes are easily treated in hospital. With opiate dependence, methadone is the most useful substitution drug because of its slow excretion and prolonged action. Withdrawal programmes vary according to preference of individual doctors, but most use methadone with or without tranquillizers. Some employ intramuscular heroin for a few days at the beginning of withdrawal. Phenothiazines are not without hazard as they may cause barbiturate withdrawal fits where barbiturate use is undetected. The opiate user who arrives in a surgery or casualty department with abstinence distress is best treated with oral or intramuscular methadone. Withdrawal from barbiturates carries the special hazard of withdrawal convulsions. In practice the simplest regime is to maintain the patient in a state of intoxication to the level characterized by slight dysarthria. Medication consists of pentobarbitone in divided doses every four hours and the dose is reduced by 100 mg every day. During any withdrawal the patient will need adequate feeding, rehydration and vitamin supplements.

Barbiturate-induced delirium is usually treated by temporary re-intoxication though this is not necessarily successful. Withdrawal from amphetamines should be abrupt. This is usually followed by prolonged sleep, after which the patient is usually depressed and irritable. Weight gain is rapid with the return of appetite.

Cocaine withdrawal is managed in the same way.

The main serious problems of withdrawal are found where there is physical dependence. This is not to minimize the pleadings, cravings and frank belligerence that often go with psychological dependence.

The most difficult problems are encountered after withdrawal. These consist in the problem of maintaining abstention. Drugs provide for the user a ready escape from the problems of everyday life, an escape which is for the user too often far more effective and immediate than many treatment methods, however sophisticated they may be. Where dependence is a symptom of an underlying depression the outlook should be better for relief of depression should reduce drug-seeking drives, but such cases are not common. The bulk of patients are suffering from personality disorders, and will initially have used drugs for pleasure or as a barrier between themselves and the difficulties of existence, so that the problem becomes one of treating a personality disorder – not an area of resounding psychiatric success. Compulsory admission may be life saving, but its universal application though superficially attractive may be a euphemism for imprisonment.

At the present time there is considerable interest in the use of former drug users in the rehabilitation of the addict. There is increasing evidence that this may be a valuable manoeuvre. Patients put in a drug-free environment and put under strong pressure to abstain, appear to respond more favourably if the pressure is exerted by former drug users. This form of rehabilitation based on self-help by reformed addicts has shown promising results in special communities in America. The former drug addict knows well the self-deceptions etc. that drug users employ and can confront the patient with these in dramatic fashion. In such communities the new entrant is given a low role and status, and is soon made aware that he has to contribute to the community and is responsible for his actions and feelings. Group encounter sessions are used and vigorous interaction is the rule. These approaches though lengthy and expensive offer promising methods of total rehabilitation. Conventional psychiatric approaches, individual and group therapy have to date not been of any lasting value. The free use of tranquillizers and anti-depressants for drug users carries the real hazard of further abuse.

A totally different approach to opiate addiction has been adopted in the United States by Dole and Nyswander. This discards a psychogenic view of drug dependence and emphasizes the importance of long-term physical dependence. Methadone is used as a pharmacological blocking agent, to reduce craving and to prevent euphoria should an opiate be taken. The method has had good results in America in centres where recidivist users maintained on methadone have been enabled to live productive and socially acceptable lives. Also the methadone programmes encourage group morale giving the user the sense of belonging to a successful venture, so that social forces play their part in the rehabilitation as well.

It is likely that in the future, pharmacological blocking agents will play an increasing part in the treatment of all varieties of drug dependence. Until then, rehabilitation of drug users should profitably include a wide range of methods.

There is little information about the rehabilitation of barbiturate and amphetamine users. Common experience suggests that severe barbiturate dependence is very difficult to treat. Amphetamine abuse also presents difficulties – the drug is attractive and relatively easily obtainable. Motivation to abstain tends to be low.

Heroin dependence may be self-limiting – the user no longer achieves euphoria with the passage of time and relies on it to avoid abstinence distress. Ageing brings psychological maturity and increasing awareness of the hazards of drug use. Therefore a patient with a relatively recent history may show less motivation to abstain than a patient with a much longer history. But this should not deter from vigorous attempts at treatment.

Drug dependence is a chronic and relapsing disorder, and the treatment of such disorders is commonplace in medicine and psychiatry. Thus, while long-term support and supervision may appear to be limited as goals – they remain for the drug user the most practical way of helping him until he is capable of achieving more fundamental degrees of change.

In the United Kingdom the maintenance

prescribing of heroin and cocaine is limited to licensed doctors. Prescribing heroin is fundamentally a social rather than a strictly medical measure, and this treatment approach is currently being evaluated. In general, however, it is unwise to prescribe dependence-producing drugs for addicts – the exceptions being the use of methadone to relieve opiate abstinence distress and the prescription of barbiturates in an emergency to the severely barbiturate intoxicated patient. This last measure will prevent withdrawal convulsions.

A recent United Nations Convention in Vienna considered the dependence-producing potential of psychotropic substances. Its main aim was to achieve international co-operation to combat their abuse. The Convention, which needs ratification by the member nations, sets up four different control regimes with graduated control measures including import and export restrictions, licensing arrangements at manufacturing and distribution levels, special labelling and careful record keeping. Four corresponding schedules based upon the therapeutic value and abuse liability of the drugs were defined. Provision is made for inclusion of new drugs on the advice of the Commission on Narcotic Drugs.

The existing schedules are shown in the table. The greatest abuse risk and the greatest control is in Schedule I and the least in Schedule IV.

Although these substances have been currently categorized, it appears that many other psychotropic drugs exhibit psychological dependence when given for prolonged periods in high dosage. It is probably wise to regard all central nervous system acting drugs as potential dependence producing, with those placed in the schedules having the highest risk element.

List of substances in recent United Nations Convention schedules

International non-proprietary name or other trivial name	Schedule
DET	I
DMHP	I
DMT	I
Lysergide LSD, LSD–25	I
Mescaline	I
Parahexyl	I
Psilocin, psilotsin	I
Psilocybin	I
STP, DOM	I
Tetrahydrocannabinols, all isomers	I
Amphetamine	II
Dexamphetamine	II
Methamphetamine	II
Methylphenidate	II
Phencyclidine	II
Phenmetrazine	II
Amobarbital	III
Cyclobarbital	III
Glutethimide	III
Pentobarbital	III
Secobarbital	III
Amferpramone	IV
Barbital	IV
Ethchlorvynol	IV
Ethinamate	IV
Meprobamate	IV
Methaqualone	IV
Methylphenobarbital	IV
Methyprylon	IV
Phenobarbital	IV
Pipradrol	IV
SPA	IV

Addison's disease

In Addisonian crises, symptoms of delirium may precede or follow coma. Otherwise the majority of patients with untreated Addison's disease show a mood disturbance: depression (q.v.) or apathy are characteristic, but euphoria (q.v.) sometimes occurs. Some impairment of recent memory is usual. All the psychiatric symptoms improve with adequate replacement treatment.

Adenohypophysis

Otherwise known as the anterior pituitary. Embryologically it is derived from an ectodermal upgrowth from the front of the primitive gut tube termed Rathke's pouch. It is one of the main endocrine glands and in addition to the growth hormone which acts direct on all metabolism the adenohypophysis secretes several trophic hormones, which control the activity of other endocrine glands. The control of the secretion of the hormones from the adenohypophysis depends on releasing hormones (factors) produced in the hypothalamus which reach the adenohypophysis through a portal blood system. Thus the adenohypophysis and much of the endocrine system is under nervous system control, the level of activity depending on a feedback (q.v.) from the circulating hormones and central factors including emotion and sleep.

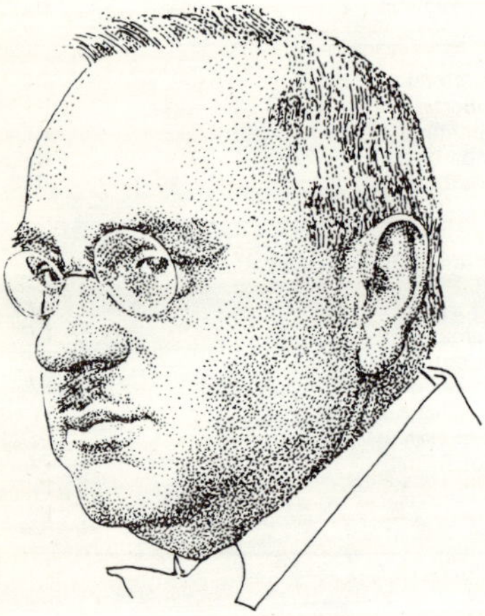

Adler, Alfred (1870–1937)

The founder of individual psychology, Adler is one of the Neo-Freudian analysts who rejected the overriding importance of sexuality and of the libido (q.v.) theory. Adler regarded current environmental influences as of greater significance in the genesis and maintenance of the mental disturbances. He considered that feelings of inferiority (q.v.) determined by genetic, organic and situational factors were of paramount importance and that neuroses or behavioural disorders were the result of the conflict between conscious or unconscious inferiority and overcompensation.
The 'life style' is determined at about 4 years of age, the child's future patterns of behaviour depending upon his relationships with authority figures in his environment. The 'masculine protest' is another Adlerian concept, i.e. that no fundamental difference exists between men and women but that any differences which are found are determined by social and cultural factors. Thus in a male society the female attempts to assert herself, her protest taking many forms, and where conflict arises, results in emotional disturbance. Adler's importance in the history of psychiatry has been much undervalued.
SEE ALSO Inferiority feelings.

Adolescence

The period from the onset of puberty to the achievement of full sexual maturity is one of enormous psychological significance yet, surprisingly, it is a period of life relatively under researched from a psychiatric point of view. Consequently, reliable figures of the incidence and prevalence of adolescent psychiatric disorder are lacking and there is a corresponding absence of information about their natural history and treatment.
Certain well-defined syndromes, schizophrenia, depressive illness, anorexia nervosa, drug addiction etc. which are discussed in more detail elsewhere, are commonly first manifest in adolescence. There are, however, no psychiatric disorders which are peculiar to the period of adolescence, and a discussion of the psychiatry of this age period inevitably centres around the specific life stresses and family patterns which exist, together with the ways in which adolescents react behaviourally to these situations.
Erik Erikson, the American psychoanalyst and anthropologist, considered each age of childhood in terms of the task the child faces and must succeed in completing before he can go on to the next phase. For Erikson, adolescence is the period where a stable concept of self-identity must be achieved. The youngster is concerned about his facial and bodily appearance, his sexual adequacy, his intellectual ability, his capacity to obtain and hold down a job, his attractiveness to the opposite sex. Thus far, his view of himself has been taken over largely from his parents, but now, in the light of his increasing independence, he must come to rely more on his own judgements and that of his age-mates.

Excessive anxiety experienced in any of these areas may result in a focusing of concern upon one particular aspect of functioning (as in the development of hypochondriacal symptoms) or it may result in 'proving' behaviour. Here, the young person reacts to anxiety by over-compensation, performing acts of physical prowess or 'showing off' in a manner calculated to quieten his own fears about his possible inadequacies.

Most adolescents face the crises of this part of their life-history well equipped to deal with them, and manage to surmount them without any long-lasting personality defects. However, certain groups of adolescents are especially vulnerable, and here the degree of emotional turmoil aroused may result in medical referral. Chronic physical illness, for example, may be well tolerated by younger children, whereas during adolescence the patient may, for the first time, come to realise that he is different from others and that life may hold fewer rewards. Juvenile sufferers from diabetes mellitus, epilepsy, asthma, etc. may first show signs of a behaviour disturbance at, or shortly after, puberty. The socially deprived youngster may also first exhibit behaviour disorder at this age. There is an association between delinquency and adverse social factors reflected in a high rate of broken homes, poverty, paternal unemployment, parental rejection, etc. The adverse effects of over-protection may also result in rebellious behaviour, first shown in adolescence. A child who has enjoyed an overclose link with his mother until puberty may react with overt emotional disturbance especially if the parent continues to make efforts to maintain his dependence.

Although the effect of family life on adolescent behaviour usually receives more attention, the reverse effect should not be forgotten. Not infrequently the practitioner is consulted by a middle-aged housewife for symptoms of depression which are found to relate in a straightforward manner to difficulties she is having in coping with or controlling her adolescent children.

Treatment of specific psychiatric syndromes, e.g. anorexia nervosa, schizophrenia, etc., will follow lines described under those headings. The less well-defined syndromes occurring more commonly in the young adolescent need further consideration.

In general the hypochondriacal, inhibited youngster who comes with a specific concern over bodily function can best be helped by being given the opportunity to discuss his worries. A short course of a minor tranquillizer, such as diazepam, may help to tide over a particularly difficult period. The aggressive or antisocial adolescent rarely consults the doctor on his own account and, more commonly, he is brought along by his angry parents or the parents may ask for advice about him in his absence.

In this situation the doctor will help most by remaining impartial, by understanding the parents' feelings of guilt, depression and anger, by stressing the importance of retaining the positive sides of the parent-child relationship even when this is most difficult, and by pointing to the chances of a good final outcome. Only a small minority of juvenile delinquents become adult criminals, although the chances of a young offender developing other social or psychological problems are not insignificant.

SEE ALSO Puberty.

Adoption of children

The need for legal adoption arises mainly as a result of the unmarried mother's inability or unwillingness to look after her child. Rarely, the need for adoption arises in other circumstances, such as when a child has been orphaned, or conceived by a married woman as a result of extramarital intercourse, the husband refusing to accept the child as his own.

The administrative aspects of adoption procedure may be undertaken by a registered adoption society, by a local authority children's department or, in the case of so-called 'third party' adoptions, by an unqualified person who is in touch with both the mother of an unwanted child and the prospective adopters. The advantages of adoption through an official body are numerous. In particular, it is helpful for the unmarried pregnant woman to have a discussion with a skilled social worker before the baby is born, to clarify her feelings about the unborn baby, and its future. The doctor may, when there is no immediate prospect of marriage to the child's father, be involved with the mother in discussions as to whether she should keep her child. There are no hard and fast rules, but in general the doctor does better to listen and to provide information than to give dogmatic advice. The emotional health of the mother is of paramount importance. In determining the mother's mental stability, appraisal of her capacity to form satisfactory relationships outside the family and the amount of realism she shows in thinking of the future are helpful guide-lines.

When application is made to the court for an adoption order by the prospective adoptive parents the magistrate appoints a member of the relevant local authority or a probation officer as 'guardian *ad litem*'. He ensures firstly that the mother's consent has been freely given, and secondly that the adoption as proposed is in the best interests of the child. The guardian *ad litem* has no responsibility to search out the putative father. In deciding whether to agree to the proposed adoption (and it is most unusual for the court to disagree), considerable weight is placed on the report provided by the guardian *ad litem*.

The doctor may be asked to advise about the suitability of a child for adoption, bearing in mind the medical history of the natural mother (and the father if this is known). He may also be asked to provide a report on the health of the baby. Finally, he may be asked to provide a reference for a couple wishing to adopt.

In assessing the natural mother's medical history, it is unusual to be provided with more than sketchy information. However, it is important to remember that the hereditary transmission of conditions such as epilepsy, asthma, diabetes mellitus is not such as to constitute a substantial additional risk to the child. An intellectually dull mother may well have a dull child, but this should not prejudice adoption into a family without academic pretensions.

It is not possible to predict adult intelligence from infant assessment, and examination of the baby as suitable for adoption should be carried out only to exclude physical disease and to ensure that the child is developing within the normal range.

Between 1 and 2% of children are adopted in Great Britain at the present time. Most adoptions are successful, especially when the child has been placed with its adoptive parents before the age of 6 months. Studies of psychiatric disorder in adopted children, however, suggest that the rate of disturbance is at least twice that in a non-adopted group. Adolescence, a time when many children go through crises of personal identity, presents special problems for the adopted child. This is an especially difficult period when the adopting couple have been unable to provide a stable home life or to communicate freely with the child about the special circumstances in which they have become his parents.

Adrenaline (epinephrine)

Adrenaline is the major hormone released from the adrenal medulla. It is also found in the brain. It is synthesized from noradrenaline (q.v.) and is metabolized to metadrenaline (metanephrine) via the enzyme catechol O-methyl transferase (COMT) and thence to hydroxy methoxy mandelic acid (VMA) by the action of the enzyme monoamine oxidase (MAO).

There are two types of receptors in the sympathetic nervous system and of these the β receptors are much more sensitive to adrenaline than are α receptors. By virtue of this activity in the β receptors adrenaline has a wide range of actions including: (a) raising BP by peripheral vaso-constriction, increased heart rate and direct myocardial stimulation; (b) the effects on blood vessels are complicated but importantly blood flow to muscles is increased; (c) smooth muscle may either be relaxed (e.g. bronchial) or constricted (e.g. spleen); (d) metabolic effects which include increased breakdown of glycogen to glucose, and release of free fatty acids. These effects are mediated by the stimulation by adrenaline of the enzyme adenylcyclase which enzyme converts ATP (adenosine triphosphate) to cyclic AMP (adenosine monophosphate). When injected directly into the cerebral vesicles in small doses adrenaline induces excitatory effects including cortical activation (via the reticular formation (q.v.)), emesis, ovulation and stimulation of the motor cortex. Large doses induce stupor and interference with release of antidiuretic hormone and thyrotropic hormone. Differing views still

exist on whether adrenaline or noradrenaline is the prime adrenergic (q.v.) transmitter within the brain.
SEE ALSO Catecholamines and Brain monoamines.

Adrenergic

A term applied to those nerve fibres whose endings liberate noradrenaline (q.v.) or adrenaline (q.v.) as the synaptic transmitter substance. These are predominantly fibres of the sympathetic nervous system, although there is evidence that certain synapses within the central nervous system itself are adrenergic. This particularly applies to some brain stem areas. The cell bodies of the adrenergic tracts are located in the locus ceruleus, the tracts being widely disseminated.
In general terms, adrenergic fibres are those which are concerned with the ergotrophic reactions of the body, i.e. those that are concerned with activity and stress.
SEE ALSO Adrenaline.

Adrenocortical function in depression

In a proportion of depressed patients, especially those with severe endogenous depression (q.v.) a moderate increase in cortisol secretion rate occurs. Plasma cortisol level and urinary corticosteroid excretion are increased. Adrenocortical activity declines to normal during recovery, whether this occurs spontaneously or with treatment.
The increased adrenocortical activity is probably secondary to the change in mood rather than its cause. It is not great enough to produce features of Cushing's syndrome but it may cause subtle biochemical changes.
Recent work has shown that pituitary-adrenal responsiveness to dexamethasone and to insulin-induced hypoglycaemia is much reduced in some depressives. These changes also disappear after recovery. Their significance is unknown, but they also occur in Cushing's syndrome.

Adult training centres

Part of the facilities which can be used to rehabilitate patients. As an extension of occupational therapy departments in large psychiatric hospitals, industrial rehabilitation units were formed where the patient re-learns habits of work, earns money for himself and improves his social contacts. After discharge the patient may have further training or retraining in an occupational centre or government sponsored industrial rehabilitation unit prior to work in protected employment or ordinary industry. In order that the patient's individual requirements are met by these varied services it is essential that a trained social worker is intimately involved.

Aerophagy

Air-swallowing. Often associated with abdominal discomfort, of emotional aetiology. In an effort to belch the patient swallows air into the oesophagus from where it is expelled.

Affect

A person's mood or inner feeling at a given moment, e.g. sadness, happiness or anxiety. Affect may be abnormal in depth, duration or setting (i.e. appropriateness of affect). Disturbances of affect are of course the primary abnormality in endogenous depression and mania but are prominent symptoms in most psychiatric conditions and the main reason for the patient seeking help.

Affective disorders

Disturbances of affect occur in almost every condition known to psychiatry, but this term is restricted to disorders in which the affective disturbance is the primary abnormality from which all the other symptoms are directly or indirectly derived. Logically, anxiety states should be included, but for historical reasons the term is restricted to conditions based on a mood either of sadness or cheerfulness, that is, to the manic (q.v.) illnesses and

the gamut of depressive (q.v.) illnesses. Affective disorders have, or are generally assumed to have, a number of features in common which distinguish them from schizophrenic illnesses and provided the basis for Kraepelin's original division of the functional psychoses into manic depressive psychosis and dementia praecox. Their most important distinguishing feature is their prognosis. Recovery from affective illness is complete; no matter how long the illness lasts or how often it recurs there is no progressive decline in function, no residual defect. It is true that some depressions, and even some manic illnesses, become chronic, but if the depression does ever lift even after many years the underlying personality and intellect are found to be still intact. Their second distinguishing feature is their periodicity. They are lifelong illnesses in the sense that one attack always implies a probability of further attacks, and over a lifetime there is an irregular alternation either between depression and normality, or between depression, mania and normality. Endogenous affective disorders may be divided into unipolar and bipolar groups, the former having recurrent attacks of depression and the latter having attacks of both depression and mania. This division into unipolar and bipolar types of disorder is further justified by their breeding true within families, a difference in sex incidence and in the natural history of the illness (q.v. depression, hypomania).
SEE ALSO Hypomania.

After care for mental patients

Help is often needed to bridge the gap for psychiatric patients between life in hospital and back in the community. This includes helping the patient to find work and shelter, helping him financially and providing convalescent and hostel accommodation. In some countries this may be undertaken by local authorities but in many areas it depends upon local charity efforts.

Aged – Behaviour in and Psychiatric disorders

SEE Psychological changes in normal and abnormal ageing and Geriatric psychiatry.

Aggression

The motor counterpart of the affect of anger, rage or hostility. It is a normal component of a subject's personality, is more pronounced in males than in females and normal variation is considerable; both excessive aggression and an undue lack of assertiveness giving rise to difficulties. Some psychopathic personalities show a marked tendency to aggressive behaviour. A change in a person's aggressivity may be due to a loss of inhibition as with alcohol or in hypomania or an arteriosclerotic dementia. Increased irritability is frequent in depression and paranoid delusions in schizophrenia may lead to aggressive behaviour to innocent people. In children temper tantrums are common, especially in the second year. Aggressive behaviour in later childhood may be a symptom of emotional disturbance.

Aggressive behaviour in the aged

Violent outbursts are often the reason for referral of an elderly patient and require careful diagnosis.

1. *Organic brain syndromes*. Acute confusional states (q.v.) may be accompanied by frightening hallucinations and patchy memory disturbances. Suspicion and uncharacteristic hostility may lead to ill-directed violence. Simple tests of orientation, attention and recent memory and a careful physical examination are indicated. In dementia (q.v.) misinterpretations and the release of underlying paranoid personality traits as a result of the brain damage may lead to violent outbursts when the patient is faced with situations which have become insoluble (catastrophic reactions).
2. *Functional psychoses*. Late paraphrenia (q.v.) can cause aggressive behaviour when an unsuspecting relative or attendant figures in a well-organized delusional system. Manic or hypomanic patients when frustrated may react with violence or abuse.
3. *Emotional crises in the non-psychotic patient*. Diagnosis and management is often difficult. There may be little to suggest psychiatric illness. The personalities of relatives or attendants and the way these interact with that of the patient must be

studied and sources of provocation on both sides assessed. Tranquillizers may be helpful, but a change in the environment may be the solution.

Agitation

This is a state of restlessness usually, but not necessarily, arising out of subjective feelings of apprehension and accompanied by an inability to relax or to concentrate. The subject's behaviour is repetitive and aimless or, if it appears to be purposeful, achieves nothing. Some degree of agitation is a common concomitant of any state of anxiety or tension, regardless of aetiology, though the movements involved are relatively restricted and inconspicuous. The patient taps his foot, adjusts his clothing, fiddles with a pipe or a pencil, shifts his position in his chair, and so on. Severe agitation is less common and is encountered mainly in depressive illnesses, particularly in involutional melancholia (q.v.). Here the whole body is involved, often to such an extent that any sustained task is rendered impossible. The patient is incapable of remaining seated, he gets up, sits down again, paces the room, wrings his hands and repeatedly starts simple tasks which he never completes. Sometimes such behaviour is encountered in the absence of any obvious tension or distress; when this occurs a dementing process, presenile or arteriosclerotic, should be suspected.

The treatment of agitation is mainly that of the underlying illness. Depressive illnesses accompanied by severe agitation usually respond to ECT or tricyclic drugs and there is some evidence that amitriptyline is more effective than imipramine when agitation is conspicuous. In the interim period before the depression is brought under control, and in dementing processes, phenothiazines may be effective in controlling even quite severe agitation while the benzodiazepines, chlordiazepoxide and diazepam are widely used to control the anxiety and mild degrees of agitation so common in less severe depressions. However, occasionally both the phenothiazines and the tricyclic antidepressants may themselves cause agitation of extrapyramidal origin. This akathisia can be controlled, to some extent, by anti-Parkinsonian drugs like orphenadrine or by reducing the dose, but sometimes there is no alternative to stopping the drug.

SEE ALSO Anxiety, Depression, Motor disturbances and Overactivity.

Agnosia

The term 'agnosia', from the Greek 'agnostos' – unknown – was coined in 1891 by Sigmund Freud (q.v.) to describe a failure of recognition.

Agnosia is classified in terms of the sensory channel affected, but implies that sensation itself is unimpaired. *Visual object agnosia* due to lesions in the occipital lobes is an inability to recognize objects which are seen. They may still be recognized in other ways, e.g. by touch. Failure to recognize faces is called 'prosopagnosia', and is often accompanied by paranoid elaboration – mirrors are covered because a strange person is seen behind them. *Auditory agnosia* is a failure to recognize familiar sounds – jingling money, running water – due to lesions in the dominant temporal lobe. *Tactile agnosia* – a parietal sign – is a failure to recognize objects by feel with intact superficial and deep sensibility. Without the latter the loss of recognition is called *astereognosis*. Agnosias are most commonly caused by vascular lesions and are usually complex. 'Pure' cases have been described in association with penetrating wounds of the brain.

Agoraphobia

A distressing disability and relatively common disorder characterized by fear of going out, especially alone. It is often associated with claustrophobic symptoms (q.v.).

Agoraphobia especially affects young women between 20–35 years of age. Neurotic traits, especially dependency and sexual anxieties, are common in contrast to patients with specific phobias such as for cats and dogs. Symptoms may occur at a time of general stress or following some emotional event when the phobia may represent a more underlying fear of the effect of 'going too far' in a sexual sense or in other ways symbolize a more fundamental insecurity.

The onset of an attack is usually sudden but the regularity of attacks and the development of a disabling inability to go to work or even to the nearby shops may take several months. The disability may last indefinitely, often fluctuating in severity, and is characterized by a well marked avoidance behaviour.
Treatment is aimed at encouraging the patient to *approach* the difficult situations and eventually to enter them without anxiety. Supportive or interpretive psychotherapy (q.v.), behaviour therapy (q.v.), either by flooding (q.v.) or desensitization (q.v.) and drugs are all useful. Tranquillizers and antidepressants may both be helpful, some authorities claiming that the monoamine oxidase inhibitors are particularly beneficial.
SEE ALSO Phobia.

Agyria
(Synonym: Lissencephaly)

A developmental defect with absence of brain convolutions. Severe mental defect occurs.

Air encephalography

Air may be introduced into the ventricles indirectly via lumbar puncture, pneumoencephalography, or directly through a burr hole, ventriculography. Pneumoencephalography is carried out with the patient sitting. At lumbar puncture cerebrospinal fluid is replaced a few millilitres at a time with injected air which passes upwards and enters the ventricular system. This procedure always carries a risk in the presence of raised intracranial pressure through the possibility of herniation of the brain into the foramen magnum and should only be performed in the absence of suspected raised intracranial pressure. If raised intracranial pressure is present ventriculography is carried out by a minor surgical procedure introducing air directly. Air once present in the ventricles can be positioned by moving the patient's head to outline the various parts of the ventricular system on radiographs. Headaches and nausea are common sequelae and the patient should remain flat in bed with analgesics and anti-emetics unless raised pressure is suspected, when the head should be elevated.

Akathisia

The term 'akathisia', literally 'inability to sit', was used by Bing to describe the minor restlessness, small changes of position and tendency to rise and sit again (*impatience musculaire*) seen in the otherwise immobile Parkinsonian patients in the wake of the epidemic encephalitis which followed the first world war. Like many of the features of post-encephalitic Parkinsonism, the symptom is now also encountered as a side effect of the major tranquillizers (q.v.) – particularly piperazine phenothiazines (q.v.) and butyrophenones (q.v.) – and occasionally with the tricyclic anti-depressants (q.v.). The patient complains of inner uneasiness or tension, and is seen hopping from foot to foot when standing or simply walking aimlessly about. It should be suspected as a sign of toxicity rather than mental agitation when restlessness associated with Parkinsonian features emerges during treatment. Treatment is by withdrawal or reduction of dose of the drug implicated and substitution of a non-piperazine phenothiazine after an interval if required.
The effect of anti-Parkinsonism drugs (q.v.) is inconsistent.

Alcoholic hallucinosis

This condition is characterized by auditory hallucinations occurring in the absence of clouding of consciousness, confusion or disorientation after the long continued abuse of alcohol. Visual, olfactory and tactile hallucinations, tremulousness and epileptic fits may occur and the condition may develop into typical delirium tremens. Usually the onset follows the cessation of drinking. The voices are frequently recognized as belonging to friends and family members. Multiple voices talking about the patient in the third person resemble the auditory hallucinations of schizophrenia. Simple clicking, 'whooshing' noises or tinnitus frequently accompany the hallucinations.
Alcoholic hallucinosis is usually a benign

transient disorder lasting a few days (occasionally weeks) and ending with full insight and no permanent sequelae. Rarely it persists and seems to merge into a true schizophrenic illness.

Alcoholics Anonymous (AA)

This organization, founded by two ex-alcoholics, has been a valuable source of help to many patients suffering from this disease. The system is based upon self-help and acknowledgement of the disability. SEE ALSO Alcoholism.

Alcoholism

The term alcoholism is regarded as synonymous with chronic alcoholism and describes the over-all picture of disability associated with prolonged excessive drinking. Acute alcoholism or simple drunkenness is a dose-related state of acute alcoholic intoxication which is characterized by predictable changes in consciousness and behaviour. Initial disinhibited cheeriness is followed by increased impairment of consciousness, co-ordination and motor function, proceeding to drowsiness, coma and death if enough alcohol is taken. Alcoholism, i.e. chronic alcoholism, is a much more extensive disorder which imposes on the sufferer physical, social and psychological handicaps often of great severity.

The World Health Organisation defines as alcoholic 'those excessive drinkers whose dependence on alcohol has attained such a degree that it shows a notable mental disturbance or an interference with their bodily and mental health, their interpersonal relations and their smooth social and economic functioning; or who show the prodromal signs of such development'. By definition then, alcoholism occurs after excessive drinking, though it is realized that there is considerable individual variation. The important point is that when a person becomes alcoholic, the amount taken is excessive for him. An important part of the definition is 'dependence on alcohol'. It can be said that while psychological dependence on alcohol is common – to the extent that many regular social drinkers may show it – for the true alcoholic psychological dependence is so extensive as to cause symptoms and above all to cause a progressive loss of control over drinking. Physical dependence on alcohol appears relatively late in the natural history of the disorder, but when it occurs indicates severe dependence.

In diagnosing alcoholism the finding of symptoms of loss of control of drinking should be regarded as paramount. These include – lying to the self and others about the amount drunk, preoccupation with alcohol and with keeping up supplies, taking extra drinks before parties or ordeals, hangovers causing loss of work and drinking earlier in the day. Once drinking is out of control dependence worsens and further symptoms emerge; these include blackouts, memory gaps, early morning shakes relieved by alcohol, feelings of nausea and weakness on standing, tremulousness and further signs of physical dependence and physical complications. It is important to stress not so much individual signs, but the necessity of finding out from the patient how much of his life is absorbed by alcohol in time, money and interest.

Jellinek proposed a classification of alcoholism based on the notion of alcoholism as a disease process in which various systems are progressively involved. He suggested, too, that the aetiology varied with the pattern of alcohol use displayed by the drinker. His classification includes alpha alcoholism, characterized by a 'purely psychological continued dependence . . . to relieve bodily or emotional pain'. Alpha alcoholism is said not to proceed to loss of control. Beta alcoholism is said to occur when organic complications, such as cirrhosis or polyneuritis, are present, but where the dependence is either physical or psychological. Gamma alcoholism is characterized by progressive development of tolerance to alcohol with cellular change, abstinence symptoms and craving with severe loss of control over the amount drunk – a truly progressive and the most damaging variety – the predominant type in Anglo-Saxon countries.

Delta alcoholism resembles gamma, but instead of a loss of control the person has total inability to abstain even for a day or so without the appearance of withdrawal symptoms. Epsilon alcoholism is episodic excessive drinking, i.e. dipsomania (q.v.).

But whether or not Jellinek's classification is employed, the basic problem to be clarified in anyone with a history of alcohol abuse is the presence of dependence, and, even more important, to find out if loss of control of drinking has occurred.
The importance of *making the diagnosis* of alcoholism cannot be over-emphasized – it is a disorder which may be missed by otherwise capable doctors. This is not just because some ignore its existence as a disease, but because of the moral overtones and social stigma which may obscure the diagnosis.
The true extent of alcoholism is hard to estimate. Jellinek's formula (q.v.), based on known deaths from alcoholic cirrhosis, though often employed, is thought by many to provide an underestimate of the true prevalence. The World Health Organisation estimates between 400,000 and 500,000 alcoholics in England and Wales using Jellinek's formula. Whatever the true numbers may be, the problem is large and an important aspect of the public health.
The aetiology of alcoholism is best described in multifactorial terms. One-factor theories of alcoholism do not account for the facts. Alcoholism is commoner in men than in women (5:1) and is mainly a disorder of middle age. Heavy drinkers tend to come from heavy drinking families – and the children of alcoholics have a higher expectation of alcoholism than do children of parents not alcoholics. Whilst no genetic inheritance has been demonstrated, it could operate, though, to date, family experience seems to be more important. Certain races show clear cultural and racial links with alcoholism. The Irish appear to be highly vulnerable, Jews and Moslems nearly invulnerable. There are wide differences between countries in alcoholism prevalence. France and Italy have wine-producing industries of equal size, yet Italy has a much lower alcoholism problem than France. This may be related to drinking habits – in Italy alcohol is linked with meals, in France it is not.
The complications of alcoholism are extensive. The alcoholic is more likely to become diabetic, to suffer from pancreatitis and to be more prone to chronic bronchitis (because of heavier smoking) than the non-alcoholic.
There are a number of clearly defined psychiatric syndromes associated with alcoholism. Derilium tremens, a state of disorganized confused overactivity, usually follows a prolonged drinking bout and is perhaps the most well known. Wernicke's encephalopathy (q.v.) and the Korsakoff psychosis (q.v.) are both relatea to thiamine deficiency in alcoholism. In the former a confusional state is complicated by oculomotor paralyses and in the latter the main manifestations are severe disorientation for time and place, gross amnesia for recent events and a tendency to confabulate answers (it is also associated with an alcoholic peripheral neuropathy). Alcoholic hallucinosis is a rare psychosis which occurs in certain alcoholics and is characterized by the occurrence of auditory hallucinations and paranoid content, in a setting of clear consciousness. This psychosis is causally related to prolonged alcohol use; it clears with abstinence.
Paranoid states (q.v.) occur in alcoholics and when they occur it is common to find delusions involving sexual jealousy. These may be related to the loss of sexual potency in the alcoholic ('brewer's droop').
Marchiafavas disease (q.v.) is a rapidly fatal form of alcoholic intoxication with demyelination of the medial part of the corpus callosum. Alcoholic dementia is an alcoholic specific dementia and like all dementias is characterized by progressive irreversible intellectual impairment.

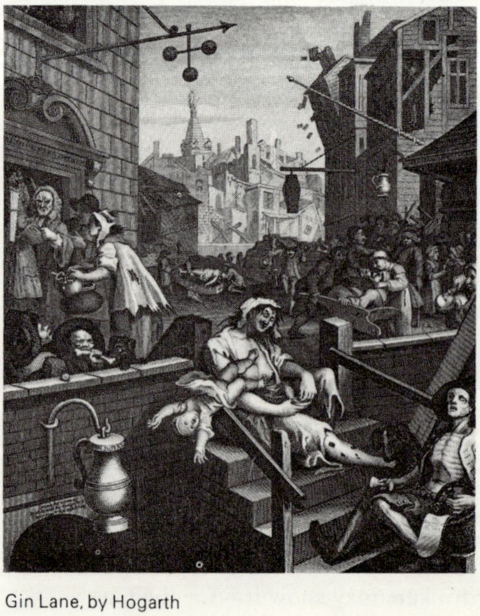

Gin Lane, by Hogarth

The treatment of the alcoholic patient starts once the diagnosis is made. Alcoholism, when recognized, commits the physician to a treatment programme which has total abstention as the main goal. The first step is to investigate fully the physical and mental status of the patient so as to treat any existing physical or psychiatric complications. For this, admission to hospital may be necessary not only for 'drying out', but also for the evaluation and treatment of impaired liver function, vitamin deficiency, diabetes and chronic bronchitis, all treatable, not irreversible conditions. In addition the specific psychiatric syndromes mentioned above will need hospital treatment. These complications, physical and psychological, are rare and their absence should not prevent the making of the diagnosis, for they are, on the whole, late events in the natural history of alcoholism. After assessment and 'drying out', it is necessary to find methods of encouraging abstention. In the case of alcoholism which is secondary to some underlying psychiatric illness – e.g. depression – the expectation is that treatment of the underlying disorder will relieve the alcoholic dependence. Unhappily this is not quite the case. Too often what appears to be 'symptomatic alcoholism is not, or if it started out as such, the process has somehow become autonomous. Thus in practice, treatment of alcoholism means treatment of a chronic and relapsing disorder. In many cases alcoholism may be related to personality disorder but this does not account for all cases without stretching to absurdity the meaning of the term 'personality disorder'. Traditional individual and group psychotherapy are of little value in alcoholism. Sedatives are to be avoided and tranquillizers used only in withdrawal. Antidepressants should be used if depression is present. Suicidal risk should always be considered – suicide is 60 times more com mon in alcoholics than in non-alcoholics. Admission to specialized hospital units is of value where the patient meets the selective admission criteria of the unit concerned. In many of these the better motivated patients respond to a vigorous group atmosphere which is positive and optimistic, no matter what idiosyncratic techniques may be applied. But the bulk of alcoholics may show poor or ill-sustained motivation. They show a high relapse rate. And for this reason, pharmacological aids such as disulfuram are employed. These drugs cause distress, often severe, if the taker drinks alcohol and are often effective where all else has failed. They should be offered to all alcoholics.

All alcoholics should be offered membership of Alcoholics Anonymous (AA) (q.v.). This organization, founded by two ex-alcoholics in America, has given help to a vast number of alcoholics; probably much more than that available from 'official' treatment sources. It is founded on self-help and acknowledgement of disability. The AA member can count on help at any time from other members and AA meetings combine esprit de corps with commitment, self-awareness and shared humility in the face of a shared problem. Perhaps the basic statement about the treatment of the alcoholic patient is that each is likely to present a long-term problem in which continued support may be the baseline though more esoteric approaches may be tried. For the severely recidivist alcoholic who faces repeated prison sentences and social dereliction, many feel that treatment is impossible, but current experience suggests that even the most grotesque derelict can improve in a well-run hostel.

Algophobia

Morbid dread of witnessing or experiencing pain. This is uncommon. However, the anticipation of pain is one component of the well-recognized fears of dentists and injections. Such patients may have abnormally low pain thresholds, at least in one part of the body, such as the teeth. SEE ALSO Phobia.

Alienation

A term the meaning of which has changed radically over the last century. It was originally used to describe insanity, the insane being regarded as basically strangers (alieni) to the society in which they moved. Their doctors were thus named Alienists. Today alienation is regarded as a more general process – an inability to identify with the culture, society, family or peer group. The outsider is sometimes an agent of change, intellectually productive and provocative, and a valuable person in society. More commonly, however, the alienated individual is unhappy and insecure, searching for security which some find in the hippie movement, the commune and other similar groups. A sense of alienation may be an early symptom of schizophrenic illness, the withdrawal of affect contributing to the feeling of strangeness in relation to the environment.

Allergy

Hypersensitivity to one or more of a great variety of agents may produce an allergic response manifest as a dermatological, respiratory or gastro-intestinal disturbance, migraine or allergic rhinitis. The relationship between allergy and emotion is a complex one, for severe emotional stress (q.v.) may precipitate a response similar to, or augment the effect of, a specific allergen.
Treatment of allergic disorders often involves the use of drugs such as antihistamines or steroids, but reduction of emotional stress by psychotherapy or tranquillizers, may play an important part in the management of individual patients.
SEE ALSO Psychosomatic disorders.

Alloerotic

Turning the erotic tendencies away from the self and towards others, and thus the reverse of autoerotic (q.v.).

Alpha adrenergic receptors

The receptor sites on which adrenaline and noradrenaline act can be divided into two types depending on their sensitivities to different catecholamine derivatives. These are termed α and β receptors. Alpha receptors in general mediate vasoconstriction. There is evidence that α receptor activation in some locations inhibits adenylate cyclase. Alpha receptors are stimulated *inter alia* by noradrenaline more powerfully than adrenaline, by metaraminol and methoxamine: they are blocked by ergot alkaloids, phenoxybenzamine and phentolamine.

Alpha enhancement
(Synonyms: alpha feedback, alpha training)

The voluntary control of occipital alpha activity by way of biofeedback training has been used in the following areas:—
(a) As a neurophysiological research tool, the biofeedback system affording a dynamic, interactive condition rather than a stimulus-response one. Valuable work has been done on the major influencing factors of alpha such as oculomotor commands, visual tracking, studies of attention, vigilance and arousal.
(b) Using alpha activity as a central physiological index of a normal relaxed state, since alpha rhythms are desynchronized at higher levels of arousal and are replaced by slower rhythms as drowsiness builds up. An increase in alpha voltage or continuity, other things being equal, has been regarded as evidence of a relaxation response which can be learned by means of biofeedback training. Applications have been attempted in chronic anxiety states and obsessional neurosis.
(c) Investigations into altered states of consciousness, based on data of unusual EEG patterns in Yoga and Zazen meditators that included large and persistent amounts of alpha activity.
SEE ALSO Biofeedback.

Alpha rhythm
SEE EEG.

Altruistic suicide
SEE Durkheim, E.

Alzheimer's disease
(Synonym: Alzheimer's pre-senile dementia)

This is the commonest of the pre-senile dementias (q.v.). A family history is found in about 15% of cases, inheritance may be multifactorial, or in a few families dominant. The onset is usually in the 50's. The duration is on average about seven years, but there is considerable variation. Memory impairment is usually the first symptom. Parietal lobe features are especially prominent. Fits occur in about 30% of cases. Dementia is progressive and eventually profound, with forced laughing or crying, forced gasping, a sucking reflex, contractures and bed sores. There is a diffuse cerebral atrophy. Histologically, there is extensive loss of neurones, mainly in the cortex but also in the basal ganglia. Senile plaques are common, and there is a general glial proliferation; characteristic is the neurofibrillary change in neurones, the so-called tangles. Although these changes are very characteristic, and enable the diagnosis to be confirmed by biopsy, they are not specific, and some or all of them may also be found in Down's syndrome (q.v.) after repeated head injuries (boxers' encephalopathy), in post-encephalitic Parkinsonism and in motor neurone disease. In senile dementia identical neuropathological changes are found, so that it is the age at which the disorder begins which is diagnostic. No treatment is known to be effective and is limited to supervision and tranquillization, maintaining nutrition, occupation, exercise and general nursing.

Amaurotic family idiocy

(Synonym: Cerebromacular degeneration)

Amaurotic family idiocy is a progressive involvement of the central nervous system with mental deterioration leading to severe subnormality and early death in cases of early onset. It is recessively inherited, and the basic pathological defect is disturbed lipid metabolism. It comprises several forms, distinguished by age of onset, but some should perhaps be regarded as separate disease entities. They are: (a) congenital, (b) infantile, or Tay-Sachs disease (q.v.), (c) late infantile or Bielchowsky-Jansky disease (q.v.), (d) juvenile, or Spielmeyer-Vogt disease, (e) adult, or Kufs disease. Loss of vision and retinal degeneration in the region of the macular are characteristic. In a number of cases a cherry-red spot is seen in the macular area on retinoscopy.
SEE ALSO Inherited metabolic defects.

Ambivalence

The co-existence of opposite feelings, ideas or wishes in regard to a person or situation. Affective ambivalence is alleged to be characteristic of manic-depressive subjects who often manifest an admixture of negative and positive feelings toward the same person. Subjects with obsessive-compulsive neurosis also show ambivalence of thought and feeling. In schizophrenia, ambivalence reflects a more profound disorganization so that contradictory feelings and thoughts are present at the same time, allowing the patient for instance to claim that her physician loves her but also that he is attempting to kill her.

Amenorrhoea

Primary amenorrhoea is diagnosed when menarche is delayed beyond the age of 18. In some cases there is a history of severe emotional trauma and a later spontaneous onset of menstruation is anticipated.
Primary amenorrhoea also occurs in anorexia (q.v.) nervosa when the illness begins before puberty.
Secondary amenorrhoea means the cessation of previously established menstruation. Psychological disturbance is a common cause of temporary amenorrhoea. It is often seen when young women are adjusting to a new environment, as after entry to nursing training or to the armed forces. Fear of pregnancy is also a well known cause of transient amenorrhoea. Psychogenic amenorrhoea is presumably due to inhibition of gonadotropin secretion by the pituitary. It usually clears up spontaneously and no treatment is needed other than reassurance.
In frank psychiatric illness amenorrhoea may be a symptom. While menstrual irregularity is a common finding in neurosis and affective disorder, persistent amenorrhoea is uncommon except in schizophrenia. It must also be remembered that certain psychotropic drugs can affect menstrual regularity.
In anorexia nervosa amenorrhoea is a cardinal feature and it often occurs before there is any significant weight loss. Menstruation often returns after weight has been regained.

In psychiatric illness generally amenorrhoea usually disappears when the psychiatric symptoms are relieved. If it persists after psychiatric recovery, menstruation can sometimes be re-established by cyclic hormone treatment or by clomiphene. Such treatment should only be given under the guidance of a gynaecologist or endocrinologist.

Amentia

SEE Mental subnormality

Amines

The main amines of interest to psychiatrists are the catecholamines (q.v.) (dopamine (q.v.), noradrenaline (q.v.) and adrenaline (q.v.)), serotonin (q.v.) (5HT), histamine octopamine and the polyamines spermine and spermidine. Dopamine is an important inhibitory transmitter in the extrapyramidal system and Parkinsonism is associated with a degeneration of the neurones containing dopamine. Noradrenaline is the transmitter of the postganglionic adrenergic nerves and also in parts of the brain (see adrenergic). In the periphery it stimulates mainly α receptors leading to a rise in blood pressure, and increased peripheral vascular resistance. The cerebral blood flow is reduced. In the brain noradrenaline is probably concerned in mechanisms underlying mood, learning reactions and reward signalling systems. At the adrenergic synapse it is stored in vesicles as a complex with ATP and is released by exocytosis, while termination of its action on the receptor depends mainly on re-uptake into the presynaptic terminal. Drugs like cocaine, amphetamine and imipramine block this re-uptake and raise effective levels of free amine at the receptors. This may explain their mood elevating effect. Monoamine oxidase inhibitors, it is thought, also raise mood by raising free brain noradrenaline by blocking the main enzyme – monoamine oxidase which destroys it. Reserpine on the other hand depletes the stores for both catecholamines and serotonin. This may be the cause of the clinical depression with reserpine.
A second enzyme involved in noradrenaline metabolism is catechol-O-methyltransferase, which O-methylates it to produce normetadrenaline and vanilmandelic acid. Therapy based on inhibition of this enzyme has not yet been described.
Adrenaline is the main hormone released from the adrenal medulla but plays little role in the brain.
Serotonin (5HT) is a neuronal transmitter in peripheral and central nervous systems, and like noradrenaline, is also affected by anti-depressant drugs. In the brain, serotonin systems are probably concerned in the control of perception, mood, sleep, thinking and behaviour. Brain serotonin mechanisms are also thought to be concerned in hypothalamic mechanisms regulating pituitary function in oestrus, ovulation and ACTH secretion. The hallucinogenic drugs such as LSD and mescaline are specific blockers of central serotonin synapses and many of them are close chemical relatives of serotonin (e.g. dimethyltryptamine, psilocybin, and LSD itself). Serotonin may also be involved in migraine, the therapeutic agent methysergide being a potent blocker of 5HT.
Much less is known about the function of brain histamine although histamine is probably a central transmitter. Antihistamics produce drowsiness, so it may be concerned with alerting functions.
Even less is known about the polyamines spermine and spermidine. Their main known function at present is in the nucleic acid mediated synthesis of proteins and it is possible that they may play an important role in brain function. Certain diseases may be associated with disorders in brain histamine and polyamines.
SEE ALSO Monoamines.
For general description see Biochemical and neuro-physiological background to mental disease.

Amine-oxidase inhibitors

SEE Monoamine oxidase inhibitors.

Amino acids in brain metabolism

Certain amino acids play an important dual role in the brain. Glutamic acid (q.v.) and gamma amino-butyric acid (GABA (q.v.)) (and possibly some related acids, e.g. aspartic acid, glycine, proline) are neuro-transmitters in brain:

glutamate being always excitatory to neurones and GABA inhibitory. GABA is found only in the brain. These two amino acids also play a role in energy metabolism since they are involved in the Krebs cycle.
There are two routes from α-keto glutamate to succinate, one direct and one via glutamic acid and GABA. The steps from glutamic acid to GABA and from GABA to succinate involve vitamin B_6 (pyridoxine) as a co-enzyme of which the first (glutamic decarboxylase) is the most sensitive to pyridoxine deficiency, which would thus lead to excess glutamate and deficient

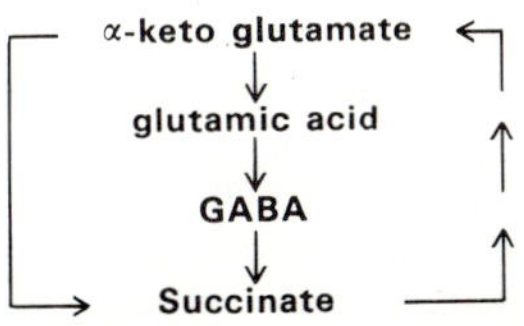

GABA production. This may explain the epileptic convulsions that follow pyridoxine deficiency, particularly in infants.
GABA and glutamate are utilized by the brain when the glucose supply fails. The levels of these amino acids fall in the brain during hypoglycaemic coma and this can arouse patients from such a coma. Glutamate and GABA are also involved in the detoxification of ammonia, the former being converted in the process to glutamine and the latter to gamma-guanidino butyric acid which has convulsant properties. This may explain why high brain ammonia e.g. (produced by feeding ammonium salts) leads to convulsions.
Amino acids in the brain are also involved in building proteins, and failures in their metabolism are a prominent cause of mental defect. Phenylketonuria (q.v.) is produced by a genetic fault which leads to a defective production of the enzyme which converts phenylalanine to tyrosine. The phenylalanine is converted instead into the toxic compound phenylpyruvic acid. Other such disorders are Hartnup disease (q.v.) where the failure is in tryptophan metabolism and amino acid transport. The normal conversion of tryptophan to nicotinic acid is blocked and pellagra results.
In maple syrup urine disease (q.v.) the fault lies with leucine and isoleucine. Other such disorders include arginosuccinic acidaemia (q.v.) and cystathionuria (q.v.).
In normal people there is a transport carrier assisted movement of nutritionally essential amino acids into the brain. The rate at which the transport occurs depends on several factors including the relative concentrations on the two sides of the blood brain barrier, saturation of the carrier mechanism and cross-inhibition of the carrier mechanism particularly among the aromatic amino acids.
SEE ALSO Biochemical and neurophysiological background to mental disease and Inherited metabolic defects.

Amnesia

Loss of memory (q.v.) may be seen in patients with organic or functional mental reactions, 'retrograde amnesia' (q.v.) relating to events before the onset of the illness or traumatic accident, 'anterograde amnesia' (q.v.) to events after it. The process of memory involves registration, retention and recall. In the psychoses – e.g. agitated depression – as in deliria and other altered states of awareness, inattention may prevent registration. In organic brain disease – due to infection, neoplasm or degeneration – the retention of short-term memory traces is more affected than that of long-term traces. The patient can recall childhood and early life but not recent events or new information, such as a test name and address. In hysterical amnesia, where the loss is most often global for the patient's whole life and even his name, by the psychological mechanism of repression, the process of recall is effected commonly in a situation of acute stress – financial or legal. Suggestion, possibly hypnotic or chemically induced, may result in the recovery of experience often with great emotion.

Amnesic syndrome

SEE Korsakoff syndrome

Amok

SEE Culture bound syndromes.

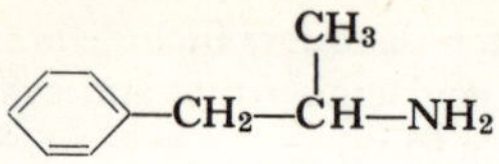

Amphetamines

Amphetamine is a phenylethylamine derivative related to adrenaline; it is the prototype of a series of compounds of which methamphetamine is the more important central nervous system active congener. Amphetamine is racemic and the dextro-rotatory compound is used. Amphetamines stimulate the reticular activating system (q.v.) and this action is the basis of the effects on arousal and vigilance. Fatigue-impaired performance is usually restored, and normal performance may appear to be enhanced, although there is conflicting evidence on whether performance is actually improved. This applies to both psychological and physical performance, and reflects a general alerting effect. Mood is elevated to produce euphoria, but as the drug wears off unpleasant let down feelings ensue. The rapid relief of let down discomfort by further dosage is the basis of the readily occurring dependency and drug abuse.
There are a number of drug interactions which are relevant to psychiatric practice. Tricyclic anti-depressants and monoamine oxidase inhibitors can potentiate amphetamines. The effects of moderate hypnotic doses of barbiturates are counteracted. Amphetamine-barbiturate mixtures have been used extensively to avoid the unwanted excitatory effects of amphetamine but such combinations show synergistic effects of the two drugs. Such mixtures do not have any advantages over amphetamines alone and are best avoided for they are extensively abused.
Amphetamines are not effective therapeutic agents in depression, and although they have been used in the past in psychoneurotic and asthenic states their value is questionable, and their use is contra-indicated because of the particularly high risk of dependence in this group of patients. Amphetamines were thought to be of benefit to some patients with aggressive psychopathic personality disorder. They have been widely prescribed as anorectics in the treatment of obesity and can be of help, but the occurrence of a group of middle-aged, overweight housewives with amphetamine dependency is a consequence. Some organic conditions are helped by amphetamine treatment, and these include narcolepsy, certain types of epilepsy, and unexpectedly the hyperkinetic hyperactivity syndrome in children. Nocturnal enuresis has been treated with amphetamines on the rationale that the reduced depth of sleep enables the patient to wake and take corrective action. Because of the high risk of drug dependence with amphetamines, their use should be carefully restricted.
Minor side effects are mainly those of stimulation, and include insomnia, anxiety, dry mouth, tremor, palpitations, irritability, headache, impotence and anorexia. Without doubt the two most serious adverse reactions are the development of drug dependence, and the precipitation of a psychotic illness which is indistinguishable from paranoid schizophrenia. Fortunately the drug-induced psychosis usually disappears when amphetamine is withdrawn. There has been extensive abuse of amphetamine by adolescents during the past few years and physical dependence to amphetamine is a major problem (see addiction).
Current medical opinion favours the total avoidance of prescriptions for amphetamines.
The phenylethylamine derivatives that are still used clinically are amphetamine average daily dose 5–10 mg), methamphetamine (q.v.), dimephenopan (q.v.), chlorphentermine (q.v.)

Amusia

The musical sense is the result of a complex amalgam of sensory impressions, and may involve musical appreciation or musical execution. Amusia may include the inability to handle an instrument, to recognize music, or to appreciate music. There are two main types – expressive amusia, the loss of the ability of musical expression; and receptive amusia, the inability to recognize melodies. Willis in the 17th century, located the musical sense in the cerebellum, Call recognized a musical organ; today, a lesion of the anterior temporal area in the dominant hemisphere is most commonly associated with an amusic syndrome. Musicogenic epilepsy is a rare type of epilepsy in which the attack is precipitated by a musical experience, sometimes of a very specific type.

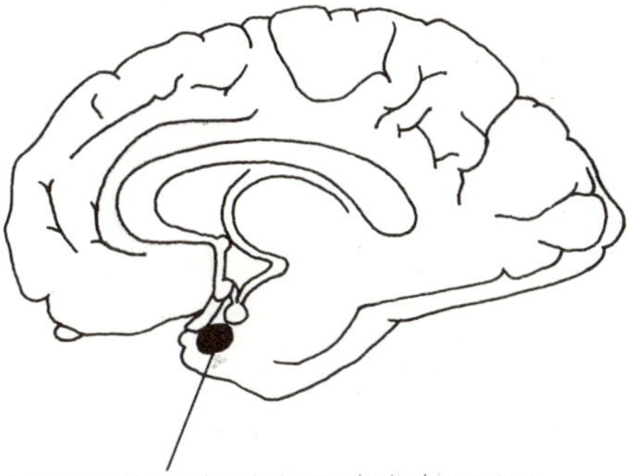

Amygdala shown in relation to the limbic system

Amygdala

This nucleus, which is situated on the inner aspect of the temporal lobe, is one of the components of the limbic system (q.v.). It is thus associated with the mediation of emotional responses.
Stimulation of the amygdala in animals leads to an attacking type of reaction (growling, piloerection, hissing, etc.). Amygdalectomy has been carried out in patients who suffer from aggressive outbursts, with encouraging results.

Anaclitic

This term defines relationships which are characterized by dependence on others Initially the infant is in this position in relation to its mother or mother surrogate. Some individuals continue to adopt this passive, dependent, immature posture throughout life. They depend on others for physical and emotional support. Anaclitic depression may be seen in infants following sudden separation from a mother figure. There is acute impairment of physical, social and intellectual development. This should be considered in all cases where infants 'fail to thrive'.
Anaclitic therapy is a type of psychotherapy in which all the patients' dependent needs are gratified in order to obtain an intense doctor-patient relationship, which is then used therapeutically.
SEE ALSO Child psychiatry.

Anaemia

Levels of haemoglobin below accepted norms are common particularly in females, and may be associated with complaints of fatigue, lassitude, breathlessness and dizziness, palpitations, anorexia and paraesthesiae. While severe degrees of iron deficiency may have a causal relationship to the symptoms described, in minor degrees the association is more probably by chance, such complaints correlating more closely to the degree of neuroticism found in the patients than to their haemoglobin levels. Suspicion as to the origin of symptoms should be entertained in the absence of systemic disease, when correcting the blood picture fails to promote symptomatic improvement, or when symptoms recur without accompanying evidence of iron deficiency.
The lack of other factors necessary for blood formation may independently underlie changes in the nervous system. Deficiency of cobalamin (vitamin B_{12}) (q.v.) causes pernicious anaemia, subacute combined degeneration of the spinal cord, and mental changes and confusional states. Deficiency of folic acid (q.v.), which causes megaloblastic anaemia, may itself cause mental change. Deficiency of thyroxine (q.v.) interferes with blood formation and results in anaemia as part of the syndrome of myxoedema which it also produces. It is then associated with marked mental change – psychoses with depression, paranoia and confusion are commonly encountered.
Finally, the treatment of epilepsy with drugs such as phenytoin, mesontoin and primidone for long periods may result in defective folate absorption and megaloblastic anaemia. Mental changes of a confusional type may be observed. The administration of folic acid to correct the anaemia may result in a deterioration of the epilepsy under treatment, but this in turn may be prevented by parallel administration of vitamin B_{12}.

Analeptic drugs (convulsants)

Convulsant drugs have found only a limited use in a psychiatric context. Some have been used to produce convulsions in the treatment of mental illness, when they are alternatives to electroplexy. Camphor,

picrotoxin and leptazole have been used in this way, but in recent years they have been superseded by pentylenetetrazol (pentetrazol) and flurothyl. Unfortunately pentetrazol induces severe feelings of fear in patients although it is an effective agent. Flurothyl is free of this disadvantage, and indeed it has been claimed to be superior to electroplexy since it causes less confusion and memory disturbance. It is an etheric substance given parenterally or by inhalation, it is unchanged by the body and is excreted in the exhaled air. In spite of these potential benefits, chemically induced convulsion therapy has not achieved any substantial general use.
Related analeptic compounds, amiphenazole, bemegride, and ethamivan have been used in the treatment of barbiturate intoxication. However, they are not true barbiturate antagonists and they may produce more difficulties than they solve. Modern practice has moved towards diuretic techniques on the reasonable grounds that it is more profitable to hasten the removal of toxic agents.

Anal erotism

The phase of anal erotism occurs after the oral phase and precedes the genital phase. It is a phase of auto erotism (q.v.) in which the child is concerned with the retention or expulsion of faeces, and derives pleasure from its control of the body sphincters. Faeces may be retained or expelled in compliance with parental wishes, or serve to express anger, stubbornness or defiance in this way. The obsessional personality is considered to be fixated at the anal level, his rigidity, orderliness, punctuality and cleanliness are interpreted as a response to conflicts emanating from this stage of mental development.
SEE ALSO Freud.

Analgesics

Analgesic drugs fall naturally into two discrete general categories, the powerful narcotic analgesics and the mild non-narcotic analgesics. Morphine is the main active agent of opium and is the standard powerful analgesic. Morphine and its derivatives, methadone and congeners, and pethidine and related compounds comprise the three main types of powerful analgesic. Without doubt effective analgesics are invaluable in relieving severe pain. The strong narcotic analgesics all show tolerance and a high liability to physical and psychological dependence (q.v.); it seems that the chemical structure required for analgesia also confers addictive properties. Psychiatric interest in these compounds is confined to the results of their addictive propensity. The main narcotic analgesics are morphine; diacetylmorphine (heroin); dihydromorphinone (hydromorphone); dihydro-hydroxymorphinone (oxymorphine); methyldihydromorphinone (metogon); codeine; dihydrocodeinone (hydrocodone); dihydrocodone; dihydrohydroxycodenone (oxycodone); morpholinylethylmorphine (pholcodine); phenozocine; methadone; levorphanol; dextromoramide; dipipanone; phenadoxone; pethidine (meperidine); anileridine; alphaprodine; piminodine; piritamide.
Mild analgesics include salicylates, anilides such as paracetamol, and phenazones, like phenylbutazone; these are free from dependence potential. Combinations of mild analgesics which include barbiturates are to be deprecated since analgesic requirement may lead to barbiturate dependence. There is an additional intermediate group of mild analgesics including codeine, dihydrocodeine and dextropropoxyphene. These compounds have a mild addictive tendency, but frank dependence on these drugs is unusual. Nevertheless excessive use of analgesic mixtures does occur, and may be related to caffeine which is often incorporated in such mixtures.

Analytic psychology

In general, this covers those psychological disciplines which use the methods of free association (q.v.), hypnosis (q.v.), abreaction (q.v.), and narcoanalysis (q.v.) to uncover mental defence mechanisms which have led to conflict and neurosis, and which are modified by interpretation in treatment.
Specifically the term refers to the hypotheses of Carl Jung. Jung rejected the biological and genetic approach, being concerned with the inner world of the individual. His brilliant insights into the

mind of the schizophrenic illumined his later work with neurosis. The collective unconscious contains the ancestral knowledge gathered over the centuries, the personal unconscious, that knowledge gained from the individual's own experience. Different types exist, the introvert and the extrovert, who handle mental activity in different ways. Jungian psychology is more profound than is commonly believed, and should not be underestimated.

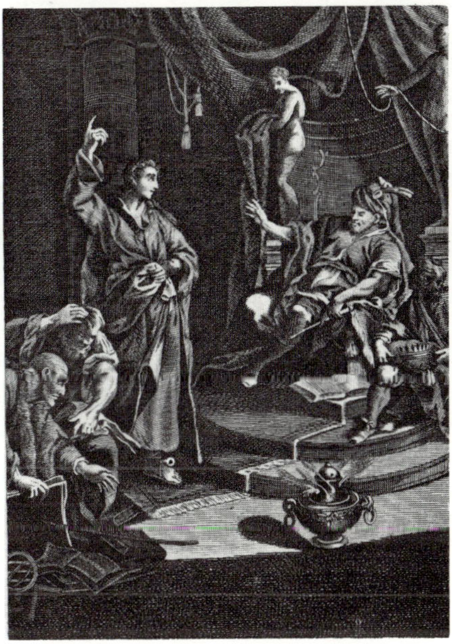

Daniel interpreting Nebuchadnezzar's dream

Analytic psychotherapy

Although subsuming a number of different analytic approaches to the mind, the term should be reserved for the particular theories and approaches of the Jungian school. Carl Jung, after his brilliant studies of schizophrenia and of word association, began to study his own mental processes, whilst at the same time treating patients in his private practice. Freud was doing much the same in Vienna, and the two men became interested in each other's work, so much so that Freud regarded Jung as the leader designate of the psychoanalytical movement. However, Jung's experience with the psychotic played an important part in the development of his ideas – so different from those of Freud, whose experience of the whole range of psychiatry was limited. The symbol (and the process of symbolization) so clearly seen in the psychotic individual was of central importance to both men – to Jung symbols were basically of two types, derived from the personal as well as the collective unconscious, whereas for Freud symbols were products of the personal unconscious. The collective unconscious, which Jung later called the objective psyche, was an accumulation of the past experiences, racial and historical, of human kind, and had a universal quality. In other words, the collective unconscious consisted of archetypical modes of thought and action compressed, as it were, for convenience in the form of symbols. Thus a wealth of past experience and feeling is condensed in the archetypical representation of the different types of women – the Witch, the Earth Mother, the Virgin Mary. There are a number of archetypes which can be recognized in the dream, symbols such as the wise old man, the dragon, the hero. Bad as well as good is represented there. The symbols of the collective unconscious have a different function to those of the personal unconscious – they express the human potential of the individual and are not the result of conflict. To seek to understand these symbols means to seek the full potential of the individual's endowments. Life thereby becomes richer and fuller, and also more realistic. Jungian practice lays much emphasis on dream analysis, for in the dream are encountered symbols of both the collective and personal unconscious. In all of us there are several aspects of the mind to be worked through before individualization can be attained. First there is the shadow, the side of the mind that is concealed in the shadows – comprising not only the unacceptable aspects of the person, but aspects which have been kept in the background as a result of strivings, desires, ambitions. Thus the shadow is not entirely negative – the attainment of one's full potential may only be realized by the understanding of what has been hidden. It is only with maturity that an individual can begin to cope with his shadow side – indeed it is in the second half of life that analytic psychotherapy offers the best opportunity of change and fulfilment.

The next stage consists of dealing with the animus and the anima, all those male and female characteristics and propensities of both the collective and personal unconscious. It is the way the individual handles his or her discoveries which is important. Acceptance and understanding paves the way for their integration into the personality so that they become part of the conscious self – and are no longer unconsciously driving the individual into false postures. When the shadow, the animus and the anima have been thoroughly analysed, then it is possible for the self – the heart of the psyche – to be fully realized, often as if a re-birth has taken place.

Jung was also concerned with the more general aspects of personality. In his book *Psychological Types*, 1921, he proposed that there were two main factors in personality – extraversion and introversion. These forces were not mutually exclusive and, in fact, could be more, or less, dominant at a particular time in life. For instance, the introverted scholar might in later life be transformed into the dedicated crusader for a cause. Four other factors were also important in this typology – thinking and feeling, sensation and intuition.

Jung's psychology is often criticized as confused and mystical, and his writings are, indeed, at times, difficult. But Jung realized that there were still mysteries, and that there was much of the mind that could not be explained. What he offers is a way of coming to an understanding of the unique individual – the self – moulded by both collective and personal experiences. It is altogether a gentler system than the Freudian, which emphasizes continual war in the psyche, the themes of fear and punishment predominating. Unfortunately it must be conceded that only a relatively small proportion of those seeking psychotherapeutic help will be able to cope with the intellectual demands of a Jungian therapy. For those able to do so, a Jungian analysis offers a rewarding experience.

Anankastic

A term used for the obsessive-compulsive type of personality, in which traits of rigidity, conscientiousness, reliability, punctuality and moral scrupulousness are found.

Anatomy of the nervous system

The nervous system is divided somewhat artificially into peripheral and central portions and these in turn are subdivided, the former into the autonomic and voluntary components and the latter into the brain and spinal cord. This is a very arbitrary split for, as the great neurophysiologist Sherrington stressed, the whole system works as one in an integrated fashion. Moreover the sections overlap anatomically.

The spinal cord extends from the caudal end of the medulla oblongata of the brain, at the level of the foramen magnum through the vertebral foramina of the cervical, thoracic and upper 1–2 lumbar vertebrae (a distance in the adult of just under 50 cm) to the conus medullaris. It shows two swellings, the cervical and lumbar enlargements where the cells of the brachial and lumbosacral plexuses are found.

The typical cross-section is composed of two posterior (sensory) horns and two anterior (motor) horns with a central transverse bar or commissure of grey matter (predominantly nerve cell bodies), surrounded by an outer zone of white matter (nerve fibres). The central commissure is pierced by the minute central canal, a continuation of the ventricular system. In the thoracic region there is in addition a lateral horn from which the preganglionic fibres of the sympathetic nervous system arise.

Thirty-one pairs of spinal nerves are present (8 cervical, 12 thoracic, 5 lumbar, 5 sacral and 1 coccygeal). Each spinal nerve carries both motor and sensory fibres. The cells for the motor fibres – the anterior root – are situated in the anterior horn. In contrast the cell bodies for the sensory inflow in the posterior root lie in the posterior (dorsal) root ganglion, within the vertebral canal, but outside the spinal cord. In the lower region of the spinal cord both the anterior and posterior nerve roots are elongated so that the spinal nerve may pass through the intervertebral foramen of the segment which it serves. This cluster of elongated nerve roots is termed the cauda equina.

The sensory fibres ascend and the motor fibres descend in the outer zone of white matter clustered into specific and named tracts (see diagram).

The dorsal columns (gracile and cuneate tracts) contain the main pathways from articular mechanoreceptive (proprioceptive) and some cutaneous touch fibres. On the periphery of the lateral white column are, dorsally, the ascending fibres of the

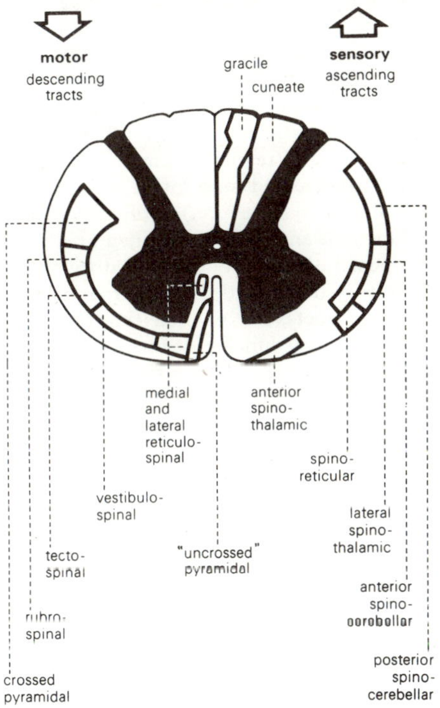

proprioceptive dorsal and ventral spinocerebellar tracts. The anterior spinothalamic tract conveys some touch and pressure sensation while the lateral spinothalamic tract conveys impulses of pain (see gate theory) and temperature (heat and cold). Deeper in the anterolateral white matter is the ascending spinoreticular tract. The dorsal column tracts and dorsal spinocerebellar tract are ipsilateral relative to the side of the peripheral input while the ventral spinocerebellar and spinothalamic pathways are crossed; spinoreticular fibres are both crossed and uncrossed.

These ascending fibres ascend to the thalamus (ventro-lateral nucleus) for transmission to the sensorimotor cortex, the cerebellum and the reticular formation for linking to other diencephalic and mesencephalic nuclei.

The main descending tracts are the 'crossed' and 'uncrossed' pyramidal motor pathways for the main transmission of impulses from the motor cortex to the opposite anterior horns and the so-called 'extrapyramidal' motor tracts: vestibulospinal; tectospinal; rubrospinal; olivospinal and reticulospinal which subserve postural, equilibration, and feedback fine control of motor activity. The arrangement of the anterior horn cells and the relationship of these cells to control of muscle is described under 'muscle tone'.

The autonomic nervous system (q.v.) can be divided into two parts, the parasympathetic derived from an outflow in cranial nerves III, V and X and the sacral nerves and the sympathetic derived from outflows in the thoracic and lumbar regions.

The brain consists of the cerebral hemispheres (q.v.), the brain stem and the cerebellar hemispheres (q.v.).

The two cerebral hemispheres, lying laterally, are joined to the brain stem via the cerebral peduncles and to each other by the corpus callosum (q.v.) and are each composed of four conjoined lobes; frontal, parietal, occipital and temporal. The surface of the cortex, which is composed of the nerve cells, is markedly convoluted (by the gyri and intervening sulci). The cerebral cortex is the highest centre for sensation, perception, memory, thought and voluntary movement decision and in consequence has a very extensive fibre connection with both the opposite cortex and the brain stem and spinal cord.

Sensory radiations flow from the thalamus and its related structures (medial and lateral geniculate bodies) to the cortex.

There is a spatial representation of primary sensory reception in the cortex. Thus, general sensations reach the postcentral gyrus, vision the calcarine fissure area on the medial side of the occipital pole, hearing in the upper part of the temporal lobe and smell and taste probably in the deeper parts of the brain around the region of the uncus or upper operculum of the Sylvian fissure. The impulses come from receptors on the contralateral side of the body and interpretation is based on a direct spatial arrangement linked to the receptors. Recent evidence suggests that perception (q.v.) involves close integration and simultaneous activity by several cortical and subcortical areas.

It appears that the prime area for the 'voluntary movement idea' lies in the precentral area in the frontal cortext. This can be linked with the main motor area (area 4) in the precentral gyrus for unlearned movements or via the cerebellum for learned movements (SEE voluntary movement). The control of the main motor pathway to the anterior horn cells via the pyramidal tract lies in the precentral gyrus of the contralateral side of the body. There is a spatial representation of different parts of the body and those portions with complex movements occupy the largest area. Like the sensory cortex the most caudal myotomes are represented just over the medial lip and the most rostral in the lowest portion of the gyrus.

The cerebral cortex also contains vast areas to which no exact function has been ascribed. Some of these are believed to be 'association areas' in which some sensory and motor interpretation and coordination occurs. There is extensive cross linking from one cerebral cortex to the other via the corpus callosum. One cerebral cortex is usually 'dominant' over the other. Thus in right eyed (handed) people the left cerebral hemisphere is dominant and the speech centre is located in that hemisphere. Dyslexia probably represents an imbalance between the hemisphere activities. The two hemispheres are not quite uniform in their function and response, the dominant hemisphere appears to be more concerned with logical, organized thought process, the non-dominant with random patterns of art forms.

In the upper part of the brain stem, the thalami are situated on either side of the third ventricle. The thalamus contains a number of separate nuclei which receive sensory impulses from lower levels of the brain and spinal cord and relay them to different parts of the cerebral cortex. These sensory impulses relate not only to exteroceptive body surface sensations but to feedback muscle control, impulses from the basal ganglia (q.v.) and the cerebellum (q.v.). The lateral geniculate body which relays sight and medial geniculate body (for hearing) may be regarded as directly related to the thalamus.

Below the thalamus lies the hypothalamus (q.v.) which integrates autonomic and endocrine functions. It receives afferent impulses directly or indirectly from most parts of the brain and sends efferents to autonomic neurones in the spinal cord and to the posterior pituitary. It affects the anterior pituitary and through trophic hormones released from the anterior pituitary, many of the other endocrine glands by releasing hormones (factors) which travel in the hypothalamic-hypophyseal portal blood system. The hypothalamus is important for emotional expression and regulates temperature, water balance and food intake.

The limbic system (q.v.), a physiological rather than anatomically defined area is composed of a variety of facilitatory and inhibitory nuclei and their interconnecting fibre tracts, that encircle the region of the cerebral peduncles. It receives its main afferent supply from the reticular formation while its efferent output is largely to the hypothalamus.

The basal ganglia (q.v.), composed of the corpus striatum, the substantia nigra and the subthalamic nuclei, lie lateral to the thalamus and surround the internal capsule, the main afferent and efferent fibre tract to the cerebral cortex. The basal ganglia are concerned with the cerebellum in the control of muscle tone and voluntary activity (q.v.).

The reticular formation (q.v.) occupying a central zone of the brain stem has an integrating effect on many body reactions, receiving collaterals from the main sensory paths and sending efferents to the cortex, the limbic system, the hypothalamus and the spinal cord.

The cerebellar hemispheres (q.v.) paired, lying on either side of the pons and covering the roof of the fourth ventricle, are joined to the brain stem by their three peduncles. The cerebellum is concerned with the learned motor responses, particularly for fine movements and the feedback control of these movements. They receive impulses from proprioceptive sites and from all parts of the cerebral cortex and the efferents return to the sensorimotor cortex via the thalamus.

Anhedonia

Loss of enjoyment in normally pleasurable occupations. It is often a striking feature of psychotic (endogenous) depressions. The patient loses interest in sex, in food, in the company of his friends and in all his favourite pastimes and does not regain it until the depression has lifted.
SEE ALSO Hedonism.

Anima

A Jungian archetype, and, as such, part of the collective unconscious; the anima is the feminine side of the man's nature and is derived from man's historical experiences with women.
SEE ALSO Animus.

Animus

A Jungian archetype, the masculine component of the female mind, derived from racial, historical experience throughout the centuries.
SEE ALSO Anima.

Ano-genital pruritus

Pruritus ani is a condition of anal irritation which leads to scratching and so to further itching. It is often seen in individuals with anxiety-prone, tense, rigid, obsessional personalities. There may be ridging of the skin, which is usually sodden, and a patch of lichen simplex on one side of the anus may result from scratching. It is commoner in men than women. The cause is unknown, and although often considered to be a psychosomatic disorder, no good evidence for this exists.
Pruritus vulvae commonly has an organic rather than psychogenic cause. Vaginal discharges due to trichomonas or monilial infections may lead to intense irritation and soreness. Psychogenic pruritus may be secondary to conflicts over sexuality, and frigidity is commonly associated. Fear of pregnancy, venereal disease, or cancer may be other causes.
SEE ALSO Psychosomatic disorders and Skin disorders.

Anomie
SEE Durkheim, E.

Anorexia

Partial or complete loss of appetite is a common symptom of either physical or psychiatric disease. It may be associated with the acute infections, in spite of the fact that the metabolic rate increases by about 11% for each degree Centigrade of fever. It may be the presenting feature of serious alimentary disease, carcinoma of the stomach or colon; and classically occurs in infective hepatitis and endocrine disorders, such as hypothyroidism or pituitary hypofunction.
In the psychiatric illnesses the affective disorders (q.v.), i.e. depression, anxiety and mania, are most classically associated with change in appetite. This symptom is therefore one of the commonest features reported in the course of history taking.
In children apparent loss of appetite may be a symptom of a special food faddiness, rather than a general loss as is often implied by the parents' description. Food faddiness is often seen in over-protected (q.v.) children and in some represents the only way they can express hostility over their experiences of the denial of autonomy and independence which can result from overprotective parental attitudes.

Anorexia nervosa

Anorexia nervosa is a disorder which characteristically occurs in young women, although it occasionally occurs in older women, and, exceptionally, in men.
The term anorexia nervosa is a misnomer as although anorexia usually occurs when the patient has lost 2 stones or more in weight, the patient may remain ravenously hungry and occasionally may have episodes when she gorges large amounts of food only to feel guilty immediately afterwards. The common feature in all cases is a fear of regaining normal weight. The anorexic may ruminate for hours after a meal about the increase in weight which may occur; the patient who has retained her appetite may fear that she may lose control of it and consequently gain weight to a state of obesity.

The patient is often a 'special' child, perhaps an only child or a child of academic parents, and it has been postulated, as in other psychosomatic disorders, that the child has had a close and markedly ambivalent tie to one parent or the other. Pre-morbid personality traits often show restricted, rigid, obsessional propensities, though a minority have gross hysterical traits.
The onset of the disorder is usually associated with some emotional conflict, the most common being conflicts about accepting the female role or, during the engagement period, if the patient had conflicts about assuming the responsibilities of marriage. Other conflicts relate to the parents, particularly the mother. Often the restriction in diet starts because the girl regards herself as too fat and may have been teased about her weight. More rarely the condition starts in the setting of a depressive illness. Amenorrhoea (q.v.) is a characteristic and often early feature. As the loss of weight becomes progressively more severe lanugo hair, dry skin, loss of normal hair and a variety of biochemical disorders secondary to starvation occur. A disturbance of oestrogen secretion and particularly disturbances of follicle-stimulating hormone secreted by the anterior pituitary gland are not directly related to weight loss and may persist when a normal weight has been regained. In all but the mildest cases admission to hospital is essential. If possible, one nurse should be made responsible for the patient's supervision and she should personally assist at every meal and by persuasion encourage the patient to eat. It is helpful if the nurse eats too. Chlorpromazine, or amitriptyline if depression is a prominent feature, are often very helpful for relief of tension and facilitating weight gain, but doses have to be much higher than one would expect in relation to the patient's weight.
Regaining normal weight is the first and essential stage of treatment, but in many patients further psychological treatment is necessary, often for a prolonged period. Relapses are common and one cannot be satisfied that recovery has occurred until normal menstruation returns.
Anorexia nervosa is a serious condition with a mortality rate up to 4%.

Anosognosia

The loss of the ability to recognize disturbed functioning in parts of the body. Thus a hemiplegic individual may not accept that there is anything wrong with the paralysed arm and leg. Lesions of the parietel lobe, or parieto-temporal areas are commonly present in such cases.

Anterograde amnesia

(Synonym: Post-traumatic amnesia)

The severity of head injury is assessed clinically by determining the extent of the antero-grade amnesia. Although islets of memory may occur, and the effects of morphia and other drugs used to alleviate post-operative distress may obscure the true length of the amnesia, none the less this is the best measure of the severity of a head injury.
SEE ALSO Amnesia.

Anti-convulsants

Anti-convulsant drugs are used in the treatment of the several kinds of epilepsy, and the spectrum of activity varies according to the drug group. The principal groups of anti-convulsants are barbiturates and derivatives (e.g. phenobarbitone and primidone), hydantoins (e.g. phenytoin), oxazolidinediones (e.g. troxidone), succinimides (e.g. ethosuximide), benzodiazepines (e.g. diazepam, clonazepam).

Drugs of choice in epilepsy therapy

Grand mal epilepsy
- Phenytoin
- Phenobarbitone
- Carbamazepine
- Primidone

Petit mal epilepsy
- Ethosuximide
- Clonazepam
- Sodium valproate

Temporal lobe and focal epilepsies
- Clonazepam
- Carbamazepine
- Sulthiame

Myoclonic epilepsy
- Sodium valproate
- Clonazepam

Status epilepticus
- Intravenous diazepam

Other compounds include acetazolamide, sulthiame, carbamazepine and phenylacetylarea derivatives, sodium valproate.
Anti-convulsant barbiturates comprise phenobarbitone and its immediate congeneric compounds methylphenobarbitone and metharbitone. Other barbiturates commonly used as hypnotics do not possess clinically useful anti-convulsant activity.
Primidone is a barbiturate derivative used solely as an anti-convulsant, and it is thought to be converted in the body to phenobarbitone. Primidone and phenobarbitone are particularly valuable in grand mal, and primidone in psychomotor seizures; they are not used in petit mal.
The adverse effects of phenobarbitone and primidone resemble those of the barbiturates in general, but primidone occasionally results in a megaloblastic anaemia.
Phenytoin is the prototype of the hydantoin group. Like the barbiturates, hydantoins are used in major and psychomotor epilepsy. However, their anti-convulsant action is thought to differ in nature from that of the barbiturates, so that combinations consisting of a compound from each group are pharmacologically sound.
Hydantoins have rather more side effects than barbiturates, but these should not obscure the value of essentially safe compounds. Minor adverse reactions include gastric discomfort, skin rashes, gum hypertrophy and hirsutism. When taken over a long period, interference with folate metabolism may result in megaloblastic anaemia. Other blood dyscrasias have been described. Neurological manifestations include nystagmus, slurred speech and ataxia. Rarely a lymphadenopathy may occur and cause diagnostic difficulty.
Troxidone is the prototype for the oxazolidinediones; the clinical use of these compounds is confined to the treatment of petit mal. Toxic effects are common and numerous; the more important ones are photophobia, skin rashes, blood dyscrasias and nephrosis.
The succinimides were introduced in an attempt to find a less toxic alternative to troxidone. Ethosuximide is the most effective member of the group and is now considered as the first choice in the treatment of petit mal. The incidence of adverse reactions is lower than with the oxazolidinediones but their nature is not dissimilar; gastro-intestinal upset, skin rashes, blood dyscrasias and lethargy are the most notable effects.
Benzodiazepine compounds possess anticonvulsant properties and are finding an increasing role in the treatment of epilepsy. Their role in the regular treatment of epilepsy has not yet been fully determined but intravenous diazepam is undoubtedly valuable in status epilepticus and clonazepam appears to have a wide spectrum of anticonvulsant activity including grand mal, temporal lobe epilepsy, petit mal and infantile spasms. The low toxicity is a factor in its favour.
There are a number of other compounds which have found a place in anti-convulsant therapy. Acetazolamide is a carbonic anhydrase inhibitor derived from the sulphonamides, principally used in petit mal. Side effects include anorexia, drowsiness and headaches. Sulthiame is also a sulphonamide derivative, but it acts rather differently and is used for major and psychomotor seizures. Adverse effects are a limiting factor and include gastro-intestinal upset, headache, drowsiness, paraesthesiae, and mental confusion which may amount to psychosis. It is perhaps most effectively combined with phenytoin.
More recently carbamazepine has been introduced. A dibenzazepine derivative related to imipramine, it is probably of most value in psychomotor epilepsy where its psychotropic action may be helpful, but it is also effective in grand mal. Carbamazepine tends to be reserved for use as an additional compound in refractory cases. Drowsiness, dry mouth, skin rashes and gastro-intestinal disturbance may occur; jaundice and aplastic anaemia have been reported. Sodium valproate is a compound chemically unrelated to any of the other groups. It is useful in generalized and focal epilepsies but side effects, including minor gastric irritation, have been troublesome particularly early in therapy. Pheneturide and phenacemide are phenylacetylurea derivatives which are effective in psychomotor epilepsy, but they are very toxic.

Anti-depressants

Anti-depressants are a group of compounds which elevate depressed mood

The effect of anti-depressants on synaptic transmission

a) Tricyclic anti-depressants

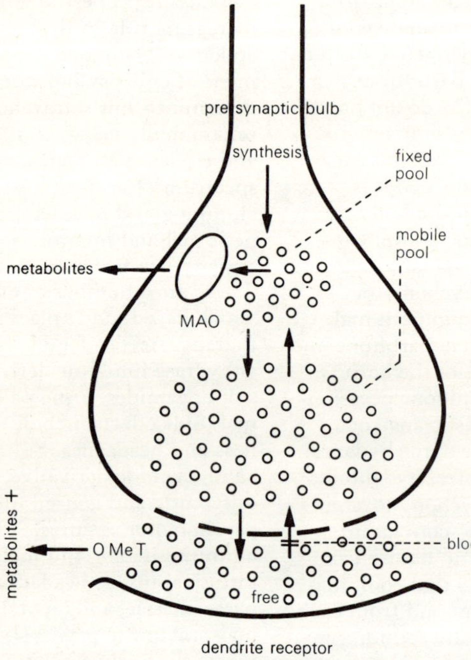

b) Monoamine oxidase inhibitors

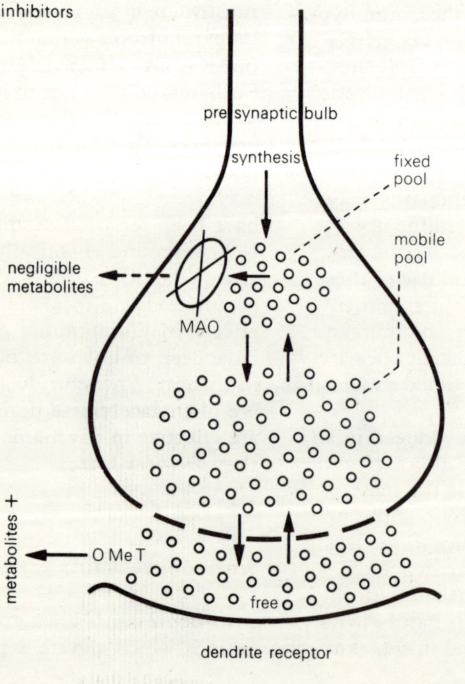

and are used in the treatment of depressive illness. Anti-depressants characteristically have a slow onset and prolonged duration of action. Unfortunately they produce a relatively high incidence of side effects, but these are usually tolerable in relation to the symptoms being relieved.

Anti-depressant drugs may be conveniently considered in two broad categories according to their mode of action. It is thought that anti-depressants act by increasing the availability of transmitter amines at central nervous system receptor sites, and this action is produced by two distinct mechanisms (see diagram). Most of the tricyclic group of compounds prevent the reabsorption of transmitter amines at synaptic junctions; imipramine and amitriptyline are examples of this group. However iprindole, chemically related to the tricyclics, may act by blocking 'masked inhibitory' monoamine receptors. Monoamine oxidase inhibitors (MAOIS) on the other hand prevent the metabolic degradation of amines. Examples of this group include isocarboxazid, phenelzine and tranylcypramine.

Tricyclic anti-depressants are of value in all types of depression, but in general response to treatment is better in psychotic depression. In children, tricyclic anti-depressants have also been found helpful in behaviour disorders and nocturnal enuresis. MAOIS are held to be of particular advantage in the treatment of some atypical depressive illnesses.

The elevation of mood produced by anti-depressant treatment is delayed in onset. Although the therapeutic response may occur in three to four days, it not infrequently takes up to ten days and may even require as long as three weeks. Unfortunately the adverse effects of the drugs are immediate and obvious, and unprepared patients may be discouraged to the point of discontinuing treatment.

The usual dose pattern is thrice daily, although some psychiatrists use a reduced dosage for the initial two or three days to minimize early adverse effects. If insomnia is a prominent symptom, then a nocturnal dose of a sedative tricyclic compound (see tricyclics) can be a particularly helpful manoeuvre. Anti-depressant drugs are frequently combined with ECT in severe or refractory depression. They have the effect of reducing the number of ECT required and the risk of relapse when ECT is used alone.

The prevailing symptomatology often provides a useful guide to the selection of a particular anti-depressant drug. Anxiety and agitation are pointers towards selecting a more sedative drug or the addition of a tranquillizer, and a benzodiazepine (e.g. chlordiazepoxide) or a phenothiazine (e.g. chlorpromazine) is often given together with anti-depressants. Conversely lethargy and anergia, without marked depression of mood, suggest the choice of a more stimulating member of the group.

Suicidal risk may increase in the early stages of treatment of retarded depression as the depressive inertia is relieved and a careful watch should be kept.

Many depressed patients suffer only a single depressive episode requiring treatment. But the natural course of such an episode is prolonged by comparison with other acute and sub-acute diseases. It is therefore prudent to dissuade patients from understandable but premature withdrawal of treatment and in patients with other than a mild depression it is worth continuing anti-depressant treatment for six months after full response has been achieved before carrying out gradual withdrawal of the drug. Relapse of depressive symptoms usually occurs within two weeks if anti-depressant treatment is stopped too soon. Nevertheless the position of maintenance therapy is still open to dispute. In other instances depressive illness is recurrent, and continuous medication is clearly appropriate in an attempt to avoid relapse. The alternative therapy in such patients is the administration of lithium salts (q.v.).

Elderly patients are not infrequently considerably more sensitive to adverse effects of the anti-depressant drugs, and in these patients the dosage must be more cautious.

The main classes of antidepressants are as follows:

A. Tricyclics (q.v.) (thymoleptics)
   1. Dibenzazepine derivatives (q.v.)
   2. (a) Iminodibenzyl derivatives (q.v.)
      (b) Iminostilbene derivatives (q.v.)
   2. Dibenzodiazepine derivatives (q.v.)
   3. Dibenzocycloheptadiene derivatives (q.v.)
   4. Dibenzocycloheptatriene derivatives (q.v.)

5. Dihydroanthracenes (q.v.)
6. Acridan derivatives (q.v.)
7. Dibenzoxepine derivatives (q.v.)
8. Dibenzothiepine derivatives (q.v.)
9. Indole derivatives (q.v.)
10. Dibenzobicyclo-octadiene derivatives (q.v.)

B. Monoamine oxidase inhibitors (thymeretics)

Anti-Parkinsonism compounds

When considering the therapy of Parkinsonism (q.v.) it is important to distinguish between the syndrome produced by the administration of major tranquillizers and that due to degenerative change in the nigrostriatal tract. In the latter group the drug of choice is levodopa but this has a negligible effect in the drug induced form. Extrapyramidal syndromes during treatment with major tranquillizers (q.v.) are rapidly relieved by parenteral administration of anti-Parkinsonism agents, or prophylactic oral doses may be given with the major tranquillizers when larger doses of the latter are used.
Drugs used in the treatment of drug induced pyramidal syndromes (see table) are mainly anti-cholinergic. They relieve extra-pyramidal rigidity and dystonic reactions, but are generally less effective for tremor and akinesia. The relief of the drug-induced extrapyramidal symptoms is rarely complete.
Anti-Parkinsonism agents have atropinic side effects, and central excitation in susceptible patients may precipitate a toxic psychosis.

Oral and parenteral anti-Parkinson agents of value in drug induced cases.

Benztropine	Amantedine
Bipenden	Benzhexol
Procyclidine	Ethopropazine
Orphenadrine	

Antisocial behaviour

No form of antisocial behaviour whether it be physical violence, pathological lying (q.v.), sexual aberration, excessive drinking, stealing (q.v.) or misbehaviour (q.v.) should be regarded as pathognomonic of a psychological illness, or as a syndrome in its own right (cf. arson and kleptomania). However, almost any type of mental disorder may result in symptomatic antisocial behaviour. In consequence a medical approach may be indicated at times. The commonest disorders manifesting antisocial behaviour are childhood behaviour disorders (q.v.) and psychopathic disorders (q.v.), whilst the two commonest forms of criminal conviction are for motoring offences and for theft, which are rarely of medical significance.
SEE ALSO Driving, Recidivism, Sexual disorders and Shoplifting.

Anxiety

Anxiety may be defined as an unpleasant emotional experience varying in degree from mild unease to intense dread, associated with the anticipation of impending or future disaster. It is related to a feeling of threat which has often little or no valid external cause. It leads to characteristic somatic, physiological, autonomic, biochemical, endocrinological and behaviour changes. It is closely related to the emotion of fear and has in common with that emotion its unpleasant anticipation of the future and its basis in past memory and experience.
Normal anxiety acts as a drive to behaviour to overcome, eliminate and resolve the threat. It has been shown that there is an optimum level of anxiety drive, the level of which depends on the complexity of the performance required and on the personality traits of the subject. Anxiety drive levels which are too low result in sub-optimal performance, whereas if anxiety becomes too great performance declines.
Pathological anxiety, where the symptoms are out of proportion in either severity or duration, should be regarded as a symptom, not as an illness or syndrome in itself. Thus anxiety may be secondary to a physical illness or a psychiatric illness such as a depressive disorder.
Persons suffering from an anxiety neurosis are often found to have previous personalities of anxious predisposition, always worriers with a history of childhood insecurity and fears and a family history of similar neuroses. The constitutional factors are important, both neurotic

traits and behaviour patterns learnt in early life where similarly affected close relatives are implicated. This predisposition may be so bad that the patient has a lifelong history of disabling anxiety which fluctuates in degree depending on his life circumstances. Other patients are less predisposed and symptoms only become manifest in response to some particularly stressful life event, and these stresses may be particularly personal to them, depending on their previous life experiences.
In any event the psychic anxiety is often accompanied by somatic symptoms stemming from physiological accompaniments of the anxiety or perhaps from some upsetting experience, for instance a close relative dying from coronary ischaemia. Thus palpitations and ectopic beats, chest constriction and a feeling of being unable to fill the lungs, dyspepsia, nausea and looseness of stools, aches and pains due to muscle tension and especially tension headaches are all common in addition to such vague complaints as dizziness, impaired memory and depersonalization. All these somatic factors may be associated with hypochondriasis and an insistence by the patient that there is a physical cause for his illness. The characteristic feature of anxiety neurosis, whatever the symptomatology, is a continuously heightened level of anxiety with fluctuations in the intensity of symptoms, the intensity building up *gradually* either slowly or rapidly. If a patient is *completely* free of anxiety between attacks and if the attacks are *unprecipitated* and *instantaneous* in onset, the anxiety is almost certainly an unusual presentation of a depressive illness.
Physiological findings are of interest, especially as a model to keep in mind when it comes to treatment. In a normal person the resting level of arousal, as measured for instance by the skin conductance level, is low but responds markedly to a stress such as a loud noise. However, if the noise is repeated over and over again the patient quickly *habituates* to the stimulus and the skin conductance returns almost to normal levels. In contrast an anxious person has a high baseline for arousal with spontaneous fluctuations in the skin conductance. An external stimulus will result in a relatively small increase in the already abnormal skin conductance. More significantly, repeated stimuli result in a very poor rate of habituation. However, if by giving such a patient a tranquillizing drug the skin conductance can be brought down to near normal levels then the response to a stimulus and the rate of habituation are likewise similar to normal. With this concept in mind treatment of the three common groups can be considered.

1. *Chronic severe anxiety neurosis*

Such patients have a life-long history of anxiety, deeply entrenched in their personality and frequently affecting personal relationships, work and other aspects of their life. Tranquillizing drugs may take the edge off their symptoms, but not reduce their state of arousal to normal or near normal levels. The therapeutic aim is necessarily limited, to keep the patient as independent as possible, at work and with an unreduced social life. This is best done with support, reassurance and advice and the use of tranquillizers to overcome bad patches. Hospitalization and frequent attendances in out-patient departments are counter-productive unless used as a very temporary measure to overcome a particular crisis. In severe entrenched cases, leucotomy may be of benefit.

2. *Anxiety state*

This describes a syndrome where a person, relatively free from anxiety traits in his previous personality, develops a state of anxiety, usually following some distressing life event. In contrast with the chronic anxiety neurosis this patient is eminently curable, though if left untreated the patient may develop chronic symptoms of anxiety. Treatment is aimed at reducing the patient's level of arousal to normal and by implication allowing normal habituation to occur. In the mildest cases simple reassurance and a sedative to ensure a good night's sleep is all that is required. In more severe cases daily tranquillizers, perhaps combined with an MAOI, are needed and sometimes an initial period of narcosis may be advised. In all cases the aim is to abolish the patient's symptoms as completely as possible. If symptoms can be completely removed and the patient is able to take up all his old activities, the medication can be reduced quickly and may even be completely withdrawn within 2–3 months. Where symptoms are not completely abolished psychological and pharmacological treatment must be continued energetically till they gradually disappear, but drug treatment should be continued for at least a year and often longer, otherwise the minor recurrences which are so common may lead to a full-blown relapse with a risk of chronicity.

3. *Chronic borderline anxiety neurosis*

These patients lie between the acute anxiety state and the chronic severe anxiety neurosis. Patients have well marked anxiety traits in their personality but are able to function well. At times, however, and usually in response to some life event there is an exacerbation of the underlying anxiety. These patients cannot be cured but it is important to prevent them slipping into chronic disability. Such patients respond quite well to tranquillizing drugs and supportive psychotherapy and these should be used, if necessary energetically, to help the patient remain at work and continue a full social life, as once these are stopped for any length of time such patients often find difficulty in getting back to their former level of activities.

When physical symptoms of anxiety are prominent (e.g. palpitation) the beta-blocking drugs such as propranolol are often beneficial either alone or in combination with a minor tranquillizer.

Anxiety hysteria

An old-fashioned psychoanalytic term for phobias. No longer in use.

Anxiety states in childhood

In the child as in the adult, painful emotions (anxiety, depression and anger) arise most commonly in response to stress (q.v.) situations. However, children differ from adults in their emotional life in a number of important ways. The stresses which they have to face are more varied and include especially those associated with biological maturation and with family life. The process of child development involves continued change – in particular the gradual relinquishing of a dependent state and the acquisition of independence. Further, for normal emotional development to occur the child must learn to experience and tolerate anxiety. The fear of strangers occurring in the second year of life is a good example of this phenomenon. Finally, the child patient is often less able than an adult to decide what is producing anxiety or depression, and therefore the doctor must more often rely on the account given by the parents and on his own observations of the child's behaviour.

Depression in childhood (q.v.) occurs only infrequently in endogenous form, and is more commonly seen as an exaggerated response to stress. Handicapping anxiety states, by contrast, occur frequently throughout the whole of childhood and merit further attention.

Within the first year of life, some babies appear fearful and unhappy whenever they are faced with any new situation, for example, when the mother tries a new food or attempts to get the child to use a spoon rather than a cup. Stella Chess has described the 'slow to warm up' baby and believes this to be a constitutionally determined temperamental characteristic. The anxiety shown by the mother, and the confidence she herself is able to display, in a new situation is another important factor. In the second year of life nocturnal anxiety, associated with frequent waking and screaming with fear, may occur, and at this age, too, excessive fear of strangers may arise.

As the child gets older, specific fears of animals, especially dogs, thunder and lightning, the dark, doctors and dentists, etc. become more common and sometimes take on a handicapping form. It is very common for children to experience multiple fears in mild form, but it is uncommon for the fearfulness to involve any serious disability to the child's life.

In adolescence (q.v.), fear of social situations and agoraphobia (q.v.) become more important.

Specific fears take on more significance if associated with other more general symptoms of anxiety, especially sleep and appetite disturbances, difficulties in concentration, irritability and tearfulness. The presence of this constellation of symptoms requires careful diagnosis of the family situation, the child's adjustment in school and other possible stresses. Symptomatic treatment, including with older children the addition of a minor tranquillizer such as diazepam, is usually effective, for these disorders generally have a benign prognosis. If the condition is in danger of becoming chronic, specialist referral should be considered.

Anxiolytic drugs

Anxiolytic implies a specificity of action which does not obtain for any drug at present in use. All anxiolytics have hypnotic effects in high doses and all hypnotics given in low dosage have the effect of alleviating anxiety. The classes of drugs in common use are the barbiturates, the major tranquillizers, such as the phenothiazines (q.v). and butyrophenones (q.v.) in low dosage and the minor tranquillizers, particularly the benzodiazepines. The usefulness of any drug is the combination of both its wanted and unwanted effects and in most cases of anxiety the balance markedly favours the benzodiazepines. In comparable dosage they are at least as effective as the barbiturates in controlling anxiety, they are less likely to induce unpleasant sedation or impairment of mental functioning, and in particular they are immeasurably safer if taken in overdose. Since anxiolytic drugs may be taken over a prolonged period of time the minimal tendency of the benzodiazepines to produce pharmacological dependence as compared with the barbiturates is also important.
Dosage must be flexible, varying the dosage in frequency and amount during the day and from one day to the next, depending on the patient's symptoms. Furthermore despite the similarity between the different benzodiazepines a patient may respond better to, for instance, diazepam than to oxazepam and vice versa.
Although the benzodiazepines are the drugs of choice for most patients on a regular day-to-day basis, barbiturates are still of use especially in severe cases of panic, for a limited period, when the patient may well be treated in bed either in hospital or under close supervision.

Apathy

A state of indifference to situations which would normally excite interest or emotion, and which occur in many psychiatric conditions. It is common in schizophrenia (q.v.), both in the hebephrenic (q.v.) illnesses of adolescents and in the residual defect states of middle age. In hebephrenics preoccupation with the phantoms of their psychotic internal world is largely responsible, but in chronic schizophrenia loss of the capacity for emotional response ('blunting of affect') is usually more important. Apathy is seen in many organic states, particularly those like Pick's disease (q.v.) where the frontal lobes are heavily involved, and when dementia is present the patient's loss of awareness may be an important contributory factor. Apathy is also common in severe depressions (q.v.) and is readily understandable in the light of the patient's loss of energy, loss of capacity for enjoyment and conviction that the future is hopeless. Finally a striking degree of apathy can be produced by long residence in a mental hospital, prison or other institution. The patient gradually becomes indifferent to events in the outside world, because he has no contact with it; his interests and wishes may be ignored by those in whose charge he remains, thus reinforcing his sense of apathy and hopelessness.
Treatment involves change in the social milieu, and participation of the patient in the change.

Apert's syndrome (acrocephalosyndactyly)

Apert's syndrome is a condition which is transmitted as a single autosomal dominant gene defect. In its usual form it shows mental subnormality, though not usually severe, acrocephalic skull, protuberant and widely set and sloping eyes, high cleft palate and syndactyly. Late paternal age is believed to be of aetiological importance

Aphasia

Aphasia, literally 'loss of speech', is used in a wider sense to mean loss or partial loss of expression or comprehension in any mode of communication – speech, writing or gesture. It is due to central conceptual or constructional difficulties and not defects in the effector or receptor neuronal pathways. It should be suspected when spontaneous or elicited speech is inappropriate, disconnected or, having regard to the educational and social background of the patient, ungrammatical; or when objects are used inappropriately. It may provide a false impression of confusion when it is present in an intellectually preserved patient, for example, after embolism, wounding, or vascular spasm, though most often, as it commonly occurs in degenerative conditions – senile dementia (q.v.), pre-senile dementia (q.v.) (particularly Pick's disease (q.v.) with temporal lobe atrophy) or generalized cerebral arteriosclerosis – it is associated with global dementia. It may be seen in children with autism (q.v.). Testing for this condition on the sensory side demonstrates an inability to grasp spoken words by questions and simple instructions; comprehend sounds, e.g. rattling keys, jingling money, rustling paper (auditory agnosia); read (alexia – sometimes congenital); to recognize objects by sight (visual agnosia) or feel (tactile agnosia). On the motor side the patient is examined as far as spontaneous conversation, recitation (aphasia) and writing (agraphia) are concerned, instructions being both spoken and written.
Finally, the patient is tested for inability to use common objects like a match or a key (ideational apraxia), and construct or copy patterns (constructional apraxia).
Common findings are nominal aphasia – inability to name while function is described ('It's a . . . for writing with . . .', i.e. a pen) and the name still recognized in a series of names (sausage, book, pen, lamp); perseveration (naming first object again when shown a second); agrammatism, e.g. telegram style of speech; paraphasia, jargon aphasia, syntactical aphasia – use of wrong words or non-existent words verbigeration – constant repetition of words or phrases; sibilation – interrupted hissing ('ss . . . ss . . . ss . . .').
Areas of the brain which when damaged result in aphasia are Broca's speech area (posterior aspect of second and third frontal convolutions), second frontal gyrus (centre for agraphia), first temporal gyrus (word deafness), angular gyrus (word blindness).
SEE ALSO Speech disorders.

Aphonia

A loss of the ability to phonate, from whatever cause. Functional aphonia may be deliberate – mute by malice, or may be a symptom of serious emotional disturbance, as in the depressive illnesses, schizophrenic disorders and neuroses. Sulking and not talking are seen in naughty children; in adults on occasions the underlying mechanisms may be very similar.
SEE ALSO Hysteria.

Apperception

This term, although of considerable historical importance, is little used in contemporary psychology. It survives mainly in the title of the popular projective technique, the Thematic Apperception Test (q.v.) (TAT).
Its original meaning implies clear perception (q.v.) accompanied by recognition or identification of the object perceived. Later, psychologists of the Herbartian School applied it to the process whereby present perceptions are linked to and interpreted in the light of the existing knowledge, the apperceptive mass, of the perceiver. Current broader usage of the term perception embraces both these usages.
SEE ALSO Thematic apperception test and Perception.

Appetite

As distinct from hunger, which has well-known physiological, biochemical and endocrinological concomitants, appetite also includes assessment of the psychological appreciation of food. It is disturbed in many psychiatric illnesses, especially affective disorders. Change in appetite, usually a diminution, is virtually universal

in moderate or severe depression. Depression of appetite in marasmus nervosus may result in extreme emaciation even in a child. Appetite may be depressed, normal or even increased during the course of anorexia nervosa, but aversion to food results in excessive purging, self-induced vomiting and disgust if bulimia does occur.
SEE ALSO Anorexia.

Apraxia

Inability to perform purposeful movements, not accompanied by muscular paralysis or sensory disturbance, caused by lesions in the corpus callosum, the parietal and possibly the frontal lobes. Apraxia may be limited to one area of the body, e.g. the face, one limb or one side of the body. In mild cases the patient may appear 'clumsy'. In more severe cases, the patient appears confused.

Arachnodactyly
SEE Marfan's syndrome.

Archetype

The archetypes are primal images of certain basic human experiences which exist in the collective unconscious, and may be made consciously manifest in the form of symbols such as the witch, the wise old man, the circle, or the mandala – a device used in the Far East for meditation. Archetypes are closely connected with instincts, are inherited and are manifested in the artistic productions of the different races of mankind.

Argino-succinic acidaemia

A rare metabolic defect characterized by the presence of large amounts of argino-succinic acid in the cerebrospinal fluid, blood and urine. It is associated with epilepsy, dysrhythmia of the EEG and mental retardation.

Arithmetical mean
SEE Mean, arithmetic.

Arousal

The term applied to the physiological reaction which occurs in the central nervous system as a result of a sudden stimulus. It involves stimulation of the cerebral cortex, hypothalmus and limbic system (q.v.). Arousal is the result of an outflow to these areas from the reticular formation (q.v.) which is itself stimulated by collaterals from the main sensory nerve pathways.

Arson

Several patterns of arson occur. In children, playing with fire is a common and normal activity, and is usually harmless. A small number of children, however, deliberately set fire to hay stacks, farm buildings and sports pavilions, usually in a group setting. The hyperkinetic child has a particular fascination with water and with fire, and may become an arsonist. In the adult there are three main patterns, the first is seen when the fire is laid out of a desire for revenge or as an act of aggression in response to some real or imagined slight. The individual may have been drinking, and decide on an impulse to burn down the factory, garage or other building. The second is deliberate arson for the sake of gain – for the insurance money – this type of arson is much more common than is generally thought. The third and by far the rarest type of arson is when the fire setting occurs as part of a sexual perversion, the individual obtaining intense sexual pleasure from the sight of the fire and the activities of the firemen. Arson is regarded as a particularly serious offence, for innocent people may be burnt to death and the damage to property may be very great. Heavy sentences are therefore often imposed.

Arteriosclerosis
SEE Cerebral arteriosclerosis.

Arteriosclerotic psychosis
(Synonym: Acute or chronic brain syndrome due to cerebro-vascular disease.)

Arteriosclerotic psychosis and senile dementia are the two most common causes of dementia in old people. Arteriosclerotic psychosis is more common in men than women and occasionally occurs in late middle age. The course of the illness averages 3–4 years but is shorter if accompanied by severe hypertension or if it is associated with a major stroke. The disorder is due to generalized occlusive disease of the cerebral arteries leading to widespread but not necessarily confluent infarction of the cortex. Extracerebral arterial disease is responsible for many cases; carotid disease typically results in cerebral damage, vertebral artery sclerosis resulting in brain-stem ischaemia.

The general features of arteriosclerotic psychosis are:

1. Memory disturbances, the defect especially affecting the registration of new events.
2. Defect of intellect resulting in impaired grasp, reasoning and judgement.
3. Disorientation for time and place occurs in severe cases or temporarily in acute episodes.
4. Personality changes are not so pronounced as in senile dementia, perhaps because the areas of cortical ischaemia are not confluent. However, emotional lability is common and with a retained insight depression is not uncommon.

In severe cases suspicion, jealousy and ideas of persecution occur, especially during or following an acute episode with confusion.

The onset of the disorder is often sudden and the subsequent course is punctuated by episodes of clouding of consciousness, presumably due to fresh infarcts. This clouding may last minutes or several days, the underlying dementia tending to increase with each episode. Arteriosclerotic changes sufficient to cause dementia virtually always result in associated neurological syndromes such as hemiplegia, hemianopia, aphasia and apraxia.

Treatment is limited to general care, management and symptom relief. Chlorpromazine and thioridazine are recommended for restlessness and agitation in episodes of confusion or mental disturbances. They may also be used at night for insomnia perhaps combined with a short-acting hypnotic such as chloral hydrate. Other drugs such as the tricyclic antidepressants and the anti-Parkinsonian drugs should be used with care as they may exacerbate the patient's mental confusion.

Art therapy

The expression of conflicts and problems in artistic activity is utilized by the art therapist in much the same way as the psychotherapist uses words. Symbols are interpreted, production encouraged, and the interpersonal relationship developed. No particular artistic ability is required, and many different techniques may be used, such as finger painting, modelling, collage, oil painting and so on. When physical disabilities exist, art therapy may be particularly useful in retraining muscular dexterity and other physical functions.

Asomatognosia

Inability to distinguish between right and left due to parietal lobe dysfunction.
SEE ALSO Body image.

Assertive therapy

The training of more assertive behaviour in situations where behaviour has usually not been assertive enough. A patient liable to excessive anxiety or tension when criticized unfairly, for example, might be taught to stand up for himself better by practice in contrived situations in which he was criticized. It is possible that 'assertive' responses are antagonistic to anxiety, in the same way as is muscular relaxation.

Association, disorders of

Associations are links between ideas, words or experiences, or between stimuli and responses, which ensure that when one of the linked elements occurs in the experience of an individual, the associated experience tends to follow. These associations derive from the previous experience of the individual and are formed in accordance with a number of well-established principles, of which the 'laws' of contiguity and similarity are the most important. Associations formed in these ways are

prominent in certain types of learning, especially verbal learning, memory and thinking. Verbal associations may be explored by means of word association tests, during which the subject is asked to respond to given words by 'the first word which comes to his mind'. Chained free association of a similar type plays a prominent part in psychoanalytic (q.v.) techniques. Disorders of the associative process are particularly prominent in the thought disorder exhibited by many schizophrenics (q.v.). Bleuler considered them fundamental to this condition and spoke of a 'splitting' and 'loosening' of associations which results in the characteristic vagueness and inconsequentiality of speech. Such schizophrenics may also show uncontrolled association by similarity, often exemplified in their talk by 'clang' associations of words which rhyme or sound alike.
SEE ALSO Thought.

Asthenia
SEE Neurasthenia.

Asthma

Asthma is typically characterized by episodic dyspnoea due to constriction of the bronchi with oedema of the mucosa. The condition may be genetically determined with a polygenic mode of inheritance, but infective, allergic and emotional factors may play a role in its precipitation. A somatic predisposition of bronchial hypersensitivity is probably necessary before psychological mechanisms can act. Although certain personality traits are often seen in asthmatics, there does not appear to be a specific personality type associated with the disease; a conditioned reflex can account for some asthmatic attacks produced by anxiety. The part played by allergy (q.v.) has been clarified by the finding of raised levels of an immunoglobulin (IgE) in some patients with a clear cut allergic history, and treatment with the immunosuppressive drugs may benefit these patients. Steroids often play an important part in treatment, but can produce psychological disturbances. If conditioned anxiety plays a prominent role in the precipitation of attacks, systematic desensitization (q.v.) in imagination may be indicated. If it is assumed that the basic problem in asthma is a variety of stimulating factors, leading to a reversible airways obstruction due to hypersensitivity, the first step in management should be to delineate these physical and psychological causes as clearly as possible, and then to treat each one without losing sight of the patient as an individual.
SEE ALSO Psychosomatic disorders and Respiratory diseases.

Astrocytes
SEE Neuroglia.

Ataractics
SEE Tranquillizers.

Ataxia-telangiectasia
(Synonym: Louis-Bar syndrome)

This syndrome comprises mental subnormality, cerebellar ataxia or choreoathetosis, and development of telangiectases which are most noticeable in the conjunctivae but may appear elsewhere in the body. The genetical transmission is probably by autosomal recessive inheritance. Hypogammaglobulinaemia seems to be a frequent biochemical concomitant.

Attempted suicide

The situation in which someone survives after deliberately endangering his or her life, either by taking an overdose of drugs or in some other way, is variously described as attempted suicide, unsuccessful suicide, a suicidal gesture, parasuicide, or self-poisoning. All five terms are unsatisfactory in that they embody implications which may be untrue but 'attempted suicide' is the most widely used. So common a phenomenon has it become in the last twenty-five years that in many general hospitals it is now the biggest single cause of medical emergency admission. A survey in 1960–61 revealed an attempted suicide rate of 1:1000 population/year, roughly ten times the suicide rate. This was probably typical of urban areas at the time and may well have increased further in the last decade.

The demographic and psychiatric characteristics of people who make suicidal attempts are different from those of 'successful' or 'completed' suicides. Attempted suicide is twice as common in women as in men, and its incidence falls rather than rises with increasing age. In fact, the majority of attempted suicides are young women between the ages of 15 and 35. The rate is higher in urban than in rural areas and in large cities the highest rates are found in areas where poverty, poor housing and delinquency are most conspicuous. As a corollary to this, social classes IV and V have higher rates than classes I and II. The means by which life is endangered also show significant differences from those used by 'successful' suicides. Overdosage with aspirin, or with assorted tranquillizers and anti-depressants, figures much more prominently, and lethal poisons like coal gas much less so. Guns and knives are brandished more often than they are used and the only common self-inflicted wounds are multiple superficial scratches on the wrists. In fact, the risk to life is often trivial, either because the drug taken was relatively harmless or the dose small, or because the subject arranged to be found soon after the event or quickly told others what he had done. In a study in Edinburgh, for instance, of 450 survivors of deliberate overdoses less than 20% had seriously endangered their lives and 50% had not taken any significant risk. The psychiatric characteristics of attempted suicides also differ from those of successful suicides. Depressive illnesses and alcoholism are relatively less prominent and the majority of the depressions are neurotic rather than psychotic in type, and often fairly mild. Personality disorders of various kinds are more prominent than in 'completed' suicides, particularly in those who make repeated attempts, while a proportion, probably 20%, have no significant psychiatric abnormality.

These facts provide ample grounds for regarding attempted suicide and suicide as distinct phenomena, and make it almost impossible to regard the former simply as a *forme fruste* of the latter. But it would be both incorrect and dangerous to draw a firm distinction between the two. For one thing, the extent to which the patient endangers his life is an imperfect indication of his intentions. Someone swallowing ten chlordiazepoxide capsules may well have believed he was taking a lethal dose and mistakes of the opposite kind are equally common, and the patient's intention to be found or not to be found, and hence his chances of survival, may be thwarted by many chance events. Even more important, though, is the fact that the patient's motives are nearly always mixed in both suicide and attempted suicide. The commonest motives are:

1. The wish to die.
2. The wish to demonstrate that one is in intolerable distress.
3. The wish to influence a particular person, usually a relative or lover. This may be to make them behave more considerately or to punish them, by making them feel guilty.
4. A Russian roulette element – deliberately hazarding life with a willingness to accept either death or survival as the outcome. (Hence the rarity of second attempts immediately after the first.)

The first of these tends to predominate in suicides and those who survive after seriously endangering their lives, and the second or third to predominate in the majority of attempted suicides.

Rational management of attempted suicide depends on establishing which were the dominant motives in each case. This can rarely be done by asking patients why they took the tablets. Quite apart from their need to dissimulate they often genuinely do not know, particularly when, as is usually the case, the attempt was made on impulse. But a careful enquiry, as soon after the event as possible, will usually make the situation reasonably clear. The most important issues are usually whether the patient took all the tablets available, whether she told anyone, how she came to medical attention, whom she had quarrelled with, whether she was suffering from a depression, or drinking, and who else was likely to be affected in what ways by the attempt.

Unlike the suicide, who is characteristically alone and friendless, those who make suicidal attempts are commonly trapped in frustrating relationships with other people; a youth whose girl friend has just left him, a woman with an alcoholic husband trying to bring up four children in a damp basement, and so on. Their main motives are usually the second or third of those listed above and, seen in these terms, their suicidal attempts are frequently successful, at least temporarily. The girl friend feels guilty and promises to return, the errant husband helps with the housework for a week or two and a social worker writes to the housing department. At times there is an element of almost open blackmail involved and, of course, if others see the situation in these terms, they react with hostility rather than guilt.

Because suicidal attempts are so often 'successful' in these important ways they are difficult to prevent, and even in cities where everyone making a suicidal attempt is routinely seen by psychiatrists with extensive psychiatric and social facilities available to them the attempted suicide rate shows no sign of falling. Nevertheless, it is probably a wise rule for all attempted suicides to be seen by a psychiatrist before leaving hospital, because many have treatable depressions or remediable social problems. Casualty officers and others are often understandably irritated by having to cope with what they regard as frivolous gestures, and advocate the substitution of less sympathetic regimes in the hope of discouraging further attempts.

It must not be forgotten that at least 10% of these unhappy people eventually do kill themselves.

There are, however, measures that could be taken to discourage overdoses. More selective prescribing of hypnotics and tranquillizers, and insistence on the disposal of unused tablets, is one obvious measure. Another would be for aspirin and similar analgesics to be sold to the public only in individually wrapped tablets, for the majority of suicidal attempts are impulsive and often the impulse would have passed before sufficient tablets had been unwrapped.

SEE ALSO Suicide.

Attention

Conscious perception (q.v.) does not embrace all the information impinging on the sense organs but is selective. Even within the perceptual field at any one time, some aspect of the situation becomes the focus of an individual's active concern, the object of his attention. Similar attentional foci within the general field of consciousness (q.v.) invariably mark the course of the more internalized processes of directed thinking. Attention may be voluntary or involuntary. The related term, concentration, refers to the ability to maintain voluntary attention over a period of time, while engaged in some goal-directed task. Involuntary attention is controlled by characteristics of the environmental stimulation such as intensity, movement, repetition etc.

Although attention at any one time can be divided or distributed within a field, there is a limit to what can be apprehended at any one moment. The attention (or apprehension) span refers to the number of objects, usually about six to eight, which can be perceived at a single glance. In such a test, the subject is merely required to report the total number. If the objects differ, and he is required to name them, the test is of immediate memory span. Clearly, attention is a necessary prerequisite for the registration phase of memory (q.v.).

Psychiatric patients frequently complain of attention and concentration difficulties and disorders of attention may also be evident in the absence of complaint. This is particularly true of patients with organic brain disease, especially when this leads to dementia. Localized brain damage may produce perceptual difficulties, sometimes referred to as 'selective inattention', when stimulation projected to the damaged hemisphere fails to be perceived when in competition with stimulation to the unaffected side. Gross distractibility is characteristic of Huntington's chorea (q.v.) and mania (q.v.) while a more subtle disorder of this nature is considered by some to be fundamental in schizophrenic thought disorder.

Attitudes

A continuing predisposition to react with a characteristic feeling or manner. Attitudes are emotionally determined and may be consciously or unconsciously acquired.

Atypical facial pain

Amongst the group of facial neuralgias are a number of patients whose symptoms do not conform to any recognized neuralgic patterns. The pain does not occur in anatomical areas, is variable and atypical, being dull, throbbing, aching or boring, and does not respond to analgesics. The recognition that the pain was a depressive equivalent (q.v.) has been a major advance, for the condition responds to anti-depressant treatment or ECT, although in some resistant cases leucotomy may eventually become necessary.

Aura

A brief subjective experience giving immediate precognisance of some epileptic (q.v.) fits. It is usually consistent within any individual. The presence of aura generally implies a focal seizure. The majority of these are temporal lobe seizures (q.v.). The aura may be obvious to the observer, though forgotten by the patient. Crude visceral sensations predominate: feelings of fear, butterflies in the stomach, sudden sensations rising to the throat. 'Indescribable feelings' in the head and throat are next in frequency. The patient's difficulty in describing the aura may lead physicians to overlook its significance. Reports of feelings in the penis, vagina, or rectum may even be withheld unless questioning is direct and helpful. Complex experiences referable to each of the special senses also occur. Most complex are 'intellectual' auras, perversions of experience of time, reality, identity, memory and especially in intensity of experience (which may objectively seem trivial). Auras of taste and smell are relatively rare (see Uncinate fits). Other aura experience depends upon the site of the cerebral lesion.

Autism

This is a relatively rare condition, which occurs in four to five per 10,000 children. The autistic child is usually apparently normal for the first few months of life. Then the child becomes unresponsive, shows little interest in auditory or visual stimulation, and resists cuddling, screaming to be put down if he is picked up. If he hurts himself he will not go to his parents to be comforted. Language delay is a common feature, indeed speech may fail to develop. By contrast, motor development is usually not delayed.

Failure to develop relationships with his parents means that the child does not go through the normal phase of separation anxiety and fear of strangers. He shows no interest in the companionship of other children. There may be ritualistic mannerisms, including walking on tiptoe, flicking fingers in front of the eyes and twiddling pieces of string or wire for hours. The child resists change so that weaning and the use of spoon and fork present problems.

Occasionally an autistic syndrome may develop later, even up to the age of 2½ years.

As the child gets older the picture may change. He may begin to lose his autistic aloofness, become affectionate to his parents and show separation anxiety. Commonly, however, the language difficulty remains, with obvious echolalia (q.v.) and prolonged confusion over the use of personal pronouns, the child referring to himself as 'he'.

About 70% of autistic children function in the educationally subnormal range of intelligence or below and the intellectual retardation may be a greater handicap than the behavioural problem. Genetic factors are probably relevant, but sibs are only rarely affected.

The causes of autism are unknown. It occurs most frequently in professional or middle class families. The view that parental, especially maternal, inadequacy lies at the root of the problem has largely been superseded. It now seems likely that autism is primarily a communication disorder, biologically determined and associated with brain dysfunction. Its similarity to developmental aphasia and the high rate of epilepsy (10–15%) shown by autistic children tend to confirm this view. Any parental abnormality is probably a reaction to the stress of having a child with such a severe behavioural abnormality.

All children suspected to be suffering from autism need expert diagnostic appraisal. Psychological testing requires patience, persistence and experience. Biochemical screening, skull X-ray and EEG studies

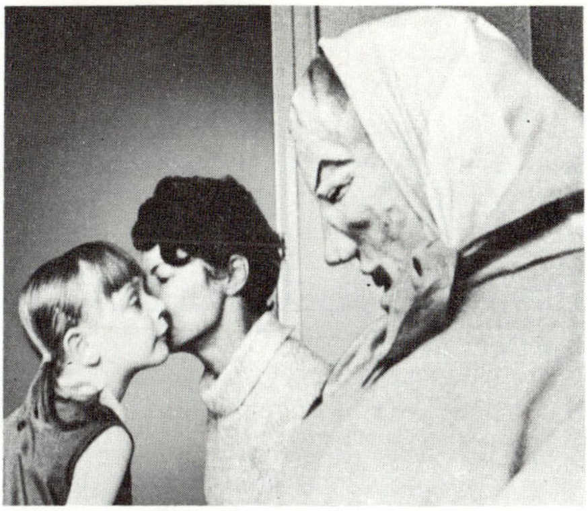

One concept of autistic reaction

should be carried out as a small proportion of autistic children will be found to be suffering from rare but well-defined conditions, such as phenylketonuria and histidinaemia.
Medical treatment is of only limited value. Symptomatic drug treatment of hyperkinesis and epilepsy may be indicated. Rarely a treatable underlying condition may be diagnosed. Appropriate educational measures offer the best hope of improvement, but even here the gains will be strictly limited. Operant conditioning (q.v.) (systematic manipulation of rewarding stimuli) is a relatively new method of treatment likely to result in small but definite gains. Guidance and counselling for parents is an important aspect of management. In many countries the parents of autistic children have formed associations and these mutual advice groups can be valuable. As indicated above, the prognosis for independent life is poor. Only about 15% of children will be able to lead anything but an institutional or sheltered existence. The higher the level of measured intelligence, the better the outlook for the child.

Autistic thinking

Introverted thought. The content of thought is related much more to fantasy than reality and the thinking results in little positive action.

Autochthonous idea

A fully formed delusional idea which appears in the mind suddenly and without any conscious preparation. It is synonymous with a primary delusion and is distinguished from a normal 'brain wave' by its content being strange or bizarre. It is one of Schneider's first-rank symptoms of schizophrenia and may be associated with a delusional mood or delusional perception.
It is to be distinguished from the much commoner delusions which the patient gradually formulates to explain his hallucinations or what he considers to be other people's unfriendly behaviour.
SEE ALSO Delusions.

Autoerotism

This roughly refers to the early infantile phase of self-love – the stage in emotional development in which sensual gratification is secured or attempted through subjective experience alone. Erotic aims are self-directed and are principally gratified in the self. This phase is pre-eminent until the phallic stage in which gratification via important external objects or persons is initiated. This earliest object-related stage for the gratification of love and erotic aims is generally termed alloerotic (q.v.).
Freud considered autoeroticism 'primordial' – it is not something which has to develop. Masturbation is a special, genital-orientated, subdivision of autoeroticism and is not synonymous with it. The autoerotic phase first becomes manifest during the oral sucking period. It is distinguished from narcissism in that autoerotism is objectless – while in narcissism the 'I' is recognized and the infant takes his own body as the love object.
SEE ALSO Anal erotism.

Autogenic training

Applying the principles of Yoga, Schultz began to treat neurosis by using muscular relaxation and exercises. The patient is taught to relax each muscle group, and eventually to be able to relax himself as a whole. The method is autogenic – that is, self-produced, although daily practice is necessary. Popular in Europe in the treatment of neurosis and psychosomatic disorders, autogenic training has links with the techniques of painless childbirth, the progressive relaxation of Jacobson and hypnosis. Autogenic training is a pleasant, effective and simply administered therapy, very suitable for group application.

Automatic obedience

Automatic obedience is the excessive compliance found sometimes in catatonic schizophrenia (q.v.). The request may promise inconvenience or pain, but is nevertheless unquestioningly carried out by the subject.

Automatism, automatic behaviour

A dissociation between behaviour and consciousness, a number of different types of behaviour are subsumed under this heading, depending on the aetiology of the dissociation. Behaviour may in certain normal circumstances be automatic, as with the repetitive movements demanded of a simple task, whilst the individual's attention is concentrated on some other subject. When pathological dissociative states occur, the results of psychological conflict, drug intoxication, or trance states, phenomena such as automatic writing, automatic painting, or sensory automatism (as with the production of hallucinations when gazing intently at a fixed object) may occur. Post-hypnotic automatism is well known, the individual carrying out complex tasks on obedience to the suggestions of the hypnotist. More important are the automatisms occurring in serious psychiatric or neurological illness. A depressive illness may manifest itself in a fugue state – the patient wandering away from home and being found 'suffering from loss of memory' days or weeks later. There is no recollection of the period involved, even when the patient is confronted with evidence of his behaviour during this time. Neurologically automatisms are nearly always manifestations of epilepsy, particularly of psychomotor epilepsy. The automatism may precede a major attack, may represent the whole attack, or occur as a post-ictal manifestation. When any antisocial activity occurs in patients with automatisms considerable difficulty may be experienced in assessing the individual's responsibility for his acts. Head injury may also be associated with automatic behaviour, the footballer who carries on with the game after being concussed being a familiar example. Rarely, diabetics may behave automatically, the blood sugar level may be either high or low, so that problems sometimes occur with regard to capability to drive a car.

Lastly the so-called hysterical fugue is regarded as an example of automatic behaviour, and has to be distinguished from the depressive and epileptic fugue states. In the hysterical fugue there is always an understandable reason for the behaviour, such as dishonesty, marital complication, personal entanglements, the fugue representing an attempt to escape from responsibility. Whether the behaviour is considered to be consciously or unconsciously determined will depend upon the psychiatrist's own convictions and attitudes. In many cases of automatism EEG investigation, the interviewing of informants, and observation of the patient in hospital are all desirable before arriving at a diagnosis.

Autonomic nervous system

The autonomic nervous system consists of those nerve cells and fibres which innervate the smooth muscle and glandular structures of internal organs. Anatomically it comprises the sympathetic trunks, large nerve plexuses, regions of the spinal cord and brain stem, some portions of the hypothalamus and certain cortical areas. The efferent pathway from central nervous system to the organ consists of two neurons, the preganglionic and the post-ganglionic, the synapse between the two being sited in a ganglion in the paravertebral chain or visceral ganglia with acetylcholine as the transmitter. Afferent fibres run from the organs to the central nervous system.

The two main divisions of the autonomic nervous system are the sympathetic and the parasympathetic, the former utilizing noradrenaline as the transmitter in most of its post-ganglionic nerve endings on the innervated organ, the latter acetylcholine. Although the two divisions appear to have antagonistic effects on visceral functions they normally act in an integrated manner; the sympathetic system exerts a widespread, general, rather coarse control while

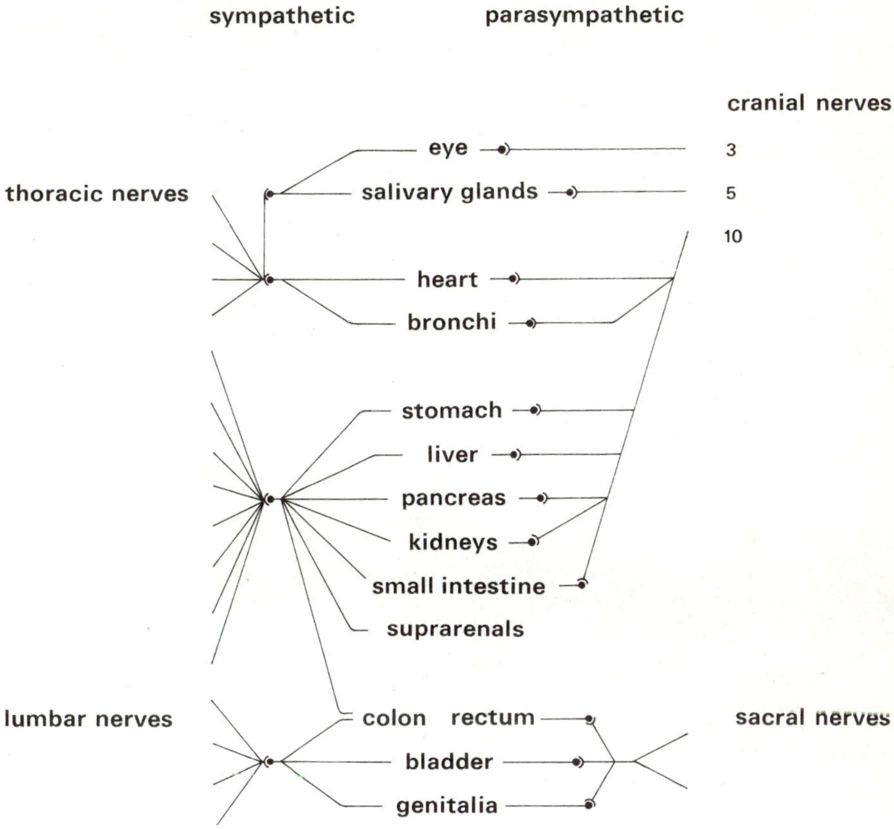

the parasympathetic fibres influence functions of individual organs in a finely tuned way. Although these functions were believed to be outside conscious control, recent research suggests that such control can be learnt.
Organs innervated by autonomic fibres include eye, lacrimal and salivary glands, heart, bronchi and lungs, liver, spleen, stomach, large and small intestines, pancreas, gall-bladder, kidney, ureter and bladder, adrenal medulla, uterus, blood vessels in skin and muscles and sweat glands. Sympathetic effects on organs may be excitatory, such as constriction of blood vessels and contraction of sphincters, and are mediated through 'α-receptors' (q.v.) on the end-organs. These effects can be prevented by α-adrenergic blocking agents, e.g. phentolamine and chlorpromazine. Alternatively, sympathetic effects are mediated via 'β-receptors' (q.v.) and are mainly inhibitory, e.g. relaxation of bronchi, stomach and bladder (but increase in heart action). These effects are prevented by β-blockers like propranolol.
Some psychiatric patients, e.g. anxiety states, agitated depressives and acute schizophrenics, have sympathetic overactivity.
SEE ALSO Hypothalamus and Synapse – transmission in.

Autosomes

Autosomes are those chromosomes (q.v.) other than the sex chromosomes. In man, the normal somatic cell contains forty-four autosomes, comprising twenty-two pairs of matching chromosomes. Certain mental subnormality syndromes with characteristic physical signs, including mongolism (q.v.) and the cri-du-chat syndrome (q.v.) are associated with gross autosomal chromosome abnormalities which can be

detected under the microscope. Many specific conditions associated with mental subnormality are, however, transmitted genetically by minute invisible changes at specific gene loci on the autosomes. These conditions are Mendelian recessive or dominant traits, and include most of the recognized inherited metabolic defects (q.v.), most of which are autosomal recessives.
SEE ALSO Genetics.

Autotopagnosia

Loss of orientation in respect to parts of the body.
SEE ALSO Body image.

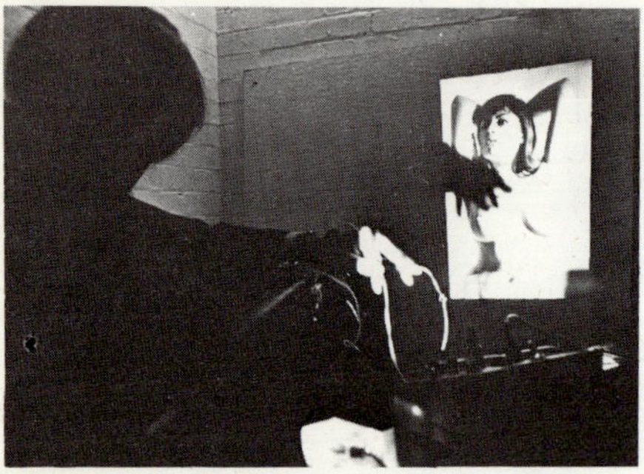

Aversion therapy

The aim of this variety of behaviour therapy is to discourage a form of behaviour which is undesired yet repeatedly performed. In the simplest way punishing a child for misbehaving can be considered 'aversion therapy', but by using the experimental findings of psychological learning theory and Palovian conditioning the techniques have been enormously refined, chiefly by the timing of the aversive stimulus in relationship either to the undesired behaviour or to the one which normally evokes it.
Aversion therapy is most often applied in alcoholism (q.v.) and sexual perversions, notably transvestism (q.v.), fetishism (q.v.) and homosexuality (q.v.). It has also been tried in drug addiction (q.v.), paedophilia (q.v.), sado-masochism (q.v.), and exhibitionism (q.v.). A variety of treatment methods have been employed. Early techniques in which nausea and/or vomiting induced by apomorphine injections were associated with the drinking of alcohol in alcoholics have largely been superseded by techniques using electric shocks as this can be accurately timed. There is no standardized way of applying electric aversion. In one successful method in transvestism the patient repeatedly cross-dresses on an electrified grid, and electric shocks just strong enough to be definitely painful are applied to the feet according to a predetermined schedule during the cross-dressing. Successful treatment might necessitate many treatment sessions and much time from a therapist with specialist technical knowledge.
The results of aversion therapy tend to be better when shocks can be delivered during the deviant act itself, as in transvestism, than when only visual representations of the problem, such as fantasies or photographic slides can be treated, as in homosexuality. The outcome with sexual deviants also depends upon the severity of the patient's personality disorder, the extent of his normal sexual interest which one hopes will replace his deviant behaviour and his motivation – patients with gross disorders of personality who lack normal heterosexual interest or contact and who are brought for treatment by others, perhaps to avoid legal consequences of their behaviour, are rarely helped by aversion (or indeed by anything else).
Even with the most suitable cases relapse is common unless the unwanted behaviour can be replaced by an alternative and acceptable pattern of behaviour – for instance normal heterosexuality. This may mean further treatment with psychotherapy or perhaps behaviour therapy of a desensitization type to counter heterosexual anxieties. It is for this reason that results in alcoholism are rarely successful unless appropriate treatment is simultaneously given for the other psychosocial problems which are normally present and the patient is helped to fill the void in his life as a consequence of his abstinence.

Axons
SEE Neurones.

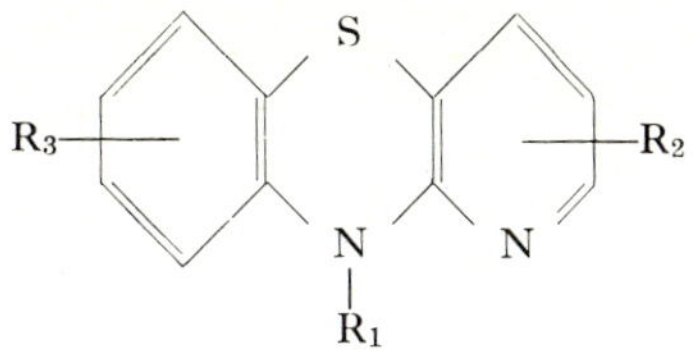

General structure of azaphenothiazines

Azaphenothiazines

Otherwise known as the benzothiazines. The chlorinated benzene ring of the parent phenothiazines has been substituted by a pyridine ring. Their pharmacological properties resemble the phenothiazines. Compounds in the series which have been studied clinically include: prothipendyl, oxypendyl, isothipendyl.

Backward children

Slowness to learn may be a reflection of a general intellectual retardation or a manifestation of specific educational disability as with children who are particularly retarded in reading.
For the aetiology and differential diagnosis SEE Mental subnormality.
Specific learning problems may be produced by innate, genetically determined, perceptual defects (as in the dyslexias (q.v.)) or they may be due to peripheral sensory defects of hearing or vision, brain damage, emotional difficulties, or inadequate teaching. Once medical conditions have been excluded, the management of these learning disorders becomes an educational problem.

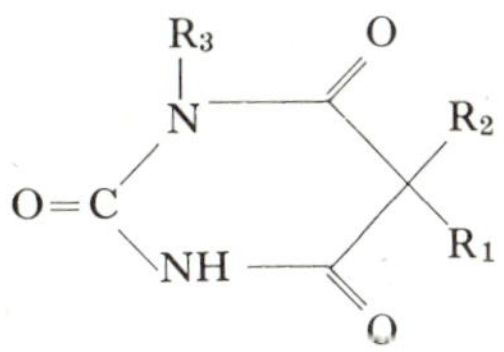

General structure of barbiturates

Barbiturates

Barbiturates were introduced into medical practice at the turn of the century, first barbitone and then phenobarbitone ten years later. Since then innumerable barbiturates have been synthesized, and today a dozen or so are established in clinical practice.
Absorption readily occurs from the gastro-intestinal tract and parenteral sites. Speed and duration of action are directly related to the degree of lipid solubility which determines the rate of tissue penetration. Metabolic degradation occurs mostly in the liver, and the various products are excreted by the kidneys alongside unchanged compound. A single dose of a short or medium acting member is cleared from the body in forty-eight hours, and proportionately longer for the long acting members. Tolerance is well recognized and is related to both increased metabolic transformation and to neuro-physiological adaptation; tolerance does not significantly increase the lethal dose.
The barbiturates are general depressants, but the central nervous system is considerably more sensitive than other tissues to their action. Central depressant effects range from mild sedation to coma according to the particular compound, the dose, the route of administration, and the degree of excitability of the nervous system at the time. The neocortex is affected first; disinhibiting effects and euphoria closely resembling the results of alcohol consumption may occur, and provide one basis for the use of barbiturate as 'soft' drugs of addiction.
Their principal clinical use is as hypnotics. While it is customary for short acting compounds to be given when insomnia is initial, and medium acting compounds to be given when sleep is disturbed during the night and early morning waking occurs, some workers suggest that prolongation of effect is better achieved by increasing the dose.
In psychiatric practice barbiturates are effective anxiolytic agents and have been used widely for this purpose in the past. During the last decade benzodiazepine compounds with some notable advantages have almost completely supplanted barbiturates in the treatment of anxiety; nevertheless barbiturates retain a very limited application in relieving anxiety although many psychiatrists and physicians believe they should not now be used. Acute and severe behavioural disturbance in psychotic or neurotic illness may call for prompt chemical constraint. Oral or parenteral barbiturate is a useful alternative to a tranquillizer, or may be used to supplement tranquillizer therapy. The early disinhibiting effect of barbiturates has found a diagnostic use in narcoanalytic techniques.
Phenobarbitone is a long acting member of the group and differs from the others in having mild mood depressant properties; for this reason it has become disfavoured in psychiatry. It holds a long established role as an anti-convulsant.
In normal doses barbiturates are comparatively free from side effects. The commonest complaint is of a mild discomfort and dullness persisting the following morning and likened to hangover. Hypersensitivity reactions are uncommon and usually take the form of maculopapular or urticarial rashes. Rarely acute porphyria may be precipitated in predisposed subjects.

Tolerance to barbiturates occurs readily and increasing doses are needed to produce the same effect. Cross tolerance to other depressants, such as alcohol, has been described. Continuing moderate dosage easily leads to drug dependence, and patients with chronic anxiety are particularly vulnerable to this. Withdrawal from dependent subjects results in severe anxiety, tremor, twitching, dizziness, nausea and vomiting and weight loss; convulsions are not uncommon and a delirious state may occur.
With prolonged heavy dosage, problems of persistent intoxication and personality changes are added to the difficulty of dependence; affect becomes labile and attitudes irritable and quarrelsome, mental function is impaired with poor concentration, dysmnesia and faulty judgement, and motor inco-ordination ensues with ataxia, dysarthria and nystagmus.
Overdosage with barbiturates has become distressingly frequent as a means of attempting suicide, and in this respect the particularly high risk of depressed patients needs to be continuously borne in mind. It has been suggested that a proportion of barbiturate overdosage is accidental and due to barbiturate automatism in which repeated nocturnal dosage occurs without realization because of confusion.
Some physicians believe that barbiturates have no place in current therapy.

Bar chart

The bar chart bears similarities to the histogram (q.v.). It expresses pictorially the absolute or percentage frequency of events and is particularly useful when the results in two or more groups are to be compared.

Basal ganglia

A series of brain stem nuclei lying close to the internal capsule. There are divergent opinions on the exact list of nuclei to be included but most would include the corpus striatum (putamen and pallidum), the substantia nigra, the subthalamic nuclei (luys) and perhaps the red nucleus.
The basal ganglia form a series of balanced excitatory and inhibitory feedback loops which are responsible for controlling the pyramidal tract, particularly for maintenance of tone and initiation of slow steady muscle activity.
Afferents from all areas of the cortex run to the corpus striatum. From the corpus striatum one loop involves the zona compacta of the substantia nigra which fires back on the corpus striatum via an inhibitory loop in which dopamine is the transmitter substance. A second loop travels via the external pallidum and the subthalamic nucleus to the internal pallidum where it meets a supply direct from the corpus striatum. The internal pallidum is the main area for efferent pathway – the ansal system that conveys its main fibres to the ventro-lateral nucleus of the thalamus and thence back to the motor cortex. There is a topical organization at each area. Other impulses leaving the internal pallidum reach the mid-brain nuclei which, via various polysynaptic tracts, influence the spinal cord ventral horn.
Damage to the nigro-striatal path and interruption of its dopaminergic transmission by neuroleptic drugs lead to Parkinsonism (SEE Extrapyramidal syndromes).

Battered child syndrome

Until just after the second world war multiple injuries in young children were mainly ascribed to mysterious bone diseases and blood dyscrasias. Now it is realized that human parents (as in many other mammalian species) can attack their children and sometimes do so repeatedly. In 1962 Kempe showed that child battering is not confined to any one socio-economic class, nor to the overtly mentally ill. Most of the parents had personality disorders (q.v.), and many are psychopaths (q.v.). Some of the parents are continuously angry and explosive, others are themselves severely emotionally damaged and demand sophisticated affection from their offspring, whilst others are rigid, controlled, fussy people who explode when their order and routine is upset by messy, demanding children. Many of the parents may have been

violently handled in their own childhood. Frequently the child is taken to the hospital or doctor with an injury (sometimes a day or two old) and the story of falling out of a cot, or down the stairs. Diagnosis may be difficult, but whole-body X-rays may show older healed injuries. A sympathetic and alert interview with the parents is essential; they should not be challenged or accused, but allowed to discuss their feelings about the child, and how he or she upsets them. More than one child may be attacked, but sometimes it is a child who has been rejected from an early age.
The risk to these children is exceedingly high. Any suspicion should lead to skilled psychiatric and social work help (e.g. from the local children's department or from special societies for child care). Police intervention may be necessary in some cases. Even after skilled attention 60% of such children were rebattered. Separation of the parents from their child may be necessary.
SEE ALSO Infanticide.

Behaviour

In its most general sense, 'behaviour' denotes the total response of an individual to a situation and usually implies that the behaviour referred to modifies the situation by its effects on the environment or the individual's relationship to the environment. Psychology is now often defined as the study of behaviour. This emphasis was introduced by J. B. Watson who argued that to make psychology an objective science, attention should be confined to directly observable and measurable phenomena. For him, behaviour consisted of integrated habit systems derived from conditioned reflexes established on the basis of innate patterns of motor and glandular response. Language habits had a special significance in that they could become 'implicit'. The behaviourist tradition, and particularly its emphasis upon laboratory experimentation, remains strong but contemporary experimental psychologists tend to specify behaviour in more molar units and are prepared to couch their theoretical explanations in terms of hypothetical covert intervening variables concerned with such processes as learning and motivation.
'Behaviour disorder' is often used in the American literature as a general term to describe any type of functional abnormality, but British psychiatric usage tends to be more restricted. There is usually an element of evaluation, on social or ethical grounds, of the behaviour or 'conduct' referred to. Thus the term may be applied to some forms of psychopathic personality and is generally used to describe one major category of psychiatric disorder in children in which unruly aggressive behaviour, stealing and truancy are common symptoms. In a narrower sense, all psychiatric illnesses are reflected in the overt behaviour of the patient, and the behavioural abnormalities, whether as specific as a 'tic' or as general as a trait of uninhibitedness, are frequently of diagnostic importance.
SEE ALSO Habit and behaviour therapy.

Behaviour disorders in children

A term used to cover the abnormal patterns of behaviour seen in children. It covers the groups of adaptation disorders, emotional disorders and antisocial or conduct disorders. A general description of these disorders will be found in the section on child psychiatry.

Behaviour therapy

This term refers to a wide variety of treatment methods, including desensitization q.v.), aversion (q.v.), flooding (q.v.), modelling (q.v.), shaping (q.v.) and positive and operant conditioning (q.v.). 'Behaviour therapy' is thus not a single entity, so that it is better to refer to 'behaviour therapies' or 'behavioural treatment methods'. These techniques have been developed by applying experimental psychological research findings in animals to human problems, and behaviour therapists sometimes claim that their treatments are derived from modern theories of learning, which are largely based on animal studies. Both these studies and behaviour therapies have developed enormously in the last twenty years, and it is now clear that the relationship between a treatment technique applicable in man and its theoretical basis in terms of animal work is often extremely tenuous. Behaviour therapists tend to regard a patient's symptoms *as* the disorder, perhaps as a maladaptive behaviour pattern acquired by learning, and ignore any possible unconscious or underlying causes or conflicts, a difference from some other psychiatric disciplines.

Behaviour therapies have been applied to two main groups of symptoms, behavioural capacities (a) which the subject has and wishes to lose, and (b) which he lacks and wishes to achieve. In the first group are sexual deviations such as transvestism (q.v.), fetishism (q.v.), homosexuality (q.v.) and sado-masochism (q.v.); alcoholism (q.v.) and enuresis (q.v.). These are treated by one or other forms of aversion therapy, aimed at producing a conditioned anxiety response towards the undesired behaviour, usually by the repeated applications of electric shocks, carefully timed in relation to the behaviour or the cues which evoke it. The second group includes phobias (q.v.), some cases of impotence (q.v.) and frigidity (q.v.) and certain obsessional symptoms. These are treated by desensitization or other types of behaviour therapy aimed at reducing the anxiety which inhibits the patient from carrying out the desired action and thus enabling him to approach and eventually to overcome the situation rather than avoid it.

In general the techniques seem to be most useful when anxiety is a material part of the problem; behaviour therapies have contributed little or nothing to the understanding or treatment of depression. They are most suitable and frequently the treatment of choice in patients with a single symptom or phobia. This is especially so with symptoms such as cross-dressing or feather phobia which can be treated directly while the unwanted behaviour is being performed and observed, though good results may also be obtained with symptoms such as impotence which must be treated indirectly (in imagination for example).

Behaviour therapies are much less effective where the symptoms are multiple or where they are associated with an underlying personality disorder when treatment with drugs or psychotherapy (q.v.) may be indicated, perhaps in association with behaviour therapy.

Although behaviour therapists are primarily interested in the patient's symptoms and psychoanalysts in the underlying emotional conflicts, the two disciplines may not be so distant as appears on the surface. Analysis implies the uncovering of abnormal emotional conflicts and the relearning, through the therapist, of normal relationships. The 'transference' and 'working through' can indeed be looked at as a process of behaviour therapy, involving aversion, modelling, shaping and, especially, desensitization. Conversely a considerable transference inevitably develops during behaviour therapy, and recently some behaviour therapists have combined the two disciplines and desensitized the patient to the conflicts which preliminary psychotherapeutic interviews have uncovered.

Behavioural sciences

All those subjects concerned with human and animal behaviour; they include psychology, sociology, biology and social anthropology.

Belle indifférence

The absence of what the observer considers to be the appropriate attitude toward a disability. Usually equated with a lack of anxiety. Nevertheless the somatic manifestations of anxiety are present if looked for.

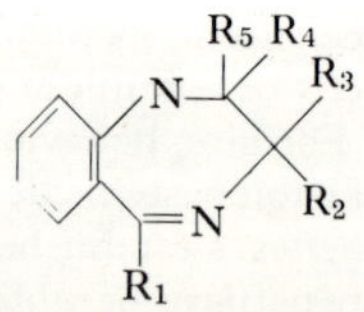

General structure of benzodiazepines

Benzodiazepines

The benzodiazepines developed first during the last part of the 1950's have become among the most commonly prescribed drugs. Chlordiazepoxide is the prototype of the series. Subsequent compounds include diazepam, oxazepam, nitrazepam, medazepam and flurazepam.

These compounds have the enormous advantage of low toxicity and therefore a wide safety margin in overdose. The pharmacological activity depends on a central heterogeneous seven-membered ring structure. Benzodiazepines are rapidly absorbed from the gastro-intestinal tract and from parenteral sites, but peak blood levels are achieved slowly and excretion is not complete for several days. Many but not all of the benzodiazepines share common metabolites. Especially important among these is desmethyldiazepam, an active metabolite with a duration of action of about 4 days. Cumulation may therefore occur. Moreover the factor of common metabolites implies that specificity of activity is not as great as is commonly suggested.
Pharmacological action may be due to an inhibition of adenosine-triphosphatase (ATPASE) responsible for the sodium-potassium pump in nerve cells or stimulation of glycine receptors.
The benzodiazepines are powerful anxiolytic agents with mild psychosedative properties. Clinically their effects are not dissimilar to the barbiturates, but their pharmacological action is clearly different; benzodiazepines exert inhibiting effects through the limbic system (q.v.) with limited action on reticular and brain stem structures. An important anti-convulsant activity has found clinical use, and muscle relaxant properties are produced through polysynaptic path inhibition.
Clinical uses are diverse, since benzodiazepines are appropriately given whenever anxiety or tension calls for symptomatic relief. The uses include anxiety neuroses; sleep disorders; alcohol and drug withdrawal manifestations; preoperative anxiety; relief of certain forms of epilepsy and/as an 'anaesthetic and anterograde amnesic' agent when given by the intravenous route prior to minor surgical procedures.
Adverse effects are uncommon; somnolence is not unexpected; paradoxical stimulation may occur, particularly in the elderly, with hyperexcitability, agitation and rage but similar paradoxical reactions occur with most disinhibiting agents, including alcohol; occasionally ataxia, headache, hypotension and vertigo may occur. Pharmacological dependence occurs infrequently after administration of high doses for prolonged periods. In addition a psychological dependence can occur, mainly in middle-aged women, who can become addicted to almost any medicament (e.g. aspirin). Despite the fact that significant dependence is unusual short courses are to be recommended and a flexible dosage schedule controlled by the patient is often beneficial with sensible patients.
SEE appendix for details of individual drugs.

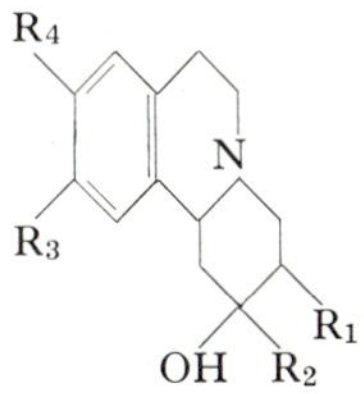

Benzoquinolizine derivatives

Tetrabenazine is the best known member of this group, and is related to the rauwolfia alkaloids. The actions are very like reserpine, but are quicker, shorter and less potent. Now little used as a neuroleptic, it has found a place in the treatment of Huntington's chorea (q.v.).

Bereavement

Bereavement is often cited as a significant cause of depression in old age. However, with increasing age, bereavement seems to play a less important part in precipitating psychiatric illness than in younger people. Where there has been an abnormal dependence and the surviving spouse has strong neurotic tendencies then bereavement is more likely to cause a psychiatric illness. Often the death or departure of a child or an active and supporting brother or sister will constitute a more important loss than that of an ailing spouse.
Even during normal mourning, help and advice from the family doctor is often required. Suffering can be relieved and in a few cases actual breakdown may be prevented. Generally excessive sedation should be avoided and the bereaved persons be encouraged to talk about their feelings, the extent of their sense of loss,

and of their love, guilt feelings, and even the hatred and anger that they may have felt for their dead spouses. There is evidence to suggest that those elderly patients who are forbidden to attend funeral or memorial ceremonies may develop more severe mourning reactions.

The acute distress of mourning is often completed in about six weeks; a return to a normal emotional state may take some months longer. Where mourning has not been adequately resolved and personal vulnerability exists (*vide supra*) then prolonged depressive reactions may occur, often with hypochondriacal symptoms which may relate to the terminal illness of the departed spouse. On some occasions severe exacerbations coincide with anniversaries of significant events. Denial of death may lead to eccentricities such as spiritualism or maintenance of a deceased person's room and belongings as a kind of 'shrine'.

Beri-beri

A nutritional deficiency due to a deficiency of thiamine in which mental changes are a common feature.
SEE Korsakoff's psychosis.

Bestiality

Bestiality, the use of an animal for sexual arousal, takes the form of vaginal or anal coitus with a cow or mare (zooerasty) or fellatio with a dog or masturbation of the animal. It most commonly occurs in adolescence in socially isolated farm workers or in relation to pets for whom the individual has strong affection. Kinsey estimated that 17% of adolescent farm workers experience orgasm with an animal at some time whilst the incidence in the total population he put at 6%. In some psychopathic, subnormal patients, acts of cruelty may stimulate orgasm (bestosexual sadism). Treatment is the encouragement of wider social adjustment through group psychotherapy and environmental manipulation. Buggery with an animal is a felony under the Sexual Offences Act (1967).
SEE ALSO Sexual disorders and Forensic psychiatry.

Beta adrenergic receptors

The receptor sites for catecholamines can be divided into two general types designated the α and β receptors depending on their sensitivities to different drugs. The β receptors are much more sensitive to adrenaline than are α receptors (see adrenaline for effects). Beta receptors have now been further subdivided into two types β_1 and β_2. The effects of β receptor stimulation are brought about by activation of adenylate cyclase with consequent rise of intracellular cyclic AMP. Beta receptors are stimulated *inter alia* by isoproterenol and blocked by propanolol and dichloroisoproterenol.

Beta blocking drugs (beta blockers)

Adrenergic receptors can be divided into two broad groups depending on their response to selected agonists and antagonists. One group is known as beta adrenergic receptors (q.v.) and hence drugs that block these receptors are called beta blocking drugs (usually abbreviated to beta blockers). The original drug in this class and the one which has been most widely studied is propanalol. Its main therapeutic indications are angina, cardiac dysrhythmias and hypertrophic obstructive cardiomyoapathies but it has also been used in anxiety particularly where there are prominent somatic manifestations. A central mechanism of action was postulated but it appears more likely that propanalol blocks the peripheral effects which tend to sustain the anxiety by positive feedback.

Beta rhythm
SEE EEG.

Bielschowsky-Jansky disease

A form of amaurotic family idiocy (q.v.) which occurs during late infantile life.

Binet-Simon test

The first intelligence test, devised by Alfred Binet and Theodore Simon. The mental age of an individual child is assessed on the results of a standardized series of test answers. The Stanford-Binet test was a later version of the test developed in the USA.

Biochemical and neurophysiological background to mental disease

The purpose of a nervous system is the provision of a feedback mechanism such that an input stimulus alters the response of the whole organism. Normal life can only exist if the response is appropriate to the input stimulus.
The input stimulus comes not only from within the body to provide internal homeostasis, but also from the external environment. Indeed, the characteristic of all but the lowest members of the animal kingdom is the power of purposeful mobility in response to the changes in the external environment.
Co-ordinated body responses demand knowledge of the surroundings through appropriate sensory receptors including both general receptors and those of the special senses. Impulses from these receptors are carried in fibre tracts within the central nervous system to higher centres. These include subcortical centres for co-ordination of muscle activity (e.g. cerebellum, reticular formation (q.v.)) and the cerebral cortex for the interpretation of conscious sensations. Other cortical centres are responsible for determining an appropriate response and for converting this intention into actual activity via integrating feedback loops through the basal ganglia (q.v.) and cerebellum and then efferent impulses to the muscles. While the direct and conscious muscle activity is under cortical control, subcortical centres are responsible for ensuring regulated muscle activity and the finesse of learnt movements with minimum conscious attention to detail.
The processes of transmission of impulses around the central nervous system involve transmission along nerve fibres (q.v.) and transmission across synapses (q.v.), the narrow clefts which separate one neurone from the next. Transmission along the nerve fibre consists of an electrochemical process depending upon ion movements, while that across the synapses involves chemical substances (neuro-transmitters (q.v.)). While there is a uniform mechanism of the nerve conduction throughout the nervous system, but with a different rate of transmission depending upon the size of the fibres, the neuro-transmitters vary from one portion of the central nervous system to another.
The physiological unit of nervous activity is the reflex arc and this is manifest at all levels of the central nervous system. In its simplest form (the monosynaptic reflex) an appropriate stimulation of the sensory receptor activates the afferent neurone which in turn affects the efferent neurone and thence the effector organ. The interposition of additional neurones between the afferent and efferent neurones of the reflex arc increases the number of synapses involved and, in so doing, makes possible the enormous complexity of reflex action of which the nervous system is capable.
The individual neurones may be either excitatory or inhibitory in type due to the liberations of either excitatory or inhibitory neuro-transmitters. The response of the next neurone depends upon the summation of the excitatory and inhibitory stimuli applied to its surface.
The response of the body to an applied stimulus not only involves the obvious motor response but changes in the internal economy appropriate to the response which is made. Such changes in the internal economy involve many mid brain centres including the hypothalamus (q.v.) the limbic system (q.v.) and the reticular formation (q.v.). The prime function of the hypothalamus (q.v.) is the control of both the endocrine and the autonomic nervous system. The limbic system, phylogenetically the oldest portion of the cortex, produces the primitive or 'animal' responses of hunger, fear, hate etc. and in the human is associated with the emotions, including the affect (q.v.). The reticular formation is the main controlling area which by virtue of numerous far ranging neurones integrates the activity of the voluntary nervous system and that of the involuntary portions.
Although some primitive responses take place naturally, a vital process in the development of appropriate responses is learning (q.v.). This involves the process of memory (q.v.). A memory is stored as engrams (q.v.) which depend not only

upon cerebral cortex integrity but also functional activity of the hippocampus (q.v.). This memory process may involve new protein synthesis within the cells. For these central nervous system processes to occur, metabolic integrity is essential. The prime energy source for the nervous system is glucose metabolism. Since no glycogen stores are held within nervous tissue and oxygen is vital for efficient glucose utilization, an intact blood supply is of paramount importance.

Many vitamins, particularly those of the B complex, are also essential for normal metabolism.

The main psychiatric diseases appear to be associated with three forms of alteration of the normal neurone physiological processes.

1. *Deranged metabolism*. Many cases of mental defect are known to be due to genetically determined biochemical disorders. These include phenylketonuria (q.v.), Hartnup's disease (q.v.), and the lipoidoses (q.v.). Moreover, since the vitamins are vital for normal metabolic activity, deficiency of members of the B group leads to mental abnormalities. These include Wernicke's encephalopathy and the Korsakoff syndrome.

2. *Alteration in cortical function*. In the organic dementias there is considerable derangement of cortical function, resulting in aberrant thought processes and problems of memory storage. Interference with the normal protein synthesis necessary for engram formation has been postulated as a possible mechanism, and hippocampal derangement is the main site of anatomical lesions. In schizophrenia (q.v.) an altered metabolism of cerebral amines may be involved.

3. *Mid brain derangement*. A regular feature in many psychiatric illnesses is an abnormality in affect. These changes in affect, and the autonomic and endocrine effects which follow (e.g. in psychosomatic disorders (q.v.)), are probably explained by alteration in the balance between mid brain centres.

Biofeedback

Biofeedback refers first to instrumentation which detects a given physiological process in the person and concurrently displays such activity back in a clear, metered form. The person thus receives additional information (feedback) about inner events that normally cannot be clearly or accurately perceived. Secondly, it implies that by means of a biofeedback system, this will result in learning to alter the regulation of visceral functions, in order, for instance, to derive a therapeutic effect. That some such effects do occur through biofeedback is supported by work in anxiety states, asthma, cardiac arrhythmias, epilepsy, faecal incontinence, hypertension, migraine, relaxation training, stroke rehabilitation, tension headaches and various other conditions.

Physiological variables used include: bloodflow, BP, ECG, EEG, electromyography, skin resistance and skin temperature.

There has been considerable controversy as to what learning principles form the rationale of biofeedback training. Operant conditioning of autonomic nervous system functions has been demonstrated in animals but only with great difficulty, using for reinforcement direct stimulation of reward centres in the brain. That biofeedback works similarly by way of operant conditioning is at best hypothetical, and the 'voluntary control' aspects of biofeedback are at variance with the notion of conditioning. Similar considerations are well known in older areas of behaviour therapy, where human factors such as cognitive mediation and complex aspects of learning beyond conditioning must operate. Their influence, as ever-present intervening variables, tends to blur the boundary between voluntary and involuntary in regard to visceral responses. Alternative biofeedback learning theories use servo-system concepts of adaptive control and patterning of skills, where knowledge of results (feedback) is an essential factor.

It remains to be seen what practical biofeedback methods will prove to work outside the laboratory, away from expensive equipment and where retention and utilization of learning in ordinary situations are the main issues. Compared with more traditional behaviour therapies, biofeedback is still a new technique and lacks standardization. The apparatus varies from computer-controlled systems to small discrete modules; the training software also varies even within the same area of application. Furthermore, the sale of elementary consumer devices, and exaggerated claims in the media have created expectations about biofeedback that are often unsubstantiated. Properly controlled trials of biofeedback methods tend to be complex and harder to implement than is the case with drug trials, so that validation studies demand expertise.

Biogenic amines

Name proposed by Guggenheim for monoamines (q.v.).

Bipolar psychosis
SEE Bipolar depression.

Birth trauma

Acute physical trauma at parturition resulting from prolonged foetal distress or prematurity may be associated with mental subnormality (q.v.), cerebral palsy (q.v.) or minor degrees of brain damage or epilepsy (q.v.). Apart from the specific disturbances due to local brain damage there are certain aspects of the brain damage syndrome which are psychologically important, such as:
1. Development difficulties – speech, hearing and sleep disturbances.
2. Motor disorders – overactivity, incoordination and involuntary movements.
3. Emotional disturbances – mood swings, impulsiveness, anxiety, temper tantrums and antisocial behaviour.
4. Learning difficulties – poor memory, poor powers of concentration and specific difficulties due to local lesions.

The success with which the child will succeed in life depends partly on the degree of the brain damage, how the child regards his handicap, and the extent of the support and understanding he receives at home and at school. In many cases the disturbed behaviour may be partly due to mishandling.

Minor degrees of brain damage are frequently overlooked and the child with a learning difficulty may be chastised for being lazy. An EEG examination should always be carried out, although the abnormality is often described as a non-specific cortical immaturity. Such records are found in 60% of children with severe behaviour disorders.

In a totally different sense birth trauma is used to denote the stressful psychological separation which occurs between mother and child at the moment of birth.

Bisexuality

Bisexuality in general biology refers to those organisms which exist in two recognizably different forms, one of which produces sperms, the other produces eggs (sexual dimorphism). In clinical use, it refers to males or females who manifest both homosexual and heterosexual patterns of behaviour to varying degrees. Kinsey estimated that 46% of the adult male population are bisexual in that they exhibit homosexual and heterosexual behaviour sometime during the course of their adult life. Bisexuality would thus correspond with Kinsey's groups 2 to 5.

Blepharospasm

A rapid, sustained contraction of the eyelids, blepharospasm is encountered in states of affective withdrawal such as stupor. It also occurs as a post-encephalitic manifestation. Frequently wrongly considered an hysterical phenomenon.

Bleuler, Eugene (1857–1939)

Bleuler's *Dementia Praecox oder die Gruppe der Schizophrenien* (1911) is one of the great landmarks in the psychiatric literature. In it he explored the inner world of the schizophrenic – and first used the words schizophrenia, ambivalence and autism. Taking issue with Kraepelin (q.v.) regarding the deterioration which Kraepelin considered to occur in cases of dementia praecox, Bleuler coined the word schizophrenia (q.v.) to describe what he considered the essential characteristic of the condition – a split in the personality which took place as a result of the disturbed thought processes. Deterioration did not necessarily occur. At a time when mental disease was equated with brain disease, Bleuler had the genius to

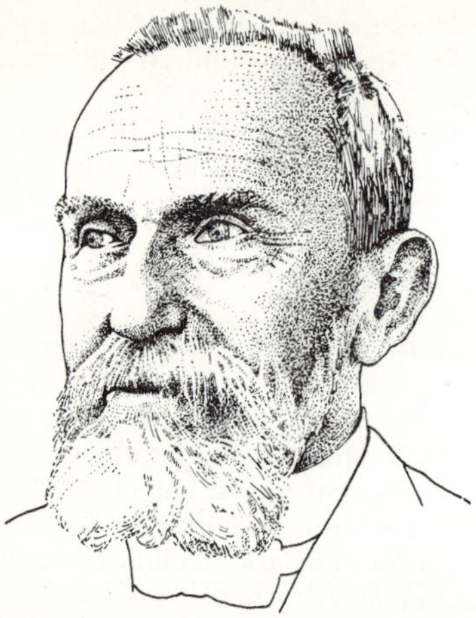

concentrate on studying the mental content of the illness and sought to understand the psychodynamics and psychopathology of schizophrenia. A brilliant group of young psychiatrists gathered under him at his hospital, the Burghölzli in Zurich – Jung (q.v.), Abraham, Eitinger and Ernest Jones, amongst others, all of whom were to make their mark in their chosen fields. Although sympathetic to Freud (q.v.), Bleuler was too broad-minded to accept the autocratic demands of the psychoanalytic core group, and his resignation had important consequences for the psychoanalytic movement, leaving it isolated from the academic world, and from the world of psychiatry.
SEE ALSO Ambivalence and Autism.

Blindness

Functional blindness is usually of sudden onset, may be partial or complete, and bilateral or unilateral when it may be associated with a functional hemianaesthesia. The functional nature of the disorder may be obvious from the patient's ability to avoid obstacles or may only be shown by the presence of intact pupillary reaction to light or by incongruities in visual field examination. The functional nature of unilateral blindness may be detected by the wearing of red and green lenses when the patient is asked to read red and green letters. If the patient can read all the letters she can see with both eyes. It is important that the blindness in these patients be regarded as a symptom when the doctor's efforts should be directed to determining and treating the underlying cause.

Blocking

SEE Thought blocking.

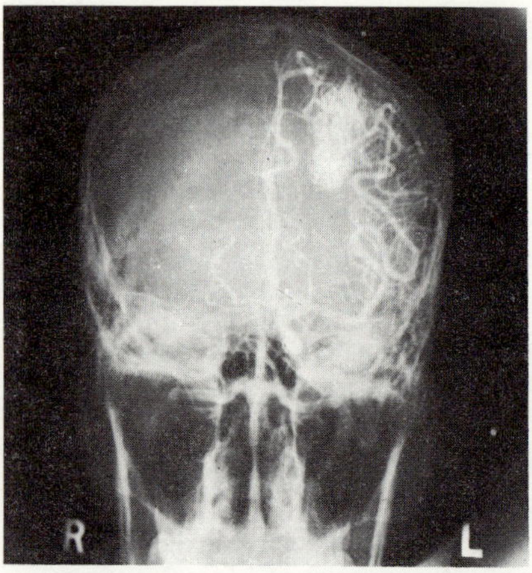

Arterio-posterior angiogram showing arteriovenous malformation supplied by both arterior and middle cerebral arteries

Blood supply to the brain

Nerve cells are more sensitive to anoxia than any other cells in the body and in consequence an adequate blood supply is essential.
The blood supply to the brain is derived from two major arteries on each side of the body, the vertebral and internal carotid arteries. The vertebral arteries join at the junction of pons and medulla to form the single median basilar artery. This divides at the upper border of the pons into the right and left posterior cerebral arteries.
The internal carotid arteries divide just lateral to the optic chiasma into the middle and anterior cerebral arteries, the ophthalmic artery and the central artery to the retina. The posterior and middle cerebral arteries on each side are joined by the posterior communicating arteries; across the mid-line arteries to the optic chiasma a further communicating artery between the two anterior cerebrals completes an anastomotic ring – the circle of Willis which surrounds the pituitary stalk. The lateral side of the cerebral hemispheres is supplied by the middle cerebral

artery; the medial surface is shared between the anterior and posterior cerebral arteries. The cerebellum is also served by three pairs or arteries, one superior and two inferior. The principal artery of the spinal cord is the single anterior spinal artery, but it is assisted by two posterior spinal arteries.
There is a generous anastomosis between the major arteries which can provide a collateral blood supply in the event of occlusion of a large artery but the arterioles to the brain substance are terminal and occlusion of these arterioles rapidly results in ischaemia and cellular damage.

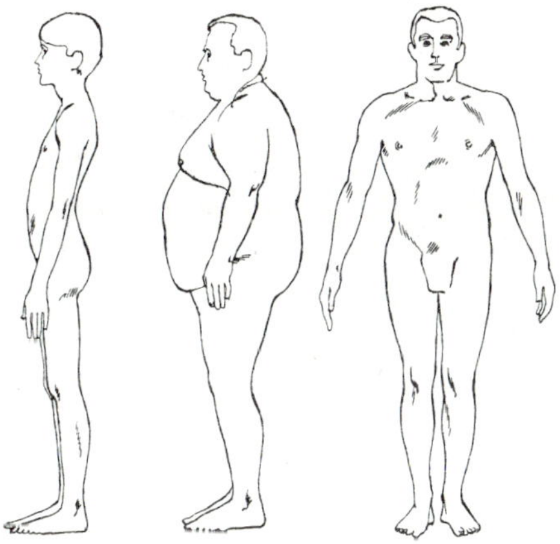

Body build

Although throughout the ages there have been attempts to link body build with traits of temperament, Kretschmer (q.v.) in 1936 first introduced this theme into modern psychiatry. He suggested that the broad, thickset pyknic build was associated with cyclothymia and a tendency to manic-depressive illness if a psychotic breakdown occurred and that the tall, narrow leptosomatic build was associated with a schizoid temperament, and with a tendency to the development of schizophrenia in the event of a breakdown.
Sheldon (q.v.) later elaborated refined techniques for somatotyping and carried out further work in correlating factors of body build with psychological variables. His three physical types of the endomorph, mesomorph and ectomorph corresponded to Kretschmer's pyknic, athletic and leptosomatic types.

Body image

At an early stage of development, the infant acquires a concept of himself as a separate entity and of his body as an agent under his own control. This 'self-concept' is progressively enriched throughout life and incorporates a detailed 'schema' or internal representation of the physical body. This is referred to as the body image.
The appropriateness of this schema naturally depends upon the integrity of the nervous system and so disorders of the body image are not uncommon in organic brain diseases, particularly when the parietal lobes are involved. There may be disorientation (autotopagnosia (q.v.)), incorrect localization (alloaesthesia (q.v.)) or failure to perceive (anosognosia (q.v.)) parts of the body. 'Phantom limb' and related phenomena result from misinterpretation of stimulation from severed nerves.
Disturbances of the body image may also be 'functional' in nature when they may involve a patient's delusional notions of how others view him. For example, the nose may be considered excessively long and an object of derision. Oversensitivity to bodily sensations is evident in certain types of hypochondriasis. Iatrogenic disturbances may result from 'spare-part' surgery.
SEE ALSO Asomatognosia.

Borstal training

A penal sentence available for offenders in Britain aged 15–21 years, who have been convicted of a crime otherwise punishable by prison. It is an indeterminate sentence in that it can be varied between six months to two years by the Prison Department depending on the boy's response. The training has been modelled on traditional British boarding school lines.

Braid cutting

A sexual perversion, the sexual pleasure being obtained by the surreptitious clipping of women's hair, usually in the cinema or theatre.

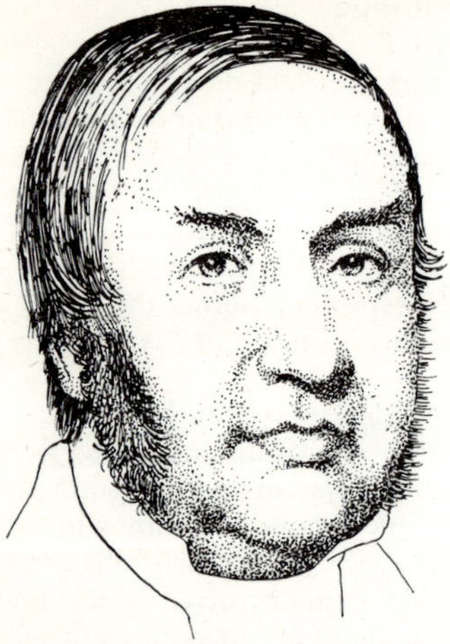

Braid, James (1795–1860)

A skilful and original Manchester surgeon, Braid was the first systematically and scientifically to examine the phenomena of magnetism. In his *Neuroypnology* (1843) he used the word hypnosis (q.v.) for the first time, disposed of the idea of a mesmeric fluid or force, and regarded hypnosis as a disturbance of attention, or, in modern terminology, a change in the state of arousal (q.v.) of the nervous system.

Brain-damaged child

The immature brain is more vulnerable than the adult brain, and it is also more plastic so that one part of the brain can more easily take over the function of another. There is evidence from animal studies that injury to the brain is most devastating in its effects at the time of fastest brain growth. The human brain grows most rapidly during the few weeks before and after birth so that it is not surprising that birth injury is one of the commonest causes of permanent brain damage. Uncomplicated toxaemia, prematurity, Caesarean section and mild degrees of anoxia have not of themselves been shown to cause brain damage, but there is some evidence from epidemiological surveys that severe prematurity (birth weight less than 1500 g.), severe degrees of anoxia, and breech delivery do, on occasions, produce deleterious effects on the child. The 'small for dates' baby, born at or near term but of low birth weight, is also at risk for abnormality in later life, perhaps because there has been insufficiency in placental blood supply to the foetus.

Serious birth injury may result in the death of the child and less serious injury in varying grades of paralysis or other disability. This has led some authorities to go further and postulate a 'continuum of reproductive casualty' with minor insults at and around birth producing relatively minor disabilities such as inco-ordination, perceptual defects and behaviour problems later in life. The evidence for slight traumata at birth having this type of effect is unconvincing. More probably socio-economic factors, linked with poor ante-natal care and consequent pregnancy complications, are also responsible for the cognitive and behaviour disabilities.

The causes of brain damage must also include pre-natal ones, such as maternal rubella, excessive irradiation and certain drugs. Obscure developmental anomalies (hydrocephalus (q.v.)), genetically determined disorders (phenylketonuria (q.v.)) and chromosomal anomalies (Down's syndrome, mongolism (q.v.)) are, with post-natal causes, discussed elsewhere.

Cerebral palsy is a disorder of motor function arising from a non-progressive defect to the immature brain. It occurs in two to three per 1000 population. The paralysis may be of quadriplegic, diplegic, hemiplegic or monoplegic type. Athetoid, ataxic and atonic types of cerebral palsy also occur. Although the cerebral palsy is often the most obvious disability, careful appraisal is necessary for the children may, in addition, be suffering from a variety of other defects, auditory, visual etc. The condition is compatible with normal intelligence, but in general the intelligence of children with cerebral palsy is lowered.

The 'clumsy child' syndrome described by Walton has not been shown to be due to brain damage, but it is convenient to discuss it here. These children manifest severe degrees of inco-ordination shown especially in bad handwriting and very poor performance at ball games. Verbal intelligence is higher than visuo-spatial ability.

Perceptual disorders in childhood can normally only be assumed to be due to brain damage where there is an associated cerebral palsy. They can, however, occur in isolation and result in defective spatial orientation, difficulty in distinguishing right from left, and incapacity to integrate auditory and visual stimuli. Some children with dyslexia (q.v.) suffer with isolated disabilities of this type. Speech and language disorders are discussed elsewhere.

Childhood epilepsy (q.v.) may occur as an isolated genetically determined condition or arise from structural brain damage, associated, for example, with cerebral palsy. The rate of epilepsy in childhood is about eight per 1000 children. When epilepsy is unassociated with other evidence of brain damage, intelligence is likely to be within the normal range.

Children with epilepsy and brain damage have a high rate of behaviour and emotional disorders, perhaps four or five times that in the general population. This does not occur solely as a reaction to the presence of a physical handicap, for children with other types of physical defect (not involving the brain), such as congenital heart disease, asthma (q.v.), etc. although showing high rates of psychiatric disorder, are not nearly as often affected behaviourally. It seems as though damage to or dysfunction of the brain results in undue vulnerability to the development of psychiatric disorders.

Drugs used to combat epilepsy may also have a potent adverse influence on behaviour. This is especially the case with phenobarbitone, which is well known to produce irritability, depression and sulkiness in some children.

Brain-damaged children can suffer from any type of psychiatric disorder though the hyperkinetic syndrome (q.v.) and childhood autism (q.v.) are commoner than in non-brain-damaged children. The more severely brain-damaged the child, the more likely is he to develop psychiatric disturbances. They are, however, particularly common with certain disorders, such as temporal lobe epilepsy (q.v.). Other factors, not directly related to the brain damage, may play important aetiological roles in the associated psychiatric disorder. These children seem particularly vulnerable to disturbed family relationships and community prejudices. These result in the child being shunned or becoming the subject of overt abuse and can affect his self-esteem and make his whole life a burden.

The main principle in diagnosis is the concept of 'comprehensive assessment'. As mentioned earlier, an obvious motor disability should not be allowed to mask a remediable language, hearing or visual defect. The practitioner should also be especially aware of the high possibility that a handicapping psychiatric disorder is present.

Psychological assessment is often helpful in the diagnosis of specific perceptual and cognitive disabilities.

The medical and surgical management of cerebral palsy will not be discussed here, and the management of epilepsy is discussed elsewhere (see Epilepsy). Most children with minor degrees of cerebral palsy or uncomplicated epilepsy can be educated in a normal school, but severe physical disability or intellectual retardation may necessitate special schooling. Physical restriction should be kept to a minimum so that the child can lead as normal a life as possible. The principles of management of behaviour and emotional disorders are the same as in children without brain damage.

Counselling and guidance of parents need to be careful and continuing. Parental guilt and anxiety may lead to over-protective or, less commonly, rejecting attitudes which may benefit from sympathetic discussion. Parents commonly blame themselves for the child's condition and find benefit and support in an understanding and reassuring doctor. Practical advice about mechanical aids etc. may be as helpful as general social support. Genetic implications of the child's condition should be carefully explained, whether or not there is an obvious genetic cause.

SEE ALSO Child psychiatry.

Brain monoamines

(Synonyms: Biogenic amines and monoamines.)

The monoamines serotonin (5HT) (q.v.), histamine and all three catecholamines adrenaline (q.v.), noradrenaline (NA) (q.v.), and dopamine (DA) (q.v.) are all found in the brain where it is thought they have transmitter function. All these

amines are formed from the corresponding aminoacids and are metabolized by the enzyme amine oxidase to the corresponding acid. A proportion of the catecholamines are metabolized in addition by the enzyme catechol O-methyl transferase (COMT) to compounds like metadrenaline and vanyl mandelic acid (VMA).
They are thought to subserve very important functions in the control of mood and behaviour. The functions of brain histamine and adrenaline are not known. The cells containing 5HT and DA are concentrated in two nuclei in the brain stem from where they send their axons to other parts of the brain. Dopamine-containing cells are concentrated in the substantia nigra, and Parkinsonism is associated with very low levels of this transmitter. Serotonin and noradrenaline or perhaps adrenaline are concerned in several functions, e.g. the control of mood, depletion of these amines leading to depression; control of sleep, serotonin seems to control slow wave sleep and noradrenaline REM sleep; noradrenaline is also concerned in rage reactions, in appetite control and in mediating signals to the brain that a positively rewarding stimulus has been received by the organism.
Thus many of the symptoms of clinical depression – the depressed mood, poor appetite, disturbed sleep, absence of enjoyment and interest in life – may be attributed directly to a disturbance of brain amines. Drugs which alleviate depression act on this system: monoamine oxidase inhibitors (q.v.) prevent the breakdown of serotonin and noradrenaline; tricyclic anti-depressants (q.v.) and amphetamines affect amine uptake and storage and potentiate their action. Rauwolfia alkaloids (q.v.) deplete amine stores and can cause depression. The phenothiazines (q.v.) inhibit central noradrenaline systems that may be overactive in the psychoses.

Brain scan

A series of compounds – chlormerodrin mercury 197 or 203, sodium pertechnetate TC 99, and indium 113m, for example, have been used by intravenous injection to demonstrate either increased uptake or an abnormal vascular bed. These radioactive compounds are all short-lived, and are

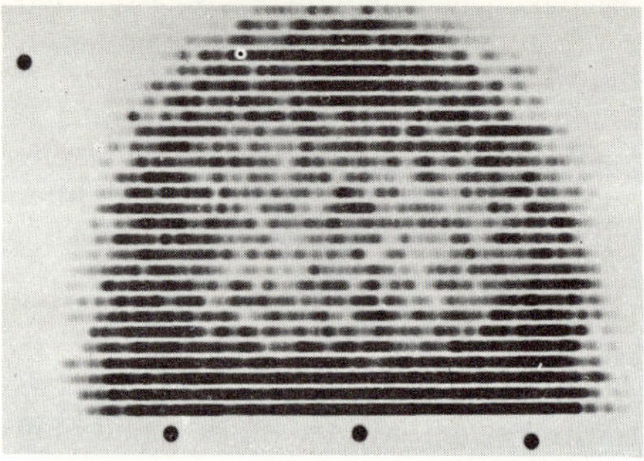

mapped over the brain using a rectilinear scanner with a sodium iodide (T1) crystal. The non-mercury compounds, apart from aiding in the diagnosis of vascularized tumours such as meningiomas with 70–80% accuracy, are also useful in demonstrating cerebro-vascular accidents and subdural haematomas. Mercury compounds may enter the nerve cell and uptake is increased in neoplasms. Finally, technetium serum albumen may be introduced intrathecally to outline the ventricles and subarachnoid space.

Brain syndrome
SEE Acute confusional state, Clouding of consciousness, Delirium, Dementia, Arteriosclerotic psychosis.

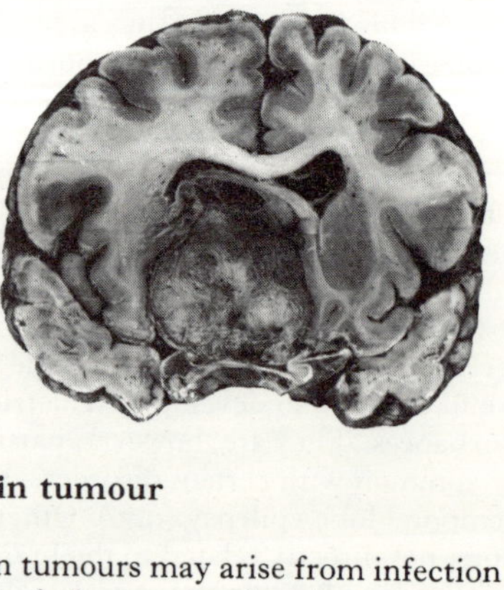

Brain tumour

Brain tumours may arise from infection – particularly parasitic (cysticercus, hydatid) from secondary deposits – the primary site being commonly bronchus but possibly breast, stomach, prostate, pancreas or kidney; or as a primary development. Tumours may occur in the coverings of the brain – meningioma; in brain tissue – glioma; within the ventricles – colloid cyst of the third ventricle; in blood vessels – angioma; or in the pituitary gland or cranial nerves within the skull – auditory neuroma. The commonest tumour of childhood is the malignant cerebellar medulloblastoma, while in adults the diffusely infiltrative glioblastoma just outnumbers the slower growing astrocytoma. Meningiomas and auditory neuromas are next in frequency – angiomas rare. The general symptoms and signs arise from increased intracranial pressure and include headache – paroxysmal, 'boring', 'throbbing' or 'bursting' – vomiting, papilloedema, generalized fits, sixth nerve palsy. Local signs – from irritation or necrosis – include focal epilepsy (Jacksonian or temporal lobe attacks), other cranial nerve palsies, pyramidal signs, aphasia, visual defects and other sensory losses. Mental changes include depression, anxiety, irritability, paranoid delusions; hallucinations and long-lasting 'functional' pictures – depressive and paranoid – have been described in slow-growing tumours. Ultimately, a more typical 'organic' picture with apathy, emotional facility, disorientation, memory loss, and intellectual failure ensues. Diagnosis is confirmed with the aid of skull X-ray (bone erosion, calcification, displaced pineal), ventriculography (deformed or displaced ventricles), cerebral angiography (q.v.) (displaced vessels, illustration of blood vessel tumours), electroencephalography (focal slow waves), echoencephalography (q.v.) (shift in midline structures), brain scan (q.v.) (differential uptake of tumour tissue).

While lumbar puncture may reveal increased intracranial pressure and increased protein in the cerebral spinal fluid, it is best performed where neuro-surgical support facilities are available. Curative treatment is surgical, particularly in meningioma and auditory neuroma. Radiotherapy has a palliative role.

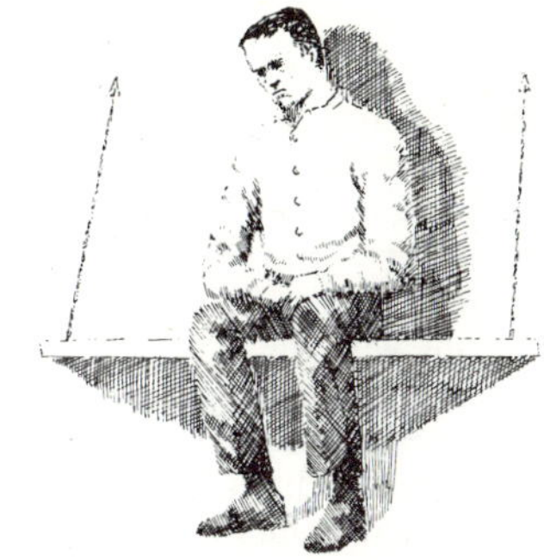

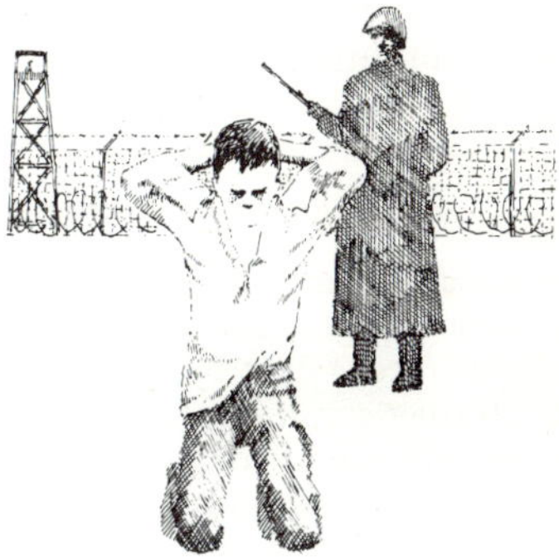

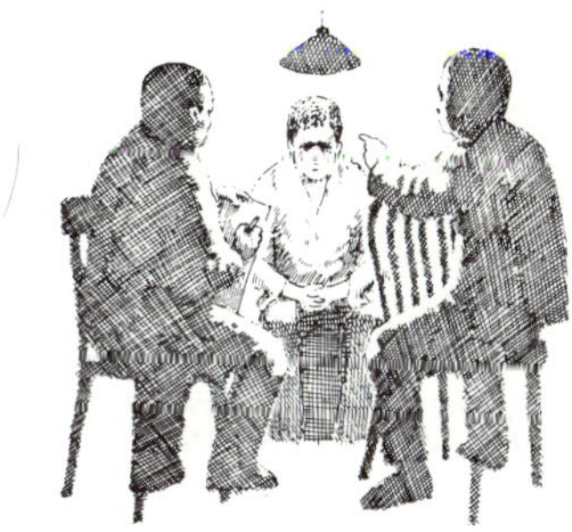

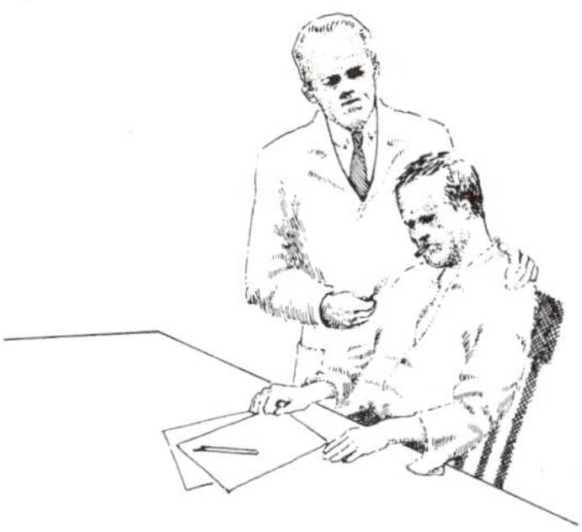

Brainwashing

A number of techniques, subsumed under the term brainwashing, are used in the Peoples Republic of China and in other Communist countries to produce mental changes in opponents of the regime. These techniques include indoctrination, repeated suggestion and the production of mental and physical exhaustion in a setting of fear and apprehension. Their aim is to produce confessions, true or false, to present to a court, or to the world, and to convince the prisoner of his heinous crime in not agreeing with the current party line. Resistance to brainwashing depends upon the prisoner's equanimity, his belief in his country or in his God, his physical health and previous instruction in resistance to interrogation.

Breath-holding

Breath-holding attacks occur most commonly after 6 months and before 3 years. In response to frustration the child usually goes into a tantrum and then suddenly stops breathing. Cyanosis occurs, and the child then takes a deep breath and often, after a further cry, resumes normal life. Very rarely cerebral anoxia may result in the production of an epileptic fit.
Treatment consists primarily of advice to the mother to ignore the attack and not to reward the child for it by giving extra attention. However, special attention should be given to the child once the attack is over, so that there is no danger of the development of secondary insecurity.

Broken home

A number of terms are used synonymously to describe a situation in which the one-parent family exists. These include broken home, single parent, parent without partner, only parent, and mother centred home. About 90% of one-parent families are headed by the mother, and this may be the result of divorce, separation, death of the spouse, or illegitimacy. Clearly the problems of the broken home will vary with the reason for the one-parent situation, and it is important to realize that it is not only marital incompatibilities which result in the consequences to the child of having, in essence, only one parent. The child reacts to his or her situation in a number of different ways: by inability to identify with happy parental figures, by anxieties stemming from divided loyalties, from economic or social restrictions, by feelings of grief and loss, and by hostility to society for the unhappiness which has been inflicted on him through no fault of his own. Children above all need security during their formative years, and when this is lacking the seeds of future life difficulties are sown, to spring up later in neurosis or disturbances of behaviour.

Bromides

The bromides were used for many years as a sedative and mild anti-convulsant, although the dangers of bromidism led to routine blood bromide estimation in centres where they were much used. Rashes and mental confusion occurred when the dosage was too high or excretion was in any way affected. No longer used today, except in the Soviet Union where bromide is used for its inhibitory properties on nervous tissue.
Carbromal is a weak hypnotic which releases inorganic bromide during its metabolism, and can thus give rise to bromidism.

Bronchial asthma
SEE Asthma.

Bronchial carcinoma

The commonest cause of metastatic carcinoma of the brain is a primary growth of bronchus with clinical effects due to increased intracranial pressure on the one hand and local destruction on the other. In 70% of patients such metastases are multiple. They are positively diagnosed by finding neoplastic cells in the cerebrospinal fluid. Discrete non-metastasized bronchial carcinoma may, however, also produce remote effects in the central nervous system in up to 16% of patients, which sometimes anticipate the discovery of the primary tumour. Sensory neuropathy was the first reported syndrome, followed by proximal myopathy, atypical motor neurone disease, subacute cerebellar degeneration, or myasthenia. Acute confusional states, particularly with visual hallucinations and possibly associated with electrolyte abnormalities due to endocrine changes (particularly excess anti-diuretic and adrenal hormones), have also been

seen. Some of these findings may be coincidental and have been reported in a similar proportion of patients with other non-malignant chest diseases. Sensory neuropathy with dorsal root ganglion degeneration and cerebellar degeneration are, however, regarded as specific associates of malignancy. Paraesthesiae, muscle weakness, fatigue, weakness and ataxia are commonly observed symptoms. Removal of the primary tumour may result in remission of the peripheral nerve but not the centrally determined signs.
SEE ALSO Organic disease producing mental disorders.

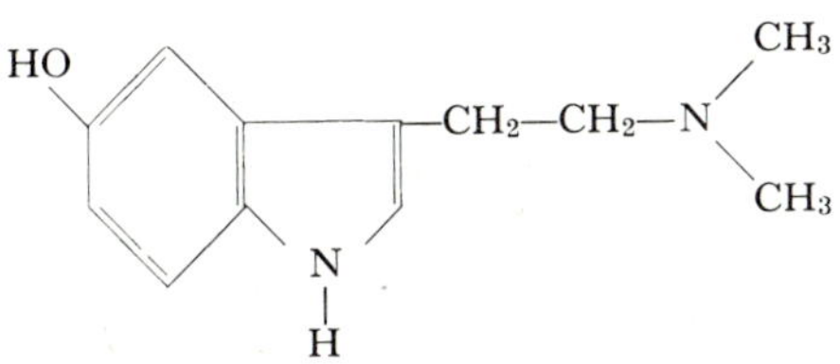

Bufotenine

A psychotomimetic indole alkaloid isolated from toadstools which is chemically related to serotonin. When administered intravenously in doses up to 70 mg hallucinogenic effects usually occur. Other effects include respiratory distress, sweating, mydriasis and nystagmus.
SEE ALSO Hallucinogenic drugs.

Buggery

Although often equated with sodomy (q.v.) (anal intercourse), in law buggery refers to both sodomy and bestiality (q.v.). It is not widely realized that the sex of the victim is immaterial, and that a man may be convicted of buggery with his wife. In bestiality no distinction is made between the anus and vagina, and the law regards as buggery any act of intercourse with an animal.

Bulimia

An excessive appetite which is a manifestation of an increased frequency of hunger sensations. It leads to bouts of overeating, which itself produces feelings of bloating, nausea, and malaise. Most commonly encountered in anorexia nervosa, it is to be distinguished from compulsive eating.

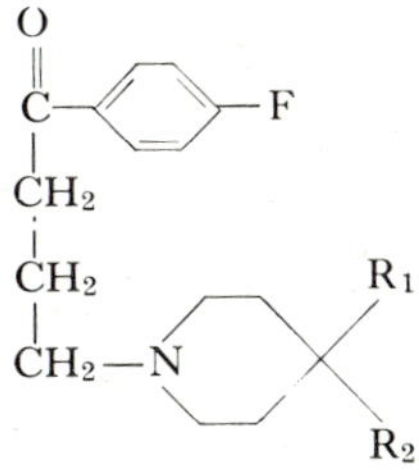

Butyrophenones

The butyrophenones are chemically related to pethidine, and their neuroleptic properties were discovered during a search for analgesic compounds. Haloperidol is the prototype of the series.
Butyrophenones are absorbed promptly and almost completely, peak blood levels occur in two to six hours and excretion is very slow. Cumulation thus occurs readily and this has important consequences on dosage.
Neuroleptic effects closely resemble those of the non sedative phenothiazines, but psychomotor inhibition is particularly well marked, and effects on the arousal system are minimal. These compounds are virtually devoid of autonomic side effects. As with phenothiazines, barbiturates are potentiated, but the butyrophenones also show specific antagonism of amphetamine and apomorphine. The butyrophenones are potent producers of extrapyramidal syndromes.
Butyrophenones are used as alternatives or in addition to phenothiazines in the treatment of schizophrenia. They find a similar alternative role in organic brain syndromes. The potent inhibitory effect on psychomotor activity has made haloperidol particularly valuable in the treatment of mania, and initial parenteral administration is the rule, normally in hospital. Haloperidol in small doses has been ad-

vocated for phobic anxiety neurosis but results are not dramatic.

Side effects are comparatively few. Like the phenothiazines the most important are the extra-pyramidal reactions and these are more likely to be of the dystonic type although akinesia is not uncommon. Correction or prevention by anti-Parkinsonism agents is straightforward and advised. Minor side effects include insomnia, blurred vision, hypotension and gastro-intestinal symptoms. Epilepsy may be reactivated. Paradoxical reactions occur, taking the form of toxic psychoses with agitation, disorientation, confabulation and visual hallucinations; depression also occurs. A disquieting syndrome peculiar to the butyrophenones has been recognized with sweating, dehydration, hyperthermia, and a dazed state of mind. It responds to drug withdrawal.

Caffeine

Caffeine is a member of the xanthine group of compounds, and together with its congeners theophylline and theobromine it is widely distributed in nature and as widely consumed by man. These alkaloids are present in various combinations in coffee, tea, cocoa and cola drinks, of which coffee in the prepared form contains the largest amount of caffeine, about 150 mg. in a cup. The origin of these beverages is shrouded in obscurity.
Caffeine is a powerful and general stimulant of the central nervous system, enhancing cortical function as well as stimulating medullary centres. Although central stimulation is the most prominent effect and the basis of its widespread consumption, there are other significant actions. The myocardium is stimulated directly; peripheral blood vessels are dilated in contrast to the cerebral circulation which is reduced; there is a mild diuretic action; gastric secretion is increased, and the metabolic rate is elevated. There is no doubt that tolerance and dependence occur but this is only mild and withdrawal produces no more than headache and irritability for a few days. Fortunately caffeine containing drinks are one of the few remaining pleasures left to man that have not been discovered to cause serious pharmacological mischief. The substance is rarely prescribed for its psychostimulant effects and it has no place in psychiatric practice. The main therapeutic use of caffeine is in the treatment of headache and migraine when it is usually combined with analgesics or ergot alkaloids respectively.

Cannabis sativa

Cannabis is obtained from the flowering tips and leaves of the cannabis sativa plant. The resin extracted from the plant or dried leaves may be used as source material. The active principals of cannabis are chemically members of the tetra hydrocannabinol group of substances. Dependence of cannabis type is characterized by psychological dependence (q.v.) – often severe but no physical dependence (q.v.) occurs. The effects of cannabis include tachycardia, raised blood pressure,

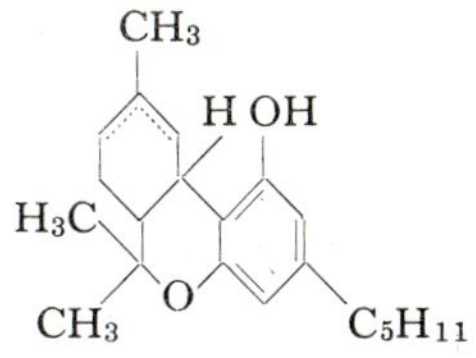

Tetrahydrocannabinol

conjunctival injection, pallor, faintness and later headache and nausea. Cannabis users look for effects such as insouciance, loquaciousness and mild hilarity, but in high concentrations excitement and hallucinosis can occur.
Acute reactions to cannabis have been described and these include unreality feelings, disorganized thinking and schizophreniform psychoses. Whether these are direct cannabis effects or whether they are reactions triggered off in unstable people is open to question but does not devalue their potential seriousness when diagnosed. Permanent long term effects of cannabis have not clearly been demonstrated, but there is evidence to suggest that in the short term it can lead people into states of disorganized inertia. In the United Kingdom it is subject to the Dangerous Drugs Act and internationally is controlled by the Single Convention of which this country is one of the signatories.

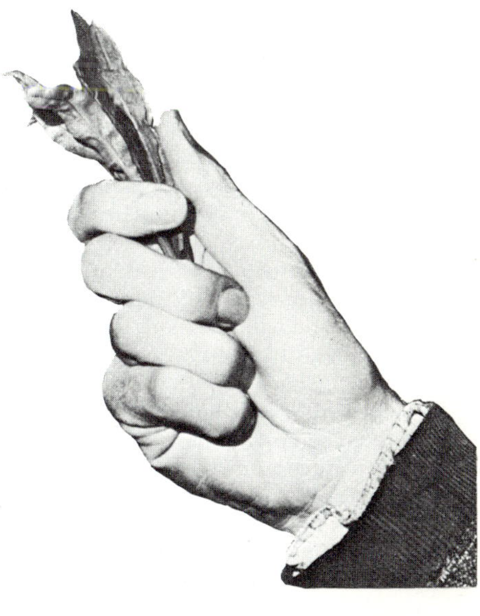

Leaves of the cannabis sativa plant

The relationship of cannabis usage to crime is far from clear. Certainly its use is common amongst delinquent subcultures in the United States, but for that matter it appears to be widely used by 'normal' individuals there. There is no clear evidence to suggest that cannabis *per se* causes violent and antisocial behaviour in unstable individuals. Again whilst there is no evidence that its use leads to progression to opiate use there is some evidence to associate its use with progression to the use of hallucinogenic drugs (q.v.).

Capgras syndrome

This is the syndrome of illusions of false recognition; it is usually observed in patients with paranoid schizophrenia, but is also present in some subjects with other chronic paranoid psychoses. The patient asserts that people around him (i.e. staff or other patients) are really relatives or friends. Less commonly patients claim that people in the ward have changed their appearance so that they will not be recognized, or are relatives who have been placed there to 'act out' the role of being patients. Variations on the central theme of misidentification may lead to very complex conceptualizations. The treatment is that of the underlying condition and the prognosis is likewise that of the underlying condition.

Carbon dioxide retention

This is associated with oxygen therapy, severe emphysema and status asthmaticus. Psychiatric symptoms occur when the CO_2 arterial tension rises to 120 mm Hg. Clouding of consciousness with headache, muscular twitchings, confusion, disorientation and hallucinations leads to coma. A coarse tremor may occur. In some cases encephalopathy with raised intracranial pressure and papilloedema occurs. Treatment comprises the administration of oxygen at not more than 1–3 litres a minute to maintain an arterial saturation of 80–85%, plus nikethamide intravenously (10–15 ml. every two to three hours). Excess CO_2 is thought to interfere with intracellular enzyme systems leading to defective utilization of oxygen.

Carbon dioxide therapy

The inhalation of 30% carbon dioxide and 70% oxygen was introduced by Meduna in 1950. Early claims for its value in many types of neurotic patient have not been substantiated. Basically it provides the means of an excitatory abreaction and as such may be helpful for removal of recently acquired hysterical conversion symptoms.

Carbon disulphide poisoning

The acute central nervous system symptoms include headache, excitement, narcosis and finally motor and respiratory paralysis. Following recovery, symptoms of neurasthenia (emotional lability, anorexia, easy fatiguability), sleep disturbance and epileptic seizures may persist for months. Chronic poisoning leads to these neurasthenic symptoms, Parkinsonism and a chronic brain syndrome. Treatment is directed towards removal of the toxin and artificial respiration.
SEE ALSO Poisons affecting mental state.

Carbon monoxide poisoning

Acute central nervous system symptoms include headache, visual disturbances, drowsiness, mental confusion and coma. Judgement is disturbed and insight is lacking. Permanent brain damage may result. At first loss of memory and a Korsakoff's syndrome (q.v.) may be prominent together with a confusional state. Neurasthenia (emotional lability, easy fatiguability, poor concentration and memory) and depression may be prolonged. Post-anoxic encephalopathy may follow an apparent recovery with features of Parkinsonism, peripheral neuritis, a chronic brain syndrome with apraxia, agnosia and aphasia. Acute organic psychoses may last for months but have a relatively favourable prognosis.
Treatment consists of pure oxygen given by a mechanical respirator or by mouth-to-mouth in an emergency.
SEE ALSO Poisons affecting mental state.

Cardiospasm (achalasia of the cardia)

The symptoms associated with cardiospasm may be mistakenly attributed to anxiety and depression, for they may come on following an emotional disturbance. A feeling of obstruction, and a burning pain substernally are complained of, and are the result of an inability of the cardiac sphincter to relax. Dilatation of the oesophagus occurs. The condition must be differentiated from globus hystericus and other types of dysphagia – organic or functional.

Cardiovascular system and psychosomatic illness

1. *The effect of emotion on the cardiovascular system*

Anxiety often has a profound effect on the cardiovascular system and can produce tachycardia, palpitations, dizziness and left inframammary pain. Many of these symptoms produce further anxiety which may lead to the patient's suspicion of heart disease. Cardiac-conditioned responses are acquired readily and are difficult to extinguish so that once a panic attack with marked cardiovascular symptoms has been experienced, there is a tendency for the attacks to be repeated with a development of further anxiety and the avoidance of situations associated with the attacks. The patient can be reassured that these anxiety induced cardiovascular symptoms will not cause any organic damage. Beta adrenergic blocking agents such as propanolol are especially beneficial in these patients, often combined with a benzodiazepine.

Driving aggressive competitive personalities are often associated with hypertension or hypertensive heart disease and the emotionally induced stress may be accompanied by a clinically elevated blood lipid level. A genetic predisposition to hypertension may be linked to certain personality traits and associated factors such as smoking and absence of exercise may be more important than the patient's temperament. There is some evidence, however, that emotional events may precipitate a cardiac infarction in patients already predisposed. For example a careful follow-up study on middle-aged widowers has shown that in the six months following bereavement the incidence of fatal coronary thrombosis is almost twice that of married men of the same age.

2. *The effect of cardiovascular disease on the emotions*

Patients who are seriously ill with heart disease often show emotional reactions. Patients who are dyspnoeic are often very anxious as are patients with myocardial infarction. The need for easy communication between the patient, the doctors and the nurses is often greater for these patients than for ill people in general. Surveys of coronary care units have shown a high incidence of anxiety among the patients and where it is absent may be explained on the basis of denial. This is perhaps the reason why some patients with a myocardial infarction will later deny that they have had a heart attack. It is now axiomatic that mental as well as physical rehabilitation is essential in patients following a cardiac infarction with an emphasis on what the patient can do and advice on leading a full healthy life.

3. *Untoward effects of drugs*

Depression is common in patients with heart disease and tricyclic antidepressants may have adverse effects in two ways. First tricyclic antidepressants directly antagonise the effect of adrenergic neuronal blocking agents such as guanethidine in hypertension. This is because drugs such as guanethidine are taken up into nerve endings through the noradrenalin pathway and of course this uptake mechanism is blocked by tricyclic antidepressants. Thus a patient's blood pressure may be controlled by guanethidine until a tricyclic is added when the blood pressure will rise to the pretreatment levels. Secondly, tricyclic antidepressants have a tendency to cause cardiac dysrhythmias and should be used with caution in patients with heart disease when perhaps a beta adrenergic blocking agent such as propanalol might be added. From the opposite aspect reserpine and to a lesser extent alphamethyldopa may cause depression in predisposed patients and excessive medication with digitalis and atropine, which may be used for the treatment of bradycardia following a myocardial infarction, may both cause mental confusion.

Care orders

In England the Children's and Young Persons' Act 1969 provides that a child or young person who is 'in need of care or control', i.e. who is psychologically disturbed, socially deprived, or behaviour disordered, can be submitted by a juvenile court to the care of the local authority for the area in which he lives. The court is not empowered to determine what type of treatment or care is required – this is left to the children's department, with the object of introducing flexibility of management.
Legislation based upon similar principles exists in some other countries.

Castration

Castration, the removal of the testes, may be carried out in elective surgical procedures, in some religious cults, e.g. Skoptics, or may be carried out by schizophrenics or transexual males as an impulsive act of self-mutilation. In some countries it is carried out on some sexual criminals, particularly rapists and aggressive paedophiles, to reduce or obliterate their sexual libido. Chemical castration is sometimes employed in this country using stilboestrol 5 mg. daily until libido is suppressed, thereafter 1 mg daily being continued. Cyproterone, a new anti-androgen, may be more specific in achieving this in the future. There is some risk of neoplastic change in the gynaecomastic tissue which is invariably induced by prolonged oestrogen therapy. Pre-pubertal castration produces failure of secondary sexual characteristics with a marked reduction in heterosexual drive and aggressivity after puberty. In adults, depressive reactions are common in the post-operative period, whilst over the succeeding one to two years, variable degrees of reduction of sexual interest and drive occur, together with some softening of skin texture and reduction in beard growth. In the older male, castration has little effects on libido or secondary sexual characteristics.
Fear of castration by the father was a central theme of the Freudian Oedipus complex, as a punishment for a boy's incestuous sexual desire for his mother. Reactivation of this repressed fear at adolescence and in adult life by another female led to impotence. The individual may then deviate to homosexual relationships which do not activate this fear or may require some symbolic penis substitute such as a fetish in order to reassure himself that the sexual partner has not been castrated.

Catalepsy

This term refers to the peculiar rigidity and alteration of muscle tone found most characteristically in catatonic schizophrenia (q.v.). The facial expression is fixed, and the body assumes immobile postures which sometimes appear uncomfortable and would be difficult for a normal person to maintain. Any attempt to alter the posture of the patient displaying catalepsy may be met with resistance (negativism (q.v.)) or by adoption of the new posture (waxy flexibility – flexibilitas cerea (q.v.)).

Cataplexy

A form of abrupt usually generalized muscular paresis leading to sudden collapse without loss of consciousness. It is generally triggered by emotion, usually laughter. Of brief duration it occurs in a high proportion of patients with the narcolepsy (q.v.) syndrome to which it is almost exclusively limited. The term is sometimes used for hypnotic sleep.

Catastrophic reaction

An emotional over-reaction of a patient with organic brain disease when exposed to a situation with which he cannot cope. A rise in pulse rate, restlessness and tremulousness may culminate in an outburst of tears or irritation.

Catatonic schizophrenia

Catatonia is the least common of the schizophrenic (q.v.) types and is characterized by alternating periods of excessive and diminished mobility. Reduced mobility or stupor can be of any degree from slowness to immobility and mutism. Even in the extreme degree the patient is fully conscious. Excitement can be extreme and violent; usually purposeless and unplanned. Other disorders of mobility are blocking, sudden arrest of movement; mannerisms, stilted, repetitive forms of expressions and behaviour; fixed postures maintained for long periods; flexibilitas cerea (q.v.) in which limbs remain in unnatural attitudes in which they are placed. Sometimes the patient is excessively compliant (automatic obedience (q.v.)) and at other times resists simple requests, e.g. soils shortly after refusing to use a toilet (negativism (q.v.)).

Language may be very disordered. A flow of unintelligible rubbish or patterned scribbling may replace communication by speech and writing.
The florid manifestations of catatonia have been greatly modified by the improvement in hygiene, freedom and occupation in psychiatric institutions.

Catecholamines

The three catecholamines of biological importance are dopamine (q.v.), noradrenaline (q.v.) and adrenaline (q.v.). These have widespread actions as neurotransmitters and hormones. They are synthesized from tyrosine (see diagram) and are metabolized by O-methylation and deamination.
Dopamine is an important central transmitter in the brain, in particular for the pathway leading from the substantia nigra to the corpus striatum. Degeneration of these cells is the prime lesion underlying Parkinsonism. There is also some evidence that dopamine systems may be pathologically overactive in schizophrenia.
Noradrenaline is the transmitter of the post-ganglionic adrenergic nerves, i.e. most sympathetic nerves, and also probably in some areas in the brain. In the periphery it stimulates mainly α receptors leading to a rise in blood pressure, and increased peripheral vascular resistance. The cerebral blood flow is reduced. In the brain noradrenaline is probably concerned in mechanisms underlying mood, learning reactions and reward signalling systems. At the adrenergic synapse it is stored in vesicles as a complex with ATP and is released by exocytosis. Termination of its action on the post-synaptic receptor depends on re-uptake into the pre-synaptic terminal. Drugs like cocaine, amphetamine and imipramine block this re-uptake and raise effective levels of free amine at the receptors. This may explain their mood-elevating effect. Monoamine oxidase inhibitors may also raise mood by raising free brain noradrenaline by blocking the main enzyme – monoamine oxidase which destroys it. Reserpine, on the other hand, disrupts the stores for both catecholamines and serotonin and this may be the cause of the clinical depression.
Adrenaline is the major hormone released from the adrenal medulla. It is also found in some parts of the brain. Dispute still exists on whether the main central adrenergic transmitter is noradrenaline or adrenaline. β receptors in the sympathetic nervous system are more sensitive to adrenaline than are α receptors. In consequence, its range of actions includes: (a) raising B.P. by peripheral vaso-constriction, increased heart rate and direct myocardial stimulation; (b) blood flow to muscles is increased; (c) smooth muscle may either be relaxed (e.g. bronchial) or constricted (e.g. spleen); (d) metabolic effects include increased breakdown of glycogen to glucose, and release of free fatty acids from depot fats; (e) when injected directly into the cerebral vesicles in small doses adrenaline induces excitatory effects including cortical activation (via the reticular formation), emesis, ovulation and stimulation of the motor cortex. Large doses induce stupor, and interference with release of antidiuretic

hormone and thyrotropic hormone. Recent histochemical methods have enabled us to trace the neurones in the brain containing noradrenaline and serotonin. The cell bodies of the noradrenaline-containing neurones are mainly located in a long narrow nucleus – the locus coerulus – in the pons and medulla and the serotonin neurone cell bodies are located in another similar nucleus – the raphe nucleus. From here the axons are distributed all over the brain and many of the terminals are distributed between neurones rather than on them. This suggests that these amines may act in a different way in the brain to transmitters like acetylcholine. For example, noradrenaline may act as a widespread signal saying 'positive reinforcement received', e.g. it would be released with pleasure-producing stimuli. Association between the external stimulus responsible for these synapses being active and positive reinforcement (e.g. food) would facilitate a chemical change at these synapses to form a memory engram (q.v.). Likewise another transmitter could similarly mediate negative reinforcement (pain) and shut off these synapses.

SEE ALSO Biochemical and neurophysiological background to mental disease and Brain monoamines.

Catechol-O-methyltransferase

This is a magnesium dependent enzyme located in the cytosol which rapidly catalyses the inactivation of the catecholamines (q.v.) by methylation of the hydroxyl group at the 3 position utilizing S-adenosylmethionine as the source of the methyl groups. There are high concentra-

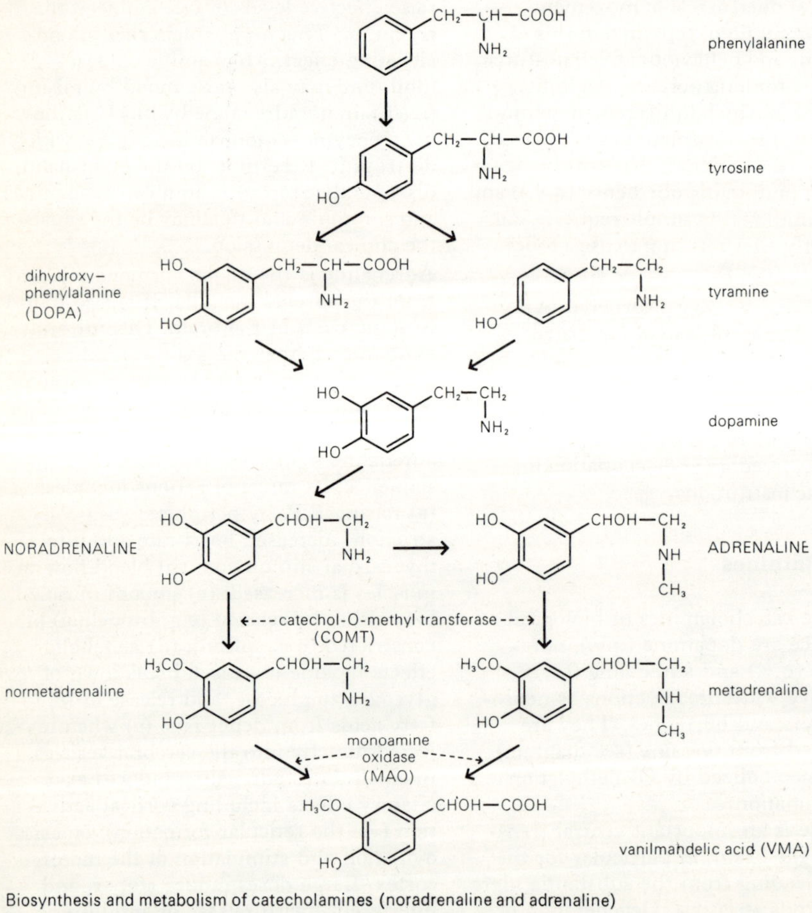

Biosynthesis and metabolism of catecholamines (noradrenaline and adrenaline)

tions of the enzyme in the liver and in relation to nerve synapses.
The first stage in the metabolism of the catecholamines can be either methylation assisted by catechol-O-methyltransferase or oxidation by monoamine-oxidase (q.v.). The noradrenaline (adrenaline) component which is bound is initially metabolized by the mitochondrial monoamine-oxidase, while the free amines are initially methylated.

Catharsis

SEE Abreaction.

Cathexis

To describe the charge of energy connected with an idea, an event, a part of the body, Freud used the word besetzung, now translated into English as cathexis. At the time, Freud was still thinking in neurological terms of a nervous energy, for the notion of a quantum of energy subject to various changes, is central to a theory of dynamic psychology. The difficulty lies in defining such energy in non-physical terms. Thus, cathexis, although much used by psychoanalysts, is an imprecise and unsatisfactory term, little used in psychiatry proper.

Causalgia

A condition caused by injury to peripheral sympathetic nerve fibres, particularly those supplying the palms and soles. It is characterized by burning pain which may be associated with vasomotor, trophic and dermal changes in the affected part.

Cephalalgia

SEE Headache.

Cerebellum

The cerebellum, joined to the brain stem by their three massive cerebellar peduncles, occupies the greater part of the posterior cranial fossa and covers the roof of the fourth ventricle.
The cerebellum consists of two lateral hemispheres joined by a median vermis. The surface grey (cellular) matter is thrown into a series of fairly regular convolutions (folia). Within its central white matter lie in each hemisphere, the large crenated dentate nucleus and the other cerebellar nuclei (fastigius, emboliformis and globusus).
Microscopically the cerebellar cortex has a regular arrangement with an inhibitory outflow from the large Purkinje cells to the cerebellar nuclei. These Purkinje cells are themselves acted upon by the basket cells and granular cells together with the parallel fibres. They receive their input from the pontine nuclei and the inferior olive via the mossy and climbing fibres respectively. The pontine nuclei and inferior olive in turn receive a rich supply of impulses derived from association areas of the cerebral cortex, collaterals from the pyramidal tract, proprioceptive and positional information and somatosensory input from many parts of the body. The main outflow from the cerebellar nuclei goes via the ventral lateral nuclei of the thalamus to the motor cortex but a supply also travels to the mid-brain nuclei that send extrapyramidal motor paths to the anterior horn of the spinal cord.
Modern theory ascribes three main functions to the cerebellum, all in association with other parts of the central nervous system: control of balance; learned pre-programmes for initiation of fine movements; feedback control influencing the finesse of movements during their performance.

Cerebral angiography

The technique of displaying the cerebral vasculature by taking serial X-ray photographs after injection of radio-opaque contrast medium into the carotid or vertebral arteries. It is employed (1) to show cerebral vascular lesions such as aneurysms, angiomas, vessel occlusions, and artheromatous plaques. (2) To demonstrate abnormal intracranial masses (e.g. tumours, abscesses, and haematomas). These will cause abnormal displacement of blood vessels, and in some cases the masses may be supplied with abnormal vessels the character of which may give clues to the exact pathology.

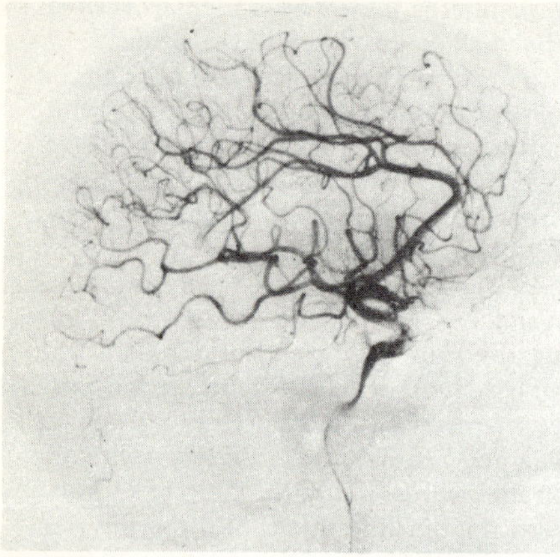

Normal lateral angiogram

Contrast medium may either be injected directly into the carotid and vertebral arteries after percutaneous passage of the needle, or these vessels may be injected with contrast from below via flexible catheters passed into the aortic arch from the subclavian or femoral arteries. In either case the procedure is time-consuming and is an unpleasant experience for the patient. In many centres, general anaesthesia is normally given. Even in experienced hands there are definite risks (greater in the case of vertebral than carotid angiography) of causing ischaemic cerebral damage from vascular spasm thrombosis or embolization. Cerebral angiography should never be lightly undertaken and should preferably only be carried out under the supervision of a physician with special experience in the investigation and management of neurological disease. With the advent of computerized axial tomography (EMI-scan) it is likely that the future use of cerebral angiography will come to be largely restricted to selected cases of cerebral vascular disease.

Cerebral diplegia

Spasticity of symmetrical distribution, mainly affecting the lower limbs, is observed in many mentally subnormal (q.v.) patients. There is no single cause of this type of cerebral palsy (q.v.), but anoxia at or around the time of birth is important in the aetiology. In some instances, cerebral diplegia together with mental subnormality follows an autosomal recessive pattern of inheritance. There is evidence also that a specific recessive syndrome exists, consisting of spastic diplegia, ichthyosis and mental subnormality.

Cerebral hemispheres

The two cerebral hemispheres, lying laterally, are joined to the rostral portion of the brain stem by the cerebral peduncles and to each other by a large transverse fibre bundle – the corpus callosum. The cerebral peduncles contain the main fibre pathways – motor and sensory – that link the cerebral cortex, the highest level of the brain, with lower centres.
The surface of the brain which is composed of nerve cells is markedly convoluted to form the gyri and intervening sulci, and within this nerve cell covering (the grey matter) lies the white matter of interconnecting fibre pathways. Each cerebral cortex is composed of four conjoined lobes, frontal, parietal, occipital and temporal.
The cortex with certain subcortical structures is the site for cognizance of the environment, interpretation, thought and for voluntary movement. Traditional theory ascribed specific areas of the cortex as subserving different functions, but it now appears likely that close integration and simultaneous activity by several parts is essential for normal cortical activity. Sensory radiations flow from the thalamus and its related structures to the cortex. There is a spatial relationship of primary sensory reception in the cortex. The general sensations lie in the postcentral gyrus, vision in the area of the calcarine fissure on the medial side of the occipital pole, hearing in the upper part of the temporal lobe and smell and taste in the deeper parts of the brain around the region of the uncus or upper operculum of the Sylvian fissure. Representation is contralateral to the receptors. Perception (q.v.) depends on the interpretation of the sensory input based upon prior experience (memory – q.v.) coupled with the existing situation and perception may thus be distorted (illusion, q.v. hallucinations, q.v. delusions, q.v.). The process of memory store, which appears to exist bilaterally and widely within the cerebral

cortex, is known as engram (q.v.) formation.

The prime area for the voluntary motor concept appears to lie in the precentral area of the frontal cortex. While unlearned movements, for example in infancy, may result from a cortical transmission to the main motor area (area 4) in the precentral gyrus, modern theory ascribes the programming and control of fine learned voluntary movements (q.v.) to the cerebellum (q.v.). From the pyramidal cells in area 4 the motor tract carries the downflow of motor impulses to the anterior horn and hence the muscles.

The cerebral cortex also contains vast areas to which no exact function has been ascribed. As a result of surgical or pathological oblation experiments some of these areas, it is suggested, may subserve 'association' activity in perception but the remaining portions are termed the 'silent areas' and are believed to be essential for the highest central process of thought and decision.

There is co-ordination of both cerebral cartices through the extensive cross-linking (e.g. corpus callosum) and one cerebral cortex is normally 'dominant' over the other. Thus in right-eyed (handed) people the left cerebral hemisphere is dominant and the speech centre is located in that hemisphere. However, the activities of the two hemispheres appear not to be quite uniform; the dominant hemisphere is concerned with the logical, well organized thought processes, the non-dominant with the random patterns typical of art form perception.

Cerebral palsy and mental subnormality

Cerebral palsy, due to a wide variety of causes, frequently accompanies mental subnormality, the same cerebral insult accounting for both effects. Neurologically, pyramidal signs are most commonly observed and may show as hemiplegia, diplegia, quadriplegia and in a variety of clinical pictures. In a number of instances extrapyramidal signs are observed, including choreoathetosis and ataxia. The clinical neurological picture depends on the anatomical site of the lesion, and in many cases both pyramidal and extrapyramidal signs are present.

The aetiology is usually environmental, anoxia at birth being an important cause; many patients with cerebral palsy and mental subnormality having a history of a difficult birth, a twin birth, etc. Cerebral palsy may appear as part of the clinical picture in many conditions associated with mental subnormality; for example, microcephaly, for which, also, there is no single cause. Choreoathetosis and mental subnormality may result from maternal and foetal antigenic incompatibility (SEE Rhesus factor). Cerebral diplegia has been attributed in a number of instances to a rare autosomal recessive gene defect. A syndrome consisting of spastic diplegia, ichthyosis and mental subnormality has been shown to follow a recessive pattern of inheritance.

The management of patients with mental subnormality and cerebral palsy depends essentially upon physiotherapy and specialized training, for example speech training, to develop to the full the physical and mental potentialities present. The prognosis varies from patient to patient and must be assessed individually; it depends largely on the degree of neurological involvement and the severity of the mental subnormality.

Cerebromacular degeneration

SEE Amaurotic family idiocy.

Character

The term character is sometimes used as if synonymous with personality (q.v.), but, more strictly, refers to those aspects of an individual's personality which are likely to be evaluated by others in relation to social, ethical or moral criteria. Thus a person's character structure represents the relatively stable and predictable, organized and integrated set of motives, attitudes, values, defence mechanisms and modes of impulse expression which determine his manner of adjustment to his social environment. The degree of organization and integration determines the 'strength' of this character.

Character structure has become an explanatory concept in relation to the aetiology of neurosis as exemplified by the distinction between character and situation neuroses. Psycho-analytic theory, in particular, stresses the importance of the neurotic character.

Character is acquired by a process of learning, but learning in a social context. Social psychologists and sociologists use the term socialization to describe the process by which an individual learns the modes of behaviour and value patterns approved of by the group. All agree that this type of learning mainly occurs in a context of social interaction with more powerful and prestigeful members of the group. Thus, although quite apt to adults adapting to new social settings, the term socialization is generally used in relation to children and, in particular, to the training imposed on children by parents and other authority figures in the society.

Behaviouristically inclined psychologists account for socialization and, therefore, for character formation in terms of normal learning processes and, in particular, the reinforcing effects of the pattern of rewards and punishments imposed by the parents. Even they, however, stress the importance of imitation (q.v.) and related, less exact copying of a social model. Freudian (q.v.) theory goes a stage further with its concept of identification (q.v.), implying internalization of the model to incorporate parental values and acquire a superego (q.v.). Psychoanalysis also stresses critical maturational stages in child-development at which the libido (q.v.) (erotic energy) becomes attached to distinctive activities and objects appropriate to the stage. Oral, anal, phallic and genital stages are described. Fixations (q.v.) the permanent attachment of some libido, may occur at each of these stages and these fixations have permanent effects on the character structure and determine the degree of regression (q.v.) (return to a more childish type of behaviour and emotional response) which is characteristic of neurotic disorder. Thus the adult of anal character structure is said to be pedantic, parsimonious, petulant and obsessional. These traits are considered to represent residual reactions to parental interference during toilet training with the pleasures associated with elimination during the anal stage of development.

Character neurosis

Another name for a personality disorder. This term is more widely used in the USA than in Great Britain where it is held that the word 'character' (q.v.) is unscientific and denotes a moral judgement.

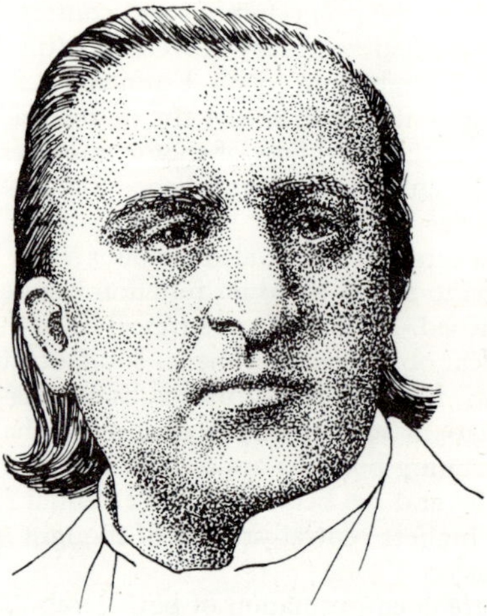

Charcot, Jean-Martin (1825–93)

The leading neurologist of his day, Charcot became interested in hypnosis, and devoted much of his time and energy to somewhat ill-conceived experiments with young and suggestible women. His dramatic demonstrations at the Saltpêtrière attracted Freud, amongst others, to Paris. Hysteria was investigated in great detail, and although Charcot's colleague, Pierre Janet (1859–1947), made solid contributions to the psychopathology of this condition, Charcot perhaps did more to retard than to advance our knowledge of hysteria.

Cheese reaction

The so-called 'cheese reaction' has become a familiar adverse effect occurring when some patients taking monoamine oxidase inhibitor drugs (q.v.) consume food substances containing indirect pressor amines. Cheese was the first such food to be identified and hence the name, but other foods include yeast extracts, such as Marmite and Bovril, and whole sliced broad beans. Certain drugs and cough medicines have a similar effect. Chianti wine and beer contain small amounts of tyramine and partly because of this reason, but mainly because of the increased tendency to get drunk, patients taking monoamine oxidase inhibitors should drink alcohol in moderation only. The crisis usually takes the form of an intense occipital and temporal headache which becomes generalized with palpitations, tachycardia, profuse sweating, and associated hypertension. Vomiting may occur, the pain may be intense, and subarachnoid haemorrhage and death may occur.

The hypertensive mechanism is due to the ingestion of indirect pressor amines such as tyramine. Tyramine is usually metabolized by monoamine oxidase in the gut wall or liver, but when this enzyme is inhibited, the amine escapes into the circulation and may excite a pressor response through the displacement of noradrenaline from binding sites.

An acute hypertensive attack is treated by intravenous phentolamine, but failing this parenteral chlorpromazine can be given. Prevention can be effected by careful dietary precautions but patients may find these restrictions irksome.

Chemical poisons, causing mental illness

SEE Poisons affecting mental state.

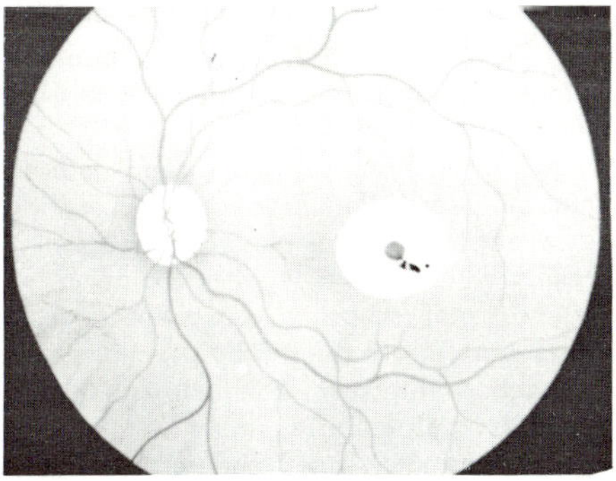

Cherry-red spot

A cherry-red spot is often seen on retinoscopy in Tay–Sachs disease (q.v.), or the infantile form of amaurotic family idiocy (q.v.). It is due to macular degeneration. Though said to be pathognomonic of the condition, it has been observed in other forms of lipidosis, and is not a constant finding in Tay–Sachs disease.

χ^2 – The chi-square test

Pronounced 'ki'. This is one of the most commonly used tests in the statistical analysis of therapeutic trials. For example, in a test of a new anti-depressant substance there may be results expressed as percentages of patients cured for groups of different size receiving either a placebo, one or more established drugs or the new drug at two different dose levels. The χ^2 test determines whether the different percentages observed can be explained by chance or probably depend on the therapy.

Child development

Child development occurs as a result of interaction between maturation (nature) and learning (nurture). When either is absent, development does not occur. A child not exposed to reading material cannot learn to read any more than can an anencephalic child, however many books are available.

The acquisition of most skills depends on both nature and nurture. Nevertheless, their relative importance can often be established; for example, it is likely that in underdeveloped countries social factors – poor antenatal and perinatal care, lack of environmental stimulation etc. – are of primary importance in determining intelligence, whereas in countries enjoying a more satisfactory standard of living, genetic factors are more significant. Comparative studies of identical and non-identical twins provide further information on this subject. One further broad generalization can be made. Rudimentary achievement is usually mainly biologically determined whereas complex skills depend more on social learning. For example, in the United Kingdom the age at which children learn to speak in three-word sentences is not related to social class, whereas later utilization of language skill is very much related to social class.

Normal development does not always occur in a smooth orderly fashion, nor are

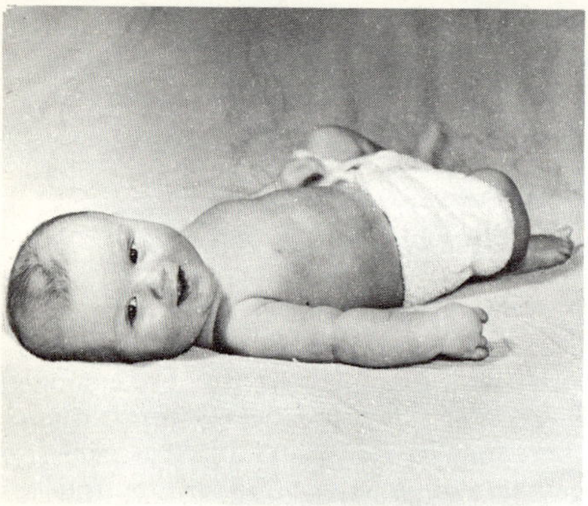

all skills achieved at the same rate. A child may be advanced in motor development but delayed in language and vice versa.
The situation is complicated when there is evidence of brain damage. Here certain functions may fail to develop because of anatomical damage (as in cerebral palsy) whereas in the same child other skills may be slow to develop because of a maturational delay, or the child may be handicapped in learning skills only because of lack of *appropriate* stimulation. A child with cerebral palsy may develop secondary problems in the area of tactile discrimination if his motor disability is allowed to prevent his gaining experience in handling common objects.
The American psychologist, Arnold Gesell, pioneered the use of developmental assessment tests, and all subsequent attempts to quantify infant achievement owe a great deal to him. Gesell divided developmental skills into motor, adaptive, language, and personal-social. Standardized information is available on norms for achievement in each of these areas.
Developmental assessment provides a good picture of how the infant is functioning in comparison with other children of his own age. Until the age of about 2 to 3 years however, it cannot provide any useful prediction of later achievement for any individual child other than the grossly retarded.
The measurement of emotional development in childhood presents more problems, because it is more difficult to find objective signs of emotional maturity. Emotional expression in the new-born infant is limited to response to frustration, deprivation and pain. Within the first two months, expression of pleasure usually occurs. By six months, it is possible to distinguish between the negative emotions of fear, anger and disgust. Jealousy may be clearly shown before 18 months. Anger responses, which are more common in boys than girls from the age of 2 onwards, become more directed and retaliatory between the ages of 2 and 5. Specific fears are most common between the ages of 2 and 3, but remain extremely frequent after this age.
In the area of language development, norms are more clearly established. Because 97% of children have acquired single words by the age of 2 and the same proportion of 3-year-olds are using three-word sentences, any child falling outside these limits of normality, is in need of careful further assessment.
SEE ALSO Child psychiatry.

Child guidance clinics

Child guidance clinics exist for the diagnosis and treatment of behavioural and emotional disorders in childhood. In contrast to child psychiatric departments in hospitals, they are usually situated in establishments closely linked to other community health and welfare facilities. The clinic team consists of psychiatrist, educational psychologist, psychiatric social worker, and psychotherapist. The director of the clinic may be the psychiatrist, but in some cases the educational psychologist is responsible for administration. The traditional pattern of working in the clinic following referral is for the social worker to make an initial contact with the family to take a history. The psychiatrist subsequently sees the child and family in a diagnostic session. Assessment of intelligence and educational attainment is carried out as necessary by the educational psychologist. Traditionally, also, the most usual form of treatment is psychotherapy which may be conducted by psychiatrist or psychotherapist on a verbal or play basis. Recommendations may be made for environmental changes, such as placement in a special school for maladjusted children. Over the past few years, there has been a considerable increase in flexibility in the functioning of many child guidance clinics. A family approach to both diagnosis and treatment with joint interviewing of family members has become more common.

Further, a wider range of treatments, including the use of drugs and behaviour therapy, is more frequently available. Staff in the clinics are spending more time in counselling other professional workers who are involved in the day-to-day care of the disturbed child.
SEE ALSO Child psychiatry.

Child psychiatry

Child psychiatry concerns itself with all aspects of disordered behaviour and emotional life during the period of maturation. Like adult psychiatry, indeed like all medicine, it has no clearly defined boundaries. Its area of interest merges imperceptibly into the fields of paediatrics, education and social welfare. Further, many of the mental disabilities from which children suffer are not pathological entities, but exaggerations of common variations in development. Some understanding of the *normal* processes of psychological maturation and of the many influences acting upon the child is therefore an essential preliminary to diagnosis and treatment of the abnormal.
There is no agreed scheme of diagnosis in child psychiatry. Some child psychiatrists indeed eschew diagnosis altogether, believing that the subject is too complex to allow for the use of simple diagnostic labels. The classification presented here does not presuppose any theoretical framework. It is a system based as far as possible on observable behaviour, and has been shown to have value with regard to prognosis and treatment.

Adaptation disorders occur in the pre-school years, and are also commonly known as 'management problems' of early childhood. Temperamental differences between children result in variation of mood, sleeping, feeding and excretory habits which are sometimes extreme. In the first few years of life both the child and its parents have the task of achieving a mutual adaptation which is both within the range of the child's capacities and is tolerable to the parents. Where this process of adaptation fails to occur and either the child or the parents are handicapped by the situation, a disorder of adaptation may be said to exist. In contrast to the position in the older child and the adult, it is often but not always futile to attempt a diagnosis 'within the child' in the pre-school years. The 2-year-old child who wakes at 5 a.m. and cries continuously until 6.30 a.m. when his parents eventually resign themselves to the task of amusing him, the 9-month-old who refuses to eat as wide a range of food as his mother would wish, the 4-year-old who clings repeatedly to his mother when she takes him to nursery school, but settles happily when she has gone – these are all children who may be brought to the doctor presenting with mild adaptation disorders characterized by the lack of 'fit' between the parents' expectations of behaviour and the child's capacity to rise to these expectations.
Emotional disorders in childhood occur when there is a handicapping disorder of affective life. The emotional state is often at least partly understandable in the light of the situation in which the child is living, but, not uncommonly, the unhappiness or anxiety shown by the child may seem disproportionate.
Emotional disorders are probably the most common type of mental disorder seen in childhood. Anxiety may be 'free floating' (q.v.), unattached to any specific object and showing itself by undue worrying, sleep disturbances (especially nightmares), enuresis (q.v.), recurrent abdominal pain or headaches, or it may be specific or phobic in character. All children show specific fears at some time or other, but in a proportion the fearfulness can prevent the child from leading a normal life. Unlike the adult, the child only rarely shows general social anxieties or agoraphobia (fear of open spaces). Specific animal phobias, of dogs, cats, spiders, etc., are more frequent, and other specific situational phobias include fear of school, fear of separation from mother, and fear of the dark. Some children have an obsessional component to their anxiety states with persistent ruminative worrying, but full-blown obsessional disorder is rare in this age-group. Depressive illness may occur in childhood but it is unusual to see the typical features of adult depression. More commonly malaise and general irritability occur without marked disturbance of appetite or sleep. Suicidal attempts are rare before the age of 15, but when they do occur they should be taken every

bit as seriously as at a later age.

Conduct disorders in childhood exist when there is a significant antisocial component to the child's behaviour. In the early school years this may show itself merely by aggressive behaviour and disobedience either at home or at school, but as the child gets older more overt signs of deviant behaviour supervene. Repeated stealing within the home has a different significance from stealing in shops or at school, but both must be regarded as evidence for the presence of a conduct disorder. Truancy (which should be sharply distinguished from school phobia or school refusal (q.v.)) involves absence from school when an attempt is made by the child to disguise or cover up the unwillingness to attend. Repeated bullying, sexual misbehaviour, running away from home, wanton destructiveness and fire-setting are also manifestations of a conduct disorder. The child may be regarded as delinquent if he is repeatedly committing offences against the law whether or not these are detected. Theories of delinquency vary in the importance they attribute to the personality of the child and the environment in which he lives. Certainly, a number of delinquent children show, in addition, a significant emotional disorder.

Developmental disorders in childhood occur as extremes of normal variations in maturation. Here there is commonly a family history of similar disorders. It has already been mentioned that enuresis may occur as a symptom of anxiety, but more commonly it arises from a delay in maturation of the neurophysiological mechanisms necessary for the inhibition of involuntary micturition. Encopresis (q.v.) or involuntary passage of faeces in inappropriate situations may also occur as a maturational disorder, but with this symptom there is frequently a significant underlying or associated emotional problem. Developmental language disorders, including developmental aphasia, are rare. More commonly, severe reading difficulties may be regarded as due to a specific developmental dyslexia, or at any rate a variant of this condition. Common features shared by all these developmental disorders is the fact that they occur preponderantly in boys and that there is a tendency (sometimes a disappointingly slow tendency) towards spontaneous improvement.

Hyperkinetic disorder in childhood is characterized by a severe degree of overactivity associated with impulsiveness, undue distractibility and short attention span. Children with organic brain dis-disorders show the syndrome quite commonly, but most children with the hyperkinetic syndrome show no evidence of organic disorder.

Psychotic disorders in childhood may be subdivided into three main groups. Childhood autism (q.v.) is a severe disorder of communication arising in infancy and associated with characteristic mannerisms and patterns of intellectual ability. Between infancy and about the age of 10, psychotic disorders are excessively rare and usually indicate the presence of organic, often progressive, brain disease. At about the age of 10, classical schizophrenia and manic-depressive psychosis, although most uncommon, do sometimes appear. These conditions arise with increasing frequency during the period of adolescence.

Neurotic disorders of adult type (psychoneuroses) are also rare before puberty. However, hysterical and obsessional disorders do occur and have their own characteristic symptomatology at this age period.

Personality disorders should only be diagnosed with great caution in childhood, for this diagnosis rests on the establishment of long-lasting patterns of maladaptive behaviour and relationships. Nevertheless, it must be acknowledged that some children present with such marked passive or aggressive traits from early childhood right through to adolescence that the term 'personality disorder' does seem justified.

In addition to the above-mentioned, there are a number of well-recognized syndromes which do not fit into this classification. Tics (q.v.) (rapid jerky repetitive movements of the body) may form part of an anxiety state, but may also occur as an isolated phenomenon. Gilles de la Tourette syndrome (q.v.) is a rare luxuriant form of the condition in which the tics take the additional form of involuntary obscene utterances. Anorexia nervosa can occur in full-blown form from the age of 10 upwards, and even before this there may be a history of extreme food faddiness.

Classification of the child's psychiatric state is only one aspect of diagnosis in child psychiatric practice. In addition, it is important to assess the relationships within the family and other possible environmental stresses acting on the child; the child's probable level of intelligence, and educational attainment, and the child's physical state.

The evaluation of family relationships always involves looking at a number of different aspects of family functioning. Clearly, it is naïve to consider that it is possible to divide families up into 'good' and 'bad' for a mother may have a splendid relationship with her husband and get on badly with her son, or alternatively may interact healthily with her whole family at one point in time, but only with irritability at another time when she is depressed. The general practitioner will often have the advantage of knowing a family over a long period of time and this will enable him to observe the development of relationship patterns within the family. He will often have had the opportunity of observing directly the warmth and affection which the parents are able to show each other at times of crisis. He will also note the amount of understanding sympathy, or hostility and rejection the couple show in talking of each other during individual consultations.

It is helpful to consider the parent–child relationship in two main areas or dimensions – the amount of control or autonomy exercised and allowed, and the degree of warmth, acceptance or their reverse that the parents exhibit. Childhood personality thrives best in a family atmosphere in which the child is accepted for what he is, and encouraged to develop independence as rapidly as the growth of self-confidence allows.

As children grow older, their social achievements may sometimes lag behind and sometimes leap ahead of their achievement in other spheres – motor, cognitive and language. For example, following the normal pattern whereby children are able to distinguish their mother from other human figures during the second six months of life, a pattern of close attachment to parents with concurrent fear of strangers supervenes. As the child develops gradual independence from its parents so stranger anxiety diminishes, and the child begins to form attachments to children of its own age.

Any crises in the form, for example, of

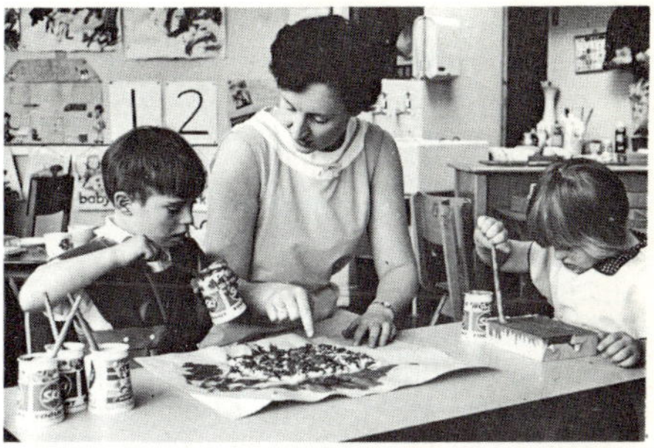

Mentally handicapped children learning through painting to gain better control of their movements

physical illness, hospitalization, etc., may result in a reversion to former patterns of behaviour, the child becoming more dependent on its mother, clinging to her and terrified when she is out of sight. Crises of this sort occur as part of *normal* maturational development. For example, when the child goes to school for the first time the challenge this presents may result in a regression to infantile habits because the child is unable to cope with the partial loss of his mother. Eventual achievement of regular school attendance represents successful adaptation to a new situation which gives the child a self-confidence on which he can build to take his next step to independence.

Amongst the stresses likely to injure personality development in childhood, great stress has been placed, especially by the British psychiatrist John Bowlby, on the effects of separation from mother. Subsequent research has shown that more commonly adverse personality characteristics arise from experiences of deprivation rather than just separation. The child who is parted from his mother but goes to the home of a familiar relative able to provide adequate substitute mothering care is much less likely to be affected adversely than the child who has to enter an understaffed institution, orphanage or children's home.

The processes of social learning cannot account for all the behaviour shown by children, for temperamental characteristics, either innate or occurring as a result of very early mother-child interaction, have been shown to exert a profound and continuing effect upon childhood behaviour. Longitudinal studies suggest that even within the first six months of life, babies show their individuality in a variety of ways, many of them persisting at least into middle childhood. Traits such as irregularity of eating and sleeping, adaptability, mood, and reaction to new situations can be traced with some degree of consistency through the early years of life. The difficult child, crying easily, unadaptable, and irregular in habits, is more difficult to rear, more prone to elicit rejecting attitudes in parents and, as a consequence, more prone to develop emotional and behaviour disorders. Some children present so few problems that a whole range of types of parental management is likely to be successful whereas a few have so many difficulties that most parents would be defeated by them.

The diagnostic appraisal must involve some assessment of the child's intellectual level and educational attainment, as inappropriate school placement and learning difficulties may well be important features in the aetiology of behaviour disorders. Interviewing the child alone, or, if he is under about the age of 8, with his mother, about his life at school, his interests, and the problem for which his parents have brought him to the doctor, will often elicit useful information about the nature of the difficulties as well as about the child's intelligence. A helpful guide to intelligence includes the complexity of language used. A specimen of handwriting will indicate any severe degree of motor clumsiness or perceptual disorder. If the child reads for pleasure it is most unlikely that he has a severe educational problem in this area.

Assessment of the child's physical state is always important, and is imperative when bodily symptoms are present. No artificial line can be drawn between so-called 'psychosomatic' disease in childhood and other forms of organic illness. Any physical symptoms may have an emotional or environmental precipitant, and any type of emotional disorder may be accompanied by bodily change. Nevertheless, certain physical disorders and symptoms are perhaps particularly prone to occur following exposure to stress situations, and certain physical disorders, especially brain damage (q.v.) and epilepsy (q.v.), render a child vulnerable to the development of psychiatric disorder.

Recurrent abdominal pain and headaches are found to have an organic basis only in about 10% of cases. In a proportion of the remainder, probably between 10% and 20% an emotional cause can be found. The child may be under stress at home or school; he may be using the pain as an attention-seeking mechanism, or his attention may become focused on his stomach or his head because of an overanxious parent.

Emotional stress has been shown to play a part in a variety of other illnesses. In asthma (q.v.), probably about a third of children have attacks precipitated by emotion, usually excitement or apprehension, but most of these children also have attacks precipitated by other situations, especially exposure to allergens. The presence of ketonuria in diabetes mellitus (q.v.) has been related to environmental stress in a diabetic adolescent. It is well known that epilepsy occurs more frequently when the sufferer is in an adverse life situation. Telemetric studies have shown that there is an increase in 4–6-second spike and wave phenomena when children are either understimulated or exposed to learning tasks just beyond their limits of ability.

In this brief general account of child psychiatric disorders, most weight has been put on the diagnostic appraisal. This is because it is only after such an assessment (which need not necessarily be so full in many cases) that the practitioner is in a position to judge whether a significant disorder is present, and if it is, what are the likely aetiological and precipitating factors. Only in this way can rational management and treatment be planned.

In many cases understanding the situation leads the doctor directly to a course of action in terms of guidance or discussion with the parent about the nature of the problem and measures which might lead to its diminution.

When, despite the measures taken by the family practitioner, a significantly handicapping psychiatric disorder persists, referral to a child guidance clinic or hospital child psychiatric department, if this is available, should be considered. In some cases, such as severe school phobia, depression to the point of suicidal thoughts or where there is a suspicion of an autistic disorder, the referral is better made early than late.

Children's and Young Persons in need of care

Most countries have in law a minimum age at which a juvenile is held to be personally responsible for his deeds. Below this age the emphasis is normally placed on parental care and discipline. However, in some children the appropriate court may be convinced (a) that he is guilty of the offence, (b) that he is beyond the control of his parents or guardians. The details vary from one country to another, but most industrially developed communities have, for such cases, systems by which the child can be cared for and kept under control within a community home or other form of institution.
SEE ALSO Community homes and Fostering

Cholinergic

A term applied to those nerve fibres whose endings liberate acetylcholine (q.v.) as the synaptic transmitter substance. These include all pre-ganglionic fibres in the autonomic nervous system, all post-ganglionic fibres in the parasympathetic system, some post-ganglionic fibres in the sympathetic system (e.g. sweat glands), somatic motor nerve fibres and some fibres within the central nervous system (e.g. cortex).
SEE ALSO Acetylcholinesterase.
For a general account SEE ALSO Biochemical and neurophysical background to mental disease.

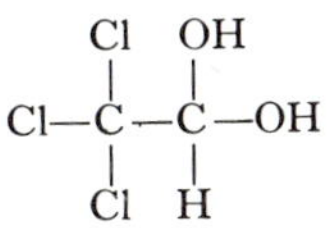

Chloral hydrate

Chloral derivatives

Chloral is the oldest member of the hypnotic group. Its popularity waned when barbiturates were introduced, for the effects and side effects are similar, but it has regained limited favour recently. Chloral is absorbed from the gastro-intestinal tract and converted in the body into the sedative trichloroethanol.
Chloral derivatives are safe and effective hypnotics preferred to barbiturate in the young for safety and less liable to produce confusion in the elderly. Chloral potentiates alcohol, indeed this mixture comprises the 'knockout drops' or 'Micky Finn'.
Chloral hydrate produces gastric irritation and a number of alternative preparations have been introduced which also liberate trichloroethanol in the body. The best known examples are dichloralphenazone, triclofos, and chlorhexadol.
SEE ALSO Hypnotics.

Cholinesterase

Acetylcholine (q.v.) must be rapidly removed from the synapse if repolarization is to occur. An important part of the process is undertaken by the enzyme acetylcholinesterase (also called true or specific cholinesterase). It is found in high concentration in the cell membranes at cholinergic nerve terminals, but is also present in red cell and placental membranes. It will hydrolyse several choline esters but has a high affinity for acetylcholine. A second cholinesterase (pseudocholinesterase, non-specific cholinesterase) has different properties.

Chromosomes

Chromosomes are threadlike structures within the cell nucleus. They are composed of desoxyribonucleic acid, the molecular structure of which carries a genetical code determining growth and metabolism. The human somatic cell has a normal complement of forty-six chromosomes, comprising one pair of sex chromosomes (X and Y in the male; two X chromosomes in the females) and twenty-two pairs of autosomes. Techniques have been developed for the microscopical examination of chromosomes to detect abnormalities of number and morphology.
Within the past decade numerous syndromes and sporadic abnormalities have been found to be associated with demonstrable chromosomal defects. Demon-

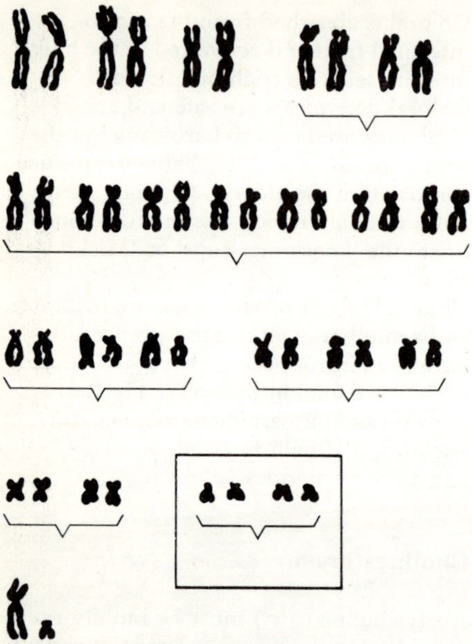

Diagram of normal chromosome pattern

strable autosomal abnormalities are usually associated with severe mental subnormality and marked anatomical changes. Mongolism (q.v.) and the cri-du-chat syndrome (q.v.) are examples of conditions associated with demonstrable autosomal abnormalities. Demonstrable sex chromosome abnormalities, which are usually a deviation from normal with respect to the number of sex chromosomes, are less often associated with marked physical malformations and severe mental subnormality, but seem to be more frequently associated with psychiatric changes, especially in the field of personality. An outstanding example is the XYY syndrome (q.v.), characterized by the presence of an extra Y chromosome in males and the tendency to criminality and outbursts of violence.

Visible chromosomal changes represent very gross defects, but it is assumed that finer chromosomal changes, or point mutations, which are undetectable microscopically, account for inherited conditions such as the inborn errors of metabolism.

SEE ALSO Genetics and Sex-linked inheritance.

Circadian rhythm

One of the innate rhythms of biological activity, circadian rhythm refers to the changes in physiological and psychological activities during a twenty-four hour cycle. There are a number of biological clocks – ultradian (seconds, minutes, hours), and infradian (days, weeks, years). Disease, time changes, drugs, and many other factors may affect these rhythms. Jet travel is the most common disturber of circadian rhythm, jet lag being experienced as fatigue, impaired concentration, anxiety and insomnia. It may take two or three weeks to adjust to the time difference involved in a journey from England to Australia, and the symptoms at times may approach the intensity of a developing anxiety neurosis. In psychiatry biological rhythms have been studied in relation to the phases of manic depressive illness, to suicide, and to menstrual disorders.

Citrullinuria

This is a rare inherited metabolic defect associated with mental subnormality. The amino-acid citrulline is found in large quantities in the body fluids. It is presumed that the enzyme deficiency in this condition is of argininosuccinic acid synthetase.

SEE ALSO Inherited metabolic defects.

Clang association

SEE Flight of ideas.

Classification of psychiatric illness

Nosological studies of disease are the bases on which rest further advances in knowledge of particular illnesses. Beginning in the eighteenth century, the taxonomy of mental illness slowly evolved until, by the early years of this century, a fair measure of agreement had been reached amongst psychiatrists regarding certain disease entities. Kraepelin had brought some order into the psychoses, splitting what he called dementia praecox into certain subgroups – a process which continued with Bleuler and other European psychiatrists. With the growth of psychiatry, particularly after the second world war, it became clear that there was a need for an international classification of mental disorders if studies of incidence, prevalence and other aspects of illness were to have any real value. The World Health Organisation's International Classification of Diseases, Injuries, and Causes of Death (ICD) became the basis for a uniform classification of psychiatric illnesses. A number of attempts were made to reach a satisfactory code, culminating in the Eighth Revision of 1968. In the United Kingdom and the United States of America, the classification was put into use, although handbooks were published in both countries, explaining the use of some of the categories, and modifying, in the case of the USA, some of the groupings so as to conform to current practices in that country. It is important that psychiatrists use the International Diagnostic Code, and use it efficiently, carefully and correctly, so that information derived from it may be of the greatest possible value.

Any system of psychiatric classification will not meet with universal approval, so diverse are the theoretical approaches to the subject. But it must be realized that classification is a tool of communication, to be used in a manner which is most productive of uniformity of diagnosis on a world-wide basis.

An internationally agreed classification is mandatory for psychiatric use, but the average doctor is, in practice, little concerned with taxonomies. What he requires is a simple classification system which can be of clinical value, particularly in differential diagnosis. There is some merit in the use of a relatively simple classification into six great clusters of illnesses.

1. Affective disorders.
2. Schizophrenic disorders.
3. Neurotic disorders.
4. Sociopathic disorders.
5. Organic disorders.
6. Mental retardation.

Each is characterized by a relatively simple underlying symptom pattern: (a) by change of mood; (b) by change of thought process; (c) by increased anxiety; (d) by social difficulties; (e) by memory disturbances; and (f) by intellectual retardation.

In the present state of psychiatric knowledge, when aetiology is, in the majority of cases, unknown or obscure, this symptomatological classification is probably the most useful frame of reference. Childhood psychiatric disorder at the present time must be regarded as a separate problem, the classificatory difficulties being a matter for the expert, and of little real relevance to the family doctor.

For detailed information the excellent *Glossary of Mental Disorders*, published by HMSO in 1968, should be consulted. The equivalent American publication is the *Diagnostic & Statistical Manual of Mental Disorders*, 2nd edn., published by the American Psychiatric Association, 1700, 18th Street, N.W. Washington, DC, 20009 USA.

Classification of psychotropic drugs

Psychotropic drugs are substances which act directly or indirectly on the central nervous system and affect mental and emotional processes; psychoactive and psychopharmacological are alternative terms, but the term psychotropic has achieved a rather more general use. The use of the prefix psycho in these names emphasizes the central importance of psychological effects amongst the various actions of drugs of this category.

Commercial pharmaceutical vigour in recent years has produced a rapidly expanding and diverse group of psychotropic agents. These new types of drugs have promoted new concepts of psychotropic activity, and a more comprehensive classification was needed to include them. The main types of newer drugs are the neuroleptics, anxiolytic compounds, antidepressants, and some psychotomimetic agents. Descriptions of these will be found under the appropriate headings.

Various classifications have been proposed for the psychotropic drugs, but one convenient one utilizes three parameters: the type of action in the central nervous system; the character of psychological effects produced; and the chemical structure of the drugs themselves (see diagram).

There is an initial natural separation into three broad categories according to the type of action on the central nervous system: central nervous depressants are inhibitory; central nervous stimulants are activatory; and psychotomimetic compounds are disruptive.

There are three main types of compound which exert a depressant action in the central nervous system: the major tranquillizers or neuroleptic compounds; the minor tranquillizers or anxiolytic compounds; and the hypnotics. These compounds form a spectrum of activity in terms of sedation, but in other ways they are disparate. The major and minor tranquillizers have important differences of action which are reflected in their clinical use in psychotic and neurotic illness respectively, but they can both be seen as depressors of affect. Hypnotics are perhaps better seen as depressors of vigilance. Narcotic analgesics and anti-convulsants could be included here, for although not used primarily for psychological effects they have some relevance to psychiatric practice.

Stimulant or psychoanaleptic compounds devolve readily into two subgroups: the anti-depressant compounds, which have an indirect activatory action and can be considered as stimulants of affect, and the psychostimulants, which act directly and tend to enhance vigilance.

Psychotomimetic or psychodysleptic drugs form a rather heterogeneous collection of compounds which have in common the effect of disorganizing mental function.

For a more extensive account of the chemical groups covered by the therapeutic group SEE Anticonvulsants, Antidepressants, Analgesics, Hypnotics, Neuroleptic drugs, Psychostimulants, Psychotaminetic drugs, Tranquillizers, Lithium.

Claustrophobia

(Synonym: Fear of enclosed spaces)

Uncommonly this occurs as an isolated specific fear, often of lifts or a locked toilet. More usually the phobias are widespread and may include crowds, shops, or even the fear of being detained talking to someone and unable to get away. The underlying fear of being trapped is frequently associated with a fear of going too far in a mixed agoraphobic/claustrophobic syndrome. As with agoraphobia, personality disturbances, and particularly sexual fears, are common. The more specific the symptom the better the response to behaviour therapy; the more widespread the symptoms the more behaviour therapy should be combined with psychotherapy or drugs.
SEE ALSO Phobia.

	Effect on C.N.S.	Psychological effects		Main chemical groups
Psychotropics Psychopharma- cological Psychoactive	**Depressant** Inhibitory	**Tranquillizers** Psycholeptic	Major Neuroleptic	Phenothiazines Butyrophenones Thioxanthines Rauwolfias
			Minor Anxiolytic	Benzodiazepines Glycol derivatives
		Hypnotics Anti-convulsants Narcotic analgesics		Barbiturates Chloral derivatives Piperidinedione derivatives Benzodiazepines
	Stimulant Activating	**Anti-depressants** Thymoleptic Indirect		Tricyclics MAOI's
		Psychostimulant Direct		Amphetamines Xanthines (convulsants)
	Disruptive Disorganize	**Psychotomimetic** Psychodysleptic Psychotogenic Psychedelic Hallucinogenic		LSD Psilocybin Mescalin

A classification scheme for psychotropic drugs. Note that lithium (q.v.), which does not fit easily into any group, is omitted.

Climacteric

This term refers to the irreversible ovarian failure that occurs in women in the fifth or sixth decade of life. Ovulation and menstruation cease, oestrogen secretion decreases and pituitary gonadotropin secretion increases in consequence. (The effects of oestrogen deficiency are dealt with in the section on the menopause.) There is no good evidence that an analogous failure in testicular function occurs in men. Most of the symptoms attributed to the 'male climacteric' are more plausibly attributable to neurosis.

Clinical trials

Clinical trials are established to confirm the value of new therapeutic procedures and to assess their problems and dangers. The widest use of the term concerns drug trials. Initial trials should be undertaken with the exact therapy known to the clinician, who assesses the dose, determines the problems and forms an estimate of the value of the new therapy.
Since such 'open' trials may be subject to observer bias, confirmatory 'blind controlled' trials are desirable. In these trials, which either compare the new therapy with existing accepted therapy or no therapy, the observer bias is avoided by concealing from him the therapy which each patient is receiving.
SEE ALSO Placebos and Controls.

Clouding of consciousness

Consciousness (q.v.) is the state of awareness implying complete contact with the external environment, and ability to comprehend it and manipulate it to the maximum capacity of the organism. Clouding of consciousness is thus any lesser state in these terms. Clouding may be physiological in the state between wakefulness and sleep. Clouding may be pathologically determined by conditions affecting the normal functioning of the brain – metabolic disturbances, toxic states, structural damage in the hypothalamic region where activating centres are sited, conditions disturbing cortical activity.
Clouding of consciousness may be established by clinical psychophysiological and electroencephalographic (EEG) (q.v.) means. Behaviourally it may be shown as a state of apathy or indifference, which may be associated with excessive drowsiness, but excitement is often marked as in delirium tremens. A periodic failure in registration will be demonstrated by patchy loss of memory. Inattention may be shown by the muddling of the order of events and by disturbances in the appreciation of the passage of time. Concentration may be tested using the 'serial sevens test', in which the patient is asked to subtract seven from a hundred and seven from the answer, and so on. Finally, clouding may interfere with intellectual function, and be demonstrated by variable loss of intellectual performance. Reaction time procedures, either of a simple stimulus-response type or involving selective responses, measure alertness and may be performed alone or in conjunction with the EEG, where slowed performance and errors are shown to correspond to slowing and abnormality in the electroencephalogram.
SEE Acute confusional states, Delirium.

Cobalamin

Deficiency of cobalamin (vitamin B_{12}) not only leads to the haematological and neurological changes of pernicious anaemia, but in some patients to a psychotic state. The mental symptoms are usually those of a depression although a confusional psychosis or a paranoid reaction is sometimes seen.
A deficiency of cobalamin, confirmed by absorption tests, may also result in a psychosis with no evidence of an anaemia or subacute combined degeneration of the cord. The possibility should be borne in mind in any patient at risk – and particularly after gastric surgery.
The mental symptoms respond well to high doses of cobalamin.
SEE ALSO Folic acid.

Cocaine

Cocaine is a crystalline white powder derived from the plant Erythroxylon coca which grows wild in certain parts of South

America. Cocaine has a powerful local anaesthetic action but when administered parenterally has a powerful stimulant effect on the central nervous system. Frequent use produces severe states of psychological dependence (q.v.) but no physical dependence (q.v.). Cocaine use may be complicated by dermatitis with intense itching, and cocaine psychosis, a drug-related psychosis, is characterized by paranoid ideas, restlessness and hallucinations. True tolerance does not occur despite the large doses taken by some cocaine users. It may only be prescribed for addicts by licensed doctors.
SEE ALSO Addiction.

Coefficient of variation

The coefficient of variation is the numerical method for expressing the degree of variability of a series of observations. A large coefficient of variation represents observations widely scattered from the mean. Mathematically it is the standard deviation (q.v.) expressed as a percentage of the mean (e.g. if the mean of a series is ten units and the standard deviation one unit, the coefficient of variation is 10%).

Cognitive

Cognition is a general term embracing all modes of knowing: perceiving; remembering; imagining; thinking; reasoning; judging. On the basis of distinctions made by Plato and Aristotle, the cognitive or noetic aspects of mind have traditionally been contrasted with the orectic aspects: conation (q.v.) (willing) and affection (q.v.) (feeling).
Cognitive structure is a term applied to an individual's organization of his past experience into a hierarchical pattern of related conceptual schemata to which current experience is related. This greatly facilitates the 'chunking' of new information and hence the efficiency of its processing. Cognitive efficiency is also greatly enhanced by the coding of information, usually in linguistic forms. The communicative aspects of language (q.v.) are also important for the transmission of information and so the relationships between cognition and language are extensive and intimate.
Disturbances of cognition frequently occur in psychiatric conditions, notably in schizophrenia (q.v.) and senility. Autistic (q.v.) thinking is a psychiatric term indicating that thinking is governed by personal needs and fantasies.
SEE ALSO Old-age.

Colitis
SEE Irritable bowel syndrome.

Coma

Coma is a state of complete loss of consciousness from which the patient cannot be roused by stimulation. It may be associated with depressed respiration, hypotension, areflexia, and loss of sphincteric control. Intracranial causes are cerebrovascular occlusion, haematoma, tumour, acute infections, abscesses, epilepsy (q.v.) and trauma. Extracranial causes include poisoning, diabetes, hypoglycaemia (from insulin or insulinoma), hepatic or renal failure, and anoxia. Although conditions of impaired consciousness are seen in certain psychiatric disorders, the term coma is hardly applicable to them (e.g. stupor (q.v.) trance (q.v.)).

Command automatism
SEE Automatic obedience.

Community care

One of the premises on which community psychiatry (q.v.) is based is that there are facilities within the community for the adequate care of its psychiatric invalids. In essence the patient is envisaged as better served by removal from a hospital environment, his care being undertaken in smaller organizations tailored to the particular need – workshops, occupation centres, hostels, day hospitals, night hospitals, and units in general hospitals. This fragmentation of services presents administrative problems and staffing difficulties, and is probably more expensive than the already heavy cost of medical care. The extent of the development of the community care concept varies from one country to another. In the Soviet

Union community care is particularly well organized. In Great Britain steps are being taken to integrate medical and social services so that community care may become a reality.

Community homes

Under more enlightened recent legislation in several countries radical improvements have been made in the handling of children and young persons who are 'in need of care and control'. In the United Kingdom, for example, some of the institutions for young miscreants are being replaced by a complex but co-ordinated system of community homes. They will cater for a wide range of children, only a minority of whom will have passed through the courts. In function they will vary from small informal quasi-family units to disciplined boarding schools of the old approved school type.
SEE ALSO Care order and Supervision order.

Community psychiatry

An ill-defined term, whose meaning varies from country to country. The isolation of the psychiatrist behind the walls of a lunatic asylum is not uncommon even today in some parts of the world. It was the reaction to this situation which gave rise to the idea of a community-based psychiatry, centred on a variety of services, general hospital, out-patient, day hospital, hostel, school clinics and so on. The psychiatrist is regarded as a pivotal figure in contact with a wide range of community facilities into which he can accommodate his patients according to their needs. The integration of social and medical services is clearly desirable if the role of social factors is as important in illness as is claimed, and the concept of community psychiatry has undoubtedly helped to bring about this integration in Great Britain. The eventual disappearance of the mental hospital will be a consequence of the success of community psychiatry, and with its disappearance problems of institutionalization will also disappear. Those psychiatrists of a sceptical bent regard many of the aspirations and claims of community psychiatry as Utopian.

Compensation

A mental mechanism operating outside of conscious awareness through which the individual attempts to offset, or to make up for, real or phantasied deficiencies. There may be actual or imagined defects in such areas as physique, performance or other skills or attributes. The term is also applied to the conscious effort made to strive to make up for such deficiencies.

Compensation neurosis

The present epidemic of road traffic injuries in the developed countries of the world and the increasing organization of workers have led to claims for compensation for injury becoming a serious problem to governments and to insurance companies. Industrial injuries benefit and social security payments may summate to provide the unemployed worker with as much, if not more, cash than he would obtain if employed, whilst the prospect of obtaining a large capital sum by way of compensation is a temptation which requires almost superhuman resistance. It is accordingly important that the doctor be able correctly to assess a man's reactions to accident, in order to do justice both to the man and to society. Problems will not arise where purely physical injuries and the well-accepted results of such injuries arise. It is when psychiatric symptoms occur, either in the absence of any signs of physical disability or accompanying physical disability, that the term compensation neurosis is likely to occur. Two schools of thought exist. The first considers that the psychiatric symptoms are nothing else but the manifestations of a desire for gain, either conscious or unconscious, which are likely to disappear once an individual has been financially satisfied. The second sees the symptoms as the genuine result of a psychiatric illness, such as a reactive depression, mixed neurosis, or hysteria, precipitated by the accident. The prolongation and maintenance of these genuine symptoms are reinforced by the legal situation, the repeated medical examinations, the legal wrangling and the ultimate court case. What is to be the family doctor's approach to a situation in which he observes leading specialists in different fields expressing directly contrary views of the same case in the witness-box? If he is asked to report on one of his patients he would be well advised to confine his report to facts – the symptoms for which he has been consulted, the dates of attendance, the progress of the patient, and the medication he has been given. It is most unwise to express an opinion unless he has had access to all the medical and legal data. Nothing is more embarrassing than to be confronted in the witness-box with unfamiliar evidence, which, if taken into account, might alter the whole complexion of the case.

For the specialist psychiatrist different considerations apply, depending upon whether he is giving a report as to fact, on one of his patients, or whether he is being asked to examine and report as an expert. His opinion as the specialist treating the patient may be given a good deal of weight by the court, although not necessarily by the expert employed by the defendant. As a result his cross-examination may be a painful experience which many psychiatrists do not appreciate. As an expert he must expect to be exposed to the cut and thrust of legal examination – the law courts are no place for the sensitive or the unprepared.

For the expert, compensation neurosis provides one of the most difficult fields of medicine, in which a knowledge of diagnosis, and prognosis, of human nature, of conditions of employment, of money, and of the law must all be taken into account. If any generalizations can be made then they are:

1. The usual course of a reactive psychiatric illness is at most twelve months: symptoms persisting after this period must be viewed with some suspicion.
2. Envy, greed and resentment are the common emotional determinants of the kind of symptoms encountered in compensation neurosis.
3. The tendency of psychiatric symptoms to remit spontaneously makes the persistence or worsening of symptoms suspect.
4. The more severe the physical injury on the whole, the less the psychiatric symptomatology. Physical factors are of little importance in compensation neurosis.
5. In cases where the injury or accident is not the subject of compensation, psychiatric symptoms are rare. It has been suggested that in countries with no compulsory insurance, compensation neurosis does not occur.

SEE ALSO Occupational psychiatry and Forensic psychiatry.

Complex

A term introduced by Bleuler and later much used by Freud to signify a constellation of emotionally charged, often contradictory attitudes and ideas, always unconscious. The individual is driven to behave in a manner dictated by his unconscious complexes – such as the Oedipus complex, the castration complex and so on – in a manner which is often unrealistic and productive of psychiatric symptoms.

Adler's inferiority complex is perhaps the best known of the complexes to the lay public; the word has proved very popular and is often used in a non-technical sense.

Compulsion

This is the recurrent urge to perform some item of behaviour which the subject has some desire to resist. Rituals (q.v.) in contradistinction to compulsions involve no desire to resist, may even be actively planned and anticipated with pleasure; by the social group as well as the individual. They are particularly common in children and are a natural aspect of their normal behaviour. Avoiding cracks in pavements, perhaps visualized as chasms descending to infernal worlds, intricate ceremonies before mounting the stairs to bed or knocking rituals before entering doorways, all for the imaginative child, serve to ward off evil influences. During development to adult life many of these features recede; some, however, persist, a situation to which the countless superstitions testify. Freudian psychodynamics stresses importance of expiation of guilt in both rituals and compulsions, often related to unconscious aggressive phantasies. Compulsive symptoms have also an increased incidence in states of fatigue, and are seen in association with oculogyric crises and encephalitis lethargica. In

schizophrenia the subject may feel himself compelled to carry out some actions under the influence of an external power. Compulsive symptoms are quite common in manic-depressive psychosis. The compulsion extends from the simplest act of rechecking to complex stereotyped behaviour patterns and it is difficult to be certain where rituals end and compulsion begins. The compulsion may be regarded as reaching the level of an illness when there is obtrusion into consciousness of undesired ideas and thoughts which may be acutely distressing. The following struggle of the patient to rid himself of the demands of these unwanted thoughts with its ensuing conflict leads to mounting degrees of anxiety, even reaching a phobic state.
SEE ALSO Obsessive – compulsive reaction.

Compulsory admission

The accent in modern psychiatric practice is placed on persuading the patient to undergo appropriate therapy whether this be as an outpatient or in an institution. Nevertheless there is a need for a procedure by which a mentally disturbed person who may do themselves or others serious harm may be legally compelled to enter a mental hospital. The exact procedure and safeguard for the patient's rights of freedom differ from one country to another but a typical system is that for England and Wales.
Under the Mental Health Act 1959 in England and Wales 'certification' was abolished, and it was clearly laid down that compulsory procedures were only to be used when permission to get a patient to enter hospital voluntarily had failed. Applications for compulsory admission may be made either for 'observation', or for 'treatment', and can be filed either by the nearest relative or by a mental welfare officer. A mental welfare officer cannot apply for a treatment order if the nearest relative objects. In an emergency, application may be made by any relative or by a mental welfare officer.
Every application must be accompanied by recommendations from two medical practitioners. One of these must be approved by the local health authority as a specialist, the other should, if possible, be the patient's family doctor. In 'urgent necessity' a seventy-two hour observation order (Section 29) can be recommended by one doctor alone.
The medical recommendations must state that the patient is suffering from a mental disorder which warrants his detention in a hospital in the interest of his health or safety or for the protection of others. He can be admitted for observation for up to twenty-eight days (Section 25) or for treatment for up to one year in the first instance (Section 26). After one month the powers of discharge rest with the nearest relative, unless the physician formally objects.
SEE ALSO Forensic psychiatry.

Conation

Conation is a term applied to those psychological processes involved in acting, willing or striving. With cognition (q.v.) (knowing) and affection (q.v.) (feeling) it makes up the triad of major psychological functions in the classification originally proposed by Plato and slightly modified by Aristotle. The conative aspect of functioning concerns the determinants and mental concomitants of action, whether purposeful or impulsive. Modern psychological theory in this area tends to be based on motivational concepts which have both conative and affective implications.
Abulia (q.v.), an inability to reach and act on decisions, is a common complaint in neurosis. Disturbances of volition, however, are most prominent in schizophrenia (q.v.). Schizophrenic patients often complain of weakening of their will and many are singularly inactive. Passivity phenomena are also very common. The patient may claim that his thoughts, actions and speech are controlled by an outside influence. Motor correlates of this type of experience are especially prominent in catatonia (q.v.), e.g. flexibilitas cerea (q.v.) (waxy flexibility: the passive acceptance and maintenance of imposed postures), echolalia (q.v.) (automatic repetition of words or phrases) and echopraxia (q.v.) (automatic imitation of another's movements). These motor symptoms also occur in certain organic conditions, especially Alzheimer's disease (q.v.).

Conceptual thinking

A concept is a general abstract idea concerning a set of objects, events, qualities, or relations. It develops by a process of generalizing from the particular. Specific events are compared, their common properties abstracted to form a concept which is then generalized to embrace all events of the same class. Thus limited experience of specific ash-trays will provide us with a general concept applicable to all ash-trays and at the same time contribute to more abstract concepts of 'roundness' or 'squareness'. Such concepts become hierarchically organized. For example, the concept 'dog' may be subsumed under the more general concept 'mammal' or broken down into subordinate concepts such as 'spaniel' or 'terrier'. In our thinking, concepts are coded by symbols, usually words. The facility with which human beings form concepts and their use of language (q.v.) enables them to internalize and deal symbolically with a world of events well beyond their immediate environment both in space and time.

It is not surprising then that disorders of conceptualization contribute a great deal to the thinking disabilities of psychotic patients. Organic brain lesions tend to impair the more abstract and flexible types of conceptualization and to limit thought to the concrete level. Sorting tests were designed to elicit abnormalities of this nature. Thus a patient, having sorted a group of blocks according to their colours might be unable to reclassify them by shape. He might classify a group of common objects correctly in terms of usage, e.g. 'all to do with eating' but fail to use more abstract concepts of size, material etc. Thought disordered schizophrenics exhibit related abnormalities and also elaboration of their conceptual systems by the incorporation of or penetration by themes deriving from the personal fantasies characteristic of their illness. The conceptual thinking of schizophrenics has been described as 'over inclusive' and as 'loose', imprecise or vague. Specific tests of these characteristics have been devised recently.

SEE ALSO Thought, Thinking, Concrete thinking, Psychoses, Schizophrenia, and Dereistic thinking.

Concordance

A term used in genetic studies implying the similarity of a twin pair with respect to the presence or absence of a characteristic, disorder or trait.

Concrete thinking

There are three stages in the development of the thought processes:

1. Syncretic thinking, the first stage of thought, in which the child endows all external objects with life in an animistic manner.
2. Concrete thinking, when objects become recognized as either inanimate or animate, but there is no generalization. For instance a table is seen as a specific table, and not one example of a whole range of tables.
3. Abstract thought, when the capacity to fit objects into a general pattern develops.

Concrete thinking may occur in both organic and functional disorders.

SEE ALSO Thought, Thinking, and Conceptual thinking.

Concussion

Concussion is the clinical state resulting from impairment of brain function following head injury, and may be due to shear forces to nerve cells or to an effect on a mid brain centre. The patient may be dazed, momentarily disoriented, but continue automatic activity. After severe trauma the patient may become unconscious, and then on recovery show evidence of an organic mental syndrome with disorientation, restlessness, impaired comprehension, perseveration, retrograde and anterograde or post-traumatic amnesia (q.v.). Personality change, psychosis, particularly depression and psychoneuroses, may follow concussion. It may be the provocative agent in some patients with pre-senile dementia (q.v.). Recovery, though slow, is usual, and treatment is by active rehabilitation after consciousness is regained.

Condensation

An unconscious defence mechanism whereby a number of elements unacceptable to consciousness are fused into a single acceptable symbol, idea, or fantasy. Condensation can best be studied in dream analysis, the individual dream symbols often representing many disparate fantasies condensed into one particular situation or symbol.

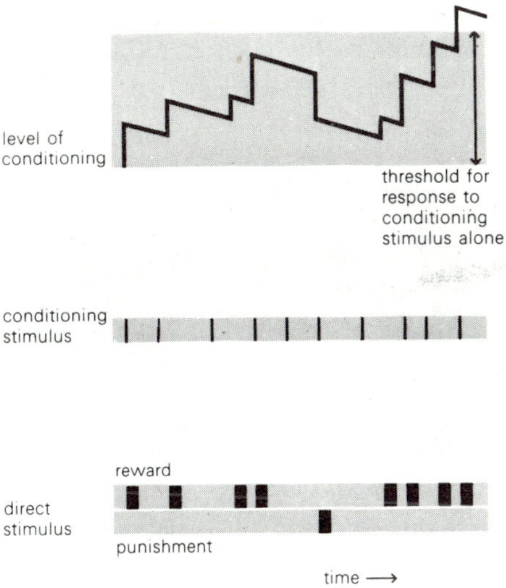

Representation of the reactions during the development of a conditioned reflex

Conditioned reflex, conditioned response

A response, acquired by a process of learning, which is dependent, conditional or contingent upon related events. In classical conditioning, which is particularly associated with the name of the Russian physiologist, Pavlov (1849–1936) (q.v.); the conditioned response (CR) comes to be elicited by an originally neutral conditioned stimulus (CS) through the repeated pairing of the latter with an unconditioned stimulus (UCS) which naturally evokes a similar but unconditioned response (UCR). The UCS may also be referred to as a reinforcer. The conditioned stimulus to be effective must precede the unconditioned stimulus. In Pavlov's well-known early experiments, he taught dogs to salivate to sound signals by presenting the sound, over a series of experimental trials, a second or two before the placement of food in the dog's mouth. Pavlov later employed this technique for his important investigations of conflict and inhibitory states. From these, he elaborated theories of brain functioning and related individual differences which he then applied to the explanation of abnormal states. Conditioned reflexes are usually involuntary responses and include a variety of acquired emotional reactions. Thus classical conditioning processes have been given considerable weight in behaviourist theories concerning the aetiology of psychiatric conditions such as phobias (q.v.). This type of conditioning is now regarded as a form of cue learning, the CS providing information concerning impending events and the CR being a form of anticipatory response.

Operant conditioning, studied intensively by the American psychologist Skinner (1904–) is concerned with the modification of voluntary or emitted responses for which the eliciting stimulus may be unknown. These operants may be contrasted with the respondents involved in Pavlovian conditioning. The basic principle underlying Skinner's influential work is that behaviour is controlled by its consequences. A response which is positively reinforced (in some sense rewarded) increases in strength as shown by increased probability of rate or recurrence. Without reinforcement the response gradually extinguishes. Negative reinforcement (punishing in some sense) produces escape and avoidance learning. Anticipatory learning is again clearly evident and discriminatory stimuli, which may be positive or negative according to the nature of the relevant reinforcers, provide cues indicating the type of behaviour appropriate to the particular situation.

These simple principles have a long history in psychological theory but Skinner and his associates have elaborated around them a detailed and precise technology which has proved remarkably effective when applied to both animal and human behaviour (q.v.). In this, great emphasis is placed on the timing of reinforcements and their contingency pattern. Different schedules of reinforcement have markedly different effects.

Behavioural modification programmes

involve a detailed analysis of the initial repertoire and the desired end point. Successive approximation techniques are employed in the shaping of the desired behaviour and the fading of redundant stimulus information.
Conditioning techniques have been widely employed in psychiatry by the behaviour therapists. The conditioning of bladder responses in the 'bell and pad' method of treating enuresis (q.v.) provides a familiar example. Operant conditioning, based on positive reinforcement, is now widely used for the modification of psychotic behaviour and provides the rationale for the token economies (q.v.) set up in many 'chronic' wards in the United States and now established in other countries. Aversive therapy (q.v.), applied to the treatment of sociopathic abnormalities, involves both classical and operant conditioning. When it provides the opportunity of acquiring effective avoidance responses it may be efficacious but when it relies largely on punishment, unavoidable strong negative reinforcement, its suppressive effect is likely to be temporary and disruptive side effects may appear.
SEE ALSO Behaviour therapy and Habit.

Confabulation

Confabulation, pseudo-reminiscence (q.v.), retrospective falsification (q.v.), and paramnesia (q.v.) are all terms used to describe the apparent recollection of imaginary events and experiences.
Confabulation commonly occurs in organic brain syndromes – Korsakoff's syndrome (q.v.), post-traumatic amnesia, limbic encephalitis – where new learning and recent memory are severely affected. It can occur in paranoid delusional states when early experience is modified to fit the delusional system. In the absence of delusions (q.v.) it is distinguished from pathological lying (q.v.) by the intactness of memory and purposive consistency seen in the latter.
SEE ALSO Paramnesia and Post-traumatic syndrome.

Conflict

The concept of conflict is central to psychoanalytic theory. With warring impulses, warring systems of thought and behaviour, the mental apparatus is continually in a state of conflict. In the neuroses this struggle is an unconscious one, the symptoms being its by-products. The fundamental conflict is a sexual one – the nuclear Oedipal complex.

Confusion, confusional states

SEE Acute confusional states, Clouding of consciousness and Delirium.

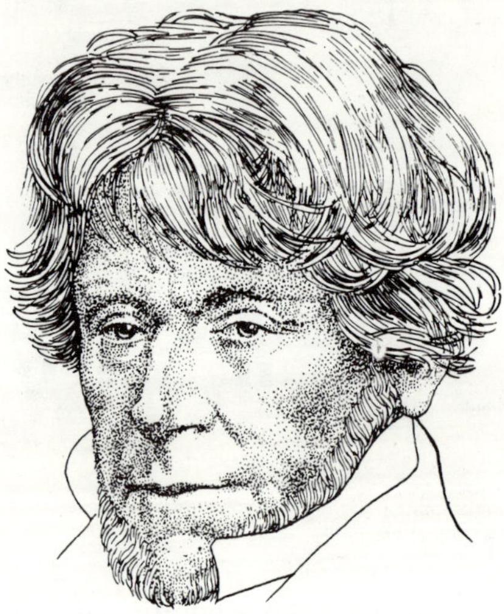

Conolly, John (1794–1866)

The abolition of mechanical restraint was put into effect by Conolly in 1839 at the Middlesex Asylum at Hanwell. Although previously introduced by Charlesworth and Gardiner Hill at Lincoln, Conolly's enthusiastic action produced a revolution within the mental hospitals of England, which spread over the next few years to Europe and to the United States. He was the author of the first comprehensive work *On the Construction and Government of Lunatic Asylums* (1847).

Conscience

Those psychic organizations that stand in opposition to the expression of instinctual actions. Parental attitudes are introjected (q.v.) by the child into the unconscious to form the superego (q.v.). This is the earliest form of conscience.
The function of conscience is to warn the subject that his ego (q.v.) is in danger of experiencing the pain of intense guilt. Conscience may become pathological if it is too rigid and powerful – as is seen in some persons of obsessional disposition; also when a breakdown and a feeling of annihilation and panic occurs instead of the usual conscience warning (this is seen in cases of severe depression); and when conscience appears to be poorly developed from the outset, allowing the feelingless, antisocial acting out of the psychopath. In the last example, however, absence of conscience as the automatic regulator of behaviour may not be the main deficit or may be more apparent than real. Psychopathic personalities can in fact experience guilt.

Constitution

The idea has existed from ancient times that some correlation may exist between somatic and psychological characteristics, particularly traits of temperament. Much attention has been paid in recent years to the role of constitution in psychiatry, great impetus being given to this work by Kretschmer and his followers. Kretschmer in the 1920's drew up somatic typologies which he correlated with psychological make-up: further notable work based on bodily measurement and psychometry was carried out by Sheldon and his colleages and later by Rees and Eysenck.
Kretschmer's original work had implications in the aetiology of mental illness; he suggested that pyknic individuals of his typology tended to have mood-swings and manic-depressive illnesses should breakdown occur, whereas the leptosomatic physique correlated with schizothymia and schizophrenia.
In addition to direct body measurements, evidence of the presence of physical constitutional factors which may correlate with psychological traits may be obtained by the use of refined techniques such as electroencephalography and biochemical and cytogenetical methods by which constitutionally determined variables can be demonstrated. This is a broad front on which many advances are being made currently.
A considerable body of evidence from twin studies shows that monozygotic (one-egg) twins have closer resemblances to each other for temperamental traits and other psychological factors than do dizygotic (two-egg) twins or ordinary sibs. This supports a constitutional basis for these factors, since monozygotic twins may be assumed to possess identical genetical make-up, whereas dizygotic twins may be as dissimilar from each other as ordinary sibs in this respect.
Family studies may be expected to yield information regarding the specificity of psychological factors and their constitutional basis. Most evidence relates to obsessional neuroses and the consensus of opinion is that the obsessional predisposition is a specific one.

Continuous narcosis

The treatment of mental disorders by procuring sleep for long periods is probably the oldest method of treatment known to psychiatry but became widely used at the beginning of this century with the advent of the barbiturates. As originally recommended, heavy and continuous sedation, sufficient to produce twenty hours sleep a day, was continued for several weeks at a time. Without the most meticulous medical and nursing attention mortality rates of up to 5% could occur from bronchopneumonia, cardiovascular collapse, suppression or retention of urine, etc. Since the conditions for which such intensive regimes were recommended, such as involutional melancholia and agitated schizophrenic states, are far better treated by other means the classical type of continuous narcosis should now be abandoned.
In acute states of anxiety and tension, particularly those resulting from continued and severe stress, a modified form of continuous narcosis for a period of five to seven days can be very helpful as an initial stage of treatment. This almost always produces marked though temporary

improvement which enables a more routine therapy to be instituted. The aim is to produce a state of drowsiness and intermittent sleep during the day and continuous sleep at night. The technique varies with different doctors but in all cases two drugs are used, one a tranquillizer to produce a continuous basic drowsiness and a short-acting hypnotic to produce a period of three hours' sleep morning and afternoon in addition to ten hours' sleep at night. The drugs should be given after breakfast and lunch so that the patient is awake enough to eat his next meal safely and attend to his toilet requirements.
In states of marked anxiety much larger doses than usual are necessary. A useful combination of drugs is chlorpromazine, 100–200 mg., t.d.s. and sodium amylobarbitone, 200 mg., given at 8 a.m. and 1 p.m. The dosage of drugs will have to be modified to suit the individual patient and usually needs to be increased after the second or third day. This treatment can be safely instituted at home for a period of five to seven days provided the patient is physically healthy and the relatives trustworthy and able to remain with the patient. As in all physical treatments safety depends entirely on meticulous attention to detail. The patient who seems able to feed himself may be left only to fall asleep with food in his mouth and in danger of inhalation and bronchial obstruction. A sleeping patient may become aware of a full bladder and in a confused state may attempt to go to the lavatory. Alternatively dehydration may occur due to neglect of fluid intake.

Contraception

The practice of contraception may influence a woman's mental health in several ways. Effective contraception will relieve symptoms of anxiety engendered by the prospect of an unwanted pregnancy. On the other hand anxiety may be increased if the method of contraception offends the patient's moral code. It is then obviously the duty of the doctor to take heed of his patient's moral views and to recommend what seems to him to be the best method for that patient.
Other women become anxious because they believe that the contraceptive method (usually an oral contraceptive or an intrauterine device) may harm them. Skilled reassurance will sometimes remove this fear. Finally, in a small proportion of women, oral contraceptives have a direct effect on mood (See Oral contraceptives).

Contract

A contract is an agreement between two or more parties which is intended to have legal consequences. Business deals, marriages, insurance agreements etc. are all contracts. Insane and drunken persons are not considered to have the necessary capacity to enter into a contract and such contracts are voidable although, so that the disordered person cannot benefit from his act, he may be liable to pay some restitution. Furthermore, a disordered person can make valid contracts involving 'necessaries', i.e. he may buy food and clothing. Two points must be proved by a person who pleads insanity: (a) he was insane at the time of making the contract and incapable of understanding the importance of the transaction; (b) the other party knew of his condition. Since the Mental Health Act 1959 compulsory patients are not certified insane but only as in need of in-patient treatment and therefore medical opinion is required on the patients' actual state of mind. A reasonable degree of mental alertness and contact with reality, together with a reasonably intact memory, must be demonstrated to permit the mentally ill individual to make a valid contract. Any contract entered into by a mentally disordered person during a 'lucid interval' is valid.
Mental disorder supervening after a contract has been made does not release either party from his obligations under the contract unless the nature of the mental disorder makes fulfilment impossible, e.g. mental disorder supervening after marriage does not of itself entitle either party to a divorce (q.v.) or to a judicial separation. Similarly, if a person who has insured his life while sane commits suicide as a result of becoming mentally ill or disordered, a contract of life insurance will stand, unless the policy contained a special clause designed to meet the contingency of suicide.
SEE ALSO Insanity, Marriage, Nullity and Forensic psychiatry.

Contracture

In psychiatry this refers to a virtually fixed contraction of a muscle or muscle group usually of hysterical origin. Wasting, deformity and gross impairment of function as a result of lack of use may be just as severe as that seen as a result of organic neurological disease.

Controls

When clinical trials (q.v.) have suggested a therapeutic value for a new procedure, it is important to assess the value more carefully by comparison with accepted therapy or no therapy. In drug trials dummy tablets ('placebos' (q.v.)) are usually administered to those receiving 'no therapy'. The comparative therapy, whether active or inactive, is termed the control. To avoid bias, the nature of the therapy received by each patient in a trial is best concealed from the observer (blind controlled trial). This is usually achieved in drug trials by the control being made physically to match the new therapy under study.

Control groups

In biological and clinical trials of therapeutic procedures it is important to compare the effect of the new therapeutic regime against a standard. The group of animals or patients which receives the 'standard' therapy is known as the control group and for valid comparison should match in all respects the group receiving the new form of therapy. Most methods of statistical analysis are based upon the groups being selected at random from the total population and a random selective procedure is therefore normally used.
The 'standard' used may be either no therapy or a widely accepted current form of therapy. In the initial stages of such a trial it is important that the physician knows which patient is receiving which treatment so that optimum dosage may be determined and unwanted or toxic effects noted. However, once an apparent action is found it is important that bias be excluded and for drug trials the later stage is preferably undertaken in a 'double blind' fashion. The control group is given an inert substance (dummy or placebo) or the reference active drug in a dosage form that is indistinguishable to either the patient or the physician from the new substance under test.
Although the control group concept is normally applied to drug trials it should be used for all therapeutic procedures under study.

Conversion

Used in two senses – the first refers to a change in beliefs, such as religious or political conversion, usually under the influence of powerful emotion. The second refers to an unconscious mechanism whereby affect is converted into a motor or sensory activity or lack of activity. Freud's studies of hysteria led him to postulate that the psychic problem was converted into a somatic problem, the result being freedom from anxiety – the belle indifférence of the hysteric. Later workers believed that psychosomatic disorders were examples of conversion – the conversion taking place along autonomic channels, instead of as in hysteria, via the sensory and motor apparatus of the nervous system.
SEE ALSO Hysteria.

Conversion hysteria
SEE Hysteria.

Convulsion therapy
SEE ECT (Electroconvulsive therapy).

Coprolalia

Coprolalia is the compulsive, shouting aloud of obscene words or statements out of any relevant social context. In association with generalized tics it occurs in adolescence in the Gilles de la Tourette syndrome (q.v.). The impulse to make coprolalic utterances is experienced by some obsessional neurotics and produces anxiety to which the individual may react by the development of some secondary compulsive behaviour. Coprolalia also occurs in schizophrenics, but the utterances are not resisted and occur in response to some inner hallucinatory experience.

Coprophagia

Coprophagia is the deliberate eating of faeces. It occurs in subnormal and psychotic children as regressive behaviour in boring and unstimulating environments and is sometimes seen in adult schizophrenics in repressed catatonic states. Rarely it is encountered as a form of male masochism, when it is associated with licking the buttocks and anus of the female partner.

Coprophilia

Coprophilia is the hoarding of human faeces or animal dung, often in parcels amongst personal belongings. It is most commonly met in socially isolated schizophrenics and in severe elderly dements. It is sometimes encountered in psychotic children where the faeces may have a symbolic significance and may be offered to the parent as a gift.

Corpus callosum

The corpus callosum is a large commissure of transverse fibres which links identical points from each cerebral hemisphere and ensures that there is a bilateral representation of the memory engram (q.v.).

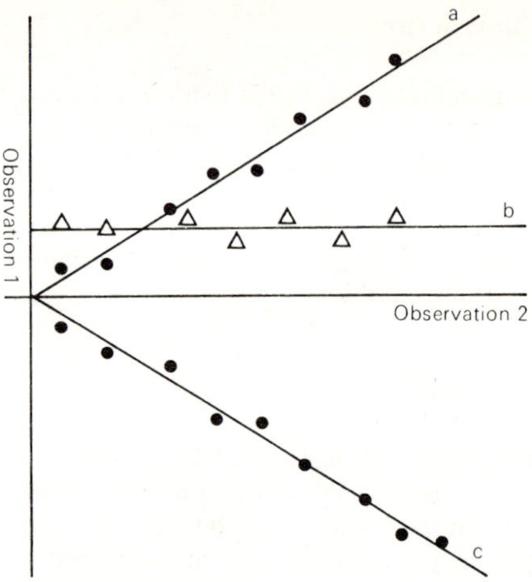

Scatter diagram showing for 3 different conditions the relationship between 2 sets of observations and the equivalent correlation curve

a. Correlation coefficient $\simeq +1$:
good positive correlation

b. Correlation coefficient $\simeq 0$:
no correlation between observations

c. Correlation coefficient $\simeq -1$:
good negative correlation i.e. g. one observation rises other is likely to fall

Correlation coefficient

The correlation coefficient is the measure of the dependence of two characteristics on each other when the relationship can be reasonably expressed by a straight line (see figure). The correlation coefficient must lie between +1 and −1. If the value is 0 or close to it, the characteristics are not interrelated; if close to +1 there is a close association between them; if near −1, an inverse relationship, i.e. as one value increases the other decreases to an equivalent degree.

Corticosteroid psychoses

Administration of corticosteroids often produces a change in mood, which is usually transitory. Euphoria is well known, but depression, tension, and emotional lability also occur. Transient depression sometimes follows cessation of treatment. In 1% or less of patients frank psychoses occur during corticosteroid treatment usually, but by no means always, after

prolonged treatment with high doses. Affective, schizophrenic and schizo-affective syndromes are seen, but frank delirium is rare. Corticosteroid psychoses are characteristically variable and lucid intervals are common.
The prognosis is good. Most patients recover if the dose is reduced or the steroid discontinued altogether. If the psychoses should persist, symptomatic treatment (electroconvulsive treatment, drugs, etc.) is effective.

Corticosteroid psychosis is rare even in patients with a history of serious psychiatric disorder. Such a history is therefore by no means an absolute contraindication to corticosteroid treatment.

Cotard syndrome

A term now seldom used to describe a mental state dominated by nihilistic delusions after the nineteenth-century French psychiatrist Cotard, who first described the condition. It is not a diagnostic entity and the majority of patients with these delusions are suffering from psychotic (endogenous) depressions (q.v.)

Counselling

Associated with the name of Carl Rogers, a psychologist, counselling is usually concerned with educational, marital, vocational and personal difficulties. The client may be advised by his counsellor – usually a psychologist, sometimes a priest – as to the best course to take in order to resolve his problem, or the treatment may be more non-directive, the interviews enabling the client to ventilate his anxieties and uncertainties and eventually to resolve his own problems.

Counterphobic mechanisms

The attraction felt for or approach behaviour made towards a feared or frightening object or situation. Persons may seek out such situations either if mildly phobic or during attempts to master their fears, repeatedly entering the problem situation. Counterphobic behaviour resembles some children's play, when frightening games are deliberately repeated. These behaviours may be performed because pleasure follows the decline in anticipatory anxiety which occurs as the behaviour proceeds while there is a progressively increasing pleasurable feeling of mastery over a difficult problem.

Counter-transference

Just as the patient transfers to the therapist the emotions experienced toward individuals in his past, so the therapist finds, in the analytic situation, circumstances relating to his own life, affecting him both consciously and unconsciously. In the counter-transference the therapist may unconsciously act out his own problems, transferring them to the patient, an obvious source of therapeutic difficulty which may seriously affect the course and outcome of the treatment.

Court Protection

In most countries with a well established modern psychiatric and legal system one section of the legislative system is charged with the duty to manage the property and affairs of persons who, by reason of mental disorder, are unable to do so themselves. The detailed procedure differs from one country to another but the procedure under English law, where the Court of Protection, an office of the English High Court acts, may be taken as a typical example. The court is only concerned with patients' property, not their persons. Usually the court operates by the appointment of a receiver (q.v.), although in simple cases it is sometimes possible to direct, for example, that a hospital shall act on the patient's behalf. The court requires medical evidence that a person is incapable by reason of mental disorder (q.v.) of administering his property and affairs. Psychopathic disorder (q.v.) is rarely dealt with by the court. It should be noted that whether a patient is in or out of hospital is not relevant to the

court's jurisdiction. The commonest disorders dealt with by the court are the dementias (q.v.) and senile confusional states.
Patients under the jurisdiction of the Court of Protection are discouraged from making wills unless there is evidence of testamentary capacity (q.v.) when a medical opinion is required.
SEE ALSO Curator bonis and Forensic psychiatry.

Courts and court procedures

The court system and procedure differ so much from one country to another, indeed from one section of a country to another in some federal communities, that it is impossible to cover the topic adequately.
The Editors have normally referred to the general principle in the English legal system where an example appeared appropriate. Readers are advised that these examples do not imply direct relevance in other countries.
SEE ALSO Forensic psychiatry.

Craniostenosis

Craniostenosis is a condition of the skull arising from premature fusion of the sutures. This abnormality of development is of diverse origin. It may lead to severe microcephaly and various distortions of shape of the skull. In the past operations were tried in craniostenosis, such as the 'hot-cross bun' operation in which a cruciform incision was made at the vertex. These operations were not successful, and no specific treatment exists. Many patients with craniostenosis have resulting neurological symptoms as well as mental subnormality, and their management is on general lines of care and training, with symptomatic treatment by physiotherapy etc.

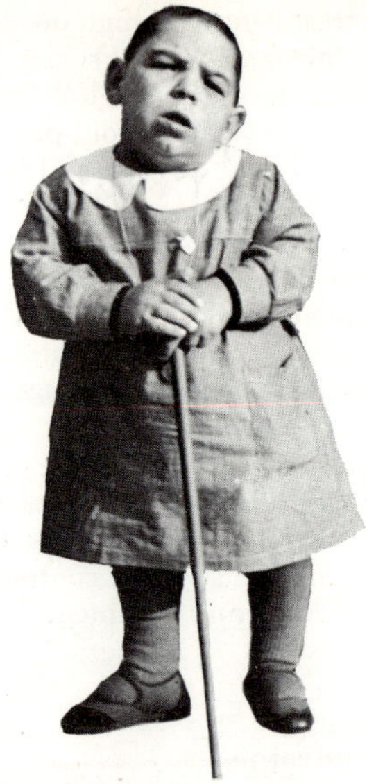

The patient is 22 years old

Cretinism

Cretinism is a type of mental subnormality, together with retardation of skeletal development, due to hypothyroidism (q.v.) in intra-uterine or neonatal life. Endemic cretinism is due to dietary iodine deficiency and can be prevented by iodine supplements in the diet. Sporadic cretinism is due to failure of foetal thyroid development. Metabolic cretinism is due to failure to synthesize thyroid hormone. A goitre is found only in endemic and metabolic cretinism.
The differential diagnosis from mental subnormality due to other causes may be difficult in the early stages for a cretin is usually normal in appearance at birth and may show no features of cretinism until the sixth month. In other cases signs may be detectable after the first few weeks of life. The child gradually fails to feed properly and becomes lethargic and constipated. The skin becomes yellow and puffy, the tongue protrudes and umbilical hernia is likely to develop. At this stage laboratory tests show thyroid hormone deficiency.
Treatment with thyroid hormone should begin as early as possible if normal development is to occur. All too often irreversible changes have already occurred, but treatment will be at least partly

effective. If the diagnosis is not made until later childhood, thyroid treatment has no effect on intelligence and may merely worsen behaviour.
SEE ALSO Hypothyroidism.

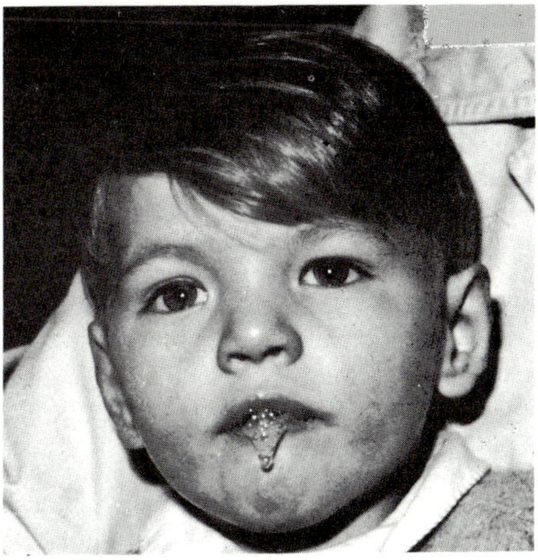

Cri du chat syndrome
(Synonym: Partial monosomy 5 disease)

This is a syndrome associated with a demonstrable autosomal chromosome defect, i.e. a partial deletion of the short arm of chromosome 5 (Denver system). It is associated with severe mental subnormality. During the first year of life the child emits a curious flat-toned cat-like wailing cry. A narrowing of the larynx has been suggested as the cause of this abnormality. The quality of the cry tends to become normal after a year. Other clinical features include hypotonia, moon-shaped face, wide-spaced eyes sloping downwards and outwards, epicanthic folds, low-set ears, prominent nasal bridge and micrognathia.
SEE ALSO Autosomal chromosomal abnormalities.

Crime
SEE Forensic psychiatry.

Criminal responsibility

A liability to punishment for transgression of the law is termed responsibility. During the past few centuries in most industrialized societies more and more people have been considered outside the usual legal framework because of their lack of this responsibility. Insanity in its grosser forms has, like infancy and deaf mutism, been an acceptable defence against conviction and/or punishment for a legal infringement, although at times certain offences have been deemed inexcusable on grounds of insanity (e.g. high treason in England in the time of Henry VIII). There are, however, in most countries a few laws of 'absolute liability', e.g. many driving laws where all that is necessary is to prove that the alleged offender committed the illegal act. Apart from these special laws of absolute liability it is frequently true that two components have to be present before full criminal responsibility is present. As stated in English law these are: (a) actus reus, i.e. the accused has to have actually committed the alleged misdeed; (b) he has to have the necessary mens rea (q.v.) or guilty mind. The burden of proof for the first component is on the prosecution whereas the burden of proof for the second is on the defence. Hence if a crime is committed unintentionally, or while the offender was insane (in the United Kingdom and some other countries this is based upon the McNaughton Rules (q.v.)) so as not to know the nature or wrongness of his act, he will be excused wholly or in part the legal consequences of his act.
SEE ALSO Diminished responsibility, Fitness to plead, and Forensic psychiatry.

Culture

The setting in which a person learns his technology, languages, religions, values, customs, beliefs, social relationships and family life and structure. Cultures vary enormously from one country to another and in each society certain members are misfits, for instance obsessional personalities are more comfortable in a highly organized society. The majority of members, however, are supported by the culture in which they live and it has been described as a protective cocoon buffering

the individual from emotional provocation and tending to eliminate sources of acute fear and anger, ensuring that each member of the society will not upset others emotionally or by abnormal behaviour.
Cross cultural psychiatry (transcultural psychiatry) is the study of psychiatric disorders in different cultures. Generally the organic psychoses, mental subnormality and schizophrenia are very similar in different parts of the world though the symptomatology may vary depending on the customs and beliefs of the country. The more psychogenically determined disorders are however more affected by cultural factors, thus hysterical conversion symptoms are more common in the underdeveloped societies in contrast to the frequency of anxiety neuroses in Western civilizations. Cultural influences are also important in diagnosis. A belief which to a western psychiatrist may appear grossly delusional might be acceptable to members of the patient's own culture.
Certain syndromes appear to be specific to particular cultural systems. (SEE Culture-bound syndromes.)

Culture-bound syndromes

Certain unusually dramatic types of behaviour in non-Europeans attracted so much attention that they have passed into the vernacular, for example – running amok, and voodoo. The alleged specificity of such behaviour to certain races or to certain countries has led to the idea that they are culture bound, although a wider acquaintance with the world shows that this is not entirely true. Amok, for instance, may be seen in Malays, West Africans, and Indians, to mention only three different types of mankind, whilst voodoo phenomena occur in South America, the Caribbean, and West Africa, and is not necessarily confined to the negro race. The incidence of these culture-bound syndromes has changed dramatically over recent years, so that once not uncommon behaviours may now appear only rarely.
Amok: is the Malay word for 'engaging furiously in battle', and describes a sudden outburst of intense, furious aggression in which the individual kills all those who may come in his path – with a knife, a sword, or other weapon. A period of brooding presages the attack, in an individual who is frustrated, and who bottles up his anger and then suddenly explodes into violent behaviour. Rarely a physical cause, such as a toxic confusional state, or a psychosis may underlie the outburst.
Latah: was also first described in Malays, and consists of two types of behaviour – automatic obedience, and a state of intense fear, in which startle reactions are prominent, and the patient may behave in an inappropriate way, talking obscenely or acting in a foolish manner. Women are most affected, and the condition has been regarded as similar to the hysterical behaviour of Charcot's female patients.
Koro: is observed amongst overseas Chinese men of Cantonese origin in Singapore and Malaysia. There is a sudden onset of anxiety affecting the genitals – the penis is thought to be shrinking or disappearing into the abdomen; clamps or ligatures may be placed on the penis to prevent this taking place. Epidemics of Koro have been described; recently in Singapore the hospitals were swamped by men convinced that, as a result of eating contaminated pork, their penises were becoming smaller.
Piblokto: or Arctic hysteria, is seen in Eskimo women who suddenly begin to scream, tear off their clothes, and run about on the ice. It is fast disappearing as is:
Wihtigo: the belief amongst certain North American Indians that they may be transformed into Wihtigo – a monster that eats human flesh.
Voodoo: is a possession state particularly associated with Haiti. Evil spirits invade the person and as a result normally unacceptable behaviour occurs in those possessed. Voodoo death, when an individual dies as a result of a spell, has been described in a number of different societies.

Cunnilingus

Cunnilingus is the erotic stimulation of the female external genitals by means of the tongue. It is practised in about 45% of marriages according to Kinsey as a form of pre-coital sexual stimulation. It is also indulged in by some female homosexuals as a method of erotic stimulation.

Curator bonis (judicial factor)

In many countries a person compulsorily admitted to a psychiatric hospital loses some of his civil rights. In Scotland a curator bonis or judicial factor can be appointed by petition to the appropriate Court if the patient cannot manage his own affairs. Many other countries adopt a similar policy by which the civil rights of mentally ill patients are protected by the courts.
SEE ALSO Testamentary capacity.

Cybernetics

The science of communication and communication-control theory, as applied to mechanical devices and to animals.
SEE ALSO Language.

Cyclothymic personality

Some people, mainly those of pyknic body build (q.v.), are subject to prominent mood changes which are not severe enough to be incapacitating, or even to be recognized as morbid, but which last for weeks or months at a time and appear to be quite independent of all environmental influences. In one phase they are full of energy and enthusiasm, optimistic, sociable and cheerful; in the other they are morose and withdrawn, lacking in energy and initiative and often preoccupied with vague somatic complaints like indigestion and headaches. These contrasting moods may alternate with one another throughout adult life, sometimes separated by periods of normality and occasionally having a predictable regularity. Those in whom the manic phase is predominant may be conspicuously successful in walks of life like politics, business management and journalism in which energy, self-confidence and sociability are at a premium. Many cyclothymics have episodes of overt manic depressive illness (q.v.) and others have close relatives who are manic depressive. Clearly there is a close relationship between cyclothymia and manic depressive illness and presumably they have a common genetic or constitutional basis. Before a diagnosis of cyclothymia is made it must be established that the mood changes are not simply responses to the disappointments, the lucky breaks and the fluctuating fortunes of daily life. The main clinical importance of the condition, apart from its implication of latent manic depressive illness, is that it is sometimes responsible for episodic and otherwise inexplicable alterations in behaviour – some cyclothymics drink heavily only in one phase of their cycle, others may be impossible to live with for months on end, and delightful at other times, and so on.
SEE ALSO Temperament.

Cystathioninuria

Cystathioninuria is a very rare inborn error of metabolism, which may be associated with mental subnormality, or other psychiatric effects. The enzyme defect is of cystathioninase, with the result that cystathionine fails to be broken down; it is excreted in large quantities in the urine.
SEE ALSO Inherited metabolic defects.

Dangerous Drugs

The British term covering both the narcotics (q.v.) and the amphetamines (q.v.) and like stimulants. In Great Britain, the main regulations affecting the practice of psychiatry are contained in the Dangerous Drugs Act 1967 which enabled the Home Secretary to require the notification of adults and to prohibit medical practitioners, except under licence (usually at an NHS clinic), from providing addicts with heroin and cocaine.
SEE ALSO Forensic psychiatry.

Daydreams

Wishful thinking, characteristic of normal adolescents and present to a small extent in normal adults (e.g. ambition). The gratification obtained by daydreams may divert the dreamer from applying her energies outwards to adapt and obtain her goals in reality. Daydreams are a marked feature in some adult neurotic patients and result both in their being increasingly dissatisfied with their lot in life and less inclined to adapt to and overcome their difficulties.

Day hospitals

In the Soviet Union the upheaval produced by the Revolution had important effects on the medical services. Shortage of medical personnel and hospital facilities, as well as ideological considerations, contributed to efforts to keep the psychiatric patient in the community, either as outpatients or, from 1932 onwards, as patients in day hospitals. All types of treatment could be carried out in this setting, the patient returning to a hostel or to his home for the night. An emphasis on work and occupation was linked with the therapeutic effort, small workshops being attached to the centres. It was not until 1946 that the first day hospital was opened, outside the USSR, in Montreal, whilst in England the social psychotherapy centre, later to become the Marlborough day hospital, is claimed to have been the pioneer, opening also in 1946. Since then the day hospital has firmly established itself as a psychiatric facility. Essentially patients attend daily, and receive all the attention which can be given in the orthodox hospital – shock treatment, pharmacotherapy, psychotherapy, rehabilitation and so on. The type of patient may vary considerably – some day hospitals take a cross section of psychiatric problems, others concentrate on chronically disabled patients. The day hospital itself may be attached to a psychiatric hospital, but be geographically separate; may be attached to a general hospital; or may, rarely and probably undesirably, function independently of other psychiatric facilities. Day hospitals may cater for other than psychiatric patients, and have proved useful for geriatric problems, and for the physically or mentally handicapped. It is claimed that day hospitals offer definite advantages – little risk of institutionalization, greater contact with the social milieu and more economical treatment. These claims are so far unproven.

Deafness

Deafness is seen more commonly among old people who become mentally ill than those who do not. This is particularly so in paranoid illnesses, whilst in paraphrenia about one-third of the patients have some degree of deafness which brings about and which is known to potentiate any tendency to suspicion or misinterpretation. To a less degree blindness shows the same relation to mental illness in old age, of which the temporary mental disturbance sometimes following cataract removal is a commonly observed instance.

Death instinct (thanatos)

The riddles of life and death have preoccupied doctors, philosophers and theologians for centuries. The organism contains the seeds of its own destruction; life can be seen as a struggle against death, activity versus the cessation of all activity. If there is this biological struggle going on, then why not a similar psychological instinctual struggle? Freud in *Beyond the Pleasure Principle* put forward the view that life is a struggle against death and that the death instinct is the dominant biological instinct. Many behaviour pat-

terns are derived from the death instinct – sadism and masochism for example, as well as so many activities hostile to the survival of the individual. The Greek word for death – thanatos – was introduced into the psychoanalytic literature by Paul Federn. The concept of the death instinct has been coolly received by most psychoanalysts, with the exception of followers of Melanie Klein. It is, perhaps, not very comforting for a therapist to believe that the death instinct is the most powerful human instinct.
SEE ALSO Freud and Instinct.

Defence mechanisms

The defence mechanisms are psychological devices to protect the being (ego (q.v.)) from conscious awareness of unacceptable instinctual (id (q.v.)) impulses and to maintain harmony with conscience (superego (q.v.)) and external reality. Freud postulated stages of psychological development during the child's first seven years of life. In each of these, specific interactions with the environment shaped the personality. At each stage of psychological development associated instinctual drives evoke characteristic defences. For example, introjection, denial and projection are defences associated with the oral phase of incorporation, whereas 'reaction formations', e.g. shame and disgust, develop in relation to anal impulses and pleasures. In this way Freud conceptualized the genesis of ego defence mechanisms. They may be classified developmentally, that is in terms of the psychological phase in which they arise; or on the basis of the psychopathology with which they are commonly asociated – e.g. obsessional defences would include denial, distortion and displacement – or whether simple (i.e. basic) or complex (i.e. a combination of simple mechanisms).
Repression (q.v.) retains the central position amongst defence mechanisms. It results in 'not being able to remember' and is particularly prominent in the inhibition of unacceptable sexual impulses.
In sublimation (q.v.) repression is operative, and energy originally invested in a sexual aim is deflected into another, non-sexual, socially acceptable channel.
Displacement (q.v.) refers to the shifting of feeling or drive from one idea or object to another that it resembles in some respect. So, for example, in the obsessional neurotic a fear of knives may be a displacement of aggressive feelings on to a potentially dangerous instrument.
Isolation (q.v.), as a defence mechanism, refers to the separation of an idea, which is remembered, from the emotion which accompanied it, which is repressed.
In rationalization (q.v.) the subject gives explanations (which may or may not be valid) to hide from himself and others the actual motives for his behaviour. The defence of intellectualization (q.v.) is closely related and refers to the excessive use of intellectual arguments to avoid the admission of emotional motivation.
Denial (q.v.) is widely used. It may operate only against an emotion associated with a particular event, or there may be massive denial of the experience itself, or its memory.
In projection (q.v.) the individual attributes his own feelings and wishes to another because his personality (ego) is too weak to assume the painful responsibility for them.
In regression (q.v.) the ego attempts to return to an earlier developmental state when pleasure was assured, in order to avoid the tension and conflict evoked at the present level of development.
Withdrawal (q.v.) is preliminary to defence. Here tension or conflict producing situations are avoided by withdrawing from the sources of anxiety instead of erecting defences against them.
In introjection (q.v.) the person turns in upon himself feelings that he has toward other people but that he cannot comfortably express to them. For example, introjection of a hate feeling leads, according to the theory, to depression.
Compensation (q.v.) is the mechanism used to combat a real or imagined inferiority; dissociation (q.v.) typical of hysterical reactions, involves the splitting off of emotionally intolerable conflicts from action which may, by the mechanism of symbolization (q.v.), be represented in dreams or in physical disorder which represent, in symbolic form, the conflict of the subject.

Degrees of freedom

This is a term used in statistical analysis of therapeutic trials, e.g. student's 't' test (q.v.) or chi-square test (q.v.). The 'degrees of freedom' is the number of values which *independently* contribute and that cannot be derived from other observed figures. For example, if in a therapeutic trial we are told that 228 improved, 27 were the same, 24 became worse out of 279 treated there are three degrees of freedom in the series for the fourth figure can be obtained by simple addition or subtraction.

Déjà vu

One of a variety of paramnesias (q.v.) or perversions of memory. A spurious sense of familiarity. A compelling feeling of foreknowledge of the events about to take place accompanied by the strange feeling that the sequence has happened before. The sensation is unlike memories evoked by re-entering a situation which has in fact been previously experienced. The feeling is more compelling, there is a slight sense of anxiety if only in wondering how so powerful an echo could be evoked from circumstances which certainty maintains are novel.
This and other paramnesias are features as the aura of a psychomotor seizure which may lead to a major convulsion. But the sensation may be the only evidence of the seizure.
Patients with phobic anxiety accompanied by depersonalization may also complain of these experiences among others which may be referred to temporal lobe dysfunction. The differential diagnosis rests largely upon the EEG findings, the absence of other seizure phenomena, and the absence of a likely aetiological factor for an epileptic disorder.
Patients with schizophrenia (q.v.) may express delusional ideas about the nature of time and their sense of foreknowledge of events. The quality of these experiences is quite different and they tend to be maintained with great persistence rather than abandoned at the least reassurance.
SEE ALSO Disorientation, Orientation and Uncinate fits.

Deliberate disability
SEE Malingering.

Delinquency

Delinquency is the term used to describe misdemeanour in children and young persons. The extent of delinquency differs within different countries and communities but the present situation in the United Kingdom may be taken as typical of many industrially developed countries.
About one boy in every five is convicted of some offence between the ages of 10 and 21 years. Delinquency is very much less common amongst girls. The earlier a boy is convicted of an offence the more likely he is to be charged again, so that about half the boys who are first convicted under the age of 14 are charged at least once more. On the other hand, persistent recidivism (q.v.) is unusual, and only about one sixth of boys convicted before the age of 21 are likely to be reconvicted after that age. There is some conflict of evidence whether the recent increase in the number of offenders represents a real increase in crime. There is probably a true increase but not as great as the figures would suggest.
Most (perhaps about nine tenths) of juvenile offences consist of offences against property: larceny, breaking and entering, etc. A small but significant proportion of young offenders commit violent and dangerous crimes.
It is possible to predict with some degree of accuracy whether a young child is likely to become delinquent. Children of low social class, from large families, with an inadequate home background are at risk. The son of a psychopathic or criminal father has a greatly increased chance of being convicted, and long-term studies have shown this effect to be transmitted (probably socially) through at least three generations. A broken home may have importance by virtue of the separation experience involved, but probably a combination of adverse social factors is involved. Low intelligence is not particularly closely associated with delinquency, but poor educational attainment (especially backwardness in reading) puts the child at greater risk. Some work has suggested

that the child of stocky build is constitutionally more disposed than the lean and angular, and various studies of adolescent personality suggest that it is the impulsive extrovert who is most likely to be convicted. A high neighbourhood rate of delinquency is important and there is some work to show that even within areas of high delinquency certain schools have better records than others.
Most classification of delinquency points to the difference between the unsocialized aggressive child who offends alone and may show many neurotic traits, and the socialized delinquent who offends with other children and in general is well integrated into a section of society whose standards differ from those more generally accepted. In practice, this distinction is not as easy to make as it sounds.
The treatment of delinquency is more a judicial than a medical matter, but the doctor may be asked to provide a report on the relevance of any associated psychiatric disorder or physical defect to the commission of an offence.
Change in legislation in several countries in recent years has led to a more enlightened approach to court procedure and subsequent care.
Whatever administrative alterations occur, the role of the medical practitioner is likely to remain largely in the area of counselling parents of pre-delinquent children and coping with the reactive neurotic illnesses occurring in the parents when prevention has failed. Counselling should involve emphasis on the importance of consistency in parental management with the maintenance of an accepting warm attitude to the child. Parental rejection and inconsistency are the family factors most likely to be associated with later conviction.
SEE ALSO Child psychiatry and Anti-social behaviour and Community homes.

Delirious mania
(Synonyms: Bell's mania, typhomania, hypermania)

An intense form of mania (q.v.) with partial or complete disorientation as the rule.

Delirium

Delirium is an organic disorder of brain function which consists of the wide range of states between mild disorientation and subtle intellectual changes through marked loss of intellectual function, fearful misgivings, and frantic restlessness to the unresponsive edge of the coma vigil.
These mental changes may be precipitated by a wide variety of severe debilitating conditions (hypoxia, heart disease, uraemia, diabetic ketosis), by salicylates, hypnotics, alcohol and exogenous poisons.
Delirium is more common in response to infection in children than adults.
The earliest phase is a difficulty in maintaining attention, changes best seen towards the evening. Emotional lability, restlessness and failure to grasp and maintain knowledge of events are apparent.
Disorientation (q.v.) in time and in place (especially when the patient has been moved from one situation to another), perceptual illusions, anxiety and overactivity ensue. Problems of management are exacerbated at night since sleep rhythm is usually impaired, information is unclear, the opportunities for illusion rife, and metabolic changes may exacerbate the underlying condition. The previous personality of the patient will to some extent influence the content of the psychosis and the amount of agitation it causes.
Physical examination may reveal coarse tremors and myoclonus. The normal EEG rhythm becomes slowed to some extent in parallel with the degree of mental disturbance, but remains bilaterally synchronous without focal abnormalities.
The management of delirium is the management of the underlying disorder. Depending on the underlying disorder, chlorpromazine may be used with caution to control the patient's restlessness.
SEE ALSO Acute confusional states, Clouding of consciousness.

Delirium tremens

A transient organic psychosis which occurs in people who are physically dependent on alcohol. This usually occurs after a long drinking bout and may be precipitated by abstinence, though this is not essential; it can be also set off by severe infections.

It is uncommon in patients below the age of 30. It may precede the onset of Korsakoff's psychosis (q.v.). Fits may occur in the prodromal period which is usually one of anorexia, restlessness and apprehension. This is followed by wakefulness and nightmares, after which the patient develops a state of true delirium with overactivity, disorientation in time and place and incoherence of speech and behaviour. The prevailing mood is one of terror, with loosely held delusions, frightening hallucinations often of a visual nature involving insects and small creatures. Coarse tremor of lips, tongue, face and upper limbs occurs and there may be pyrexia. Though delirium tremens is self-limiting, appropriate medical treatment includes vitamin saturation, fluid replacement, antibiotics if infection, e.g. pneumonia, is present. Tranquillizers with a pharmacological cross tolerance to alcohol such as the benzodiazepines or chlormethiazole, should be used to control restlessness and insomnia.
SEE ALSO Alcoholism.

Delta rhythm
SEE EEG.

Delusions

Delusions are false beliefs, which are unaffected by a reasonable demonstration of their untruth or improbability and are out of keeping with the cultural and educational background of the subject. These qualifications are necessary because not all false beliefs are delusions. They may be mistakes or errors of information which can be corrected by demonstration or persuasion. To determine whether they are delusions such beliefs must be assessed against the cultural background of the subject.
Delusions vary in content, duration and intensity from one individual to another and in the same individual at different times. Content often reflects the patient's mood. Thus a depressed patient may show delusions of unworthiness and guilt and of nihilism (q.v.). An elated mood may be reflected in grandiose delusions. Likewise fear, suspicion or jealousy may be shown by delusions of persecution or infidelity. There is sometimes a considerable disparity between the content of the delusion and the mood displayed, as when the end of the world is cheerfully assured or a personal disaster related with indifference. The intensity or degree of conviction with which a delusion is held can vary from indifference to anger and indignation, and this will affect the patient's behaviour in response to the delusion. As conviction about a false belief lessens, the patient may gain 'insight', i.e. the realization that the belief has been incorrect, and there may be a stage of partial or fluctuating insight. As to duration, delusions can be fleeting; very characteristically in mania (q.v.) where events in immediate experience may touch them off. In schizophrenia (q.v.), particularly of paranoid (q.v.) type, they more often persist.
The multiple delusions of an individual patient may have no relation to one another (unsystematized) or may closely cohere (systematized). In systematized delusions the connection may be reasonable and logical if the original assumption is granted, e.g. if a patient believes his thoughts are being read he may come to believe that a piece of medical apparatus is the instrument by which this is accomplished.

Dementia
(Synonyms: Organic dementia; chronic brain syndrome)

A global deterioration of mental functioning is implied, intellectual, emotional and volitional, but the first of these is the essential feature. The onset, except after a gross trauma, is insidious, and the course usually but not necessarily progressive and irreversible. The central symptom-triad consists of intellectual deterioration, defective memory for recent events and disorientation in time and place, which persists in the absence of clouding of consciousness. The loss of judgement and disinhibition (due to release of control) may result in outbursts of temper, sexual indiscretions and other socially unacceptable acts. Unpleasing traits of personality tend to be caricatured. The family may suffer materially and morally. Delusions of being robbed, poisoned or maltreated are common and may cause the patient to retaliate. In the earlier stages systematized

paranoid illnesses or sustained depressive psychoses may occur, accompanied by suicide or suicidal attempts. The affect which at first is anxious, irritable or labile, becomes shallow and fatuous, and emotional responses are blunted. Eventually, if the process cannot be halted, simple activities become disorganized, speech incoherent, habits deteriorated and existence vegetative.
Among the commoner causes of dementia in young adults are head injury and encephalitis; in middle age, cerebral tumour, syphilis, myxoedema, alcoholism, pernicious anaemia, or one of the pre-senile dementias (q.v.); and in old age senile degenerative or cerebro-vascular disease, tumour or subdural haematoma. Normal pressure hydrocephalus should also be considered.

Dementia infantilis

A condition with an onset usually in the first five years of life characterized by severe speech disturbance, restlessness and anxiety, and rapid deterioration within months to a state of dementia. It is probably not a clinical entity but one presentation of a whole range of degenerative cerebral disorders.

Dementia praecox
SEE Schizophrenia.

Denial

One of the defence mechanisms, denial is an unconscious process whereby painful thoughts and feelings are repressed. Thus in denial of illness, the acknowledgement of a serious illness and its possible consequences are avoided, with the advantages such a position entails. Elation may be the result of denial of that mental pain we call depression; in the Capgras syndrome, or in nihilistic delusions, denial is an important psychopathological mechanism. In the non-technical sense of the word, denial is a universal and normal conscious activity.

Denver system

In 1960 a meeting of fourteen experts in human cytogenetics in Denver, Colorado, devised a standard system of nomenclature for the human chromosomes. They numbered the autosomes in sequence according to length, the longest No.1, and the shortest No.22. The sex chromosomes X and Y were not numbered. In addition to numbering the autosomes, the chromosomes were grouped (designated A to G) according to the position of the centromere (the constriction at which the spindle is attached during cell division).

Dependence (drug dependence)
SEE Addiction.

Depersonalization syndrome

Feelings of unreality related to the self (depersonalization) or to the world around (derealization); whereas the former may occur alone, derealization is almost always associated with feelings of depersonalization. The onset is often sudden with associated feelings of faintness and fear of impending disaster (or insanity). Sometimes the subject says he feels mechanical, like an automaton; others describe the feeling of being shut off by a glass screen. In some phobic patients hyperventilation appears to act as an intermediate mechanism, while the relationship to migraine and non-specific cerebral dysrhythmia has also been noted. Depersonalization occurs in obsessional subjects with phobic anxiety states and in depressive reactions; in young schizophrenic subjects depersonalization is often associated with derealization and passivity feelings. In temporal lobe epilepsy it is associated with déjà vu phenomena (q.v.). In subjects taking LSD (q.v.) depersonalization is usually associated with visual perceptual and body image changes. The treatment is that of the underlying syndrome, i.e. depression or schizophrenia; some phobic subjects with depersonalization do well with phenelzine 15 mg. t.d.s. and chlordiazepoxide 10 mg. t.d.s.

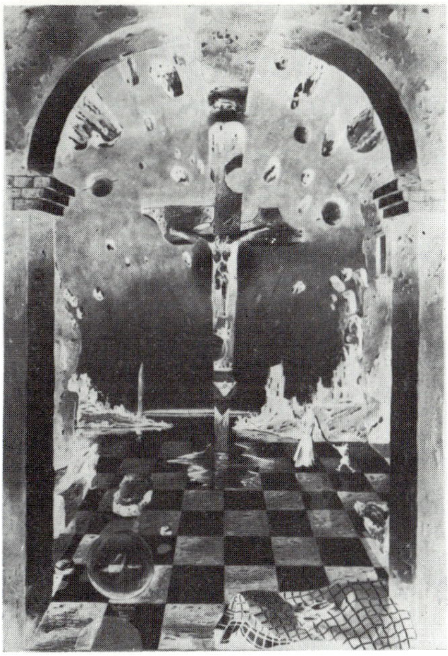

Depression

This word is, unfortunately, used in at least three different senses to describe a mood, to describe a syndrome, and to describe an illness. As a mood, depression is part of universal human experience, usually developing in response to the frustrations and disappointments of life but sometimes 'coming out of the blue' for no apparent reason. The syndrome of depression consists of a depressive mood together with some or all of a number of other symptoms – insomnia, weight loss, inability to concentrate, suicidal ideation, and so on. The illness depression involves the presence of this syndrome and also implies that the state is not transitory and that it is associated with significant functional impairment – the patient is unable to work or is only able to do so with reduced efficiency, or has lost his capacity for enjoyment.

Depressive illness is common and must rank close behind coronary artery disease, hypertension and chronic bronchitis as one of the major causes of serious morbidity. (Its major complication, suicide, also ranks high in mortality tables with between 5000 and 6000 deaths per year.) Depressive psychoses account for 35 to 40% of all mental hospital admissions in Great Britain. Including in-patients and out-patients, the incidence of new episodes of depression is about 500 per 100,000 population per year. This implies that in an average general practice of 3000 patients there would be at least fifteen patients with new episodes of depression every year – probably many more if mild cases not referred for a psychiatric opinion are included.

Depressions vary widely in their symptomatology and in their course and response to treatment, and although numerous attempts have been made to classify them none of the many suggested schemata has won wide acceptance. It has often been claimed that there are two distinct types of depression, variously known as psychotic or endogenous depression (which includes the depressive phase of manic-depressive illness) and neurotic or reactive depression. The evidence for this dichotomy is tenuous but it is widely used, if only for lack of anything better.

Endogenous depressions are subdivided into unipolar (recurrent depression) and bipolar (manic-depressive) types which have distinctive genetic and sex differences. Endogenous depressive illness often develops without apparent cause, though they may equally well develop in the aftermath of some obvious stress. They tend to deepen rapidly and the patient's mood varies little from day to day. It may, however, show a distinct diurnal variation, being at its worst in the early morning and improving steadily as the day progresses. Disturbances of sleep, appetite, and weight are usually prominent. The insomnia is worse in the second half of the night and typically the patient has no difficulty getting to sleep but wakes after three or four hours and lies awake thereafter. Loss of appetite is often profound and accompanied by a weight loss of 10 lb. or more, by constipation, amenorrhoea, and by loss of libido. Many patients show a characteristic psychomotor retardation; their speech and bodily movements are slowed down and restricted in scope and often all spontaneous speech is lost. Other patients are apprehensive and agitated, pacing aimlessly up and down and asking the same questions again and again. The depression of mood is often profound and accompanied by a complete loss of interest in work and normal pastimes. The patient stops reading because he cannot concentrate enough to take in what he reads, and stops watching television because it no longer interests him. Almost always he is emphatic that there is no enjoyment left in life, and this conviction, allied with an inability to believe that there is any possibility of recovery, leads almost inevitably to thoughts of suicide. To make matters worse he is often tormented with guilt and self-reproach, blaming himself for peccadilloes committed long ago or for his moral weakness in allowing himself to lapse into inactivity. Sometimes these guilt feelings become delusional in intensity and may be accompanied by hallucinatory voices accusing him of further crimes.

The typical clinical picture of neurotic or reactive depression is less well defined and characterized more by the absence of typical psychotic features than by positive features of its own. The depression either begins after some crucial loss or disappointment, like being passed over for promotion or the break up of an engagement, or, perhaps more commonly, develops in a setting of chronic frustration and dissatisfaction. Often the onset is insidious and there is considerable fluctuation from day to day with occasional 'good days' of near normality interspersed amongst periods of gloom. Weeping may be prominent and often the patient is anxious, tense and irritable to such an extent that these symptoms may overshadow the depression. Insomnia and loss of appetite may be complained of, but a more detailed enquiry often establishes that the patient is gaining rather than losing weight and that, although she may well have difficulty getting off to sleep and sleeps less soundly than usual, she eventually oversleeps and then wakes still feeling tired. Self-pity is usually more prominent than guilt and eventual admission to hospital is often preceded by a suicidal attempt which the patient has no difficulty in surviving.

Psychotic depressions tend to occur in people who are energetic and extroverted and who, except for a variable number of obsessional features, do not have obvious neurotic traits. They often have a history of previous episodes of depression or mania and their illnesses clear up completely with treatment, or even without it. Neurotic depressions, on the other hand,

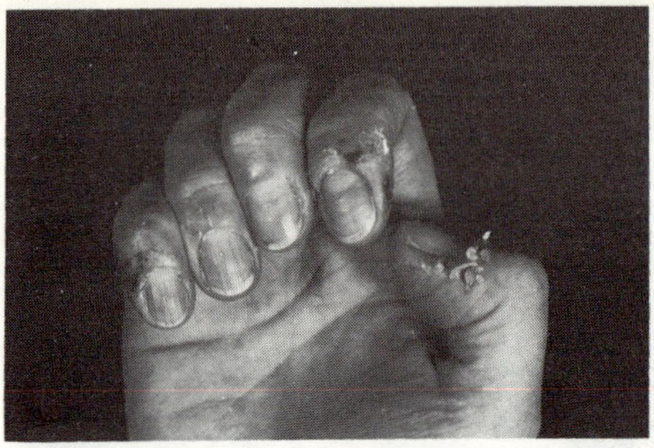

are typically encountered in people with lifelong neurotic traits of one sort or another and, although they are usually not so severe as psychotic illnesses, they often last longer and recover incompletely.

These are the two classical stereotypes, but in fact few patients fit neatly into one or other of these pigeon-holes. Psychotic and neurotic features co-exist in all manner of combinations and patients exhibiting a mixture of both are probably more common than pure forms of either kind. None the less the stereotypes are useful abstractions, and the nearer the symptomatology of an individual patient is to the psychotic stereotype the more likely is that patient to respond to ECT or tricyclic drugs. Given such a situation, the most appropriate solution is probably to regard depressions as a continuum with the typical psychotic stereotype at one pole, the neurotic stereotype at the other and the majority of patients ranged in between.

There are other depressive syndromes, however, which are not adequately portrayed by this means. Involutional melancholia (q.v.) must be mentioned here, if only to be dismissed. This condition used to be regarded as a distinct entity, on the grounds that its poor prognosis, its obsessional pre-morbid personality and its clinical picture of agitation, depersonalization and hypochondriasis distinguished it from manic-depressive illness. In fact, there is no genetic evidence for its being a distinct condition, its response to treatment is the same as that of other psychotic depressions and an obsessional pre-morbid personality is common to the majority of depressions, whatever their symptomatology.

Depressions as a whole are twice as common in women as in men, but this female preponderance is largely due to the high frequency of relatively mild neurotic depressions in women between the ages of 25 and 45; after the age of 60 there is little difference between the two sexes. Neurotic depressions predominate in young adults and show a strong female preponderance. The more severe psychotic depressions become increasingly common in middle age and show a less-marked sex difference. Parkinsonism and incipient cerebral arteriosclerosis (q.v.) in particular are often accompanied by depression, and there is some evidence that the incidence of occult neoplasms is higher than chance expectation in patients becoming depressed for the first time after middle age. Whatever the eventual explanation of these relationships they emphasize the necessity for a meticulous physical examination of all elderly depressives. Although these are the classical presentations of moderate and severe depressions, it is important to appreciate that many anxiety states overlie and obscure depressive illnesses. Moreover many present with somatic symptoms (see Depressive equivalents) and may tempt a diagnosis of neurasthenia (q.v.). Careful history taking reveals at least some depressive symptoms. Depression may also present as alcoholism, particularly dipsomania (q.v.).

The biochemistry of depression has attracted increasing attention in recent years, though most research has been concentrated on the relatively well-defined psychotic or manic depressive depressions. The clinical observation that endocrine disturbances of various kinds are often associated with depression led to a search for hormonal abnormalities and it is now established that most severe depressions are accompanied by elevated serum cortisol levels which revert to normal as the depression recovers. What is uncertain is whether this increased cortisol production is aetiologically important or whether it is simply a non-specific response to emotional arousal: probably the latter, for typical endogenous depressions may still occur after adrenalectomy and the therapeutic administration of steroids is more often associated with euphoria than with depression.

More likely to lead to real advances in understanding are reports of abnormalities of cerebral amine metabolism in depression. There is evidence that severe depression is accompanied by a depletion of local amine concentrations in the hypothalamus and brain stem and there are many indications that this may be directly or indirectly responsible for the mood change. The Rauwolfia alkaloid reserpine causes a similar depletion of brain stem amines and is notorious for its liability to precipitate depression; conversely both groups of antidepressant drugs, the tricyclic group, the monoamine oxidase inhibitors, cocaine, amphetamines and ECT, all have the effect of increasing these local amine concentrations. Most investigations have shown decreased concentrations of either 5-hydroxyindole or catecholamine metabolites in the CSF of depressed patients. It is still unclear which group of amines, the catecholamines (noradrenaline and dopamine) or the indoleamines (5-hydroxytryptamine), is the more important and research is hampered by a lack of any experimental animal prone to depression and by the anatomical and moral inaccessibility of the human brain stem, but it does seem that we are at last approaching some understanding of the chemical basis of mood. There are also reports that endogenous depressions (and also manic illnesses) are accompanied by abnormally high intracellular sodium levels which revert to normal on recovery. The effectiveness of lithium salts in the treatment of manic depressive illness suggests that these electrolyte disturbances may also be aetiologically important, rather than simply a secondary consequence of increased mineralocorticoid activity.

One may seek to 'understand' or 'explain' depression in psychological terms just as one may seek to explain it in physicochemical terms. Indeed, the two approaches are complementary. The most widely accepted psychological explanation is the classical Freudian view that depression is the result of a turning inwards upon the self of aggressive impulses previously directed externally. Anyone familiar with the clinical manifestations of depression can hardly fail to be struck by its close associations with hostility and there is some epidemiological evidence to support the view that depression and outwardly directed aggressive behaviour are alternatives to one another. However, some psychotherapists now see the aggressive feelings of depressives merely as a secondary reaction to the depression and regard a loss of self-esteem as the crucial factor precipitating the mood change.

The treatment of depressions, particularly in general practice, has been transformed by the introduction of effective anti-depressant drugs. The most important of these are the tricyclic group (q.v.), of which imipramine and amitriptyline are the most widely used. It is characteristic of all these drugs not to exert their anti-depressant effect until they have been taken regularly in adequate dosage for at least two weeks. In consequence they must be taken for at least three, and preferably four, weeks before it can be decided whether or not the patient is responding. They also have prominent atropine-like actions (causing dryness of the mouth, constipation, increased sweating, etc.) which are dosage dependent. To minimize these side effects it is customary to start with a small dose (25 mg. t.d.s.) of either imipramine or amitriptyline, to double this after a week and sometimes to increase it further to 200 mg./day if the depression is not responding and side effects are not troublesome. When prescribing any of these drugs it is important to explain to the patient that he will probably not feel better until he has been taking the tablets for some time and that the side effects he may experience will get less troublesome as time goes on.

These tricyclic drugs are considerably more effective in psychotic than in neurotic depressions, but even in the latter they often prove beneficial and they should probably be used as the drug of first choice for both. The differences between one member of the group and another are small, although amitriptyline may be somewhat more effective than imipramine, particularly in agitated depressions. Because depression is so frequently accompanied by anxiety it is often helpful to prescribe chlordiazaepoxide 10 mg. t.d.s. or diazepam 5 mg. t.d.s. as well until the depression begins to respond, but if agitation is severe a phenothiazine (e.g. thioridazine 100 mg. t.d.s.) is preferable. Once the depression has responded the tricyclic drug should be continued in all bar the milder cases for at least six months and then cautiously tailed off. In patients who suffer frequent recurrences of depression attempts at prevention can be made with continuous tricyclic medication (unipolar type) or with lithium carbonate (unipolar or bipolar types).

The status of the other group of anti-depressants, the MAO inhibitors, is much more equivocal. Several well-controlled trials have demonstrated that they are of little value, but others have suggested that they are just as effective as the tricyclic group. In so far as there is a consensus of opinion it is that they are most likely to be effective in neurotic depressions, particularly in those with prominent phobic anxiety. Like the tricyclic drugs their anti-depressant effect only becomes apparent after a lag of ten to fourteen days. In all other respects, though, they are very different. Their side effects, instead of being common but trivial, like those of imipramine and amitriptyline, are rare, but potentially serious. By blocking the normal degradation of ingested amines they create a situation in which amine-containing foods, like cheese and yeast extracts, may produce violent headaches and dangerous hypertensive crises and in consequence these foods must be rigorously avoided while the drug is being administered. Similarly, MAO inhibitors interfere with the breakdown of drugs containing amine groups, which means that they cannot be given to asthmatics as both adrenaline and isoprenaline are amines. The effect of other drugs, especially alcohol and the barbiturates, may be potentiated, and occasionally dangerous reactions may occur with morphine and pethidine. The hydrazine type of monoamine oxidase inhibitor may cause a severe toxic hepatitis.

Partly because of these side effects, and partly because the evidence for their efficacy is so equivocal, the MAO inhibitors are much less widely used than the tricyclic group, but they probably ought to have a limited role in the treatment of neurotic depressions that have failed to respond to a tricyclic drug. The most widely used members of the group are isocarboxazid, phenelzine and tranylcypromine. The latter is probably more effective but is rather more liable to cause hypertensive headaches.

Amphetamines and their derivatives are widely used for the treatment of relatively mild neurotic depressions, in spite of being regarded with disfavour by most psychiatrists. Their advocates maintain that the depressions encountered in general practice are very different from those seen by psychiatrists, and doubtless this is true, but the controlled trials conducted by the British College of General Practitioners also found amphetamine preparations to be no more effective than placebos and, in view of their addictive potential and their widespread abuse, they probably ought not to be prescribed, except perhaps in the elderly depressive where, used with care, they appear to be valuable.

The indications for ECT have shrunk considerably since the introduction of effective anti-depressant drugs, but it still has an important role in the treatment of patients with psychotic depressions which have failed to respond to an adequate course of a tricyclic drug, or in whom past experience has shown drugs to be ineffective. It is also still the most effective treatment for patients with severe retardation verging on stupor, or with widespread delusions. Occasionally patients with intractable depression are submitted to some form of modified leucotomy. This should only be done as a last resort, for the results are both irreversible and not totally predictable, but there is no doubt that it can be dramatically effective.

Regardless of the symptomatology of the illness it is always important to obtain as full an understanding as possible of the social and psychological situation in which it arose, for by tactful intervention it will often be possible to alter this situation in small but important ways. The patient's relatives or employer may be helped to understand her predicament better and to alter their own behaviour accordingly; social agencies may be able to ease the familiar problems of poor housing, loneliness, and debt, and the patient herself may be helped to take some crucial step, like separating from an alcoholic husband, which she had previously lacked the courage to carry through. A kindly and confident supportive role is nowhere more important than in the management of depression, for the patient has frequently lost all self-confidence and often fears that she is beyond treatment. At the very least the doctor's demeanour will determine whether the patient actually takes the tablets prescribed for her. Even in severe endogenous depressions which are often regarded as being inaccessible to, or not in need of, any form of psychotherapy it is well worth assuring the patient, confidently and repeatedly, that she is going to recover. She may not be able to believe this at the time, but to hear it is still a considerable comfort. Neurotic depressions are more likely to be accessible to, and in need of, interpretative psychotherapy, and sometimes dramatic improvements can be effected by this means. But on grounds of economy alone it is probably wise to confine oneself to drug treatment and general supportive measures initially and only to embark on more time-consuming therapies after it has been proved that simple remedies have failed. In patients with chronic depressions arising out of severe personality disorders neither drugs nor interpretative psychotherapy has much to offer, but a patiently maintained supportive role may still produce slow but definite changes as the patient gradually learns that the world is not universally hostile, and that this relationship at least is dependable and constant.

SEE ALSO Affective disorders.

Depression in childhood

Most unhappiness occurring in childhood is situational and temporary in its nature. Children vary in their readiness to suffer discouragement and show tearfulness as one of the characteristics of their temperament. The threat of the loss of a love object is a constant factor to be found in these negative moods. Children should not be regarded as suffering from 'depressive illness' if their mood is understandable in the circumstances and not handicapping in its severity.

Some children, however, show more profound degrees of withdrawal and depression in response to adverse circumstances, while others, particularly in adolescence, show endogenous mood swings similar to those occurring in adulthood. Some institutionalized infants deprived of adequate maternal care show a syndrome which has been called 'anaclitic depression' characterized by apathy, failure to thrive, developmental retardation and irritability. Such syndromes are socially preventable by the provision of substitute maternal care.

Older children may show mental states

characterized by feelings of boredom, irritability and lability of mood as part of an emotional disturbance characteristic of adolescence. In some, however, more serious endogenous depressive states occur, with loss of appetite and weight and sometimes suicidal thoughts. Inability to concentrate at school, with a falling off in school work, and lack of interest in social or peer contact are more common symptoms.

The use of anti-depressants should not be regarded as a substitute for an enquiry into the child's life stresses. However, increasing use is being made even in early adolescence of the tricyclic agents (q.v.), such as imipramine and amitriptyline, and of the monoamine oxidase inhibitors (q.v.).

Depression in the elderly

Depression is at least as common a reason for admission to hospital as dementia. The clinical picture resembles in the main that found in the younger age groups, but guilt and gross retardation are less common and hypochondriasis, agitation, obsessional symptoms and preoccupations with poverty more so.

Recurrent depressive illnesses which started in earlier life show certain differences from those beginning in the senium.

History and clinical aspects	First illness before senium	Onset in the senium
Family history of depression	Often found	No significant association
Current physical health	Average for age	Significant increase in physical ill health
Immediate response to treatment	Good	Good
Long term response	Good	Frequent relapses

Treatment of depression in the aged is with anti-depressant drugs of the tricyclic group, often starting with 10 mg. t.d.s. of imipramine or amitriptyline in order to avoid postural hypotension, ataxia, urinary retention and acute glaucoma. A failure to respond to an average dose of anti-depressants strengthens the indication for ECT, as does refusal to eat or drink, regressed and withdrawn behaviour, and evidence of severe suicidal risk. Elderly depressives can die of starvation, dehydration and the effects of decubitus if adequate treatment is too long delayed.

Depressive equivalents

Occasionally patients are seen with an insistent somatic complaint, most commonly chronic pain in the face or head, which does not correspond in character or distribution to any familiar syndrome, nor respond to measures directed at suspected local pathology, but is cured, sometimes dramatically, by a course of an anti-depressant drug or ECT. The existence of such patients has given rise to the concept of 'depressive equivalent'. In some ways it is an unfortunate term, because although these patients do not have classical depressive symptoms, like retardation and guilt, they do have other depressive symptoms if a proper history is taken. They are moderately depressed (though often they attribute their low spirits to the pain), have difficulty sleeping and concentrating, are lacking in energy, and have lost interest in their normal pastimes.

Depressive illness should always be considered in the differential diagnosis of atypical facial pain or intractable headache, but it is equally important to appreciate that if depressive symptoms are genuinely absent, anti-depressive measures will probably prove futile.

Deprivation, emotional

SEE Emotional deprivation.

Deprivation, sensory

May be produced by a variety of methods such as immersing the patient in a tank of water at body temperature. After 24–72 hours the subjects crave for stimulation, become abnormally restless, perceptual distortions and visual hallucinations may occur, and occasionally fleeting paranoid delusions. Paradoxically, schizophrenics appear to be more tolerant to sensory deprivation which may actually reduce the intensity of their hallucinations.

Derealization
SEE Unreality – feelings of.

Dereistic thinking

Thinking which is not directed towards reality situations. It is determined by affectively and instinctually set goals and characteristically disregards any contradictions with reality, logic or experience. Dereistic thinking occurs in fairy tales, daydreams, pseudologia phantastica, and a whole range of morbid psychiatric states. SEE ALSO Conceptual thinking, Schizophrenia and Thought, Thinking.

Derived activities

The tendency of repressed impulses to use any opportunity for indirect discharge gives rise to 'derived activities' or symptoms. The energy of the deflected impulse is displaced on to another with which it is associatively connected. Such substitute impulses and activities are known as derivatives; most neurotic symptoms are thus derivatives.

Dermatitis artefacta

The deliberate self-production of blisters or sores on the skin by a variety of means which may often elude detection. Dermatitis artefacta occurs in individuals seeking escape from an unpleasant situation or as a masochistic phenomenon akin to the self-mutilation of the adolescent girl.
The diagnosis is usually suggested by the nature and site of the lesions (i.e. accessibility to method of damage), their recurrent nature and the permeability of the patient. However, occasional cases of the disorder may remain undiagnosed for long periods.

Descriptive psychiatry

A system of psychiatry based on a detailed study of symptoms and phenomenology; by contrast dynamic psychiatry is concerned with those unconscious drives and conflicts which are presumed to determine behaviour. The term 'descriptive psychiatry' is sometimes used in a reductionist, derogatory way. The great era of descriptive psychiatry was the latter half of the nineteenth century. Emil Kraepelin (q.v.) is probably the best known protagonist of descriptive psychiatry; his text-book exerted a great influence over generations of psychiatrists.

Desensitization
SEE Systematic desensitization.

Detention centres

Under English legislation an offender aged 14–21 can be sentenced to stay in a detention centre for three or six months. There are junior centres for boys aged 14–17 and senior centres for the older ones. The regime in these centres was originally designed along military lines and officially described as 'brisk and firm'. There are no detention centres for girls.

Diabetes mellitus

Emotional stress often aggravates diabetes and temporarily increases insulin requirements. Indeed the emotional reactivity of children and adolescents may partly explain the difficulty in stabilizing young patients.
Diabetics may show psychological reactions to their illness varying from total denial to elaborate overconcern.

Dibenzazepine
SEE Tricyclic anti-depressants of which it represents an important group; subdivided into iminodibenzyl derivatives (q.v.) and iminostilbene derivatives (q.v.).

Dibenzobicyclo-octadiene derivatives

There are two members of this chemical group in clinical use: benzoctamine (q.v.) which is primarily sedative and anxiolytic, and maprotiline (q.v.) which is anti-depressant.

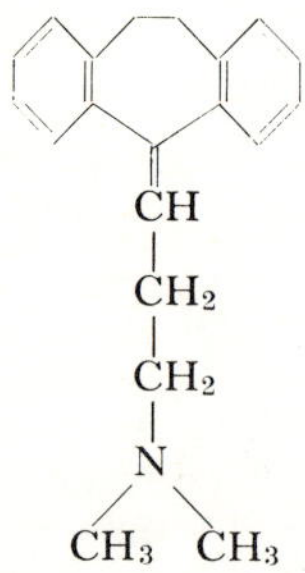

Amitriptyline

Dibenzocycloheptenes (including dibenzocycloheptadiene and dibenzocycloheptatriene) derivatives

Dibenzocycloheptadiene compounds are tricyclic anti-depressants. Amitriptyline (q.v.) is the prototype of the group. This drug is sedative and has the general properties of the tricyclic anti-depressant (q.v.) compounds in addition to the sedation. Nortriptyline (q.v.) is closely related to amitriptyline from which it is derived metabolically. It may act fractionally more quickly than its parent compound and has similar actions although it is claimed to have a lower incidence of side effects and to be less sedative. A closely related dibenzocycloheptatriene compound protriptyline (q.v.) is now in use which has some direct stimulant as well as anti-depressant properties.

Dibenzothiepine derivatives

A group of tricyclic antidepressants represented in clinical use by prothiadene.

Dibenzoxepine derivatives

One of the groups of tricyclic antidepressant compounds of which the sole representative used clinically at present is doxepin (q.v.).

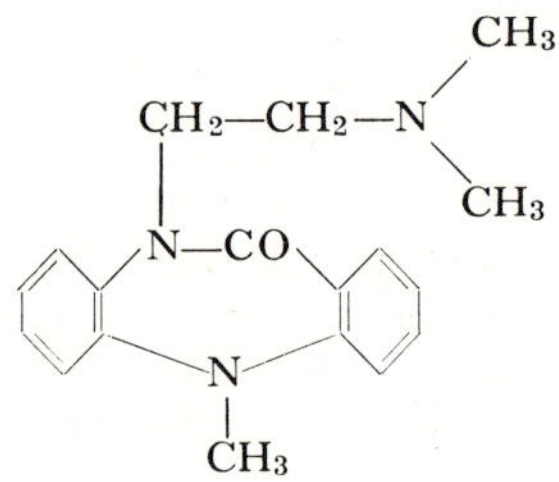

Dibenzepin

Dibenzodiazepine derivatives

One of the groups of tricyclic compounds with thymoleptic properties. The only clinically used member of this group is dibenzepin (q.v.).

Diencephalic autonomic seizures

A type of seizure in which the manifestations are autonomic – vasodilation, lachrymation, sweating, salivation, pupillary alteration, slowing of pulse rate and respiration, and hiccoughing.
SEE ALSO Epilepsy.

Diencephalon

The diencephalon is the most rostral part of the brain stem and is embedded between the cerebral hemispheres. Within the diencephalon lie *inter alia* the thalamus of each side with its related structure the medial and lateral geniculate bodies, the hypothalamus, the pineal body and related structures, the posterior pituitary; and the fibre tracts to and from the cerebral hemispheres.

Diffuse sclerosis (cerebral)
(Synonym: Schilder's disease)

A rapidly progressive demyelinating disease which affects large areas of the cerebral white matter. The signs depend on the sites of the lesions, but typically a homonymous hemianopia rapidly develops, with confusion and bewilderment. At times a fit ushers in the development of the condition. Space-occupying lesions must be excluded. The condition is usually progressive and ends fatally.

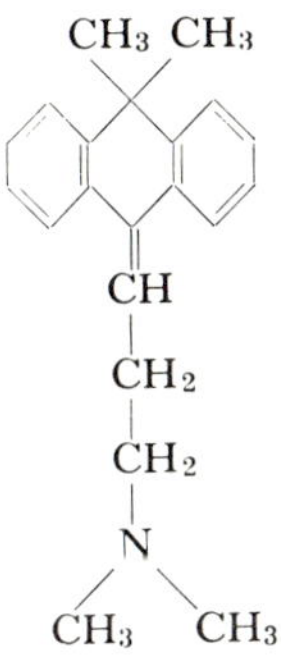

Melitracene is an example of a dihydroanthracene

Dihydroanthracenes

One of the groups of tricyclic compounds with thymoleptic properties. The only one which has been extensively studied is melitracene.
SEE appendix.

Diminished awareness
SEE Clouding of consciousness.

Diminished responsibility

Recent legislation in many countries (including the United Kingdom and most of Europe) embodies the principle of diminished responsibility for homicide where a mental defect substantially impairs responsibility. Thus, for example, the relevant portion of the English Act states: 'Where a person kills or is party to the killing of another, he shall not be convicted of murder if he was suffering from such abnormality of mind (whether arising from a condition of arrested or retarded development of mind or any inherent causes or induced by disease or injury) as substantially impaired his mental responsibility for his acts and omissions in doing or being a party to the killing.' The onus of proof for diminished responsibility rests (as with insanity) on the defence. If such diminution is proven then the accused is liable to be convicted of manslaughter (q.v.) instead of murder (q.v.).
This concept is much broader than the definitions of insanity laid down in the McNaughton Rules (q.v.) and gives the court greater flexibility for sentence and disposal of the unstable murderer. It has been clearly established that psychopathic disorder may substantially impair mental responsibility within the meaning of the Act.
SEE ALSO Criminal responsibility and Forensic psychiatry.

Diphenylbutylpiperidines

A recently introduced group of antipsychotic drugs of which the commercially available members are pimozide and fluspirilene (the latter drug also existing in long-acting form). It has been shown that they have a powerful selective inhibitory action on brain dopaminergic synapses. They are relatively low in autonomic side effects but produce extrapyramidal syndromes.
They are effective in the treatment of withdrawn schizophrenics.

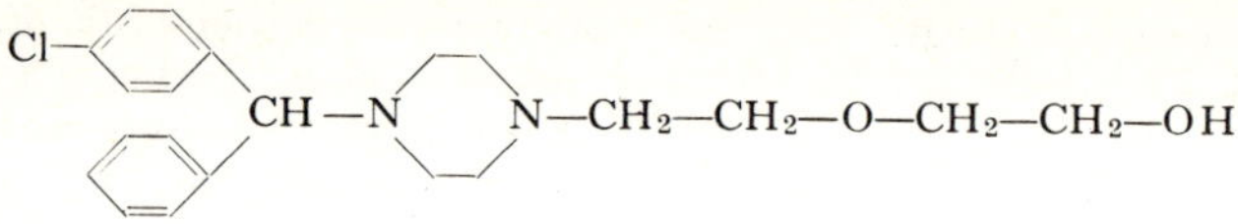

Diphenylmethanes

Diphenylmethane derivatives

The diphenylmethane derivatives are pharmacologically heterogeneous, showing *inter alia* clinical activity as anxiolytics, anti-Parkinsonism agents, and anti-histaminics.
Hydroxyzine benactyzine and captodiamine have had limited use as anxiolytics but have been superseded. Benztropine and orphenadine are widely used anti-Parkinsonism agents. Other compounds include the anti-histaminics diphenylhydramine and cyclizine of which the latter also counteracts motion sickness. Azacyclonal was thought to antagonize the psychotomimetic effects of lysergide, but trials in the treatment of schizophrenia were disappointing. Pipradol is closely related to azacyaclonal and is a central stimulant.

Dipsomania

True dipsomania is characterized by episodic or periodic excessive alcohol abuse between periods of relative abstention. It corresponds to Jellinek's (q.v.) 'epsilon alcoholism'. It is to be distinguished from 'mania à potu' (q.v.), where acute psychotic excitement follows ingestion of relatively small amounts of alcohol. Though rare, dipsomania is likely to be associated with quite severe personality disorders. It can occur in patients who drink to excess in periods of schizophrenic excitement though probably its clearest psychiatric association is with episodic mood disturbance – e.g. in recurrent depressive states or in the cycles of manic depressive psychosis (q.v.).
SEE ALSO Alcoholism.

Disablement Resettlement Officer

A specialist of the British Department of Employment and Productivity, responsible for placing both physically and mentally handicapped people in employment. Every large employer is legally obliged to take on a percentage of workers who are registered as disabled; at present this is 3%. However, there are never enough of these places and except at times of greatest prosperity, the Disablement Resettlement Officer tends to have an uphill task. One study showed, however, that schizophrenic men discharged from hospital who settled successfully in work generally found their jobs themselves. Rightly or wrongly, many patients feel that the 'green card' of the registered disabled person is more of a hindrance than a help with prospective employers.

Disorientation

Disorientation is a loss of bearings in terms of time, space or identity, and is recognized by the observation of behaviour and the responses to test questions. Orientation for time is checked by asking the day, date, month and year; for place, by asking about the patient's present whereabouts; for person by asking the patient's name, address, job, doctor's name etc. A failure to discriminate between right and left (as in Gerstmann's syndrome) is called right-left disorientation. Disorientation is found in all organic brain syndromes – due to arteriosclerosis, senile and presenile dementias, infections, intoxications, neoplasm, metabolic disturbance. It is, however, also met in acute psychoses – oneiroid or dreamlike states – where it is due to inattention; in the Ganser syndrome (q.v.) of approximate answers; and in other hysterical reactions.

Displacement

Displacement is a normal, conscious activity, whereby emotion is discharged onto a less powerful object for the security of the individual. The domestic cat or dog is familiar as the recipient of displaced violence toward society. In psychoanalytic theory, however, displacement is one of the unconscious defence mechanisms. Affect is displaced from one object to another, the two being linked by a chain of associations, and the affect attached to the original object too intense to be acceptable to consciousness.

Disseminated lupus erythematosis

A collagen disease occurring predominantly in young and middle-aged females. It presents in a variety of ways, including dermatitis ('butterfly rash'), lesions of mucous membranes, myopathy, arthritis, renal, cardiovascular, pleural or pulmonary lesions, and constitutional disturbances. A quarter of the patients show neurological or psychiatric change. The latter are usually those of a confusional psychosis. The diagnosis is suggested by an episodic history involving a number of systems, and is confirmed by a positive LE cell, fluorescent antibody or complement fixation test.
SEE ALSO Organic disease producing mental disorders.

Disseminated sclerosis
SEE Multiple sclerosis.

Dissociation

In mental as in physical functioning the nervous system exerts an integrative action which enables a multitude of separate processes to work harmoniously and smoothly in relation to one another, and to whatever demands the internal and external environment imposes on the organism. It is when a particular mental activity or group of activities becomes split off from this whole, losing its place in relationship to other psychological and physical functions, that we speak of dissociation. Thus, loss of memory, of sensory functions such as hearing or vision, of speech, or of muscular functions may occur, as may a dissociation between purely psychic activities, such as that between affect and reality. Many psychiatrists wrongly equate dissociation with hysteria. In fact dissociation is a normal mental process, and may be observed in the everyday examples of forgetting, or in the changes in awareness which occur during intense concentration. In psychiatric illness an accentuation of the process is seen, so that whole areas of mental and physical function may become split-off from consciousness, as in the fugue (q.v.) states or the functional paralyses. The dissociative phenomena are only symptomatic of some underlying disturbance and must not be given a diagnostic significance *per se*. It is an all too common error to assume that dissociation equals conversion hysteria (q.v.), a diagnosis which in any case is under increasingly critical scrutiny. In fact dissociation may occur in any psychiatric disturbance, as well as in those organic conditions leading to psychological disturbance.

Distortion

The dream work alters and distorts the latent content of the dream, so that sleep is maintained.

Diurnal variation

A pronounced diurnal variation in mood is a characteristic feature of endogenous or manic depressive depressions (q.v.), though it is only exhibited by a minority of patients. Typically the depression is at its worst in the morning and improves steadily as the day goes on. Other symptoms like retardation and difficulty in concentrating fluctuate in parallel with the mood change. Sometimes this deep depression only descends five or ten minutes after the patient wakes in the morning, and occasionally the rhythm is reversed and the depression is at its worst in the evening. Whatever the precise pattern it is important to establish that the variation is not simply a response to environmental changes, like the return of the patient's husband from work.

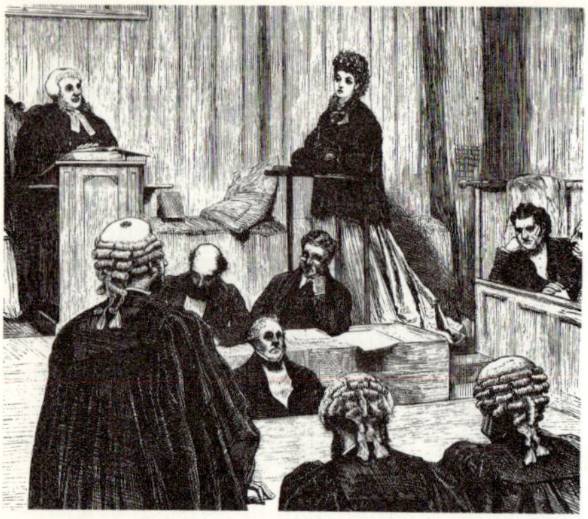

Divorce Court, 1870

Divorce

In Britain, under the Divorce Reform Act of 1969 there is only one ground for divorce – irretrievable breakdown of the marriage (q.v.). There are five proofs of such breakdown: (a) one party has committed adultery and the other finds it intolerable to continue the marriage; (b) the behaviour of one partner is so bad that the other cannot reasonably be expected to continue cohabitation; (c) desertion for two years; (d) separate living for two years and mutual consent for a decree; (e) separate living for five years.

There is no mention of insanity in this new Act, but it is clear that if the five years' separate living has been caused by insanity then this will be a valid ground. It will require court interpretation to determine what sort of behaviour will constitute the second ground, but serious mental disorder will no doubt be considered.

The views and laws relating to divorce differ markedly from one country to another and generalized statements are not possible.

SEE ALSO Nullity.

Dopamine

This compound is an important central transmitter in the brain in particular for the pathway leading from the substantia nigra to the corpus striatum. Degeneration of these cells is thought to be the lesion underlying Parkinsonism and the administration of levodopa, the aminoacid precursor of dopamine, improves many Parkinsonism patients. There is also some evidence that dopamine systems may be pathologically overactive in schizophrenia. The butyrophenones (q.v.) most active in schizophrenia are specific blockers of dopamine synapses. Antabuse, which exacerbates schizophrenic reactions, blocks the conversion of dopamine to noradrenaline and hence raises brain dopamine levels. Dopamine is metabolized by the enzyme anine oxidase, and catechol O-methyl transferase and monoamine oxidase inhibitors are known to exacerbate schizophrenic reactions.

SEE ALSO Monoamines and Catecholamines.

Double bind

First formulated by Gregory Bateson and his co-workers. This is a situation existing between two or more persons, in which inter-personal communication is seriously distorted. Repeated experience of the situation, together with a primary negative injunction, followed by a secondary injunction conflicting with the first, and no prospect of escape are all necessary conditions for the double bind situation. Usually there is a dominant but emotionally disturbed mother and a weak father; marital conflicts and hostility also provide the child with contradictory messages – to love, to be kind and gentle contrasting with the battles between mother and father. The double bind has been considered a significant aetiological factor in the development of schizophrenic illness. The inability to discriminate between mutually contradictory stimuli may result in serious disturbance in the experimental animal: the double bind has been regarded as an analogous situation in the human. However, it is a mechanism which may occur in a multitude of situations, even the psychologist himself must beware lest he find himself involved in a double bind situation with his patient – perhaps on the one hand exhorting the patient to mature, and to behave more responsibly and on the other hand fostering the patient's dependency for his (the psychiatrist's) narcissistic gratification.

Doubts

Obsessional doubts are part of the symptomatology of obsessive-compulsive neurosis. The questioning obtrudes on to consciousness and, even though they are regarded by the subject as unreasonable, cannot be banished. The subject may question whether he really put out his cigarette in the cinema or whether it may not be burning to the ground; whether he did really lock the back door, etc. Obsessional doubts are almost always associated with phobias (q.v.) and rituals (q.v.). Philosophical doubts (i.e. the persistent thought 'why am I?') are sometimes seen in young schizophrenics.

Down's syndrome

SEE Mongolism.

Dreams

Dreaming is associated with rapid eye movement (REM) or paradoxical sleep, which occurs four to five times a night, lasting about twenty minutes each period, and accounts for 20–25% of sleeping time. The EEG at this time is similar to that of a drowsy state and is made up of 4–10 c/sec. waves.

In contrast to orthodox sleep, patients when wakened from REM sleep more often state that they have been dreaming and the descriptions of these dreams are lengthier, more vivid and detailed. Associated with REM sleep is an increased brain temperature and blood flow, penile erection and the heart rate, respiration and blood pressure are subject to sharp and frequent fluctuations. It has been suggested that REM sleep is associated with protein synthesis in the brain and brain regeneration. Thus the proportion of REM sleep is increased in neonates, after head injury or drug overdose and is decreased in subnormality and old age.

It is obvious from the above that REM sleep is a time of considerable physiological activity and it is not surprising that there is associated mental activity though people recall only a fraction of their dreaming experience. The significance of the content of dreams has always been a matter of controversy, and nowadays

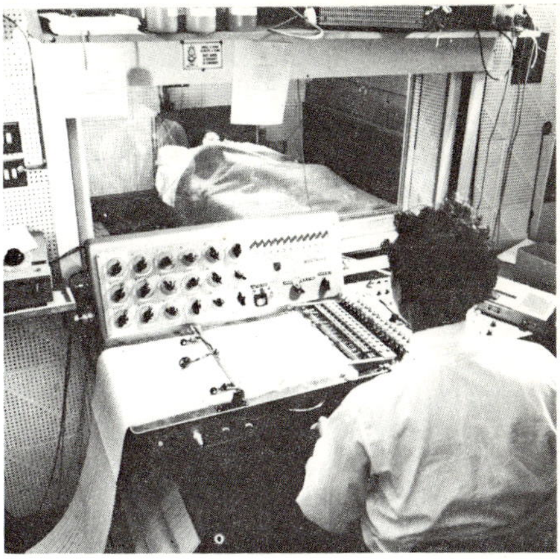

'Sleep Laboratory', Edinburgh University

can be expressed as extending from those who hold that dreams are a random selection of mental processes to those who think they all stem from material which has been repressed from conscious thought. This is largely a question of belief or otherwise in psychoanalytic theory. Scientific study has not confirmed an early suggestion that dream deprivation is of special psychiatric significance over and above its physiological importance (see sleep deprivation). Emotions can, however, influence dreams content, and states of anxiety, depression, etc. are reflected in anxious and depressive dreams. Similarly outside stimuli, such as noises or communications played on tape, can influence or be incorporated into the dream material, frequently disguised by symbols. These influences and their effect on dreaming are neither surprising nor altogether unexpected. In these respects they contrast strikingly with the more esoteric tenets of psychoanalytical dream theory and dream interpretation. While it is true that sexual emotions and experiences may determine and influence the content of the dream, the importance of the part they play is still in doubt. No theory of dream interpretation is free of valid criticism. Many can be safely rejected with frank disbelief. In recent times psychiatric thought has been substantially influenced by the analytical dream theories of Freud, Jung and Adler, which have attempted to utilize the dream both as a diagnostic tool and as an agent in therapy.

Hynotics such as barbiturates may initially result in apparently dreamless sleep, while others such as nitrazepan may provide vivid memories of the night's dreams. Dream deprivation in normal subjects eventually results in the occurrence of features common to the psychoses, e.g. hallucinatory experiences.

Drive

Motive is the most general term applied to a state which arouses and maintains an individual's behaviour in the direction of some end or goal. Drive is sometimes used synonymously with motive but more frequently is reserved for the primary drives, with a known physiological basis and shared by humans and animals, such as hunger, thirst, the sex drive and the drive to escape from noxious stimulation. These drives are instinctual in nature, universal and derive from some condition of physiological deficit or excess. The behaviour associated with a drive is directed towards the re-establishment of physiological stasis and usually culminates in consummatory behaviour, such as eating or copulation, concerned with an environmental goal object or incentive. The biological function of these primary drives is the physical preservation of the individual or species.
The expression, even of these primary drives, is greatly modified by learning. Other secondary or acquired motives are the products of learning and are of major importance in human motivation. Many of these are related to social aspects of behaviour and particularly to the preservation of the individual's social status. Others may be linked to a person's self-concept and the preservation of his self-respect. The psychologist, Maslow, proposed a hierarchy of human motivation with the animal drives at the bottom and self-actualization at the top. He suggests that any one level in this hierarchy can only become active when drives at the lower levels are satisfied.
Psychiatric disorders frequently involve abnormal variations in the intensity or expression of motivation.
SEE ALSO Instinct.

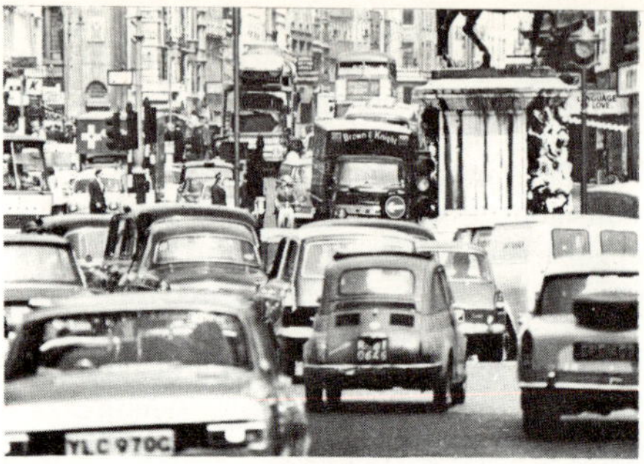

Driving

Skill and attention are essential for fault-free driving. Both are diminished by any form of sedative drug and it is an offence to drive in any sort of intoxicated state. With prescribed sedatives (barbiturates, tranquillizers, anti-depressants etc.) the patient should be warned that his driving skill may be impaired and that if this is so he must not drive. With regard to alcohol the British law has been strengthened recently in the Road Safety Act 1967 by stipulating that driving a vehicle with 80 mg./100 ml. of alcohol in the blood is an offence.
Until recently epileptics were debarred from holding a driving licence, but under new regulations an epileptic will be granted a licence if he has been fit free whilst awake for three years and is deemed unlikely to be a source of danger (any nocturnal fits in the past three years must not be a new phenomenon). The patient's GP will have to furnish a report, and it is recommended that before doing so consultant opinion should be sought. Driving heavy grade and public vehicles is not allowed.
Patients receiving in-patient treatment for mental disorder or suffering with severe abnormality are not entitled to apply for a driving licence. A licensing authority may revoke a licence in circumstances when disease or physical disability is likely to cause danger to the public.
The more serious and persistent motoring offenders are often persistent offenders in other areas. Some people may be specifically aggressive and violent in their cars, and the largest category of homicide offences in Britain is causing death by dangerous driving.

Drug addiction
SEE Addiction.

Drug dependence
SEE Addiction.

Drug-induced depressions

The administration of some drugs is known to be associated with a higher than chance incidence of serious depression and a similar relationship is suspected for others. The best known example is the Rauwolfia alkaloid-reserpine. When used in large doses as a tranquillizer in the 1950's as many as 30% of patients became depressed and several suicides were reported. Whether the smaller doses now widely used in the management of hypertension cause depressions is less well established, but it is widely believed that they do. For this reason preparations containing reserpine should not be given to patients with a history of depressive illness or continued in those who become depressed while receiving the drug.
Several other drugs are suspected of precipitating or causing depressions, including oral contraceptive preparations, alphamethyldopa, levodopa, phenobarbitone, and phenothiazines of the piperazine group when used in high dosage in the long term treatment of schizophrenia. For 'the pill' the evidence is quite strong and there is a suggestion that the risk is particularly high for preparations with a high progesterone content; for the others the evidence is mainly limited to clinical impressions. As with reserpine, it is probably advisable to avoid these drugs in patients with a history of depression and to stop them if a depression develops during their administration.
Finally, the acute psychotic reactions sometimes precipitated by steroids may be depressive in type, in spite of the fact that these drugs are normally associated with a mood of euphoria.

Durkheim, Emile (1858–1917)

Durkheim's monograph *Le Suicide* (1897) remains one of the most stimulating contributions to the subject. As a sociologist he regarded suicide as a social phenomenon, each society had a collective inclination to suicide, and the suicide rate was an indication of the integration of the individual with society. Thus large families and well integrated societies had low suicide rates. There were three types of suicide, the altruistic, the egoistic, and the anomic. The altruistic suicide was best exemplified by hara-kiri – self-killing for a cause or a belief. The egoistic suicide occurred when society's control over the individual was impaired; the individual behaved selfishly by killing himself – to escape from an unbearable situation. Lastly, anome was a state of normlessness, of inability to integrate in a society which was changing very rapidly. Very popular today, the concept of anomie is used to explain the alienation of youth from a society which is said to be cruel, heartless, devoted to pleasure and the exploitation of group by group. Sociological theories of suicide have not appealed to those who have to deal with suicidal individuals – the theories being based on outmoded and simplistic concepts of human psychology.

Dysarthria

Dysarthria is the term applied to difficulties in articulating words and, in contradistinction to aphasia (q.v.), is due to an imperfect motor or effector pathway – nervous or muscular. Cerebellar incoordination causes explosive speech or scanning in which syllables are unduly separated. Changes in the level of consciousness will also produce ataxia of speech. Thus alcohol, drugs and hypoglycaemia result in slurring. Increased muscle tone, for example, in motor neurone disease results in spastic slurring, while the rigidity of Parkinsonism results in slow, mumbled, monotonous reproduction. Muscle weakness due to myopathy or lower motor neurone destruction leads to difficulty with labials, dentals and gutturals.

Dyslalia

This is a defect of articulation occurring in childhood in the absence of abnormalities in the movement of tongue, lips or palate. The defect is primarily one of consonant substitution and consonant omission, especially the latter. For example, the child who says 'Ang oo wewy mu' for 'Thank you very much' is showing dyslalia.

The defect may arise as part of a general delay in intellectual development, as a persistent habit of faulty articulation, as an imitative phenomenon, or as a regressive pattern of behaviour in a disturbed child (baby talk being part of a wish to remain a baby). There is an association with other language defects including reading retardation.

Treatment depends on the underlying cause, but the advice of a speech therapist is always required where faulty articulation results in the child having difficulty making himself understood.

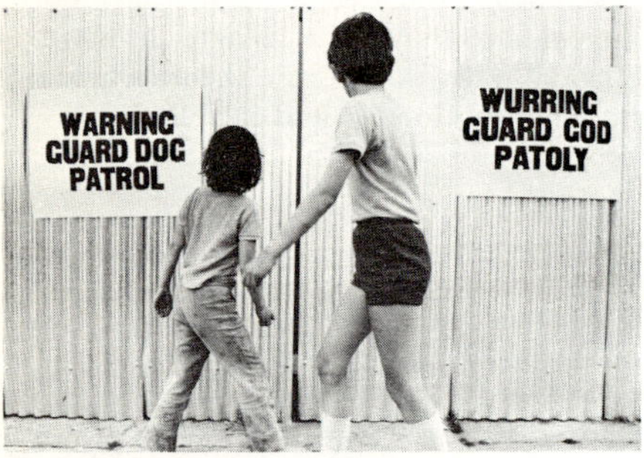

Dyslexia (word blindness)

Severe difficulty in reading occurs in about 5% of children of normal intelligence. There may be a family history of reading problems and delay in the acquisition of speech. The child may show clumsiness, poor right-left discrimination, reversal of letters, motor impersistence, and a tendency to write letters in mirror image fashion. Neither left handedness nor contralateral hand-eye dominance predispose to this condition as is often stated.

Although all these features do occur in the background of children with reading problems, only very rarely does any single child show more than a small number of them. Some authorities therefore question the existence of a single dyslexia syndrome. Other causes of severe reading difficulty include poor visual or auditory acuity, low intelligence, emotional disorder, and inadequate teaching.

The management of the disorder is primarily an educational and not a medical problem. Individual or small group tuition with an experienced teacher is often helpful. An important task is the prevention of secondary behaviour problems, especially antisocial disorder, arising out of the child's frustration.

Dysmenorrhoea

Cramping menstrual pain may be due to pelvic disease. Primary dysmenorrhoea is related in a complex way to progesterone secretion and can often be relieved by pre-menstrual progestogen administration. In any painful condition psychological attitudes influence a person's reaction to the pain. Thus women of vulnerable personality may overreact to their periods and any associated pain. Nevertheless surveys of normal populations fail to show a clear association between dysmenorrhoea and neurosis, so that severe dysmenorrhoea can occur in psychologically healthy women. Such patients will be helped more by analgesic or hormone treatment than by psychotherapy.

Dysmnesia

A term implying impaired or disordered memory (q.v.). It occurs most commonly in organic brain disorder. The Korsakoff syndrome (q.v.) is otherwise known as the dysmnesic syndrome.

Dysmnesic syndrome

SEE Korsakoff's psychosis.

Dyspareunia

Dyspareunia is difficult or painful intercourse in the female. When it occurs at the first attempts at intercourse it is commonly due to a vaginismus, resulting from contraction of the perineal musculature and spasm of the outer vaginal barrel with absence of vaginal lubrication. Although a rigid hymen may be responsible,

anticipatory fear or revulsion at penetration by the penis is common.
The patient frequently has an anxious and immature personality; occasionally the dyspareunia may be a symptom of a more marked personality disorder. A joint interview with the sexual partners should clarify any misunderstanding on sexual technique and hygiene. Thereafter desensitization of the conditioned anticipatory fear is carried out, sometimes using vaginal dilators passed while the woman is in a state of relaxation, and in most cases improvement is rapid. In more disturbed personalities, latent homosexual problems with repressed aggressive feelings to males may require prolonged psychotherapy.
Where dyspareunia occurs after a period of previous normal sexual adjustment, pelvic pathology must be excluded, e.g. perineal, vaginal or cervical scars, endometriosis, chronic pelvic infections, infective or degenerative vaginitis.
SEE ALSO Frigidity.

Dysphagia – functional

Difficulty in swallowing in the absence of any organic disturbance is found in conditions of severe anxiety, or in depressive illnesses, when it may be the expression of a hypochondriacal delusion. Cardiospasm, and hiatus hernia as well as oesophageal lesions must be carefully excluded.

Echo encephalography
(Synonym: Sono-encephalography)

Echo encephalography is a useful technique adapted from industrial flaw detecting to determine shift in midline structures. An ultra sound wave is transmitted from and received by a probe containing a pair of barium titanate crystals. The wave is reflected by the midline structures of the brain, which produce a strong and persistent echo. If these structures are central then the echo is equidistant from the probe placed successively on each side of the head. If the midline structures are displaced the echo will be nearer the probe on one side than on the other. In cerebral atrophy echoes may be obtained from the subarachnoid space and the ventricles may be measured as proportionately enlarged when compared with each hemisphere. Finally, subdural haematomas tend to prevent the appearance of midline echoes.

Echolalia

The echoing of phrases, usually those spoken by members of the patients entourage, but sometimes of the patient's own thoughts (echo de la pensée). It is almost invariably a sign of schizophrenic illness (q.v.) to be distinguished from perseveration (q.v.) and palilalia (q.v.).
SEE ALSO Echopraxia.

Echopraxia

The immediate imitation of the behaviour of those around the patient, it is a manifestation almost exclusively of a schizophrenic illness (q.v.), but may be found in some severely mentally subnormal patients.
SEE ALSO Echolalia

Ecology

The study of the interaction between an organism and its environment, ecology may properly include any aspect of this interaction, the individual, the colonies of individuals, the relationship between other individuals of a different species, the physical environment and so on. Psychosomatic medicine has contributed a great deal to the concepts used in human ecology. In general more attention is paid by ecologists to the physical external environment than to the psychological internal environment.

Ecstasy state

A rare condition in which the patient falls into an ecstatic mood, feeling uplifted, joyous, peaceful and utterly calm and happy. Religious ecstasies are well documented in the lives of the saints or mystics; in psychiatry it is difficult at times to differentiate between a schizophrenic experience and a mood change occurring in a manic-depressive illness. Ecstasy in response to hallucinatory voices, or visions will usually be of a schizophrenic origin. The influence of drugs such as heroin or LSD must always be excluded.

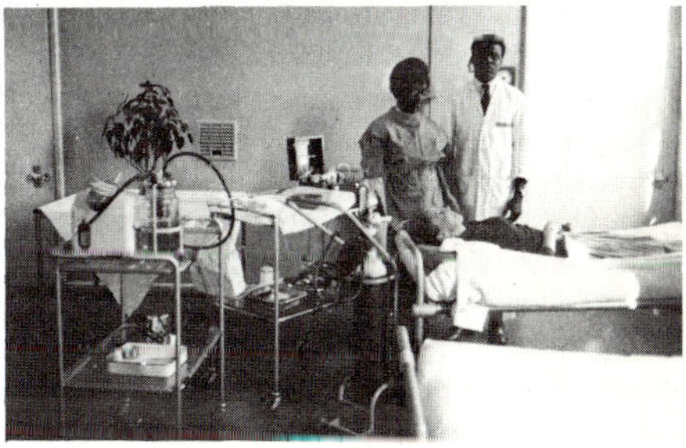

ECT (electroconvulsive therapy)
(Also known as Electroplexy)

Convulsion therapy was reintroduced into psychiatry by Meduna in 1933 for the treatment of schizophrenia and in 1937 Cerletti and Bini showed that electrically induced fits were therapeutically just as effective but at the same time more reliable and less disagreeable than the earlier chemically induced convulsions. ECT is a completely empirical form of treatment.
The mechanism of action of ECT is unknown. The only certainty is that the fit is the essential part of the treatment. Increases in noradrenaline and 5-hydroxytryptamine metabolism have been shown as short-lived effects following ECT. More significant may be a report that

ECT increases the sensitivity of the receptor site to neurotransmitter amines.
Convulsion therapy was first used in the treatment of schizophrenia but when given alone and before the advent of the phenothiazines, the results were not good.
In combination with the phenothiazines or other major tranquillizers, however, it is again becoming increasingly popular not only for catatonic states, where the response is often dramatic, or in patients with a strong affective component, but also in most cases where the onset or exacerbation is an acute one and even in more chronic paranoid schizophrenias resistant to treatment with medication alone.

The main indication for ECT is depression of a mainly endogenous type. In suitable cases, ECT results in a complete cure of the illness though, of course, it does not prevent a recurrence. It is particularly effective in those endogenous depressions characterized by marked agitation which occur for the first time in the involutional period of life. ECT, however, is of no benefit in the neurotic types of depression however severe they may be.

In practice ECT must bear comparison with the anti-depressant drugs. On the one hand, in suitable cases, ECT will result in a complete cure of the illness whereas anti-depressants will provide only symptomatic relief and will need to be continued for perhaps many months until a natural remission is encouraged and brought about. On the other hand, ECT involves the inconvenience of repeated anaesthetics and at least a halfday off work once or twice a week even when given on an outpatient basis. In practice the anti-depressant drugs are of most use in mild to moderate degrees of depression where the patient can be treated at home or in the out-patient department of the hospital.
ECT should be reserved for the more intractable cases or for more severely depressed patients in whom anti-depressants are less likely to succeed. In severely depressed patients there is no doubt that where depression and agitation are causing physical distress because of difficulties in eating or from exhaustion through insomnia or general agitation and restlessness, most psychiatrists would prefer to start treatment with ECT rather than wait for a trial of the anti-depressants.
This again holds for patients with suicidal feelings as although both methods of treatment have a latent period before improvement occurs there is no doubt that ECT is much more likely to benefit the severely depressed patient and such a risk to life should not be prolonged by a trial of a less-effective treatment.

Rather than choosing between ECT and anti-depressant drugs, it is becoming increasingly common for drugs such as imipramine to be given concomitantly with ECT particularly in patients with considerable environmental or personality problems, in order to prevent a relapse which might otherwise occur with ECT by itself.

Although primarily of use in depressive illnesses, paradoxically ECT can be useful in states of mania. It is indicated in cases which are inadequately controlled by the major tranquillizers, or in those cases where the illness is protracted. In both instances, the attack can often be terminated by a course of ECT when the treatments are usually given rather more frequently, e.g. three or four times in the first week reducing to twice weekly.

ECT is an extremely safe treatment when given by an experienced team and fatalities should be no more than one in several thousand patients; in other words, little more than the dangers of giving an anaesthetic. Fifty per cent of fatalities are due to adverse effects on the cardiovascular system and the only complete contra-indication to ECT are a recent cardiac infarction. Other contraindications are relative. For instance, in cases of pulmonary tuberculosis or congestive heart failure, and in states of physical debility, one should weigh the disadvantages of an anaesthetic and modified convulsion against the continued restlessness of the depressive illness.

ECT is usually given twice weekly initially, but this may be decreased to once weekly towards the end of treatment. In favourable cases, improvement begins after the third or fourth convulsion, when six or seven treatments may suffice. If improvement is not apparent after six or seven convulsions, it is rarely advisable to continue.

A partial amnesia as a result of treatment is common, especially in elderly patients.
The amnesia increases with the frequency and number of convulsions and in the elderly can be reduced by decreasing the

treatment to once weekly as soon as the clinical condition permits. The amnesia is practically always temporary, but in elderly patients may last for several months. It is rarely serious in degree, but rather an inconvenience, particularly for a patient who relies upon his memory in his job. Such memory disturbances have often been thought to be an integral and necessary part of ECT, but recent work suggests that this may not be so.

Technically, ECT may produce transient cardiac irregularities and therefore atropine should be given, either subcutaneously half an hour before treatment or perhaps preferably intravenously with the anaesthetic. It also reduces bronchial secretion. The patient is anaesthetized with intravenous thiopentone or methohexitone and this is followed by a muscle relaxant which, by reducing muscular activity, virtually abolishes the risk of fractures and dislocations and also reduces cardiovascular disturbances especially that due to the Valsalva effect.

The electrodes are usually placed one each side of the temporofrontal regions (bilateral ECT). Recently unilateral ECT where the electrodes are applied to the non-dominant side if the head has been advocated as being therapeutically as effective, but producing less post-treatment confusion and impairment of memory than the bilateral method. Recent work also suggests that a stimulus consisting of brief high-voltage pulses (bidirectional) leads to less confusion and memory loss. Convulsions induced by inhalation of flurothyl (hexafluorodiethyl ether) are being investigated and are also said to minimize confusion and memory disturbances.

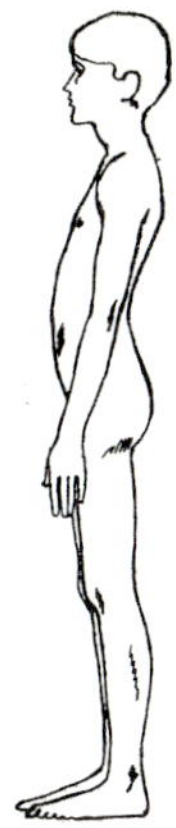

Ectomorph

An ectomorph is an individual displaying features of one of the three main types of body-build in Sheldon's classification of somatotyping. Characteristics include a tall narrow structure, long limbs and little subcutaneous fat.

SEE ALSO Constitution.

Educationally sub-normal

SEE ESN.

Edwards' syndrome (trisomy E)

This syndrome is associated with trisomy of an autosomal chromosome in the E group (see Denver system). The syndrome comprises severe mental retardation together with obvious gross physical malformations which occur in different patients in various combinations. The main specific malformations are of the face, hands, feet and heart. A defective falx cerebri has been reported as a feature and hypoplasia or agenesis of the corpus callosum is not infrequently seen as part of this syndrome. The chances of survival beyond infancy are poor. There is marked retardation in growth and a failure to thrive.

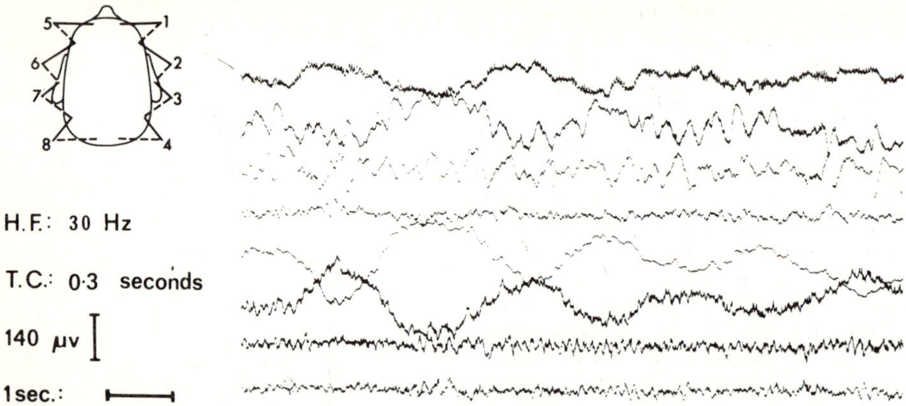

E E G following massive right-sided cerebro-vascular accident. Normal alpha activitv is seen on the left (Channels 7 and 8) but is absent on the right where instead slower theta and delta components are present.

EEG (electroencephalogram)

The EEG is a recording of the electrical activity of the cerebral cortex obtained from the surface of the scalp. Occasionally recordings are made directly from the exposed surface of the brain at operation (electrocorticogram). The signals are of extremely low amplitude (typically 10 to 100 μv), lying mainly in a frequency range of 1 to 50 Hz, and are of extremely complex wave form. The EEG changes markedly with age, particularly during childhood, and is also sensitive to small changes in state of awareness. These factors have therefore to be taken into account in clinical interpretation.
In the neonate slow waves in the delta (less than 4 cycles per second) and theta (4–7 cycles per second) bands of irregular and asynchronous occurrence predominate. Alpha rhythms (8–13 cycles per second) gradually displace the slower rhythms so that by 15 years the EEG is alpha dominated.
The EEG is markedly influenced by the patient's alertness. In sleep the EEG is dominated by slow waves and different stages of sleep can be classified by EEG patterns.
Some types of psychopathic personality have EEGs which are markedly immature for their chronological age and in states of confusion from metabolic or other organic factors the EEG has generalized, bilateral slow wave activity reflecting the patient's decreased state of awareness. Local or general areas of abnormal slow wave activity may be caused by local or generalized brain pathology such as tumour or dementia.
In epilepsy, paroxysmal activity may be seen and a diencephalic or cortical type diagnosed and, if the latter, the particular area of diseased cortex from which the epilepsy originates.
The EEG is used for clinical diagnostic purposes in the investigation of epilepsy, early detection of suspected intracranial lesions such as tumour, etc., in the investigation of some diffuse cerebral infections and degenerations and in assessing the effects on the brain of systemic disorders, notably hepatic failure and anoxia.
It must be emphasized that a normal EEG does not exclude an organic brain lesion.
SEE ALSO Grand Mal, Petit Mal, and Temporal lobe epilepsy.

Effort syndrome (Da Costa's syndrome)

(Synonym: Neuro-circulatory asthenia)

Seen particularly in soldiers in wartime, the condition is encountered very rarely in peacetime or in a civilian population.
Symptoms include breathlessness, left infra-mammary pain, and anxiety, with tachycardia, palpitations and an exacerbation of all symptoms on exercise.
Iatrogenic factors play an important part in delimiting the syndrome, whilst discharge from military service also provides an incentive to the production of this stereotyped clinical picture.
SEE ALSO Psychosomatic disorders and Cardiovascular system and psychosomatic illness.

Ego

The ego is that part of the personality structure which deals directly with the external and internal environments. It modifies the instinctual drives of the id (q.v.) into socially and emotionally acceptable channels. The various mechanisms involved include: perception; motor action; appreciation of reality and a desire to ensure safety and self-preservation. Memory, affect, thinking, and a general synthetic function are all involved. Its development depends on physical and cerebral maturation, and upon experiential factors beginning at birth, when stimuli from the external world first impinge upon the individual. Controlling and modifying the ego is the superego (q.v.) or conscience. Conflict between superego and ego may result in guilt feelings, or often painful emotions. The ego has at its disposal various psychological mechanisms to defend itself from being overwhelmed by 'id' (instinctual) impulses, and to protect itself from reality demands too powerful for the individual ego. Repression, denial, projection, regression, displacement, reaction formation, rationalization, intellectualization, sublimation, etc. are such mechanisms.

Ego-ideal

The ego is that part of the mental organization concerned with reality testing. The ego-ideal is one component of the ego, based on identification with loving parents, and the striving for attaining what one wants to be. The ego-ideal may change during maturation, but represents in general an ideal object with which the individual hopes and tries to identify.

Ego syntonic

Ideas or impulses which are acceptable to both the ego and, incidentally, to the super-ego, and which conform to the ego-ideal, that image of the self held up as free from criticism.

Eidetic imagery

50–60% of children up to the age of 12 are able visually to hallucinate previously perceived objects. In adults vivid visual imagery occurs just prior to falling asleep. In some individuals this ability is so strong as to be a feature of personality – the eidetic personality.

Elaboration, creative

As a Freudian psychoanalytical concept, specific instinctual conflicts arouse anxiety which may be disguised in dreams, phantasies, or stories. This is a psychic defence mechanism, with gratification in imaginative processes substituted for the satisfaction of the original instinctual aim. In creative elaboration the important feature of the dream is elaborated, expanded and distorted as part of the disguise of what it actually represents. It is thus somewhat the converse of condensation (q.v.). This mechanism differs from sublimation (q.v.) in that it is not necessarily related to social values. Creative elaboration often involves mechanisms of symbolization (q.v.) and identification (q.v.).

Elation

The characteristic mood of mania (q.v.), although it also occurs in some schizophrenic illnesses, in intoxication and in normal people as a temporary response to unexpected good fortune. Manic elation has a characteristic infectious quality. The patient is sociable and amusing and the onlooker feels tempted to join in. In many manic patients, however, elation is less conspicuous than overactivity and irritability and the fundamental elevation of mood only becomes apparent when the patient fails to be discomfited by bad news.

Elective mutism

A condition occurring in childhood when despite normal language development the child is mute in one situation but is known to use speech in other situations.

Electra situation (complex)

Electra was the daughter of Agamemnon, who, on his return from the siege of Troy, was murdered by his wife, Clytemnestra. Electra hated her mother and incited her brother Orestes to kill their mother to avenge their father's death. Afterwards Electra became overwhelmed with guilt. The Electra complex refers to analogous situations in the relations between the girl and her parents. The girl blames the mother for her lack of a penis and as she grows out of the mother-dependent stages of development, turns more to her father. The attitude of the parents determines whether there is a satisfactory resolution of this female Oedipus complex.

Electrolyte distribution in depression and mania

Electrolytes are fundamentally important for the transmission of electrical impulses in the nervous system, for the maintenance of resting electrical potentials across cell membranes and are important in the metabolism of neurotransmitter substances.

Studies in depressed patients measuring exchangeable body sodium, isotopic sodium retention or external balance (strict diets) show that sodium retention is greater during depression and is diminished with recovery. There is some evidence that the distribution of sodium in the body may also be altered. It is suggested that intracellular (non-exchangeable) sodium is abnormally high in depressed patients and remains so even after recovery and even greater changes in the same direction were found in mania.

Electromyography

In neurology, valuable information regarding muscle function has been obtained using needle-recording electrodes inserted into the muscle. In psychiatry, surface electrodes have been used to investigate the activity of muscle masses beneath the skin. Both anxious and depressed patients have elevated levels of muscle activity. The technique is also useful in monitoring the effectiveness of relaxation therapy.

Electroplexy

SEE ECT (electroconvulsive therapy).

Electro-oculogram

The electro-oculogram is a recording of the changes in electrical potential over the front of the head produced by eye movements. There is a standing potential of about 70 mv between the front and back of the eye and changes in orientation of the eyeball therefore produce detectable signals. Apart from its use in research applications, the electro-oculogram is chiefly used for the study of nystagmus (electronystagmorgraphy), either spontaneous or induced by caloric tests.

Eliminative functions

The toddler is proud of his ability to micturate and produce faeces, the products of his own body holding obvious fascination for him. By contrast, parents feel it is their duty to instil a disgust reaction to faeces in their children and to train them to achieve bowel and bladder control as early as possible. There is no good evidence to show that training alters the age at which these skills are acquired, and there is some suggestion that enuresis (q.v.) and encopresis (q.v.) are less frequently found in populations with a more relaxed attitude to toilet training in the early years.

Embryology of the nervous system

The nervous system is derived from the embryological ectoderm. The central nervous system first appears as a mid-line thickening of the ectoderm known as the neural plate. The fringes of the neural plate grow more rapidly than the intervening portion and rise up to form the neural folds which enclose between them the neural groove. The folds continue to grow and then gradually fuse from the middle of the embryo caudally and rostrally, to form the neural tube open at either end – the anterior and posterior neuropores. At the same time, a further group of ectodermal cells are budded off lateral to the neural ridge to form the neural crest. This neural crest subsequently develops into the posterior root ganglia, the neurilemmal sheaths of the peripheral nerves and the ganglia of the autonomic nervous system.

The proliferating cells within the wall of the neural tube arrange themselves in three layers, ependymal zone innermost, mantle zone next and marginal zone outermost. The neuroblasts, which will be converted into the neurones (q.v.); the spongioblasts, which form the majority of the neuroglia (q.v.) are derived from the ependymal zone.

During the fourth week of foetal life the anterior and posterior neuropores fuse to convert the tube into a closed hollow structure. The rostral part of this hollow tube now shows three swellings, the forebrain, midbrain and hindbrain vesicles. The forebrain vesicle expands and from it develops the telencephalon (the cerebral hemispheres) and the diencephalon (the thalamus and related nuclei, the hypothalamus, the pineal gland and related areas and by a downgrowth the posterior pituitary. From the forebrain vesicle optic evaginations arise to form the optic cups and ultimately the optic nerves and neural portion of the retina. The cavity of the forebrain vesicle provides the third ventricle and by outgrowths the lateral ventricle within the cerebral hemispheres.

The midbrain vesicle develops into the mesencephalon (the midbrain) while from the hindbrain vesicle are derived the metencephalon (the pons and cerebellum) and the myelencephalon (the medulla oblongata).

The spinal cord develops from the neural tube lying caudal to the fourth somite with the tube reduced to the minute central canal of the spinal cord. Its cells form into an anterior (motor) group which grow out towards the myotomes and a posterior group (sensory) into which grow the cells derived from the developing posterior root ganglia.

The cavity of the midbrain becomes the aqueduct of the midbrain, that of the hindbrain becomes the fourth ventricle.

During the fourth to sixth week of foetal life three more flexures appear in the neural tube, the midbrain, cervical and pontine flexures which align the growing brain into its definite adult spatial relationship.

Embryopathy

Embryopathy is a general term used for a disturbance in embryonic development leading to pathological changes. Important amongst known causes are environmental insults, including maternal infections that may affect the embryo, e.g. syphilis, rubella and toxoplasmosis; maternal-foetal antigenic incompatibility, e.g. rhesus incompatibility; teratogenic agents including various drugs and harmful irradiation. The developing central nervous system seems to be particularly vulnerable to noxious influences, especially during early intrauterine life, probably accounting for the high prevalence of mental subnormality in these patients.

Emergencies, psychiatric

It is as well to recognize that psychiatric emergencies are related not only to the disturbed behaviour of the patient, but also to the anxiety this behaviour engenders in others.

Panic attacks or lesser degrees of acute anxiety may present as emergencies, especially if there is a disease phobia or particular somatic expression of anxiety (i.e. palpitations or a psychic dyspnoea). If the patient is well known to the practitioner, firm reassurance (i.e. on the telephone) may suffice; this should emphasize that the panic will pass (it always does) and that the nature of the condition is understood by the doctor. If an appropriate sedative is available in the house a stat dose should be advised; sodium amylobarbitone 200 or 300 mg. is particularly effective for this purpose. If the patient is not known, a home visit is usually necessary to make sure that no serious organic illness is present. Admission to a psychiatric unit is seldom justified but may be required because of pressure from relatives or to persuade the patient that 'something is being done'.

If acute intoxication (with alcohol, amphetamines or LSD) is causing such a degree of behavioural disturbance that the family doctor is called, then the appropriate response is usually to refer the patient by ambulance to the casualty department at the general hospital. Attempts to contain such problems within the domestic setting usually only result in a further call in the early hours of the morning.

Acute psychotic excitement, whether hypomanic or schizophrenic, demands a parenteral phenothiazine (e.g. chlorpromazine 50–100 mg. intramuscularly) and referral to the appropriate psychiatric clinic by ambulance. Discussion by telephone with the duty doctor at the psychiatric clinic may clarify the alternatives, i.e. if the patient refuses to go to hospital it may be better to arrange for his admission accompanied by nurses from the hospital the following morning. For the intervening hours the relatives may be instructed to administer further doses of a phenethiazine by mouth.

Suicidal threats, even when they have a fairly obvious manipulative function, must be taken seriously. The patient is sedated (e.g. a benzodiazepine) and arrangements made for an early appointment at the psychiatric out-patient department within the next forty-eight hours. An attempt at suicide justifies the prompt referral of the patient by ambulance to the local general hospital. Current psychiatric opinion is that all such patients who have made suicidal attempts require medical and psychiatric assessment and that this can only be effectively achieved in the hospital setting.

Psychiatric emergencies in adolescence usually relate to 'bad behaviour' (i.e. staying out all night, drug taking, etc.) and the so-called 'identity crisis' (the symptoms are those of depersonalization perplexity and sometimes passivity feelings in which the subject feels that he is being controlled by some external power or mechanism). All problems with adolescents require that the doctor be prepared to spend a lot of time, listening both to the patient and to the parents. Drug problems usually indicate the need for referral, while 'identity crisis' nearly always requires specialist opinion because of the difficulty in discriminating this syndrome from a schizophrenic illness.

Psychiatric emergencies in old people are usually ignored in text-books, but such problems can be very real for the practitioner. Typical examples are of the old lady who starts wandering at night, the old man who turns on the gas but does not light it or sets fire to the rubbish (but in the middle of the sitting-room). The most effective move is to call out the consultant psychiatrist for a domiciliary visit to let him see directly the problems raised by the patient's behaviour.

EMI scanner (computerized axial tomograph)

Axial tomography is an advanced radiological technique which allows detection of small variations in density of tissue to the passage of X-rays which are not apparent in conventional films. The X-ray source and detector are moved in a plane at right angles to the longitudinal axis of the body. A computer-based system calculates the density to X-radiation of the tissue at each point in the plane scanned and presents the results as a cross-sectional view.

The technique appears likely to revolutionize neurological and neurosurgical diagnosis, as it provides a non-invasive method for reliable detection and localization of soft tissue lesions in the head (tumours, abscess, haematoma, etc.) and could therefore largely replace cerebral arteriography and air encephalography.

Emotion

The term emotion is commonly used synonymously with affect to imply the feelings or mood of the individual. It is probably more accurate to use emotion to specify the consciously perceived feelings and affect to include the basic drive energies that produce both conscious and unconscious feelings.

The emotional component of a reaction to an impulse is believed to be derived from reactions within the limbic system (q.v.). This receives collaterals from the main sensory pathways via the reticular formation.

The emotions are in their turn perceived by the subject but also manifest themselves as changes in autonomic and endocrine activities via the links which exist between the limbic system and the hypothalamus.

Emotional deprivation

For normal emotional and intellectual development, a child needs a satisfying and lasting relationship with one or more adults to look after him in a caretaking role. Despite the obvious nature of this statement, the sad fact remains that this simple need is not met for many children in present-day society.

During the first six months of life the child's needs are primarily physical, he becomes able to discriminate his mother's voice. Within the second six months he becomes more fully aware of his mother, and from this time up to about the age of 5 years he is especially vulnerable to deprivation experience. Deprivation must be distinguished from separation. A brief separation from a mother to the care of another relative known to him does not produce deprivation. The adverse effects of deprivation on personality arise as a product of the frequency and duration of the traumatic experience, the amount of emotional deprivation involved, and the temperament of the child.

Characteristically, the young deprived child in an institutional environment is impulsive, distractible, impersistent and craving for attention and material rewards. He may be cheerful, but is unable to tolerate frustration, and is likely to be somewhat retarded in intellectual development. This mental retardation is probably not solely a result of adverse genetic inheritance but also the lack of environmental stimulation.

Emotional deprivation may occur in 'family' children as well as the institutionalized, especially where family size is great or when maternal depression or inadequacy leave the mother with inadequate emotional resources to care for her children.

Empathy

Understanding the expression of thought and feeling of others is greatly enlarged by the extent to which we can enter into and compare it with our own; that is the extent to which empathy is possible. Degrees of emotion, such as grief or fear, which are beyond what we have experienced can nevertheless be appreciated by extension from experiences we have had and in this way symptoms, such as those occurring in depressive illness, are understandable. Some psychiatric manifestations are not comprehensible to normal experience in this way, for example schizophrenic thought disorder which has no parallel in ordinary experience. The ability thus to empathize with a patient is often regarded as differentiating schizophrenia from affective disorders and more generally psychoses from neurotic and personality disorders.

Empathy is obviously of great importance in the therapist's relation with the patient in the course of psychotherapy (q.v.), particularly in its most concentrated form, psychoanalysis.

Employment

Lack of suitable employment may be a problem for people with various forms of psychiatric illness and handicap. Those who have had a severe schizophrenic illness tend to be slow in movement, unable to take initiative or responsibility and socially withdrawn. They often need a long and patient process of rehabilitation, starting in a hospital industrial therapy unit and perhaps going on to an intermediate rehabilitation unit or special factory. With epileptic patients of working age, 50% had job difficulties and about 10% were unemployable. Many old people find retirement and idleness irksome, particularly when they have not developed leisure pursuits. Stopping work is often associated with loss of social contacts, a fall in income and a feeling of no longer contributing to the business of society. Similar problems occur with the mentally subnormal, particularly from the steady shrinkage of unskilled employment, such as agricultural labouring or domestic service. However, higher-grade patients are often capable of surprising levels of skill, if suitably trained.

SEE ALSO Old age and Unemployment.

Encephalitis lethargica

Described by Von Economo in 1917, it was epidemic in the next decade but has gradually disappeared since then. 'Sleepy sickness' refers to the peculiar somnolence which was a frequent feature of the acute phase. Mental symptoms were also frequent but CNS signs were often slight and easily overlooked.
Parkinson's syndrome may develop during the acute stage or after a variable interval and compulsive thoughts, often associated with oculogyric crises and muscular tics may also be a sequel. Personality change in children or adolescents may occur, characterized by emotional outbursts and antisocial behaviour.

Encopresis

The involuntary passing of faeces in inappropriate circumstances occurs for a variety of reasons, but is relatively uncommon as a symptom of disturbance in childhood. At the age of 7 years about 2% of boys and at age 12 about 1% of boys are encopretic. Girls are affected less frequently.
One common cause of encopresis is severe mental retardation. Another common cause is constipation. When the lower bowel becomes impacted with faeces increase in bowel contents no longer results in afferent stimulation of nerve endings in the colonic submucosa, so that no 'call to stool' is experienced. Overflow incontinence of liquid faeces results. Removal of the impacted faecal mass by laxatives or bowel wash out is an essential preliminary to other treatment.
Encopresis in the absence of constipation or mental retardation is a much more difficult problem and is often a sign of quite serious psychological disorder in the child, sometimes associated with rejecting parental attitudes. Simple training procedures have had some success, although psychotherapy is more commonly employed in treatment. The prognosis for the symptom must be good as encopretic adults are practically unheard of. However, there is a suggestion that other adult psychopathology may not infrequently become substituted for childhood encopresis.

Encounter group

SEE Newer group therapies.

Endocrine disease

Psychiatric symptoms are common in all types of endocrine disease, partly because of the effect of excessive or inadequate hormone production on the brain. Major psychiatric disorders are well-known (although by no means constant) complications of excess or deficiency of cortisol, thyroxine and parathyroid hormone in the adult. Excess of insulin, exogenous or endogenous, rapidly impairs cognitive function. In foetal and neonatal life thyroid deficiency is, of course, a cause of mental subnormality.
Manfred Bleuler and his colleagues in Zurich have studied a large number of patients attending an endocrine clinic. As well as the restlessness of the hyperthyroid and the torpidity of the hypothyroid patient etc., they found a very frequent occurrence of the 'endocrine psychosyndrome' – a state of fluctuating and dysphoric depression and tension such as is often seen in 'reactive' depressions. Symptoms of this kind are not unusual in other physical illnesses, particularly chronic and painful disorders.
If the endocrine disease can be successfully treated, any psychiatric symptoms may disappear. If the endocrine disease cannot be effectively treated, or if the psychiatric symptoms persist in spite of treatment of the endocrine disorder, symptomatic psychiatric treatment is indicated and is sometimes gratifyingly successful.
SEE ALSO Organic disease producing mental disorders.

Endocrine system and the brain

Most endocrine activity is under hypothalamic control. The posterior pituitary direct by a nervous pathway, much of the rest through trophic hormones produced by the anterior pituitary. The anterior pituitary is itself controlled in large measure by releasing and inhibitory factors, formed and released in the hypothalamus which travel through the hypothalamic hypophyseal portal blood system. These releasing factors are poly-

peptides and the composition of some of them is now known.
The production of the hypothalamic factors is partly controlled by feedback from the blood level of the trophic hormones and the peripheral hormones and partly by the effects of higher brain centres (including the limbic system, q.v., and reticular formation, q.v.).

Endogenous depression

Depression where the constitutional factors are predominant in contrast to reactive depression where environmental circumstances are the most important aetiological factor. Such a constitutional predisposition may show itself in the family history, previous personality and in various symptoms pointing to a diencephalic disturbance such as early wakening, marked loss of weight, diurnal variation of mood and amenorrhoea. The more pronounced the endogenous features, the more likely is the depression to respond to physical methods of treatment such as tricyclic antidepressants or ECT.
SEE ALSO Reactive depression.

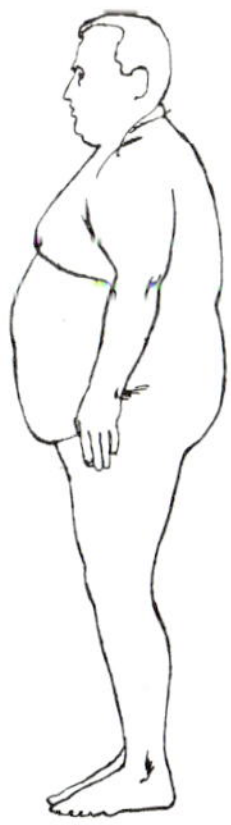

Endomorph

An endomorph is an individual displaying features of one of the three main types of body-build in Sheldon's classification of somatotyping. Characteristics include a short, thick-set stature with deep body cavities and a tendency to be well padded with subcutaneous fat.
SEE ALSO Constitution.

Energy

The force or vigour of expression, especially physical activity. Characteristically it is low in people with a depressive constitution and to a more variable extent in patients with a neurotic personality.

Engram

The term engram was first used by Lashley. It is applied to the hypothesized permanent or semipermanent change in nerve tissue which results from excitation. Hence it is the unit of memory. It is still unclear exactly what the change consists of in biochemical terms.
SEE Memory.

Enkephalin

A recently synthesized endogenous polypeptide found in nervous tissue which may be concerned with pain suppression. It is not clear yet whether it is itself a transmitter substance in specific areas or activates other transmitters. Enkephalin is in some tests more potent than opiates but its relationship to the problems of addiction is currently unknown.

Enuresis

Most children gain bladder control both by night and by day between the ages of 18 months and 4 years. Involuntary micturition (enuresis) beyond the age of 4 years is, however, not an uncommon problem. It occurs at least weekly in about 5% boys and 2½% girls at the age of 5, and even by the age of 10 and above over 3% of boys and 2% of girls are wetting their bed or pants at least once a month. Most enuresis does not have a pathological cause but it is important to exclude those conditions which are, on occasions, responsible for its presence. The urine should always be examined to exclude urinary infection and diabetes mellitus. No further investigation is indicated unless there is definite, associated symptomatology. Dysuria and haematuria are indications for repeated examination of the urine with further investigations as

necessary. Difficulty in starting the stream also calls for urological assessment. Dribbling between episodes of micturition usually has no pathological basis, if unaccompanied by other symptoms. X-ray of the spine for spina bifida occulta is not indicated as this is not a cause of enuresis. In the great majority of cases, physical investigation is negative. Usually, the child is suffering from an isolated developmental disorder involving delay in the maturation of nervous pathways responsible for the control of micturition. This view of causation is supported by the generally benign prognosis, by the frequent presence of a family history of enuresis, by the sex differences found (developmental disorders generally occuring in boys more often than girls) and by the frequent absence of organic or emotional factors to account for the condition. Emotional factors may, however, be important in aetiology and it is important to be aware of this. When enuresis occurs after a period of satisfactory control of micturition, when the child shows associated soiling (encopresis, q.v.), when there is evidence of deliberate wetting, and where the enuresis is diurnal as well as nocturnal, emotional stress is more likely to be playing a part. More commonly rejecting family attitudes and the child's feeling of failure at his incontinence lead to secondary emotional disorders. Diagnosis therefore involves a full appraisal of the symptom and of the family attitudes to it. Whatever other specific measures of treatment are instituted, it is important to help the family take up a non-punitive and sympathetic attitude to the symptom. Comments by the doctor that the child is 'just lazy' do not help in this respect. The parents should be encouraged to ignore wet nights and reward dry ones. Imipramine or amitriptyline 25 mg. nocte in children aged 6–12 and 50 mg. nocte in older children is often effective in stopping nocturnal enuresis, but the child usually relapses on stopping the drug. The 'bell and pad' conditioning method of treatment properly applied is effective in about two thirds of cases. Again, there is a significant relapse rate, but if relapse occurs a second trial is worth while. This method of treatment involves placing a metallic pad connected to an alarm bell under the child's sheet. When the child starts to wet the bed the alarm goes off and wakes the child. The patient then goes to the lavatory, finishes emptying his bladder and returns to bed after resetting the alarm. If it is going to be effective, this method of treatment has usually resulted in dry nights before a fortnight is up.
Where it seems likely that emotional factors are prominent, or with enuresis that is resistant to physical methods of treatment, a further assessment of the child's mental state and family attitudes is indicated. Psychotherapeutic intervention may be necessary in these circumstances.

Environment

SEE Ecology.

Environmental modification

Doctors commonly advise their patients to change their job, leave home or to carry out certain environmental modifications, in the belief that psychiatric symptoms are related to a current social situation. This manipulation of the environment is rarely effective for it so often rests on a very inadequate base. When careful psychosocial investigation and assessment of the individual's personality and psychopathology have been carried out, it may be justifiable to recommend or effect environmental modification. In an institutional setting environmental changes based on careful study may be of much therapeutic value.

Ependyma

The ependymal zone is the innermost of the three layers of the embryonic neural tube (q.v.) and is the zone from which the majority of nervous tissue is derived. The term is also applied in the adult to the cells which line the cavities of the ventricular system.

Epilepsy

Epilepsy connotes a wide variety of paroxysmal behaviours associated with altered consciousness and with cerebral dysfunction as reflected by paroxysmal electrical discharges in the EEG. It is not a disease, since its age and mode of onset, its course and prognosis depend critically upon the conditions which underlie it, such as cerebral degenerations or malformations, encephalitides, brain tumours, metabolic disorders. Nor can it entirely be regarded as symptomatic, since most often its cause is uncertain or unknown. The form of the seizure, the degree of altered consciousness, and the nature of the EEG are not always reliable indications of the aetiology or the prognosis. The range of phenomena subsumed under 'epilepsy' is so large as to make any generalization about 'epilepsy' meaningless. The epilepsies and their medical and social implications are best considered ontogenetically.

The incidence of *seizures in the newborn* is from five to ten per 1000 births. Seizures in the first month account for about half the incidence in the first year of life. Local or generalized twitching (rather than tonic/clonic seizures), cyanosis, and a 'cerebral' infant are observed. Birth injury cerebral malformation and infection, hypoglycaemia (due to failure to feed the newborn) and hypocalcaemia (due to excess phosphate in cows milk) cover most known causes. Mortality is up to 50% and many survivors are mentally subnormal. *Infantile spasms* are episodically recurrent, jack-knife, whole body flexions (or extensions) usually associated with hypsarrhythmia (q.v.) in the EEG. Two thirds of all cases start in the first six months of life. Males preponderate 2:1. Mortality is 15%; most survivors are mentally subnormal. Severe cerebral abnormalities are known to underlie both the seizures and the mental subnormality in half the cases. Despite disappointing results, treatment in hospital is a matter of urgency because there may be some cases for whom this is critical.

95% of all *febrile convulsions* appear between 6 months and 4 years. Mostly they are brief and non-recurrent generalized seizures. Prolonged convulsions must be stopped since they damage the immature brain and may lead to serious sequelae (hemiparesis, mental subnormality, hyperkinesis, temporal lobe epilepsy (q.v.)). Febrile convulsions also identify some children who are at risk for epilepsy. Young age, female sex, lateralized seizures, long and recurrent seizures all worsen the late prognosis. *Akinetic attacks*, sudden drops to the floor, and *myoclonus*

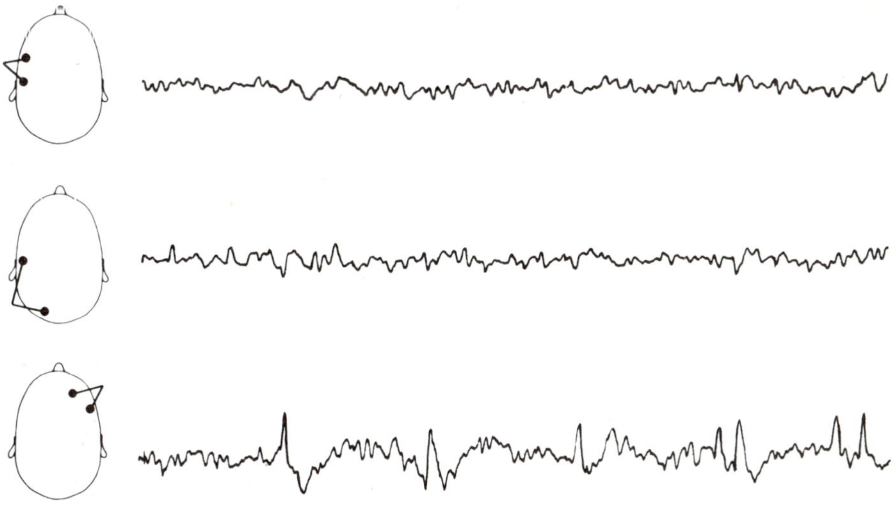

Typical EEG in Psychomotor Epilepsy.
The right anterior temporal region shows a staccato of sharp waves and spikes.

brief shock-like muscle group jerks, are also early manifestations of some severe chronic epilepsies.

Petit mal (q.v.) absence attacks often begin in the early school years. Their frequency may be considerable but often the attacks are unnoticed. One third to half the patients later develop major convulsions. The likelihood increases with late development of the petit mal. Mental deterioration is exceptional but educational performance is often below expectation.

The over-all prevalence of epilepsy in school children is about six per 1000. The prevalence of five per 1000 in the whole population reflects the net effect of remission or death in patients with early onset epilepsy and the occurrence of epilepsy of late onset in adults. In adults too it is usual for no cause to be found, but the effects of head injury (q.v.), brain tumours, metabolic disorders, and cerebro-vascular disease must be considered (SEE Fits).

Epilepsy is compatible with normal function. This is the goal of management. But problems may arise in any sphere of life due to abnormal cerebral function, socially incapacitating seizures and prejudice. Most serious problems arise in the group whose chronic epilepsy extends from childhood. Drug therapy to control seizure frequency also implies unwanted effects upon mood, behaviour and motor functions. Phenobarbitone for example, depresses some adults and makes many children uncontrollably overactive. The cerebral dysfunction may be apparent in subnormal intelligence but may subtly reduce the expected school or work performance in those of good intelligence. Personality development may be variously distorted depending upon the age of onset and the milieu. No specific 'epileptic personality' emerges but behaviour disorders, overactivity, sensitiveness, and depression are common. The suicide rate is high. A specific chronic, paranoid, hallucinatory psychosis of onset in middle life occurs in a small proportion of patients, especially those with psychomotor epilepsy (q.v.).

Epileptic attacks are frightening to both the patient and to witnesses. Fear leads to restriction and to prejudice. Undeclared epilepsy is still grounds for nullity in marriage although, provided sound genetic advice is given, epilepsy should be no bar. In most countries the law prohibits epileptics from driving motor cars, but newer legislation often eases the situation of those under good seizure control. There is little evidence to support the belief that epilepsy is associated with criminality.

Epilepsy, biochemistry of

Epilepsy can be induced by pyridoxine deficiency. This vitamin is a co-factor in enzymes concerned with the conversion in brain of glutamate to gamma aminobutyric acid (GABA). As the former is an excitatory transmitter and the latter an inhibitory one, any block in this conversion will lead to excess excitation, i.e. convulsions. Acetylcholine, another cerebral transmitter may also be involved as the CSF of epilepsy contains free acetylcholine not found in normal CSF. Neurones from epileptogenic foci have excess levels of intracellular sodium and low potassium. However, the difficulty in all these investigations is to distinguish possible causes of abnormal neuronal excitability from the metabolic results of the excess activity itself. Thus it cannot yet be claimed that the biochemical basis of idiopathic epilepsy is known.

Epilepsy in the aged

This is often due to cerebral ischaemia. Primary and secondary neoplasms and neuro-syphilis must not be overlooked. Epilepsy may present as attacks of delirium of sudden onset, sometimes with incontinence, in a well-preserved person, or as paroxysmal unilateral pain when it may be ascribed to psychogenic causes, or if there is transient hemiparesis, to strokes or vascular spasms. Diagnosis may be aided by the EEG. Treatment with phenytoin or sulthiame may control the fits. Phenobarbitone should be avoided in the elderly.

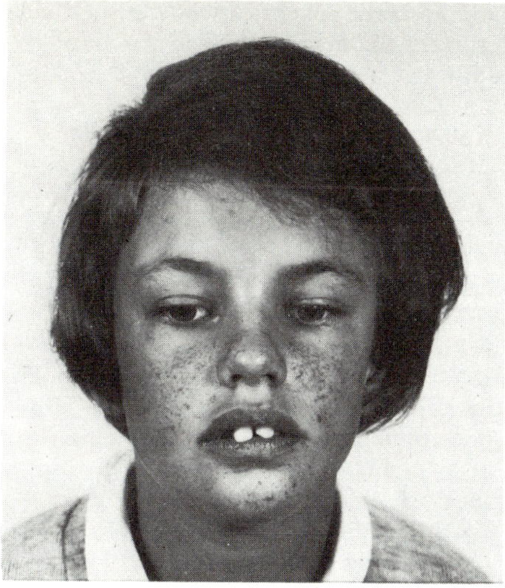

Epiloia
(Synonym: Tuberous sclerosis)

In this condition multiple tuberlike nodules are scattered throughout the body including the nervous system. Among a variety of skin lesions the 'butterflyrash' on either side of the nose, is a cardinal feature of the condition. This usually appears about the age of 4 to 6 years and is permanent.
Epilepsy and mental subnormality, often severe, are other components of the clinical picture.
The condition is inherited as a Mendelian dominant with variable expressivity.
SEE ALSO Mental subnormality and inherited syndromes.

Epinephrine
SEE Adrenaline.

Erection

Erection or tumescence is the stiffening and enlargement of the penis (or clitoris) due to vascular distension of the corporal venous sinuses. Changes in the dimensions of the flaccid penis can be measured by a phallograph and used as an indication of sexual arousal. Penile erection occurs intermittently during sleep, particularly during dreaming, and is manifest as the 'morning erection'. Priapism is persistent painful erection and is due to some local irritative lesion in the pelvis or to a blood dyscrasia producing thrombosis of the venous sinuses. It can be due to cantharides poisoning. Sexual arousal commences in the cerebral cortex and in the subcortical tracts of the limbic system. Nervous impulses then descend through the hypothalamus to the spinal cord close to the pyramidal tracts finally emerging in the pelvis in the nervi erigentes to the genitalia. Stimulation of first, second, and third sacral nerves produces erection through the parasympathetic fibres. Subsidence of erection is brought about by stimulation of the sympathetic roots from the second, third and fourth lumbar nerves.

Erotic

Erotic is the adjective pertaining to the mental state which anticipates sexual excitement. Erotic stimuli are most commonly visual, tactile or olfactory and are manifest through clothes, cosmetics and mannerism usually in relation to the erogenous zones of the body, *viz*. mouth, anus, genitals and breasts.
The capacity for erotic arousal in man is uniform compared to the periodic arousal in the oestrus behaviour of many mammals.

Erotogenic zones

Erotogenic zones are areas of the body usually around the orifices, e.g. mouth, anus, genitals, breasts, which on stimulation produce sensuous and sexual excitement. According to Freud's theory of sexual development, sucking and biting in the infant are the first manifestations of the libido (q.v.) (oral stage). This is followed by a transfer of pleasurable activities to the anus (anal stage), finally culminating in transfer to the genital region (genital phase) between the ages of 5 and 7 years. Thereafter follow the Oedipal (q.v.) conflicts ending in genital latency. Fixation of the libidinous energy at one of these stages due to some psychic trauma during development or later regression to one of the earlier stages was in Freudian terms thought to predispose the individual to the different forms of neuroses and sexual perversion.

Erythroblastosis foetalis
SEE Kernicterus.

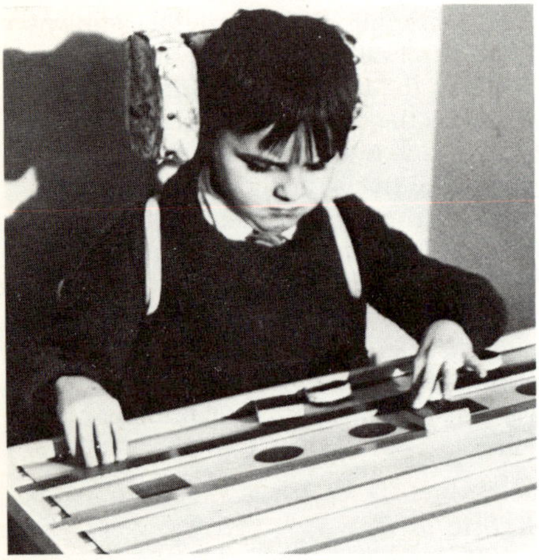

ESN (educationally subnormal)

The English term educationally subnormal (ESN) was deliberately contrived to be flexible in order to cover a wide group of children so consistently backward in scholastic progress as to require special education outside the curriculum of ordinary schools. Prior to 1944 such children in England and Wales came under the auspices of the Mental Deficiency Act then existing, but they are now provided for by the education authorities. ESN facilities vary considerably from one local authority area to another. ESN schools may be run on a residential or day basis. Peripatetic teachers are provided by some local authorities for children whose physical condition keeps them at home. A few progressive ordinary schools are able to provide special classes for children unable to benefit from the ordinary curriculum.

Esquirol, Jean Étienne Dominique (1772–1840)

Best known for his two-volume work *Des Maladies Mentales Considérées sous les Raports Medical, Hygiénique et Médicolégal* (1838), Esquirol was an important influence on contemporary psychiatry. He emphasized the importance of emotion and of social change in the development of mental illness; reorganized hospital administration; kept careful statistics and founded the first psychiatric teaching clinic in Paris.

Ether sniffing
SEE Inhalant addiction.

Ethical problems

Ethics is the subject dealing with the rules of conduct in various situations. The first ethical code in medicine is the Hippocratic Oath (470–360 BC), which has been slightly altered to be embodied in the 1949 Declaration of Geneva of the World Medical Association. Subsequent Declarations have been made in Helsinki 1964 (experimentation), Sydney 1968 (death), Oslo 1970 (abortion) and Tokyo 1975 (arrest and detention). No universal declaration deals with psychiatric ethics, although the power of compulsion entrusted to the psychiatrist makes it particularly necessary for a set of rules to be available. Psychiatric patients must have their civil rights protected; experimentation must be particularly carefully controlled when dealing with insane patients. In general the rights of the individual must be balanced against the rights of society. When acting as a public servant, the doctor may have to take measures depriving an individual of certain liberties – for instance, the suspension of a driving licence. He may even have to allow a prisoner on hunger strike to die. Advances in medical technology have brought with them serious ethical problems for the medical profession and for society; who, for example, is to determine the point when a deliberate cessation of treatment should occur, to allow a patient to die? Medical ethics has, so far, been of more concern to theologians, philosophers and retired physicians and its teaching is comparatively neglected in many medical schools. In many countries no mental health legislation exists and in those countries where legal codes are in effect, then supervision and control may leave much to be desired.

Ethology

The study of behaviour, particularly in its natural setting, ethology is a new name for behaviourism, and for instinct psychology. The ethologist is concerned with the behaviour of bird, beast, insect and fish, and is usually a zoologist. From the behaviour itself is deduced the meaning of the behaviour. Important concepts are imprinting (q.v.) (the time-specific development of certain patterns of behaviour) releaser (a specific stimulus for specific behaviour), and displacement activity (inappropriate behaviour in response to a stimulus).

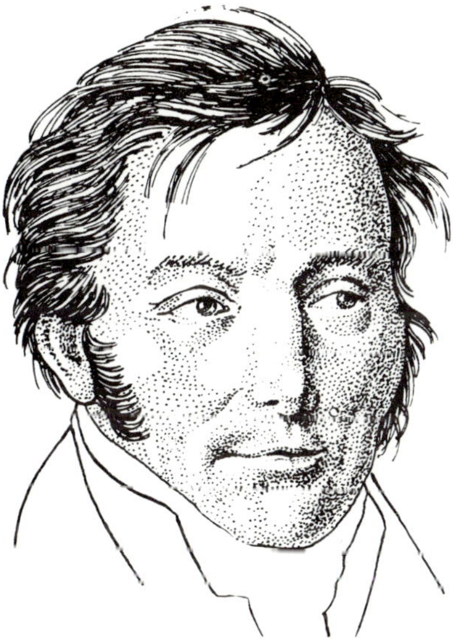

Jean Esquirol

Eugenics

The control of reproduction in order to increase the number of individuals with good genetical endowment and to reduce the number of those with poor or adverse genetical endowment in the population. Eugenic measures have been considered and applied mostly in connection with intelligence in efforts to reduce the prevalence of mental subnormality. Wholesale negative measures such as segregation, sterilization and abortion have not been successful in producing the large-scale effects in the community envisaged by their protagonists; this is due mainly to the fact that the vast majority of mentally subnormal individuals of all grades are offspring of parents who themselves are not mentally subnormal. Moreover, the most severely mentally subnormal patients, those most easily distinguished and selected for subjection to these measures, are in any case infertile. In individual cases, on the other hand, negative eugenic measures may be of social as well as genetical benefit. For example, it has been asserted, with justification, that the sterilization of feebleminded parents is beneficial to the children already born to them. Genetical counselling is of increasing importance as our knowledge of the genetic disorders increases.

The idea of positive eugenic measures is also based largely on the crude and not altogether true assumption that like breeds like, and it is unlikely that spectacular results would appear in the population if those thought to be especially well endowed genetically were encouraged to breed.

SEE ALSO Genetics.

Eunuchoidism

A eunuch is a pre-pubertal castrated male, although the term is frequently extended to those males whose testes have never functioned. Less severe degrees of failure are known as eunuchoidism. Here the testes and penis are underdeveloped at puberty, whilst the beard and body hair are sparse and sexual libido remains reduced. Eunuchoids are tall (due to delayed union of the epiphyses) whilst the face is lean and angular. There is a reduction in testosterone levels in the blood and androgen excretion in the urine is low. Whilst eunuchoidism may be due to local testicular damage, e.g. trauma, mumps, torsion of the testis (primary eunuchoidism), it is more commonly due to hypothalamic failure (secondary eunuchoidism). Eunuchoidism may occur in Klinefelter's syndrome (q.v.) (XXY), when it is associated with gynaecomastia and sterility. Full neurological and endocrinological investigations of patients with eunuchoidism should be carried out before testosterone replacement therapy is commenced.

Euphoria

A mood of contentment and wellbeing. Euphoria in psychiatric terms always has a pathological connotation and is often an important early sign of organic cerebral disease. It differs from elation in subtle but important ways. It has no infectious quality and no element of gaiety, for its bland contentment is based on lack of awareness and inability to experience sadness or anxiety rather than on anything positive.
It may be seen in any condition involving extensive cerebral damage, particularly if the frontal lobes are involved. It occurs sooner or later in senile and arteriosclerotic dementias (q.v.), in disseminated sclerosis and in Huntington's chorea (q.v.) and is often seen also after severe head injury and old-fashioned forms of leucotomy (q.v.). Euphoria is sometimes seen in Addison's disease (q.v.).

Examination of the mental state

This is the most important part of the psychiatric assessment. It is the equivalent of the physical examination of an organic disorder and all the doctor's senses must be used to elicit information.
Behaviour and talk
Abnormality of general behaviour and appearance is usually the first sign to the relatives that the patient is not well. The facial expression, walk, dress, mannerisms, etc. are often clear indications of the underlying illness. The nail bitten or tobacco-stained fingers of the tense anxious patient, the egg stains on a dementing bank manager's waistcoat, and the fatuous grinning or stereotypes of the schizophrenic are obvious examples.
Talk can be excessively fast or slow. Hesitancy, discursiveness, etc. are common in states of anxiety and depression. Neologisms and abnormal association of ideas are characteristic of certain forms of schizophrenia and may lead to incoherence which is also common in states of dementia. Sudden changes of topic may occur in mania and schizophrenia or simply because the subject provokes too much anxiety. The form of talk may vary with the topic and give a clue to emotionally charged subjects.
Mood
This may be of happiness, sadness, anxiety, perplexity, irritability, or indifference. It is important to assess the depth of a patients depression in order to assess the risk of suicide. A shallowness of affect may be due to an organic or schizophrenic deterioration. The constancy of mood may shed light on the aetiology of the condition. A reactive depression would be suggested if the mood responded easily to changes in the environment or topic raised by the doctor. In certain schizophrenics the mood may be incongruous and an abnormal lability of mood is characteristic of hypomania and is common in dementias.
Preoccupation, morbid beliefs, and disturbances of perception
Cues from the history are important in eliciting these phenomena, which include obsessive compulsive phenomena and depersonalization; ideas of reference and other paranoid ideas which may be of depressive or schizophrenic origin; passivity feelings and auditory hallucinations which are commonest in schizophrenia; or illusions and visual hallucinations which are suggestive of an organic state with clouding of consciousness.
Sensorium
True disorientation only occurs in organic mental states, orientation for time being most vulnerable. Loss of memory for recent events is typical of dementia and can be confirmed by simple testing. A complaint of 'poor memory' is frequent in states of agitation, but this is due to lack of attention and concentration and must be distinguished from a true memory loss. Grasp is characteristically disturbed in dementing disorders but may suffer in any psychiatric disorder secondary to the lack of attention, etc.
Intelligence can be assessed from the school and work records and the general history but is more accurately done by special tests.
Insight and Attitude to Illness
Does he regard himself as ill?
What does the patient himself think is wrong?
Has he an appreciation that it is a psychiatric illness?
Does he understand the nature and extent of the disorder?
Does he think he can get well?

The relationship between patient and doctor
The patient's co-operation, suspiciousness, demanding or passive behaviour, and any change in relation to the interview is important as also are the doctor's own reactions to the patient. Excessive feelings of irritation or sympathy by the doctor are often important cues to the nature of the patient's (usually neurotic) disorder.

Examination, psychiatric

In all cases an attempt should be made to answer the following questions:
1. Why has this particular patient developed psychiatric symptoms at this particular time?
2. Why has he developed this particular type of disorder?
3. What methods of treatment are indicated?
4. What is the prognosis for the present disorder and for the future?
This is done by taking a careful history from the patient and a close relative or friend, examination of the mental state and by a thorough physical examination.
The skill of interviewing seems to reside in the early establishment of rapport with the patient and taking the role of participant observer. The psychiatrist must know clearly the order in which he wants the data, but must let the patient talk about things in their natural order, redirecting the topic at times and sometimes going right back to an earlier phase to clarify some point. The patient is reassured if the psychiatrist understands what he is saying and indicates clearly when he does not understand the patient's meaning. The interview, which may need to be extended to two sessions, covers the history (present illness, previous health, personal history etc.) and provides cues as to what areas to focus on in the detailed examination.
Certain disorders, such as a classical schizophrenic illness or an organic dementia, can be diagnosed from the history of the present illness and examination of the mental state. In the majority of neuroses and affective disorders, however, greater attention must be paid to the patient's previous personality and life history. The essential point to remember is that anxiety, depression, etc. are symptoms, analogous to pyrexia in an infective illness, and diagnosis depends on the underlying cause. Mistakes in diagnosis and hence treatment of psychiatric disorders are generally due to assessing symptoms and ignoring aetiology.
The doctor should approach the problem of aetiology by asking himself what sort of personality the patient had before he became ill.
1. Is the patient a man who has never been able to make more than precarious adjustment in life? In such a case the life history will reveal the occurrence of psychiatric symptoms arising as a response to many events, some more stressful than others. If so, are his present symptoms applicable in terms of a personality disorder?
2. If his previous personality was a good one, has some stress occurred so out of the ordinary that he is now unable to cope, where he had always been able to do so before? These stresses may be physical, endocrine, or psychogenic and the latter may be non-specific or specific, where the patient is especially susceptible to the particular stress concerned. Furthermore, these stresses may be cumulative and additive. Thus a woman who is anaemic because of menorrhagia associated with the climacteric and looking after an ailing mother may break down following the additional stress of her husband's death.
3. Although the patient's personality is, on the whole, stable, he may be genetically predisposed to psychiatric illness, e.g. depression, so that a relatively mild stress will precipitate such an illness, often with characteristic features. Evidence of such a genetic predisposition may be found in the family history or in certain characteristics of the personality.
If after a search as has been outlined above no really convincing explanation can be found to show why this patient developed this particular disorder at this time, the case should be left *sub judice*. Further investigation may reveal some unsuspected organic disorder which is the underlying cause for the patient being unable to cope and for the consequent development of psychiatric symptoms. In essence, psychiatric diagnosis must be a positive one as diagnosis by 'exclusion' of an organic cause can be dangerous.
Similarly, while physical examination is always important, cues from the history indicate which bodily system requires the

most attention. Physical examination in young adult patients is quite often negative, but this information can be used to reassure the patient; likewise the fact of the examination reminds the patient that the psychiatrist is also a doctor.
SEE ALSO Forensic psychiatry.

Exhibitionism

Exhibitionism is the deliberate exposure of the male genitals, usually of the erect penis, to a passing female. It is carried out at a window, on some secluded pathway or close to a public toilet. Whilst the act has to induce surprise or even fear in the female subject to fully sexually excite the male, the exhibitionist is rarely if ever, intent on any form of physical or sexual assault. The practice commences in adolescence as a method of enhancing weak sex drive and becomes habitual, occurring after marriage during a wife's pregnancy, or when the individual has pent up aggressive feelings, or is sexually humiliated by his wife. Aversion therapy in phantasy situations, group psychotherapy and marital counselling are the most useful treatments. In recidivists chemical castration with oestrogen may be of value.

Existential psychiatry

Beginning with the phenomenological approach pioneered by Brentano and Husserl, which sought to distinguish between physical and mental phenomena, and particularly to study the latter, existential psychiatry has developed via the work of Jaspers, Binswanger, Medard Boss and Jean Paul Sartre. There is a strong philosophical background derived from Kierkegaard and Heidegger, and this, together with the fact that much of the literature is in German, has made existentialism and existential analysis a relatively closed book to many Anglo-American psychiatrists. Essentially the individual is seen as uniquely living a particular form of existence, an existence which includes moral and spiritual values and experiences, as well as inter-personal or intergroup relationships. Thus to understand the person, the therapist has to understand that person in relation to his mode of his existence – his being in the world (dasein). Existence may be stupid and meaningless to Sartre, or pathogenic to Laing – who sees the schizophrenic as a sane person in an insane world. Only by an analysis of modes of existence can the individual hope to change or come to terms with that existence; perhaps in the majority of cases inner calm is a matter of accepting existence, of giving up striving and futile desires, of making peace with God, and with the demands of society.

Exogenous depression
SEE Reactive depression.

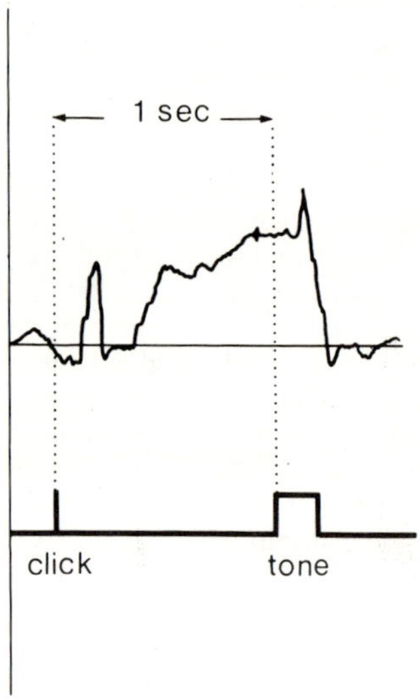

Expectancy wave

The expectancy wave or contingent negative variation (CNV) is a change in the electroencephalogram preceding a voluntary act. Typically it is elicited by presenting two stimuli about one second apart and requiring the subject to respond to the second one. A negative potential builds up at the vertex following the first stimulus and collapses as the subject responds. Abnormalities of the CNV may occur in anxiety states and psychoses.

Exposure, indecent
SEE Exhibitionism.

Extrapyramidal syndromes

These syndromes are related to abnormal functioning of the extrapyramidal motor system, the basal ganglia. An imbalance between cholinergic (q.v.) and dopaminergic (q.v.) neurones is probably involved in most cases. This commonly results from temporary or permanent interruption of the dopaminergic nigro-striatal pathway.

The commonest form is Parkinsonism characterized by the classical triad of akinesia, tremor and rigidity together with other features such as the festinant, shuffling gait, loss of associated movements, drooling of saliva, seborrhoea and sometimes oculogyric crises. Akathisic patients show great restlessness and agitation, tapping their feet, repeatedly standing up and sitting down or pacing to and fro. In dystonic states, muscle groups go into repeated spasms resulting in torticollis, opisthotonus, or retrocollis Dyskinesias consist of a group of related syndromes with repeated tic-like movements, especially of the tongue and mouth region. Other syndromes include chorea, ballismus and athetosis.

Extrapyramidal syndromes may be caused by vascular lesions, degeneration of the basal ganglia, and toxins such as carbon monoxide poisoning. Frequently, reversible syndromes occur during treatment with major tranquillizers such as the phenothiazines and butyrophenones. Acute dystonic reactions may occur after a few doses whereas Parkinsonian reactions are delayed a few weeks. Dyskinetic syndromes, usually irreversible, may occur in a few elderly patients after years of phenothiazine treatment.

Levodopa with or without a decarboxylase inhibitor is the most effective current therapy for Parkinsonism but is not effective in the drug induced condition. Other anti-Parkinsonism agents (q.v.) should be used if the dosage of the drug causing the disorder cannot be reduced.

Extrasensory perception (ESP)

Paranormal sensations, that is perceptions based on no recognized end organ stimulation, fall into four types of phenomena.

1. Telepathy – thought transference from person to person.
2. Clairvoyance – the perception of objects without sensory stimulation.
3. Precognition – the perception of a future event.
4. Psychokinesis – the influencing of an external event by mental concentration.

There are a number of psychologists who consider that evidence exists to suggest the reality of ESP; the majority, however, regard these phenomena as non-proven.

Extraversion

An extravert is an individual whose characteristic interests and modes of behaviour are directed outwards to other people and the physical environment. He is sociable, active and impulsive. By contrast, the introvert is inwardly directed to his own thoughts and feelings and his interests are theoretical rather than practical. Jung (q.v.) saw these as two distinct personality (q.v.) types but psychological testing of large groups indicates a continuous dimension of extraversion-introversion with most people falling within the central ambivert range.

Falsification, retrospective

Some degree of falsification of memory is normal; it is the degree and type of falsification which transforms it into a pathological condition. It occurs then in psychopathic personalities, particularly pathological liars, in organic states such as Korsakoff's syndrome, and in functional psychoses such as schizophrenia. It may be extremely difficult clinically to establish just where truth ends and falsehood begins. SEE ALSO Confabulation, Ganser syndrome, Hysterical pseudo-dementia, Memory, and Pseudo-reminiscence.

Family

The family is part of a total social structure made up of a number of systems: marriage, family, kinship, religious, ethical, economic and so on. Within this complex structure the family itself is composed of many elements. First, there is the nuclear family, consisting of two different sexed adults, in a socially approved sexual relationship, with one or more children resulting from the union, or reared within this nuclear unit. In certain societies the joint or extended family includes within it the nuclear family, but is a larger kinship group living in the same area, patrilocal or matrilocal, with certain mores and maybe related by blood in the male or female lines. Marriage and parenthood may follow certain rules – endogamy or exogamy (marriage within or without the group), monogamy, polygamy, or polyandry. All kinship ties spring from the family, their strength depending on the social norms and patterns of the particular society. The family may be studied in a number of different ways, anthropologically, legally, economically, socio-psychologically, psychoanalytically, or from the viewpoint of religion. It is thus apparent that the subject is enormously complex, and that a true understanding of the family must be based on many frames of reference. In psychiatry, a relatively new and, as yet, ill-defined field of family psychiatry has been established largely by child psychiatrists who hope that an understanding of family dynamics may shed light on the behavioural and other disturbances of children (q.v.). The broken home (q.v.) may specifically play an important part in the aetiology of delinquency. For all mental illness, however, it is important for general practitioners to consider not only the effects of the family situation on the patient, but also the effects of the illness on the other members of the family.

Family therapy

The sick person can be regarded in a number of different ways, as a sick individual, as a sick member of society, or as a sick member of the most important sub-group of society, the family. Increasing awareness of the strains and the tensions within families, the analysis of sick roles, and the contributions of child psychiatry have all turned many psychiatrists away from the treatment of the individual, to the treatment of the family. The family is considered to have a dynamic all of its own, produced by the complex interactions of its members, all related one to the other, and by societal norms for family behaviour. Thus family therapy differs from group therapy, when the group comes together as a group artificially created by the therapist. A knowledge of the family structures and behaviours acceptable to the particular society must underpin the therapist's understanding of personal and inter-personal dynamics, for the goal of therapy is to create a healthy family, that is, a family able to cope with the internal and external problems confronting it, and so to establish the basis for what might be called a happy family life. Therapy may be carried out in the home itself, and the therapist may be assisted by a co-therapist, usually of the opposite sex. The commonest indications for family therapy are conflict between man and wife, or between parents and children, although it is often used as a blunderbuss prescription for all types of psychiatric disturbance.

Fantasy
SEE Phantasy

Fatigue

A state of weariness resulting from bodily or mental exertion which is of medical significance if its severity is disproportionate to the setting. It is a common symptom of many physical illnesses, but psychological factors may be an important contributory element and are sometimes predominant. It may also be a conspicuous feature of depressions and chronic anxiety states. In some individuals it is prominent and enduring in the absence of physical illness, depression, or anxiety.
SEE ALSO Neurasthenia.

Fear

The emotional response to consciously recognized and external sources of danger. The subjective experience ranges from mild apprehension and uneasiness to intense dread. Somatic and physiological concomitants are mediated especially by the autonomic nervous system and endocrine glands. There is an immediate rise in serum catecholamines, e.g. adrenaline, and a later rise in serum cortisol. Dilated pupils, cutaneous vasoconstriction with increased muscle blood flow, increase in heart rate and stroke volume, sweating and tremor prepare the subject for a fight or flight reaction.
Fear may be distinguished from anxiety for in the latter the source of danger is largely unknown or unrecognized and is primarily of intrapsychic origin. In free floating anxiety there is lack of a consciously recognized source of danger for attachment of the anxious feeling. Phobic reactions are pathological fears. Some situation, person, object or creature is invested with special significance and the subject becomes fearful on confrontation.

Feeblemindedness
SEE Mental subnormality.

Feedback mechanisms

A process within the body by which the activity of a control area is itself governed by the substance or activity it controls. Thus, within the endocrine system, the secretion of hypophyseal trophic hormone is inhibited by raised levels of hormone derived from the target endocrine gland. Feedback is also a common feature in central nervous system control, for example, the use of proprioceptive information from the muscles in the control of finesse of movement by the cerebellum.
SEE ALSO Biofeedback

Fellatio

Fellatio is the stimulation of the male genitals by the mouth. The male penis is inserted into the mouth of the female partner. As a form of pre-coital stimulation fellatio occurs in about 50% of normal, well-adjusted marriages. Fellatio is also commonly practised by some homosexuals, and may be the preferred mode of sexual activity.

Fetishism

Fetishism, from the Portuguese for a charm, is the sexual perversion whereby an animate or inanimate object, not usually regarded as sensuous, becomes the fixed and exclusive stimulus for sexual arousal. Common fetishistic objects are mackintoshes, furs, hair, shoes, rubber garments, cigarettes and leather handbags, and the fetishist may involve himself in criminal acts in order to obtain them. Many fetishists marry and are potent, providing their wife partakes in the fetish (sexual piquantism). The condition is sometimes aetiologically related to brain damage, especially to temporal lobe epilepsy. Treatment is by aversion therapy (q.v.) and counselling psychotherapy with the marital partners.

5-hydroxytryptamine
SEE Serotonin.

Fitness to plead
(Synonym: Insanity on arraignment)

If an accused is so mentally disordered that it would be unjust to proceed with the trial, it may be postponed, sometimes indefinitely. Such a decision is normally

only taken in the presence of severe mental disorder and of a serious charge, for the result may be compulsory detention in a mental hospital without trial. The issue depends on different definitions in different countries but a typical example is that the accused should be capable of: (a) instructing counsel; (b) appreciating the significance of pleading 'guilty' or 'not guilty'; (c) challenging a juror; (d) examining witnesses; (e) understanding and following the evidence and court procedure.
SEE ALSO Forensic psychiatry.

Fits

One of a wide variety of terms used to designate the visible behavioural expression of epileptic disorders. Perhaps better reserved for the behavioural syndrome, typified by what (in common belief) an epileptic seizure looks like. In this way it expresses a presenting complaint, the basis for differential diagnosis.

Fixation

The arrest or cessation of psychosexual development at some given point in the maturing process. It may be a transient, temporary and normal block in maturation or become more permanent and pathological giving rise to neuroses or personality deviations. The term was used by Freud in his scheme of psychodynamic personality development so that fixation may occur at oral, anal or phallic stages of development. Fixation at one of these stages is then held to account for sexual deviations in which the organ of the particular stage is the focus of the abnormal sexual interest and activity.
SEE ALSO Infantile sexuality.

Fixed postures

Fixed postures are the immobile, statuesque, attitudes adopted for long periods by catatonic patients. Such positions as standing with arms elevated, on one foot, or lying with the head lifted from the pillow, would not be sustained in normal people because of the discomfort. The phenomenon is a rare but dramatic manifestation of catatonic schizophrenia (q.v.).
SEE ALSO Flexibilitas cerea.

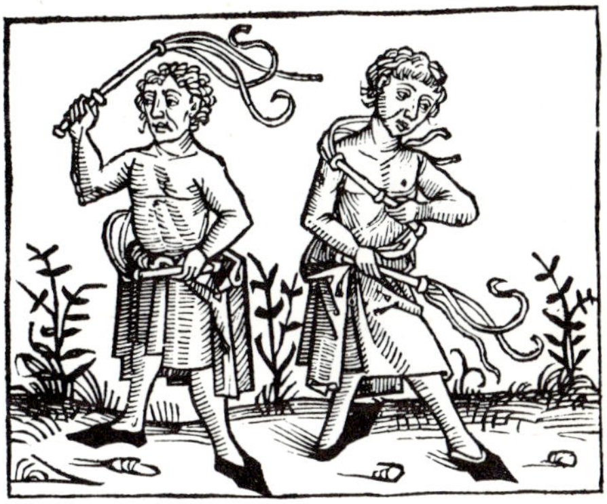

Flagellation

Flagellation is a common form of sadomasochistic perversion in which sexual excitement, orgasm and ejaculation are induced through whipping the trunk, buttocks or breasts. The whipping is usually performed by the woman, but the man may also be the active flagellator. Self-flagellation is practised as a group activity in some societies. The whip is a penis symbol inducing contortions of pain resembling orgasm in the recipient. The weak sexual drive of the patient is enhanced through summation with emotional excitation of pain. Much erotic literature deals with flagellation; it is said to be a particularly English perversion.

Flexibilitas cerea

Flexibilitas cerea is a manifestation of automatic obedience (q.v.) in which the subject allows his limbs to be placed in uncomfortable postures which he retains. While being moved in this way a smooth, uniform, mild resistance can be perceived similar to that of wax. The condition is characteristic of schizophrenia (q.v.) but also occurs in diffuse brain disorders.
SEE ALSO Fixed postures.

Flight of ideas

A characteristic feature of the speech of manic (q.v.) patients. As the pressure of speech builds up the patient's train of thought starts to change almost from one phrase to the next and it is these changes which constitute the 'flight of ideas'. They are often based on irrelevant similarities in the pronunciation of unrelated words ('clang associations') and may be genuinely if unintentionally witty: 'Of course I'm not ill. I'm not even illegitimate. My mother was a nice girl, at least until she grew up. Right up. Right up yours. Mine's a double Scotch, if you get round to asking. Are you Scotch too? Or just a psychiatrist? I know a joke about psychiatrists . . .'

Flooding

Or 'implosion'. In desensitization (q.v.) the subject approaches feared situations gradually without anxiety, usually in imagination but sometimes also in reality. In flooding, on the other hand, the patient is confronted in imagination or reality with his most feared situation at once, and encouraged to remain in contact with that situation until the evoked anxiety subsides.
Animal phobias are the most common phobias treated by flooding when anxiolytic drugs during the first one or two treatment sessions make the treatment more acceptable.

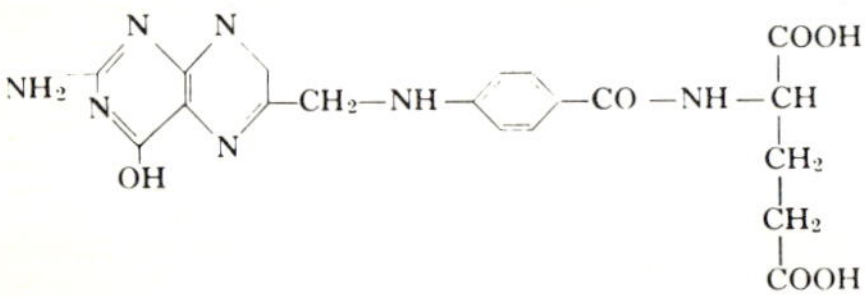

Folic acid

The mental symptoms associated with folic acid deficiency resemble those seen in cobalamin (q.v.) deficiency. Although macrocytic anaemia is usually present, some cases occur without the anaemia or bone marrow changes and the only confirmatory finding may be a low serum folate.
Drug-induced folate deficiency is particularly liable to occur in epileptic patients.

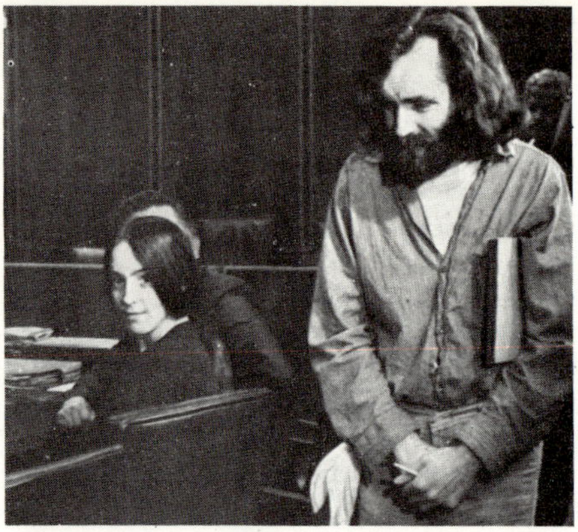

Charles Manson and Susan Atkins on trial in Los Angeles for multiple murder.

Folie à deux

This term refers to the phenomenon of two closely associated people suffering similar mental illnesses simultaneously. Usually the affected subjects are members of a family, husband and wife, or are at any rate living in close association. Although affective disorders can occur in this way, the term refers more to paranoid states (q.v.), particularly where delusions are shared and acted on by both partners. Sometimes more than two people are affected. In a recent widely reported case in America some members of a group of people living together were induced to commit random, purposeless murders; they were described as being 'hypnotized' by the dominant member of the group and acted on remote, eccentric beliefs propagated by him. It is usual to find in 'communicated insanity' of this kind that one member of the partnership is dominant and that if they are separated (e.g. by hospital admission) the illness of the acquiescent partner abates rapidly.

Folie circulaire

SEE Manic-depressive psychosis.

Folie de doute

A form of obsessional thinking; persistent doubting. The subject remains unsure if he has turned off the gas, extinguished a cigarette or put the gramophone records

back in the right order; he may have to check several times.
SEE ALSO Compulsion.

Folie de toucher

The compulsion to touch objects is observed in subjects with obsessive compulsive neurosis (it is also seen in normal children). Dr Samuel Johnson is reputed to have felt compelled to touch every second railing in certain London streets.

Forearm blood flow

This physiological measurement, recorded by means of intermittent venous occlusion plethysmography, has been used in psychiatric research as a measure of blood flow through muscles. Anxious patients have high blood flows especially during panic. Retarded depressed patients have normal or even low levels.

Forensic psychiatry

The application of the principles of general psychiatry to a population that comes into conflict with the law, plus a degree of knowledge sufficient to give useful specialist advice within a court of law. Medical advice in relation to marriage (q.v.), divorce (q.v.), testamentary capacity (q.v.), contract (q.v.) etc. all fall within the broad forensic heading. The forensic psychiatrist is mainly concerned with personality disorders (q.v.), psychopathic disorder (q.v.), alcoholism (q.v.), sexual disorders (q.v.) and sometimes drug addiction.
The role of the psychiatrist in court procedure is discussed under legal aspects of psychiatry (q.v.).
The psychiatrist is under increasing pressure to treat as medical problems individuals, who formerly were regarded solely as penal problems. Attempts have been made to offer medical treatment to the psychopath, the most difficult problem the forensic psychiatrist has to face. Many hospitals other than the special hospitals (q.v.) are reluctant to become involved with antisocial patients, unless they are psychotic, owing to the structure of the mental hospital, the open door policy, and the difficulties in controlling antisocial patients in such situations. The Prison Medical Department of England and Wales has established small psychotherapy clinics at many of the larger prisons, and set aside one establishment – Grendon Underwood – as a psychiatric prison (q.v.) with a medical officer as its governor.
SEE ALSO Criminal responsibility, Diminished responsibility, and Legal aspects of psychiatry.

Formication

SEE Paresthesia.

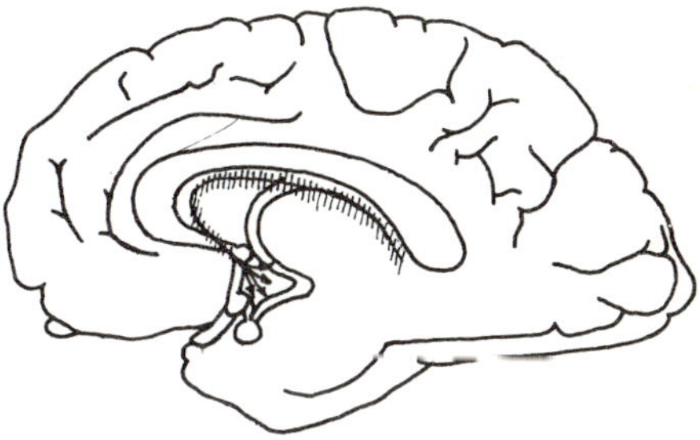

Fornix

The fornix arises from the hippocampus and forms one of the direct conducting systems from the primitive cortex to the hypothalamus. Its fibres end mainly in the mamillary bodies and the tuber cinereum. It is thus an integral connecting area within the limbic system (q.v.).

Fostering

Fostering is the process of arranging for persons not related to a child to care for and support that child by taking the child into their home and family. Under recent English legislation the definition of a foster child has been broadened to include all children of compulsory school age whose care and maintenance are undertaken by an unrelated person, irrespective of whether that person is financially rewarded or not. It differs from adoption (q.v.) in that the natural mother's rights with regard to the child are not irrevocably supplanted. Children's departments can board out (q.v.) juveniles to foster homes when they are given the special powers of a care order (q.v.) by a juvenile court.

Free association

This gives rise to trends of thought or chains of ideas which spontaneously arise into consciousness when restraint and censorship on logical thinking are removed and the subject reports orally everything that passes through his mind. It is a fundamental technique of modern psychoanalysis, initially used by Freud when he discovered the disadvantage of attempting to use the hypnotic techniques of Charcot to bring forward basic psychic material and make it available to analytical interpretation. The associations are determined by material, held unconscious by repression which may be released by this technique.

Free floating anxiety

A nameless dread or apprehension where the anxiety is unfocused or is attached to obvious trifles. This is in contrast to specific anxieties where the fear is of insanity, cancer or other bodily illness or of an external situation as in a phobic reaction of spiders or closed spaces.

Frequency distribution

The frequency distribution is the table constructed from a series of measurements of individuals, see table. This table shows the frequency with which some defined characteristic is present in the group under consideration. This frequency of observations can also be expressed in graphical form, e.g. histogram (q.v.).
SEE ALSO Mean, Median, Mode, Range, and Normal curve.

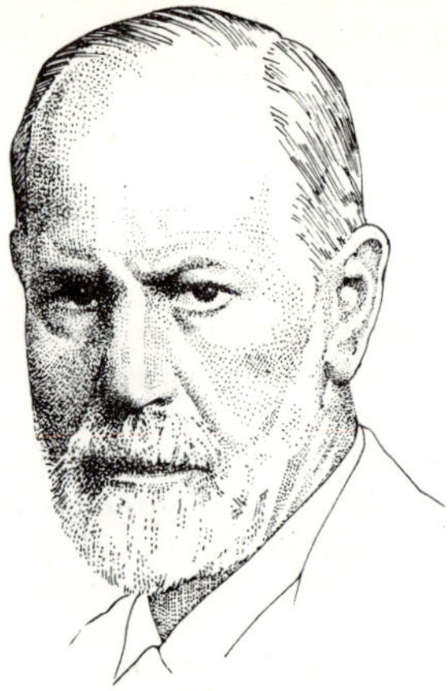

Sigmund Freud (1856 – 1939)

Freud, Sigmund (1856–1939)

Graduating from the University of Vienna in 1881, Freud had already spent some time in Brücke's physiological laboratory studying the histology of nervous system. As Privatdocent in neuropathology in Meynert's department of psychiatry he published studies on the acoustic nerve and the cerebellum and two important neurological books. Although not greatly attracted to the practice of medicine, Freud had to earn his living by seeing patients, many of whom were neurotics. Dissatisfied with the available therapeutic methods, chief of which was electrotherapy – Freud decided to visit Charcot's Clinic to learn about hypnosis. After about four months at the Saltpêtrière, Freud returned to Vienna and set up in practice. Patients were slow in coming and his fellow neurologists were critical of his overenthusiastic acceptance of Charcot's teaching. Freud began to collaborate with Josef Breuer (1842–1925) one of the most successful physicians in Vienna and co-discoverer of the Hering-Breuer reflex. Their book 'Studien über Hysterie' (1895) described the treatment by catharsis of female hysterics, but Freud also described the

Categories (in ascending order)	1	2	3	4	5	6	7	8	9	10	11	12	13	14	15
Number of observations	2	1	0	0	1	3	5	6	8	11	12	15	14	10	4

A hypothetical frequency distribution table showing a skew arrangement and outlying observations. These figures are also used for the diagrams showing mean, median, mode range and the histogram.

new method of 'free association' (q.v.) which had been suggested to him by one of the patients. By 1896 Freud was using the term psychoanalysis to describe his new technique. During the years 1894–9, Freud suffered from a number of psychiatric symptoms – anxiety, hypochondriacal and depressive in type. He began to analyse himself and to confide by letter in Wilhelm Fliess, a Berlin oto-rhino-laryngologist, who had some strange ideas on human psychology. Out of this period of turmoil, psychoanalytic theory was born. The 'Traumdeutung', (1900) – a book Freud always regarded as his major work, marked the end of his illness. In it Freud described some of the mental mechanisms concerned with both normal life and neurosis – repression, forgetting, symbolization, secondary elaboration, screen memories and so forth. The Oedipus complex, the id, the super-ego, the ego, and the castration complex – all came flowing out of Freud's fertile mind over the years. A devoted, albeit small, band of followers of great capacity spread psychoanalysis beyond the confines of Vienna, the Nazi persecution later dispersing many of them to the United States and England. Freud left Vienna in 1938 and found a home in London, where he died a year later.

Frigidity

Frigidity is the inability of the woman to become sexually aroused and experience orgasm in heterosexual intercourse. Primary frigidity (existing from the first attempts at coitus) is commonly found in patients with immature, hysterical personalities and is often associated with neurotic symptoms and may be a manifestation of underlying homosexuality (q.v.). Secondary frigidity (occurring after previous normal sexual responsiveness) is most commonly due to loss of sexual attraction for the husband due to his excessive demands, alcoholism, personal hygiene or simply to disenchantment.
It may also be secondary to long-standing dyspareunia. Frigidity after pregnancy may be symptomatic of a chronic puerperal depression. There is no evidence of a biological decline in orgasmic responsiveness after the menopause, although this does occur in later life.
Speed of sexual responsiveness has a normal distribution in the population. Some females are constitutionally predisposed to slow orgasmic response and may require many months or even years of a warm, stable, relationship with their partner to achieve speed of orgasmic attainment compatible with the partner. This difficulty will be further increased if the husband suffers from premature ejaculation (q.v.).
Counselling psychotherapy with both partners aims to promote mutual tolerance of the disorder, to educate and to release mutual fear and apprehension. Associated personality disorders and homosexuality may require more prolonged individual psychotherapy. Male sex hormones are known to stimulate female sexual responsiveness but often have undesirable masculinizing effects.
SEE ALSO Dyspareunia and Vaginismus.

Frontal lobe syndrome

The mental symptoms secondary to damage to the frontal lobes, e.g. from trauma, neoplasm, syphilis, Pick's presenile dementia and occasionally as an untoward effect after pre-frontal leucotomy. Change in personality is the characteristic feature with irresponsibility, facetiousness and perhaps antisocial behaviour, leading in more severe cases to apathy, anergia and even mutism.

Frotteurism

Frotteurism is the deliberate rubbing of the male's genitals against some unsuspecting female's clothed buttocks in order to provoke orgasm. It usually takes place in crowded public places such as trains, lifts or railway platforms.
Mutual erotic arousal may occur between a male and female rubbing elbows or legs together, again in some crowded, public place. The anticipatory fear of being discovered greatly contributes to the over-all sexual excitement.

Fugue

A condition of altered consciousness in which the subject wanders away from his home or work. Often a fugue occurs in the setting of a depressive illness and sometimes appears to be a symbolic equivalent to suicide. As part of the spectrum of automatic behaviour seen in epilepsy (psychomotor seizures) a fugue is associated with mental clouding, feelings of unreality or déjà vu (q.v.) hallucinations and mood changes (fear, rage, depression etc.). An hysterical fugue (dissociative reaction) is related to an intolerable situation from which the subject feels compelled to escape; there is often partial or complete amnesia for the event. A fugue may also occur in organic brain damage, e.g. after a head injury.

GABA
SEE Gamma aminobutyric acid.

Galactosaemia

Galactosaemia is inherited as an autosomal recessive trait. The specific biochemical defect is lack of galactose-l-phosphate uridyl transferase activity. It is primarily a disease of early infancy; acute symptoms include vomiting, diarrhoea, jaundice, failure to thrive. Some patients show mental retardation. The diagnosis is made biochemically by an abnormal galactose tolerance curve and by presence of galactose in the urine. Biochemical demonstration of the missing enzyme gives confirmatory evidence. Symptom-free cases have been described, or isolated signs may appear late in life, such as cataracts and cirrhosis of the liver.
Treatment is dietary, based on lactose and galactose restriction. This should be started as soon after birth as possible; children treated later may still improve but some effects (e.g. cataracts, mental subnormality) may then be irreversible.
SEE ALSO Inherited metabolic defects.

Gall, Franz Joseph (1758–1828)

The founder of phrenology, Gall began his career as an anatomist with a special interest in the nervous system. He attempted to correlate personality traits with the shape of the skull, which was supposed to mirror the anatomy of the brain beneath. This early attempt at cerebral localization fascinated the contemporary medical world, but led to extravagant claims eventually discrediting what was originally a serious study of brain function.
SEE ALSO Phrenology.

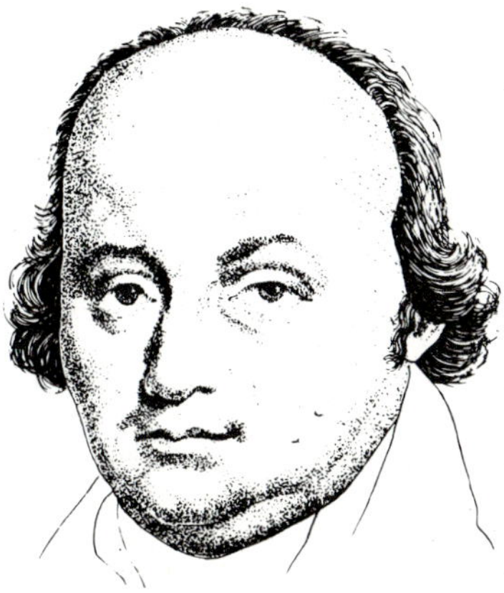

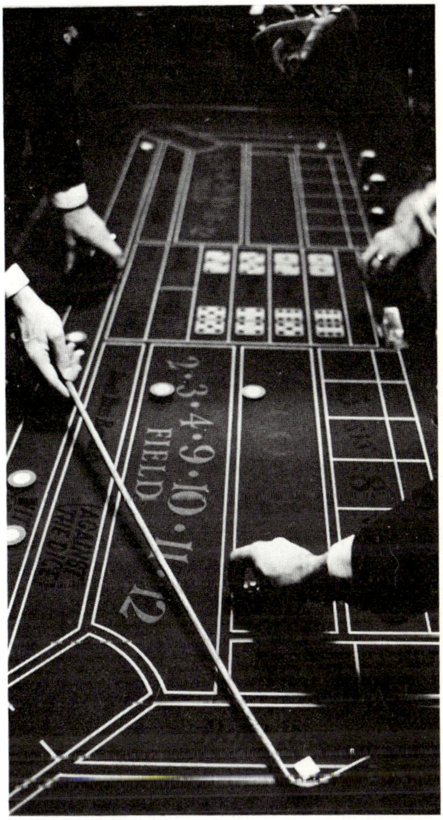

Gambling

Gambling is sometimes regarded as a psychiatric symptom; certainly the form (i.e. horse-racing, football pools etc.) and the intensity of the habit, which is socially acceptable, are tied to the culture. It is commoner in males and certain nationals (i.e. Irish, Italians etc.). Freud suggested that gambling was a masturbatory equivalent and others a form of sado-masochism. Recently its relationship to 'fate' and attitudes to external control have been emphasized and the high incidence of suicide in gamblers is of interest in relation to similar attitudes to external control found by some authors in accident proneness and patients with suicidal potentiality.

Successes have been claimed with behaviour therapy (q.v.) and referral to Gamblers Anonymous or some similar organization may be helpful.
SEE ALSO Forensic psychiatry.

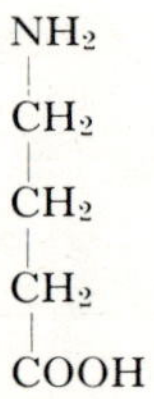

Chemical structure of γ aminobutyric acid

Gamma aminobutyric acid (GABA)

This simple aminoacid is a peripheral neuronal transmitter in some animals and it is almost certainly a brain transmitter in man. Its action is always inhibitory. Blockade of its action leads to convulsions. It is formed from glutamate by decarboxylation by an enzyme which has pyridoxine as a co-factor. This may be relevant to the epilepsies associated with pyridoxine deficiency, particularly those in infancy.
SEE ALSO Biochemical and neurophysiological background to mental disease.

Gangs

Younger children tend to play or be delinquent mainly as individuals, but towards puberty, gregariousness becomes stronger. The larger social unit of the gang then becomes established, particularly in working-class areas and particularly where other social opportunities are lacking, such as in large housing estates. Whether or not a gang exists mainly for delinquent purposes, or mainly for social support and joint activities, depends both on social conditions in its home district and on the personality of the leader(s). At different periods, gangs tend to take up a prevailing fashion.
Towards the end of adolescence, most members tend to break away and courting or marriage takes the place of gang activities.

Ganser syndrome

In 1898 Ganser described a condition occurring in prisoners characterized by disturbances of memory, hallucinations, and behavioural changes which appear calculated to impress the observer with the subject's madness. Thus, when asked 'How many legs has a cow?' the reply may be 'Five'. Despite the apparently simulated nature of the symptoms, their gross nature and simplicity, the possibility of an underlying schizophrenic illness should not be underestimated. The condition most probably represents a simple-minded delinquent's response to his environment whilst experiencing the internal psychological changes of a developing mental illness.
SEE ALSO Hysterical pseudo-dementia and Malingering.

Gargoylism

The term gargoylism embraces two conditions in the group of mucopolysaccharidoses. These are Hurler's syndrome and Hunter's syndrome. Both are usually associated with severe mental subnormality and with multiple skeletal changes, dwarfing of stature, hepatosplenomegaly and cardiovascular deficits. Biochemical investigation of the urine shows excessive amounts of chondroitin sulphate B and heparitin sulphate.
SEE ALSO Inherited metabolic defects and Mental subnormality.

Gastro-intestinal psychosomatic disorders

SEE Psychosomatic disorders.

Gate theory of pain

This is the most recent theory of pain and includes some of the previous theories of receptor specialization and patterning. It incorporates the newer concepts of feedback and central control.
Under the gate theory, stimulation of the skin evokes nerve impulses that are transmitted to the central nervous system via A (fast) fibres and C (slow) fibres. There the impulses affect three spinal cord systems: cells of the substantia gelatinosa

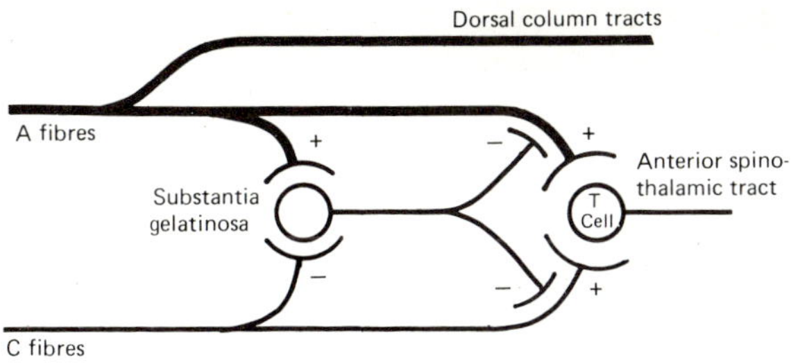

Gate theory of pain

in the dorsal horn; dorsal column fibres; T cells of the dorsal horn.

The combination of input determines by which route impulses reach the central nervous system and thus which sensations they evoke. Unmyelinated C fibres are non-selective and may respond to modalities other than noxious stimuli so impulses transmitted by them do not specify the nature of the stimulus; the small myelinated A fibres on the other hand are modality specific.

Gating is a device for combining the two inputs to distinguish pain from other stimuli. A fibres enter the dorsal columns via the medial divisions of the dorsal roots but also have excitatory terminations on the T cells and substantia gelatinosa cells of the dorsal horn (see diagram). C fibres also terminate via excitatory endings on T cells but are inhibitory on substantia gelatinosa cells. The substantia gelatinosa cells in turn exert a presynaptic inhibitory influence on T cell afferents. The T cells themselves send fibres to the anterolateral spinothalamic tract.

If C fibres are active the substantia gelatinosa cells are inhibited, there is no presynaptic inhibition of the T cells and the resulting transmission of impulses through the anterolateral system is interpreted as pain. If A fibres are active there is transmission in the dorsal columns but the T cells are inhibited via the substantia gelatinosa cells.

Whether a stimulus gives rise to pain or another modality of sensation depends on the relative number of the A fibres that are stimulated and also the inherent properties of these fibres, i.e. C fibres tend not to adapt while A fibres do.

It appears that the T-cell output must reach a certain threshold before pain is produced and descending fibres (probably reticulospinal fibres) affected by emotion and attention etc., exert control over the sensory input.

At higher areas of the central nervous system pain gives rise to a complex sequence of behaviour which cannot be accounted for simply by a pain centre. A major portion of the higher brain centres, triggered by input from the T system, and probably activated by collaterals to the reticular formation, is implicated in this perception and behaviour pattern.

Gaucher's disease

Gaucher's disease is a disorder in infancy and childhood of lipid metabolism resulting in the accumulation of cerebroside in the cells of the reticulo-endothelial system. Clinical signs include hepatomegaly, splenomegaly, neurological and intellectual impairment with progressive deterioration. About one third of reported cases have been familial; there is good evidence that it is transmitted by an autosomal dominant gene.

SEE ALSO Inherited metabolic defects.

Gender role

Gender role is all those things a person says or does to disclose himself or herself as having the status of a boy, man, girl or woman. It is primarily determined by the presence or absence of the Y-chromosome in the genetic constitution.

The Y-chromosome directly influences the type of foetal gonad whose intrauterine hormone secretion is responsible for the sexual dimorphism of the internal and external genitalia and the ultimate sexual responsiveness of the brain.

In normal individuals this sexual anlage is

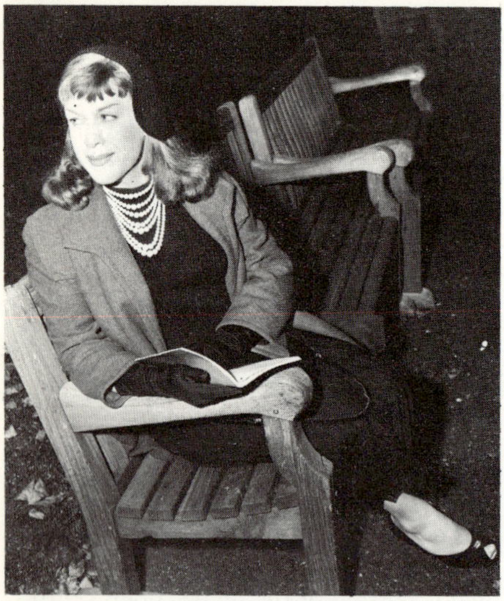

Gender role – transexualism

congruous with the sex of assignment at birth, sex of rearing, and the subsequent gender role. In cases of pseudo-hermaphroditism (q.v.) the true sex may be wrongly assigned at birth resulting in the individual being reared and having the gender role of the opposite sex. Gender role can (contrary to what was previously held) be successfully changed in these cases even in adolescence. Male intersexes have an increasing dissatisfaction with their wrongly assigned female gender role in adolescence and often require surgical and social change to their true sex. Transexualism (q.v.) is a psychological cross-gender identification where a true male or female is convinced they are a member of the opposite sex and are only at ease in the gender role of that sex.
They not infrequently demand surgical cosmetic procedures to their genitalia etc. to allow them completely to indentify with what they feel is their correct gender role. There is, as yet, no uniform psychiatric or surgical opinion about the advisability of these mutilating procedures upon the normal genitalia.

General paralysis of the insane (GPI)

Kraft-Ebing's dictum that general paralysis is a product of syphilization and civilization is no longer true in that the disease has virtually disappeared from the Western world.
This disease was eradicated by malaria inoculation, massive penicillin therapy (in courses of 10–20 million units), sex education, and the early treatment of syphilis. GPI appears ten or more years after primary infection. The whole cortex is atrophied and a progressive dementia with a psychosis develops – classically with grandiose delusions, but now more often depressive or confusional – associated with dysarthria, trombone tongue, spastic paraplegia, fits, and the Argyll Robertson pupil. Disease activity is determined particularly by a cellular response in the cerebro-spinal fluid as well as a 'paretic' curve in Lange's colloidal gold test, increased globulin and total protein, and a positive Wasserman reaction. General paralysis may be associated with tabes dorsalis (q.v.), (taboparesis).
SEE ALSO Syphilis and Infections, Mental symptoms due to.

General systems theory

A theoretical concept that considers events as interacting organized components ('systems'). The behaviour of the system depends on the interaction of its constituent parts and the systems themselves interact to form suprasystems. The systems theory as applied to psychology stresses the approach to the individual in totality as a balance of the interrelated and interdependent systems that affect human behaviour. It is related in principle to the Gestalt (q.v.) theory.

Genetics

The gene is a hypothetical basic unit of heredity corresponding to large and elaborately constructed molecules of desoxyribonucleic acid (DNA) which are transmitted from one generation to the next unchanged unless altered by mutation. This hereditary material exerts effects through its control of biochemical reactions, accelerating some and retarding others. It is necessary to think of the genetic constitution (genotype) as acting as a whole, the cumulative effect of minor influences of many genes of small effect

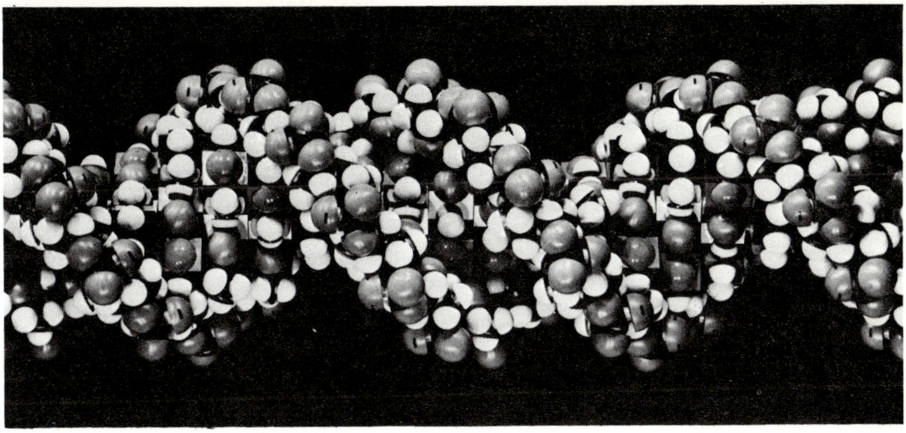

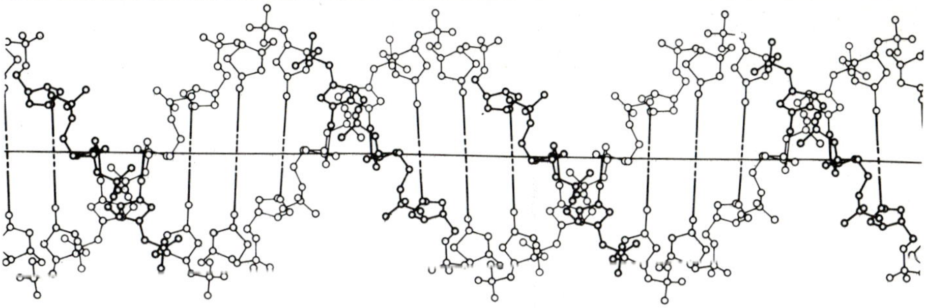

Model of the DNA molecule

being important as well as the major effect of single genes. Genes may be influenced by the external environment, the internal environment of the body, and the effect of other genes, the observable manifestation (phenotype) being the result of the interaction of all these factors.

The classical methods of genetical research include the statistical, genealogical proband method. This involves taking a random sample of patients suffering from the disease to be studied and ascertaining the incidence of the disorder in the relatives. A higher incidence than that among the general population will suggest that the disorder is familial, but a particular distribution among the generations of relatives might be suggestive of a specific genetical mode of inheritance. For example a manifestation of a condition among 50% of offspring in successive generations will suggest a dominant gene of full expressivity. A recessive condition would be suggested by an increased rate of consanguinity amongst parents, apparent clinical normality in the parents, and a manifestation of about 25% in the children with sharp segregation between normal and affected sibs. Another classical genetical investigation is the study of twins. This assumes that whereas uniovular twins have identical genetical make-up, binovular twins are genetically no more alike than ordinary siblings. Thus, a higher concordance rate for any trait or disorder in uniovular twins is strong evidence for it having a strong genetical basis.

Observations made along these lines have shown that specific psychiatric conditions and subnormality syndromes, personality traits and many psychosomatic disorders have a marked genetical basis.

In addition to these classical types of investigation, genetics can be used for the specific classification and indentification of psychiatric syndromes. Thus involutional melancholia has been demonstrated by genetical studies to be basically the same illness as other endogenous depressive disorders. On the other hand, there is now strong evidence that the bipolar manic-depressive disorders are genetically distinct from the unipolar recurrent depressions. Furthermore since genes act bio-

chemically this suggests that these are biochemically distinct illnesses and may eventually respond best to different types of therapy. In fact far from being therapeutically sterile, a genetical identification of a disorder stimulates research into its biochemical cause and hence treatment, e.g. phenylketonuria (q.v.) and galactosaemia (q.v.).
Genetical studies may also be used to identify non-genetical, e.g. psychological, factors of importance. Thus in uniovular twins with identical genetical make-up and who are discordant for the illness under study there is a strong inference that some environmental and perhaps psychological factor was important in precipitating the illness and a series of such cases can be very useful in identifying the types of stress which may be relevant.
Finally pharmacogenetics are assuming increasing importance. It is well known that approximately 50% of the population are slow inactivators of isoniazid, that this is genetically determined and that such patients have a higher incidence of side effects such as peripheral neuropathy. Recent work on plasma levels of tricyclic anti-depressant (q.v.) drugs suggests that genetical factors are important in their metabolism and may thus affect the patient's response and the dosage required.

Geriatric psychiatry

People aged 65 years or over now constitute a significant proportion of the population of most industrially developed countries (e.g. about 12% at present in England and Wales). The effect of the fall in birth rate is now nearly over, but the reduced mortality among the young will cause a permanent ageing of the population. In addition old people themselves are now living longer. The importance of these trends for psychiatry lies in the fact that degenerative changes in the brain and its vessels, and the mental disorders due to them, become progressively more common after 60 and reach their highest incidence in the eighth and ninth decades. Geriatric health and welfare will therefore increasingly need to be geared to the requirements of the very old, which are not identical with those of the younger aged, among whom non-organic disorders are of more importance.
There is no sharp dividing line between the psychiatry of the young and the old, and many disorders which begin earlier in life may persist or recur in old age, when they tend to be modified by the psychological (q.v.) and physical changes of ageing. The following scheme refers to disorders that begin in old age. It is basically descriptive, but embodies what is known about aetiology, and is useful for prognosis and management.

Organic psychoses	Dementias (chronic brain syndromes) Acute confusional states (delirium, acute brain syndromes) Late paraphrenia (chronic delusional psychoses)
Functional disorders	Affective disorders of late onset (depression mania) Neurotic (psychogenic) reactions and personality changes (q.v.).

The dementias of old age are generally progressive and have a high mortality. Some 6–7% of those aged 65 or over suffer from dementia of at least moderate severity, 1–2% living in institutions, the remainder at home. After the age of 80, some 20% are affected. Arteriosclerotic and senile dementia (q.v.) are the most important forms, and may be distinguished from each other by the occurrence of cerebro-vascular accidents in the former. Acute confusional states (q.v.) due to generalized brain dysfunction from diverse causes are common; unless there is also an underlying dementia, the mental state, if the patient survives, generally returns to normal. Late paraphrenia (see Persecutory states in the aged) has a good prognosis for life but requires indefinitely prolonged treatment. Affective disorders (q.v.) are far commoner; they generally respond well to treatment but tend to relapse; suicide or associated physical illness may shorten life. Neurotic reactions may be set off by physical illness in previously stable people, and may prolong convalescence. 15–20% of old people have functional symptoms that give rise to some restriction and disability.
As in geriatric medicine, multiple diagnosis is often appropriate. For example, patients with senile dementia may also suffer from cerebro-vascular disease.

Emotional disorders are common in the early stages of dementia or after a stroke; and unlike the organic illness they are amenable to treatment. Depression may lead to dietary deficiencies with secondary avitaminosis or electrolyte disturbance which in turn may produce an organic syndrome.

An important point is that drugs often have unwanted, even dangerous effects in the aged. Neuroleptics may cause ataxia or hypotension, with a tendency to fall, or urinary retention or acute glaucoma. Treatment of physical diseases may also bring about psychiatric complications. During anaesthesia hypotension may result in cerebral anoxia with residual mental impairment. Anti-hypertensive drugs such as methyldopa, can cause depression, and the use of purgatives or diuretics without dietary supplements may result in potassium deficiency with general weakness, and, perhaps depression. Barbiturates, bromides, benzhexol and anti-diabetic agents may cause confusional states, and sudden withdrawal from heavy barbiturate medication may cause fits. The aged, in fact, run a special risk of iatrogenic disorder.

Old people who are depressed or demented are not likely to press their claims for medical help, and since their relatives may regard them as old rather than ill, their condition may be unreported until a late stage. Some form of registration of the aged, and regular visiting of them is therefore desirable. The general practitioner may find it helpful to have a health visitor or social worker attached to his practice to keep him informed at least of his 'high risk' patients, who include the very old and physically ill, the recently discharged from psychiatric treatment and the bereaved or isolated.

As people grow older they tend increasingly to rely on the support of others, and it has often been shown that the single, the childless widowed, the poor and those living alone make disproportionate demands on the Health and Welfare services. It is important to realize, however, that a failure to cope, which may appear to be indication for social support, may actually be due to physical or mental illness and be remediable by treatment. Effective medical services to which they have ready access, are among the essential social needs of the aged if they are to continue to be viable in the community.

The aged often need the services provided by different authorities and general practitioners are in a good position to co-ordinate these services to provide continuity of care. They need, however, to know what domiciliary services are available from their local authority and how to obtain them.

The relative merits of domiciliary as opposed to residential care and of mental and geriatric hospitals and welfare homes are being debated. Patients with acute affective or paranoid psychoses can and should be treated in ordinary short-stay psychiatric units but follow-up is specially important, because of relapse and suicide, and more use could be made of out-patient and day departments both for follow-up and for diagnosis.

The dementias are the main cause of difficulty. It is generally agreed that the patient must be kept at home for as long as possible, but to avoid rejection (q.v.) by the relatives some relief must be offered before the burden becomes too severe. This may take the form of day attendance, short-term admission for holiday or other purposes or a month-in, month-out system. The patient's condition should be reviewed regularly, and the effects on the family carefully gauged. Patients who live alone may be supported for a time by domiciliary services and help from neighbours, but residential care can be delayed too long. Welfare homes adapted for the 'elderly mentally infirm' (dements of advanced age without gross management problems) may be suitable for some, but those who are immobile, incontinent or disturbed need the facilities of a hospital. Patients with severe emotional or behaviour disturbances need mental hospital treatment.

Gerontosexuality

The choice of an old person – usually female – as a sexual object is encountered most often in criminal practice, a youth assaulting and raping a woman, or a number of women whose ages may range from 60 to 80 years. It may rarely occur in civil practice when a young man marries a woman in this age group. The causes lie in the particular type of relationship the individual has had with older women during his formative years, mental illness being rarely encountered.

Gerstmann's syndrome

Acalculia, right-left disorientation, agraphia and finger agnosia, either for the patient's fingers or the examiner's fingers, are found in patients with lesions of the left angular gyrus, and comprise Gerstmann's syndrome.

Gesell, Arnold (1880–1961)

Noted for his observations of children's behaviour at different stages of their development, he wrote many works on child psychology, and helped to popularize the subject in the United States. He founded the Clinic of Child Development at Yale University. His behavioural observations of children in a somewhat artificial setting led to an undervaluation of the effects of social and cultural factors on development.

Gestalt psychology

The German noun Gestalt is translated literally as form, structure, pattern or configuration but also implies an integrated whole which is more than the sum of its parts. This name and concept is closely associated with a school of psychology of which the main exponents were Max Wertheimer, Wolfgang Kohler and Kurt Koffka who, early this century, reacted strongly against the atomistic, analytic approaches of the contemporary behaviouristic and introspectionist schools. The basic argument of the gestalt psychologists was, and is, that mental processes and behaviour (q.v.) cannot be analysed into elementary units without neglecting the important organizational features related to the whole. The initial emphasis, was on the psychology of perception (q.v.) and stress was laid on 'figure-ground' relationships, 'gestalt' laws of organization, and field theories of cortical functioning. Later investigations extended into the areas of learning and thinking. Kohler's studies of insightful-problem-solving by apes are particularly well known.

Gilles de la Tourette syndrome

The aetiology is uncertain but organic factors are probably important, e.g. Sydenham's chorea. Symptoms are (a) complex convulsive tics, (b) compulsive utterances, often of obscene nature and associated with respiratory dyskinesia. Symptoms appear between 10 and 15 years, usually in males. Successes have been claimed for treatment with butyrophenones and behaviour therapy.

Globus hystericus

A feeling that there is 'a lump in the throat' may occur in conditions of anxiety or depression. This feeling usually interferes with breathing, which may come in sighs or gasps; at times it may be a manifestation of hyperventilation or of tetany.

Glucose-6-phosphate dehydrogenase

Glucose-6-phosphate dehydrogenase deficiency is an inborn error of metabolism transmitted often as a sex-linked recessive trait. Its mode of inheritance, however, together with the other features such as incidence, severity and clinical implications may vary in different racial groups. It is rare amongst northern Europeans. It is responsible possibly with other factors for severe neonatal haemolytic jaundice-kernicterus (q.v.) and subsequent mental subnormality. The ingestion of certain drugs and beans may lead to haemolytic anaemia in children with G-6-PD deficiency.
SEE ALSO Inherited metabolic defects.

Glue sniffing

Inhalation of industrial solvents to produce euphoria has been widely reported in America, rarely in the United Kingdom. The list of solvents employed is large and includes toluene, benzene, acetone, ethyl acetate, diethyl ether and hexane. Toluene is most commonly used because of its cheap availability in model aeroplane glue. The glue is squeezed into a rag and the vapour inhaled or concentrated by inhalation from a plastic bag. Its main use has

been by children and produces acute intoxication rather like simple drunkenness. Ataxia and dysarthria are common and the user may explode into excited behaviour. Hallucinations may also occur. This is followed by a hangover. Chronic glue sniffers are usually youngsters with early evidence of severe personality problems.
SEE ALSO Addiction.

Glutamic acid

An amino acid which is found in high concentration in the brain. Its function within the central nervous system is still unclear, but it may be an excitatory neuro-transmitter (q.v.) or be involved in the transport of potassium across the cell membrane. It also acts as a detoxifying agent for ammonia within nervous tissue.

Glycine

Glycine (an amino acid) is present in high concentration in brain tissue. Its exact function is unknown but it may act as an inhibitory neuro-transmitter (q.v.).

Glycol derivatives

The glycol derivatives or propanediols are minor tranquillizers derived from the muscle relaxant mephenesin. The principal members are meprobamate, tybamate and phenaglycodol.
The propanediols are mild central sedatives with muscle relaxant and some anticonvulsant activity, acting by depression of the thalamus and limbic system. The clinical spectrum resembles that of the barbiturates, but with less hypnotic potency.

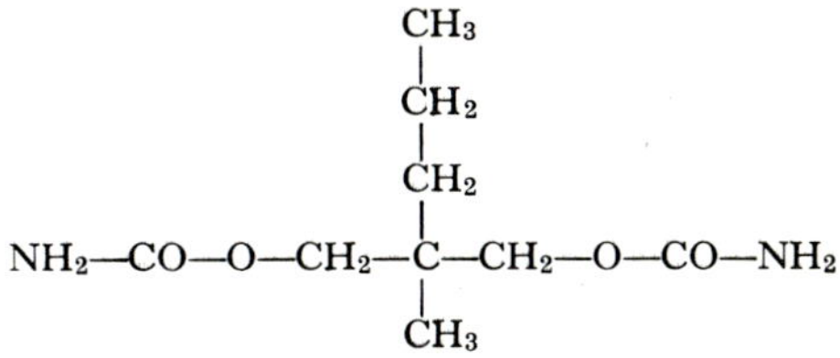

Chemical structure of meprobamate, a glycol derivative

Meprobamate was extensively used as an anxiolytic agent but has been largely superseded by more effective drugs. The advantages, if any, of the more recently introduced derivatives have still to be established. The main side effects are drowsiness, anaphylactoid reactions, ataxia and drug dependence.
SEE ALSO Anxiolytic drugs.

Grand mal

The major convulsive seizure is characterized by loss of consciousness and loss of posture followed by a phase of tonic flexion or extension with severe inhibition of respiratory movements. The seizure may terminate at this stage or pass to the stage of repetitive clonic movements. The eyes may be open, the face suffused and purple. Urine and faeces may be voided. Foamy saliva tinged with blood issues from the mouth. Gradually the violent movements

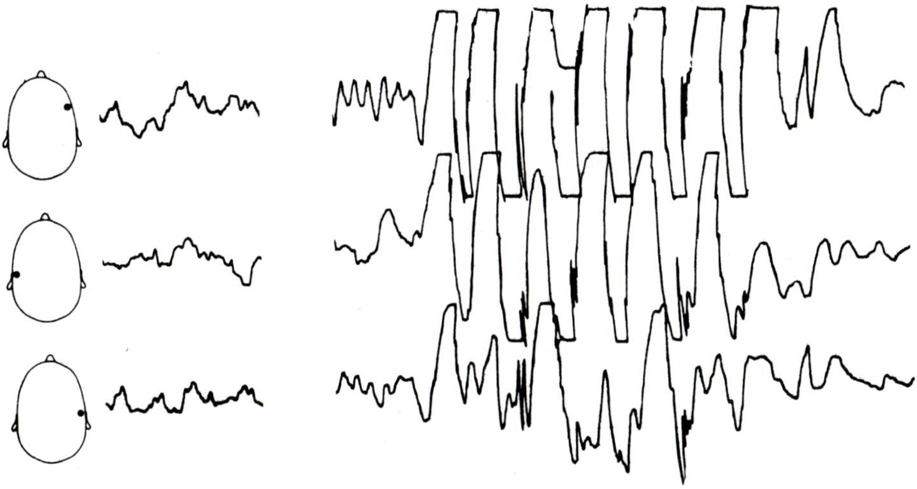

die down and relaxation ensues accompanied by an inspiratory groan. Unconsciousness persists for a variable period but prolonged coma or the reappearance of seizure movements suggests status epilepticus (q.v.). Post-ictal sleep frequently follows a brief phase of recovery of consciousness. A cry, shout or scream may precede the initial loss of tone. Restlessness and irritability occur in the post-ictal phase and interference by attendants at this time may precipitate an assault. Post-ictal automatisms (q.v.) are usually self-orienting. Recovery after sleep may be accompanied by depressed mood, but some persons wake refreshed.

The EEG obtained during a grand mal is usually heavily obscured by muscle artefact and is somewhat superfluous. A generalized rhythmic discharge of high amplitude spikes in the alpha/low beta range is usually generalized and symmetrical and synchronous in all surface leads, Post-ictal slowing into the delta band with suppression of the voltage precede the reappearance of normal or sleep rhythms.

First aid during the seizure should be confined to guarding the patient from dangerous items within his immediate compass. Tight clothing may be eased at the neck. Less damage to the mouth occurs if this is left alone, but oxygen may be administered.

SEE ALSO Epilepsy and EEG.

Grasp of general information

This part of the mental examination relates to (a) ability to assess the current situation and behave appropriately, (b) insight (q.v.) into the status of 'being a patient', and (c) comprehension of the wider context, i.e. events in the world. Tests for these components come under the headings 'orientation' (time, place and person); 'insight' (i.e. acceptance/non-acceptance of status as patient); and 'general information' (i.e. what was in the newspaper yesterday).

Grief

A painful emotional state occurring as a normal response to bereavement. Its severity and duration are very variable but a number of components can usually be recognized:

1. Somatic distress – sighing respiration, weakness and intermittent feelings of tension and unreality.
2. Disruption of normal behaviour patterns, resulting in lethargy or aimless activity. (This is, understandably, most prominent where previous behaviour patterns were largely dependent on the deceased).
3. Guilt feelings – inappropriate feelings of remorse for having been unsympathetic or neglectful towards the deceased person, or even for having caused, or contributed to, his death.
4. Hostility – angry outbursts directed at friends trying to offer comfort or at anyone associated with the death. Physicians and nurses sometimes bear the brunt of this hostility and it is important for them to recognize it for what it is, an irrational but essentially normal part of the emotional response to bereavement.
5. Preoccupation with an idealized image of the dead person and also difficulty believing that he is really dead.
6. Sometimes there is an element of identification with the dead person – taking over his interests, his mannerisms and sometimes his symptoms.

Normally these all begin to subside within a few weeks, though they may persist much longer. It is important to realize that the extent of the outward expression of grief and its duration varies between the different races. In the early stages it is nearly always beneficial for the bereaved person to weep and to express his feelings, including those of guilt and anger, and he should be gently encouraged to do so. It is often helpful initially to prescribe hypnotics, but the routine prescribing of tranquillizers and anti-depressants is to be deplored. Usually they are ineffective in this setting, they discourage the patients from expressing their grief openly, and they may sow the seeds of future dependence.

Grief reactions may become morbid either by being unduly prolonged or by developing into overt depressive illnesses with weight loss, agitation or retardation and suicidal impulses. This occurs most often in women widowed in middle age. The predominance in women may be because they lack the careers and outside interests

which help to sustain widowers, though depressions as a whole are commoner in women anyway. The dividing line between 'normal' and 'morbid' is necessarily arbitrary, but the latter should be assumed if definite signs of restitution are not developing after six months. Psychotherapeutic exploration of the patient's feelings about her husband and the circumstances of his death, together with encouragement and assistance in rejoining the life of the community, are usually the basis of management, but sometimes amylobarbitone interviews are necessary before the patient's feelings emerge, and if severe depressive symptoms are present tricyclic drugs (q.v.) or ECT (q.v.) may be required.
In the last decade evidence has accumulated to suggest that the mortality from a wide spectrum of physical illnesses, especially coronary artery disease, is raised in the first year after bereavement. The explanation for these findings is still obscure, but it seems likely that a complex and indirect, but none the less causal, relationship is involved.

Group psychotherapy

Any form of psychotherapy in which several persons are treated simultaneously, usually by one psychotherapist. Group therapy over the last twenty years has exerted a profound effect upon general psychiatry. Pioneered by S. H. Foulkes, Joshua Bierer and Maxwell Jones in the United Kingdom, group methods have spread to include a wide range of activities covering all types of patients. Group analytical psychotherapy is based on psychoanalytic principles established in individual psychoanalysis. Eight to ten patients discuss their problems in the presence of a passive therapist who makes use of transference interpretations. The group meets once a week, the session may last for ninety minutes, and the total period of therapy may encompass a period of two years. A group may be open or closed, meaning that new entrants may be taken in as members leave, or that the whole group is preserved intact until therapy finishes.
Directive group therapy is used for didactic or educational purposes, and may be of value in social groups such as ward patients, staff, or other professionals.
Activity group therapy is carried out with children or psychotic patients, the patients taking part in various forms of activity such as play dance, or art therapy.
Recently an explosion of group therapeutic activity has been seen in the United States, where 'sensitivity' groups act out these feeling problems in physical contacts and living activities. Various forms of group therapy are part of the cultural milieu of a society – religious groups, initiation groups, men's societies and so on.

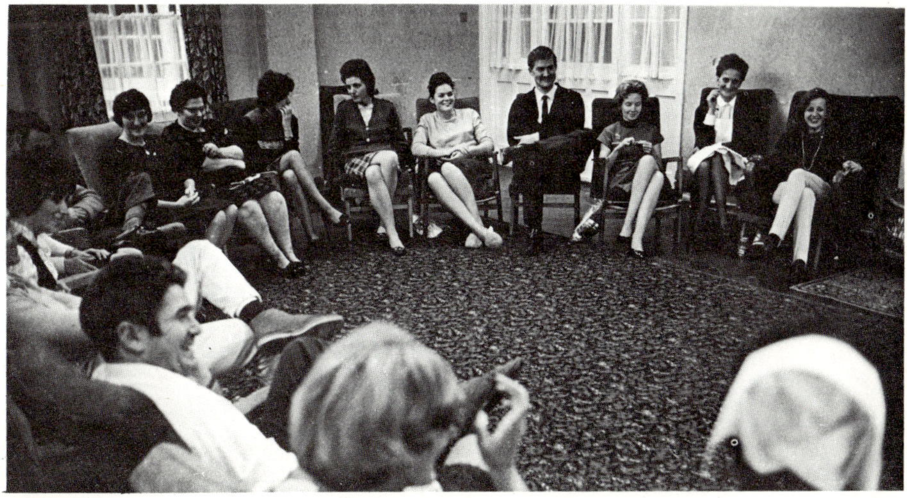

Guardianship

As with compulsory admission to hospital (q.v.) a guardianship application may be made in respect of a patient on the grounds that he is suffering from mental disorder and that it is necessary in the interests of the patient or for the protection of others. There is a similar limitation of its use as applied to patients suffering from subnormality or psychopathic disorder, who must be under the age of 21. A local authority can act as guardian. Applications can be made by the nearest relative or by the relevant and defined social worker and must be supported by two medical recommendations. If a private person is nominated as guardian, he or she must be approved by the local authority. The powers conferred are those which would be possessed if the guardian were the patient's father and the patient was under the age of 14. A person received into guardianship has the same right of access to a mental health review tribunal (q.v.) as that given to a patient sent compulsorily to hospital for treatment.
SEE ALSO Boarding out and Forensic psychiatry.

Guilt

A painful emotional state derived from awareness of having flouted personal or social ethical standards. It is a characteristic and often prominent feature of psychotic (endogenous) depressions (q.v.). Guilt is, of course, not necessarily pathological but in this setting it usually is, either because it is excessive (e.g. the woman tormented with guilt because once, years ago, she travelled on a bus without paying), or because it is uncharacteristic (e.g. the husband who has indeed been unfaithful to his wife but is normally quite untroubled by the fact), or because the crime concerned is imaginary (e.g. the daughter with a delusional conviction that she was responsible for her aged mother's death).

Habit

Habit as a technical term refers to a customary pattern of behaviour (q.v.) predictable from the conditions affecting an individual at any particular time and acquired by a process of learning. A stricter application refers only to the underlying acquired tendency to respond in the characteristic fashion. Apart from habitual overt activity, reference may be made to habits of thinking or of emotional response. Habits are contrasted, on the one hand, with pre-programmed reflex or instinctual reactions and, on the other, with behaviour governed by conscious decision and choice.

In recent years the concept of habit has become closely linked with the behaviourist school of psychology and refers to the acquired links between stimuli and responses established either by temporal association, as in classical conditioning (q.v.), or by the reinforcing properties of reward or punishment, as in operant conditioning (q.v.). These principles find psychiatric application in the planned re-educational habit-formation and habit-breaking of behaviour therapy (q.v.).

Habit disorder

A deterioration in a person's previously settled disposition or tendency to act in a certain way. Often a presenting symptom in dementia.

In children it is used to describe such symptoms as thumb-sucking, nail biting, head rolling, enuresis and other behaviour disorders. They may be primarily auto-erotic or represent a regression to infantile sources of satisfaction in response to environmental frustration.

Habituation

Psychological habituation refers to the rate at which a patient's response to a stimulus lessens with repeated exposure. This usually refers to mild anxiety provoking stimuli presented at approximately one-minute intervals and response is measured by the psychogalvanic response (q.v.) (PGR). Normal people and patients with specific phobias habituate quickly, compared to patients with anxiety states and agoraphobia. Treatment with a tranquillizer increases the habituation rate in the latter types of patient.

Drug habituation (WHO, 1967) was defined as distinct from addiction in that there was no compulsion to continue the drug, no tendency to increase the dose and no physical dependence. In 1964 the WHO recommended the term 'drug dependence' to include habituation and addiction as there was so much overlap.

Hallucinations

A hallucination is a false perception having no external stimulus. It should be distinguished from the other common disorder of perception, illusion (q.v.), in which there is a distortion of perception. The most common hallucinations in mental illness are 'voices', which occur most frequently in schizophrenia (q.v.). These may address the patient, converse about him, echo his thoughts or be inarticulate. They may be attributed to an internal or external source and the subject usually has a strong conviction of their reality.

Hallucinations can occur in other sensory modalities than hearing and are thus classified as visual, tactile, olfactory and gustatory. Some sensations are difficult to attribute or occur in more than one modality (e.g. having strength drained away; being sexually stimulated) and may be indistinguishably merged with delusions (q.v.).

Behaviour and mood may be noticeably affected by hallucinations, particularly auditory. The patient may be preoccupied and show expressive changes; may answer abusive comment in kind or may act impulsively in response to a command or imputation.

Hallucinations are experienced among normal people (e.g. hearing a telephone bell, noticing a smell of burning) particularly when falling off to sleep (hypnapompic (q.v.) or between sleep and waking (hypnagogic (q.v.). Hallucinations occur in many mental illnesses and brain disorders. The setting varies from clear consciousness without other disorder (hallucinosis), vividly described by Evelyn Waugh in his autobiographical *The Ordeal of Gilbert Pinfold*, to the general clouding

of consciousness and perception occurring in delirium. Hallucinations which are highly organized and detailed, like watching a play, are commonest in hysteria.
SEE ALSO Perception.

Hallucinogenic drugs

These are substances which have as their most striking property that of producing severe perceptual disturbance including hallucinations (q.v.). A number of names have been applied to this group including psychedelic (q.v.), i.e. 'mind altering', and psychotomimetic, i.e. 'able to mimic the manifestations of psychosis'. Experimental studies, however, suggest that the term hallucinogenic by no means accounts for the bulk of the activity of these drugs, though hallucinogenic activity may be most striking. In fact the activity of such drugs is influenced not only by the user's personality structure but also by his mood and his expectations of the drug effect. This is true of all 'mind altering' drugs – including alcohol, the opiates, barbiturates and the amphetamines.
The use of naturally occurring substances with hallucinogenic properties is frequently recorded in history. The taking of hallucinatory mushrooms by tribes in northern Siberia and the use of the sacred mushroom by Mexicans – the latter in the setting of religious observance – are well documented. Also the suggestion has been put forward that the state of 'berserk' – described in Nordic myths – may well have been caused by intoxication with amanita muscaria which contains the hallucinogen bufotenin.
The actions of hallucinogens are dramatic and remarkable. They include profound affective change, with feelings of fear, anxiety, dread and tremor, followed by disturbances in perception. These take the form not only of hallucinations but also quite bizarre changes in the quality of perception – intensification and distortion of images, and considerable preoccupation with the nature of the perceptual experience. In addition to this there are found feelings of altered reality of the self (de-personalization) and of the environment (de-realization) and the subject's thinking is altered – thought processes becoming more diffuse and perhaps showing a dreamlike quality.

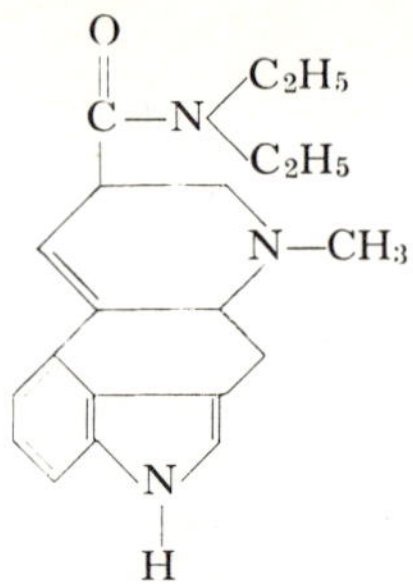

LSD

A convenient classification of hallucinogenic drugs would include:
1. The tryptamine group. This group contains substances which are straightforward tryptamine derivatives and substances which contain the tryptamine nucleus in a complex ring structure. The simple tryptamine derivatives include dimethyl tryptamine, diethyl tryptamine, serotonin (q.v.), bufotenin (q.v.) and psilocybin (q.v.) (the active principle of the sacred Mexican mushroom). Other hallucinogens with the basic tryptamine nucleus in a complex ring include LSD (q.v.), harmine (q.v.), and ibogaine (q.v.). Harmine is found in Peganum harmala, Banisteria caapi and Haemadictyon amazonicum – used by South American Indians. Ibogaine is the active principle of the plant Tabernanthe iboga – used in West and Central Africa.

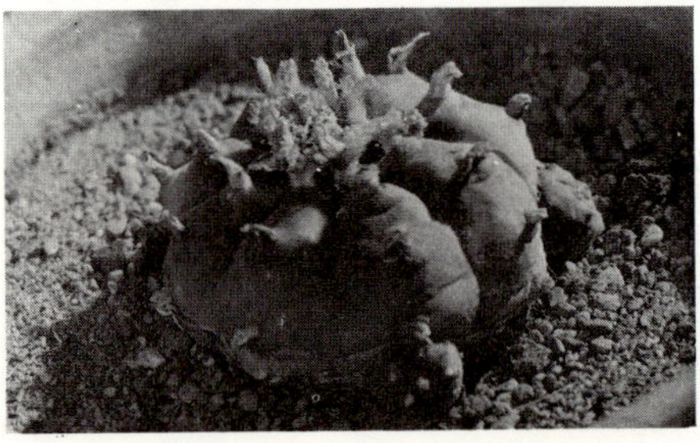

Cactus lophophora williamsii, from which mescaline is derived

2. The phenylethylamine group. These are all related to the sympatheticomimetic catechol amines – of which the best known is mescaline (q.v.), the active principle of peyote derived from the leaves of the cactus Lophophora williamsii – used in tribal and religious ceremonies in America. Other substances in this group include TMA –

trimethoxy amphetamine – and MDA – methylene dioxyamphetamine.
3. The third group is mixed and includes ditran (q.v.) which causes total loss of contact with the environment and total amnesia; also tetrahydrocannabinol – the active principle of cannabis (q.v.) – and phenyl cyclidine (sernyl (q.v.)) – which may cause marked loss of skin sensation, body image disturbance and confusional states. Of all the hallucinogens, LSD 25 is the most widely known, and it has been used in psychiatric treatment and research, although there is little consensus of agreement about its place in therapy. Many claim it as a useful treatment for alcoholism, but its real place in treatment is not clearly defined. Research interest in the hallucinogenic-induced states is based on their resemblance to psychoses and they were called 'model psychoses'. Though it was thought that investigation of model psychoses might throw light on the aetiology of psychoses such as schizophrenia, it is a fact that as yet there is no clear evidence linking the action of hallucinogens to the causation of psychoses, though tantalizing similarities between the syndromes exist. The casual self-administration of hallucinogenic drugs has found favour amongst young people, but informed medical opinion rightly deplores such use as being yet another example of the use of drugs for hedonistic purposes in situations where the illusory gains of spurious insight are offset by the hazards of adverse reactions which are unpredictable in onset and duration and sometimes tragic in outcome.
SEE ALSO Addiction.

Hanging perversion

Sexual gratification may be perversely obtained by binding in such a way with ropes as to produce repeated partial self-strangulation. When death occurs by accident, murder may be suspected. This perversion is often associated with sadomasochistic (q.v.) practices.

Harmine

Harmine is an alkaloid obtained from Peganum harmala, Haemadictyon

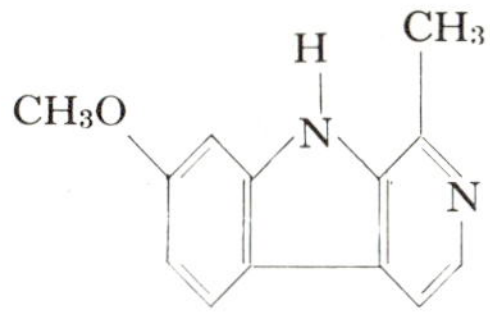

amazonicum and Banisteria caapi, South American plants. Orally or intravenously, hallucinations are produced together with disagreeable autonomic effects such as nausea and ataxia. The stimulant action of harmine may be connected with its inhibitory effects on monoamine oxidase.

Hartnup disease

Hartnup disease is an inborn error of metabolism: evidence points to its inheritance as an autosomal recessive trait. It is characterized by bizarre biochemical features, the most constant being generalized aminoaciduria. Abnormality in nicotinamide utilization has been postulated. Psychiatric effects vary from case to case, and are episodic. They may accompany the appearance of a pellagra-light sensitive skin rash with transient neurological disturbance characterized by variable cerebellar signs. Mental confusion is a frequent concomitant. A more permanent effect in some patients is mental subnormality.

Hashish

SEE Cannabis sativa.

Hay fever

An allergic rhinitis produced seasonally by various allergens, especially wind-born pollens from, for example, timothy grass. It is usually constitutionally determined and may be associated with non-seasonal vasomotor rhinitis (q.v.), asthma, or eczema. Psychological factors, although affecting the condition, are not primarily responsible. Treatment should include avoidance of the allergen, attempts to increase resistance to it, and palliative medication if necessary.
SEE ALSO Allergy.

Headache

It is necessary to distinguish headache due to local organic lesions (or dysfunctions)

from headache due to systemic illness, and to distinguish both from headache due to or associated with psychological factors.
In many cases there is understandably an overlap between local physical and psychological factors. Local organic lesions include cerebral tumour, subdural haematoma, temporal arteritis, sinusitis, vasomotor rhinitis and migraine. Systemic causes of headache include hypertension, renal failure, emphysema, eyestrain (due to refractive errors), and constipation.
Tension headaches are probably the commonest variety seen in clinical practice. The pain is usually frontal, sometimes occipital, and sometimes extending right over the cranium. It has been suggested that the intermediate mechanism is spasm in the occipito-frontalis muscle. Sufferers are reputed not to show much overt anxiety as if the headache were an adequate release symptom. Environmental stress and fatigue are precipitating factors. One of the differential diagnoses of tension headache is migraine (q.v.).
Headache, or more precisely abnormal and unpleasant cranial sensations are described by patients with depressive illness. Some patients describe it as a feeling of pressure on the top of the head, while others experience a feeling like a tight band encircling the head.
Some patients with chronic hypochondriasis complain of headaches but these usually consist of bizarre sensations in the head. Sometimes the description is couched in electrical, sometimes in physiological terms, i.e. 'a feeling of waves of blood washing over the brain'.
The treatment of the physical group is primarily that of the underlying disorder though symptomatic relief may be indicated. Tension headaches are usually relieved by tranquillizers such as chlordiazepoxide. At the same time, however, psychiatric management should include an assessment of personality and environmental stresses with directive psychotherapy aimed at achieving a better handling of situational pressures and a more effective discharge of tension before symptoms ensue. The purely psychiatric syndromes (i.e. depression and hypochondriasis) require adequate treatment of the underlying condition (i.e. ECT, pharmacotherapy, etc.)
SEE ALSO Psychosomatic disorders.

Head injury

Head injury may be associated with penetrating wounds of the brain, with depressed fractures of the skull, or with bleeding into or around the brain. The clinical picture depends not only on the severity of the trauma, but also on the presence of such complicating factors. The immediate effect of trauma is concussion (q.v.) – when slight, associated with a dazed, vague mental state; when severe, with unconsciousness. Most patients recover consciousness rapidly and with no complications. Minimal concussion, with the restoration of lucidity followed by a progression into confusion or unconsciousness, suggests intracranial bleeding or subdural haematoma. Delayed recovery is occasionally encountered with semiconscious restlessness, perseveration, or meaningless cries with incontinence, and total dependence on nursing care persists for months. Shorter periods of post-traumatic delirium may also be observed. Most often amnesia (q.v.) for a period before and after the accident is a permanent residuum; occasionally more extensive mental deficits, both organic and functional, are observed. Dementia affects both memory and intellectual performance. A dysmnesic syndrome (Korsakoff's psychosis) (q.v.) sparing intellectual performance is occasionally seen. An epileptic fit shortly after head injury, intracranial haematoma, and a combination of depressed fracture and prolonged post-traumatic amnesia are all bad prognostic signs pointing to late epilepsy. Repeated minor injuries, as sustained by boxers, may have just as devastating effects as isolated major trauma. The resulting 'punch drunk' syndrome includes ataxia, dysarthria, personality change, and dementia. A common neuro-pathological finding is a torn septum pellucidum.
The post-concussion syndrome, of headache, giddiness, poor concentration, and anxiety, follows a proportion of head injuries. Depression, schizophrenia-like states and personality changes are also seen.
Investigation after head injury may include X-ray – demonstrating fractures; lumbar puncture – showing blood in cerebrospinal fluid; electroencephalogram – for monitoring recovery and showing focal damage; and in the chronic stage, psychological

tests. Tests of intelligence may indicate poorer global performance than the patient's work record and educational achievements suggest, or may show discrepancies particularly between verbal and abstract performance, using, for example, the Mill Hill vocabulary and progressive matrices tests. Low verbal performance points to focal damage, while in more diffuse disturbance abstract ability tends to be impaired while verbal scores remain satisfactory. Memory and visual and auditory learning may also be tested – the latter by teaching the definitions of words not properly known in the Mill Hill vocabulary test.
SEE ALSO Post-traumatic dementia and Epilepsy.

Hebephrenia

Hebephrenia is one of the most common types of schizophrenia (q.v.); it is usually insidious and has an onset between 15 and 30 years. It may appear to arise from adolescent difficulties, career, making friends, or sexual worries. Difficulty in concentration is noticeable in pupils or students. Psychic life is widely affected; will power, direction, thought, and emotion are all disordered or impaired and this is reflected in behaviour. Thought disorder shows itself by: incongruous association of ideas; answers which are beside the point, although evidencing that the question has been grasped; by vague preoccupation with pseudo-religious and philosophical notions. Grandiloquent but fatuous statements will occur. Auditory hallucinations are common. Increased sexual drive with flagrant promiscuity may occur.
Depressive or neurotic symptoms can appear at an early stage giving confusion in diagnosis.

Hedonism

A philosophical doctrine in which pleasure seeking is the supreme goal. In the psychiatric sense, the term hedonism implies the seeking of certain goals merely because of the pleasure that ensues, rather than as ends in themselves.

Hepatolenticular degeneration

This inborn error of copper metabolism is inherited as an autosomal recessive trait. Copper is deposited in the tissues, leading to pathological changes in the liver and brain. The basal ganglia especially are affected, leading to extrapyramidal rigidity, athetosis, tremor, dysarthria, and dysphagia. Dementia usually supervenes. The Kayser-Fleischer ring, greenish in colour, at the limbus of the cornea, is a curious diagnostic feature. The age of onset varies widely, from childhood to advanced adult life. Some clinical improvement may follow the administration of a chelating agent, such as British anti-Lewisite or penicillamine.

Heredity
SEE Inheritance.

Hermaphroditism
Hermaphroditism is the rare condition of androgyny where an individual possesses both male and female sex organs. The chromosome constitution is usually XX although degrees of mosaicism may be present. Psychosexual constitution is flexible and the gender role (q.v.) is congruous with sex of assignment at birth and sex of rearing.
Pseudo-hermaphroditism (q.v.) or 'inter-

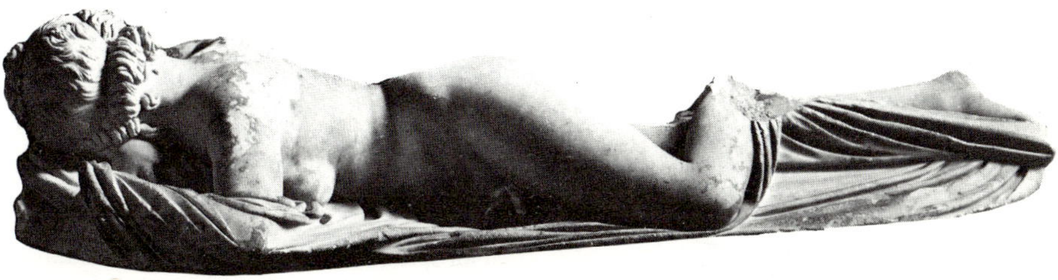

Hermaphrodite, National Museum, Rome

sex' is more common particularly in the male where the constitution is 44–XY. There is testicular feminization due to the enzymic failure of the somatic cells to respond to the masculinizing action of androgen.
The undescended testicles and rudimentary penis are mistaken for female genitalia at birth and the child is reared in the female gender role until adolescence when masculinization makes the mistake evident. Sex may then have to be reassigned.
Female pseudo-hermaphroditism is rare and usually due to an adrenogenital syndrome. High androgen output from the female adrenal results in a hypospadiac penis, the child being wrongly assigned and reared as a male.

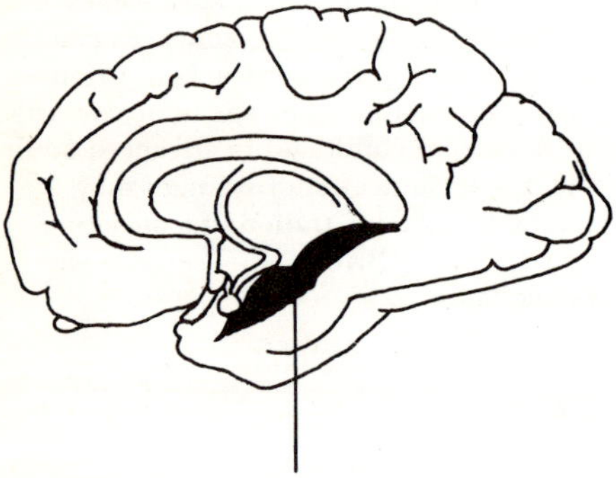

Hippocampus

The hippocampus lies in the floor of the temporal horn of the lateral ventricle. It consists of archecortex, of simpler structure than the neocortex elsewhere. Afferent fibres run in the fornix (q.v.) to the mamillary body (q.v.) and anterior thalamic nucleus and also to the hypothalamus (q.v.). The hippocampus is part of the limbic system (q.v.) and is concerned in the integrative control of attention and alerting responses and of some visceral and sexual responses. It is involved in the setting down of the memory trace as lesions of the hippocampus and related structures may result in severe disturbances, e.g. the Korsakoff syndrome (q.v.).

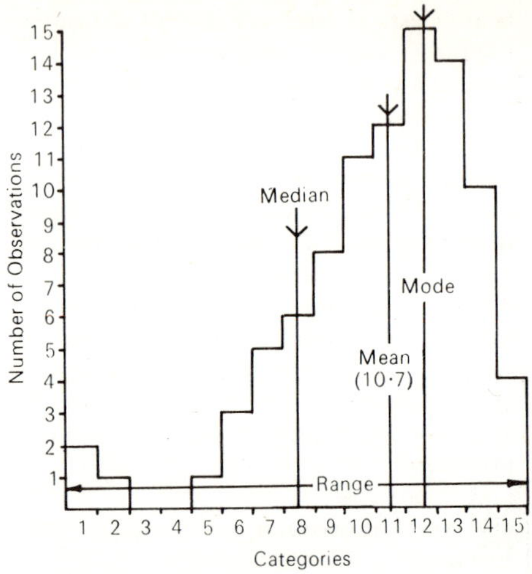

A histogram presentation of the hypothetical data presented in 'Frequency Distribution' –showing range, mean, mode, median. This shows a skew distribution with outlying observations.

Histogram

The histogram is a chart showing the frequency of observations in each of several groups. The frequency is shown as a bar (see figure). The histogram has its greatest value when the grouping is by time interval, e.g. number of deaths in an age group.
SEE ALSO Bar chart.

History taking

This is basically the same as for any other medical patient, but as the nature of the patient's disorder and mental state may influence the account he gives of his illness and past history it is important to get an independent account from a close relative or friend. The doctor should not be satisfied with a simple diagnosis obtained from assessing the development and symptomatology of the present illness. Rather he should attempt to make an assessment of the strength and weakness of the patient's personality and his ability to adjust to the usual stresses of life. Second, a search should be made for any genetic factors which may predispose to psychiatric disorder and for any stresses, particularly those to which the patient might be unduly susceptible and which might be of aetio-

logical importance. In this respect dates of events are often of importance. For instance the date of the mother's death may suggest emotional deprivation in early childhood or suggest an 'anniversary' factor as playing an aetiological role in the patient's illness.
The order in which the information is obtained will depend on each individual patient and experienced doctors will take each subject as it develops naturally, leaving subjects to which the patients may be sensitive until later in the interview. It is important to realize that psychiatric patients are frequently very sensitive to the first impressions the doctor makes and for this reason the first interview is important from a therapeutic point of view as well as from the point of view of general assessment and diagnosis.

Homoeostasis

The basic principle of homoeostasis was stated by Claude Bernard: 'La fixité du milieu intérieur est la condition de la vie libre, indépendante'. A wide range of functions such as level of blood sugar and body temperature are continuously monitored and any excessive drift operates mechanisms which counteract these tendencies. Such systems are referred to in cybernetic jargon as 'negative feed-back' controls and often as in the central nervous system there are several levels of control. These reflexes occur without awareness or purposiveness. Nevertheless, adaptive alterations in bodily functions can occur in response to changing requirements when maintenance of the *status quo* would be biologically disadvantageous.

Homicidal threats

Homicidal threats must always be taken seriously, particularly if the doctor himself is their object. Morbid jealousy leads to murderous thoughts towards spouse or lover, schizophrenia to threats to prominent public figures, or others unrelated to the patient. Threats to children are particularly disturbing – the depressed mother is a particular risk, but obsessive patients, and schizophrenics may create justifiable anxiety. These thoughts are often confided to the doctor, either personally or by letter. Threatening letters which hint at killing or injury must be taken seriously; if the doctor himself is threatened he would be well advised to discuss the matter with the local police. Drug addicts and criminals may threaten medical personnel in an attempt to bribe them to supply drugs, or as a medical excuse for their activities.
SEE ALSO Infanticide and Murder.

Homicide

In British law there are four categories of criminal homicide: murder (q.v.), manslaughter (q.v.), infanticide (q.v.), and causing death by dangerous driving (see Driving). A disproportionate degree of interest and emotion is invested in the small subcategory murder. The most economic and rational approach to reducing the death rate from homicide in the United Kingdom would be to attack the large problem of causing death by dangerous driving. Current United Kingdom legislation has created a distinction between capital murder and non-capital murder and introduced new grounds on which a conviction could be reduced to manslaughter (q.v.). Under one part of the current United Kingdom Act 'Where a person kills or is a party of the killing of another, he shall not be convicted of murder if he was suffering from such abnormality of mind (whether arising from a condition of arrested or retarded development of mind or any inherent cause or induced by disease or injury) as substantially impaired his mental responsibility for his acts and omissions in doing or being a party to the killing.' Capital murder includes murder done in the furtherance of theft, by starting an explosion, in resisting arrest, assisting an escape, murdering of a police or prison officer, or a second killing. The death penalty for capital murder was subsequently abolished. The law relating to homicide varies widely from one country to another.
SEE ALSO Manslaughter, Murder, and Forensic psychiatry.

Homosexuality

Homosexuality, sexual activity between members of the same sex, is a universal human phenomenon. Kinsey found that 37% of the male population in the United States had had physical contact with another male to the point of orgasm at some time in their lives; only 4% of males or females are exclusively homosexual. The reasons for homosexuality are unclear; chromosomal sex is normal, and a genetic factor is uncertain. Gender role (q.v.) may play a part, and the manner in which a child is brought up, in particular the relationship with the mother, seems to be very important. A dominating, overprotective, and basically 'male hostile' mother, together with a weak, absent, or affectionless father, is often encountered in the life history of the homosexual. Early imprinting mechanisms may also play their part. The role of sexual seduction and of mutual sex play at school have been much exaggerated, and many false generalizations have been made as a result of the highly selected material which comes to the notice of doctors.

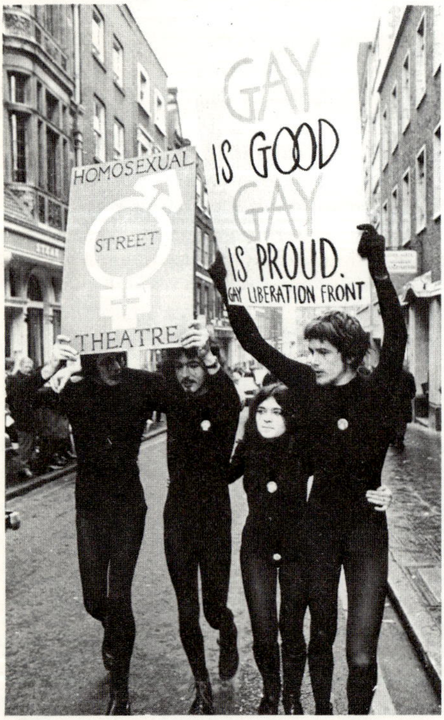

Members of Gay Liberation Front

Homosexuality may be 'latent' and manifest itself in aberrant forms of heterosexual behaviour such as promiscuous seductions (Don Juanism), strong affiliation to male groups, e.g. weight-lifting, wrestling, or in early onset impotence. So-called 'homosexual panic' is an abnormal psychogenic reaction of intense anxiety occurring in males whose repressed homosexual tendencies are suddenly inadvertently activated by another male. Some latent homosexuals seek solace in alcohol. The content of some paranoid delusions, particularly in alcoholics, is produced by reaction formation of homosexual attraction for a male into feelings of hostility and persecution by the same individual. Promiscuity is common in homosexuals. About 30% of all venereal disease in males is acquired through homosexual relationships.

There is a divergence of law from one country to another on homosexuality. The United Kingdom, for example, about ten years ago removed from the ambit of the criminal law homosexual acts between consenting adults in private over the age of 21. Treatment of homosexuality by intensive psychotherapy or psychoanalysis is uncertain in its efficacy. General psychiatric treatment is primarily concerned with improving personal and social adjustment rather than with the deviation itself.

Hormone therapy has no place in treatment, although surgical or chemical castration may be necessary in the case of the homosexual paedophiliac offender. Behaviour therapy treats homosexuality as a learned pattern of sexual behaviour capable of modification by electrical or chemical aversion therapy or by avoidance deconditioning procedures. Homosexuals who are well motivated for treatment are most appropriate for behaviour therapy and encouraging results have been reported, although to date the series of cases has been small and with comparatively short follow-up.

Hormone treatment of sexual deviations

Virtually the only deviates who request or accede to this form of treatment are sexual offenders, chiefly paedophiliacs. Homosexuals whose sexual desires are in danger of getting out of control and leading them into an offence such as importuning in a public lavatory may also be suitable for treatment on a temporary basis.

The standard treatment depends on counterbalancing the output of male hormone by giving oestrogens either orally or by depot injection. Nausea and feminization, particularly breast enlargement, are common side effects. Recently cyptroterone acetate has been introduced. This is an antiandrogen and also inhibits gonadotrophin production. Side effects are less than with oestrogen but include inhibition of spermatogenesis, initial lethargy and fatigue and some gynaecomastia.

In either case, while the intensity of sexual drive is diminished, its direction in unaltered and concomitant psychotherapy is advisable. In every case the patient should consent to treatment of his own free will or if the responsibility for a patient is vested in some other person, such other person must without fail be consulted.

Hospital orders

Under recent British law mentally disturbed people who have committed offences can be admitted to hospital for treatment if a hospital is willing to take them.

SEE ALSO Compulsory admission, Mental health review tribunal, Probation, and Psychopathic disorder.

Hunter's syndrome

SEE Gargoylism.

Huntington's chorea

Huntington's chorea is a pre-senile dementia with a dominant mode of inheritance. The mean age of onset is about 35 years, but there is wide variation and in a few cases the disease appears in childhood. Usually the patient is well advanced in the reproductive period, and has already transmitted the gene to at least some of the offspring before the first signs appear. These are not infrequently psychiatric, and widely diverse in nature, e.g. apathy, moodiness or depression, disorder of attention, paranoid ideas or delusions. These psychiatric changes usually precede the neurological signs by some interval. The disease progresses relentlessly, with the appearance of choreiform movements beginning with small jerking movements of the extremities, face and shoulders, but leading eventually to grotesque writhing of the whole body. The patient becomes dysarthric, ataxic and more neurologically disabled, in addition there is a progressive dementia. The duration of the condition is variable, averaging about ten or fifteen years from the onset.

There is no specific treatment apart from general management and nursing care, although tetrabenazine may reduce the dysarthria. Genetical counselling to families of Huntington's chorea patients is of the utmost importance.

Hurler's syndrome

(Synonym: Hunter's disease)

SEE Gargoylism.

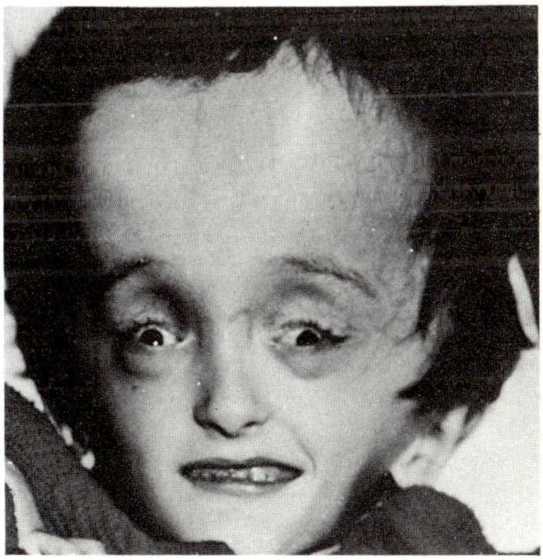

Hydrocephalus and subnormality

Internal hydrocephalus is produced by obstruction to the free circulation of cerebro-spinal fluid which is produced by the choroid plexus within the ventricular system of the brain, passes down the aqueduct of Sylvius, through small fora-

mina to the subarachnoid space, where it is absorbed. Obstruction can occur through congenital malformation of the brain, e.g. congenital narrowing of the aqueduct of Sylvius, transmitted by sex-linked inheritance; spina bifida cystica (the Arnold Chiari malformation); malformation of the cerebellar vermis (the Dandy-Walker syndrome). Post-meningitic adhesions may block the outflow of cerebro-spinal fluid from the ventricular system, and infection is in fact the commonest cause of acquired hydrocephalus. Intracranial haemorrhage at or around birth may lead to hydrocephalus. Rare causes are tumours and cysts in childhood. In a number of cases spontaneous arrest soon occurs, but in others this does not happen and progressive neurological involvement, mental impairment and sometimes blindness due to pressure on the optic nerves may occur.
In surgical treatment an artificial shunt is inserted between the lateral ventricles of the brain and the right atrium of the heart, via the jugular vein. Through this, the excessive cerebro-spinal fluid is drained off, passing through a valve.
SEE ALSO Mental subnormality.

Hyperaesthesia

Exaggerated sensitivity to tactile stimuli; this is chiefly found with disease or injury of peripheral nerves. Hysterical hyperaesthesia is often bizarre and usually affects the head, abdomen, or one half of the body; the diagnosis rests on the absence of signs of organic illness and the presence of a continuing psychopathology.

Hyperkinesis

Children show temperamental differences in their level of activity. In a small minority, overactivity is so pronounced as to constitute a clinical entity. The hyperkinetic syndrome is characterized by extreme, poorly regulated overactivity, associated with a short attention span and marked distractibility. Aggressive behaviour and destructiveness are commonly present. In addition, the child is likely to be of below average intelligence with immaturity of speech, and to show absence of anxiety in social situations which most children would find inhibiting.
Overactivity of this degree of severity commonly makes an impact on family life when the child becomes mobile about the age of 18 months to 2 years. It may reach a peak or first come to notice at school entry, when the child is expected for the first time to sit still for a long period. There is usually a reduction in the level of activity before puberty but other problems may supervene.
The overactivity is characteristically independent of the social situation, the child not being able to sit still for more than a minute or two under any circumstances. Some children become more active in anxiety-provoking situations.
The aetiology is probably mainly constitutional, but there is an inconstant association with minimal brain damage.
Treatment is symptomatic. Dexamphetamine sulphate has a paradoxical quietening action in childhood and is sometimes effective. Haloperidol and chlorpromazine have also been successfully employed. Recently, techniques of behaviour modification have shown promising results.
SEE ALSO Child psychiatry and Motor disturbances.

Hypermnesia

An unusual degree of the ability to retain and recall the details of past events. In children this may be associated with eidetic (q.v.) (extremely vivid) imagery, and a recent intensive study of an adult stage

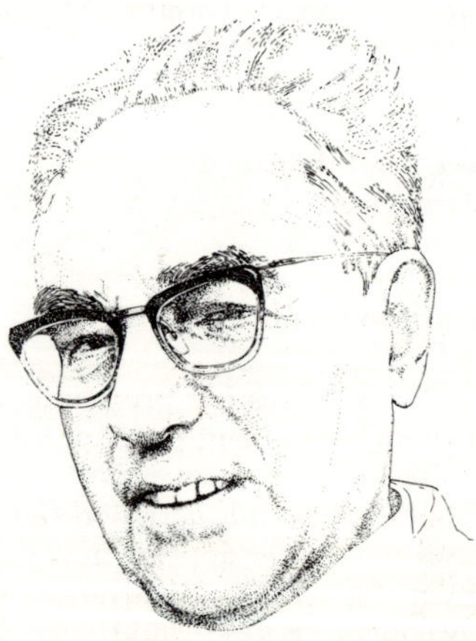

Luria. Russian psychologist

'memory-man' by the Russian psychologist Luria indicated the importance of synaesthesia (q.v.) (sensations in one modality accompanied by associated sensory impressions in other modalities, e.g. coloured sounds) in his memory processes. Hypermnesia may occur during hypnosis and in some pathological states, such as hypomania (q.v.) and paranoid psychosis (q.v.).
SEE ALSO Memory.

Hypertension

Hypertension is a constitutional disorder in which, among others, hereditary and environmental factors are important. In the benign phase of the disease hypertension is often labile and considerable increases in blood pressure may be produced by anxiety. It has been suggested that transient increases in blood pressure produced by stress may later become persistent.
While hypertension is usually relieved symptomatically by antihypertensive drugs, it is valuable to determine and treat any precipitating emotional disorder. The personality profile of hypertensives often reveals a great deal of conflict with anxiety and inability to express aggression directly. Hostility may be intense and chronic, and as it accumulates it requires further inhibition to keep it repressed. Treatment should thus include evaluation of the underlying psychopathology and an attempt to alter the patients life-style if this is having an adverse effect on his blood pressure. Knowledge of the disease may increase anxiety further and may need treatment with a benzodiazepine such as chlordiazepoxide or diazepam.
Serious depression may result from the use of reserpine, which should seldom be used because of this effect. Methyldopa, which also depletes cerebral noradrenaline, is now widely used and can also cause depression. It is important to appreciate that the administration of tricyclic antidepressant drugs (q.v.) blocks the therapeutic effect of guanethedine type antihypertensives.
SEE ALSO Psychosomatic disorders.

Hyperthymic personality

Within the spectrum of normal healthy personality structures, a group is found whose mood is usually set at a higher level than the average and these are characterized by the term 'hyperthymic personality'. They are exuberant and cheerful by nature, radiate good humour and are consequently popular with their colleagues.

Hyperthyroidism

Typical psychological features are anxiety and emotional overreactivity. Differentiation from anxiety states can be difficult and sometimes, in patients with undoubted hyperthyroidism, anxiety symptoms persist in spite of effective antithyroid treatment.
Occasionally hyperthyroidism is accompanied by the appearance of a major psychosis, usually agitated depression and less often mania or schizophrenia.
SEE ALSO Endocrine disease.

Hyperuricaemia (Lesch–Nyhan syndrome)

This syndrome appearing within the first few months of life in males (sometimes in sibs), is characterized by high blood uric acid levels, urinary calculi, severe involvement of the central nervous system, self-mutilation, severe mental subnormality, and death at an early age. It is possible that this rare syndrome is transmitted genetically as a sex-linked trait.
SEE ALSO Inherited metabolic defects.

Hyperventilation syndrome

Anxiety associated with either an increase in respiration rate with frequent sighing, or, in the severe form, breathing which is rapid, shallow, irregular; often leads to lightheadedness, giddiness, pallor, paraesthesiae, blurring of vision and occasionally tetany. Patients often express the fear that they will not be able to get enough air into their lungs. Treatment should concentrate on the underlying anxiety (q.v.).

SEE ALSO Psychosomatic disorders and Respiratory disease.

Hypnagogic hallucinations

Hallucinatory experiences which occur on the edge of sleep, usually visual, often of patterns, shapes, colours; they may be more grotesque. They are commonly experienced by normal persons, especially during periods of tension and anxiety. The subject often denies dreaming or being asleep. They are frequent in narcolepsy (q.v.) and those under the influence of drugs. They are complained of more by anxious persons, who may seize upon them as a symptom of morbid significance.
SEE ALSO Hallucinations.

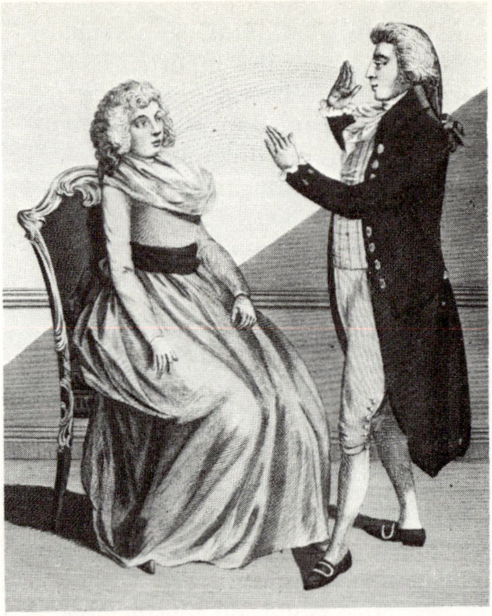

Hypnopompic phenomena

The brief persistence of the imagery of a dream into the waking state. Thus in waking there remains a hallucination (q.v.) of slightly altered quality from the dream state. The hallucinatory phenomena on the edge of waking are better described as hypnagogic (q.v.) and the term hypnopompic reserved for those experiences which remain though the eyes are open. They have no special significance.

Hypnosis

Hypnosis as a therapeutic tool was introduced by Mesmer and was used by Freud to treat hysterical patients before he developed the technique of psychoanalysis by free association.
It may be defined as a state of semi-conscious suggestibility and the technique of hypnosis is that of increasing the patient's innate tendency to suggestibility. The doctor should explain the idea of hypnosis to the patient to rid him of unwarranted anxieties derived from gossip and theatrical demonstrations. Hypnosis can be carried out sitting in a chair or lying on a couch, whichever is preferable to the patient and provided always that he is relaxed. Techniques vary from those where the patient's co-operation is paramount, such as asking him to concentrate on his fingers and by repeated suggestion inducing levitation of the fingers, hand, and finally the whole arm, to those techniques where the doctor induces the heightened suggestibility by powerful suggestion through the force of his own personality. In all cases the suggestion is made that the patient becomes increasingly relaxed and drowsy and in suitable subjects and perhaps after several sessions, passes into a state of hypnotic sleep. One of the most important characteristics of this hypnotic state is post-hypnotic suggestibility.
Hypnosis has three main uses:
1. To promote relaxation, e.g. for behaviour therapy.
2. To make strong suggestions, for instance to remove early hysterical symptoms prior to more formal psychotherapy. Simple habits such as finger picking in cases of recurring warts may also be treated in this way.
3. To uncover hitherto repressed memories, particularly in states of hysterical amnesia, after an acute stressful experience.
A few people are very easy to hypnotize, but it is not always easy to detect these in advance and an attempt to hypnotize a patient which fails undermines his confidence. Furthermore many doctors are not temperamentally suited to use hypnotherapy and some are put off by the possibility of producing dependence if symptoms are removed by suggestion without the underlying cause being properly resolved. For these reasons the use

of drugs, such as methohexitone sodium or thiopentone, is usually preferred as being a quicker and a surer method of inducing relaxation, heightening suggestibility, and uncovering repressed material.

Hypnotics

The term hypnotic designates the sleep-inducing properties of a drug while sedative indicates a rather milder activity producing quietness and drowsiness. This difference is a quantitative one, and soporific drugs are capable of producing either effect according to the dosage used.
Hypnotic compounds are given to correct insomnia, a frequent concomitant of psychiatric illness. It is a distressing complaint, particularly if persistent, and hypnotic agents are widely used. They are valuable therapeutic agents, but their wide use is in part the result of underuse of other psychotherapeutic measures.
The existing hypnotics alter the quality of sleep; the proportion of paradoxical sleep (q.v.) is initially reduced. Return to normal after discontinuing hypnotics may take several weeks and the first few nights are likely to be disturbed, with vivid dreams. Consequently patients may be reluctant to discontinue their hypnotics and dependence and chronic hypnotic medication ensue all too quickly.
Overdosage with hypnotics has now become a favourite method of attempting suicide, and this risk is particularly high in patients with a psychiatric illness. It may be difficult to reconcile requirements of effective dosage and safety in disturbed patients; recruitment of a responsible relative to control tablet supply is one solution of this problem.
There is a wide range of hypnotics available. Of the more important ones, barbiturates (q.v.) have been popular over the years but have been discredited recently due to the suicide risk and dependence problems, and chloral derivatives (q.v.) continue to be a valuable alternative particularly in the young and elderly. Piperidinedione compounds (q.v.) are also well established hypnotic agents. More recently benzodiazepines (q.v.) have become a strong contender in psychiatric practice because of their wide safety margin. Methaqualone has had a vogue, but there may be serious difficulties in treating overdosage and it has been misused by psychopaths.

Hypochondriasis

This term is used imprecisely in a number of different though related ways: (a) to describe people who are constantly preoccupied with their health, whether or not they believe or suspect that they are ill; (b) to describe those who, in the absence of reasonable evidence to that effect, either worry that they might have, or are convinced that they do have, some serious illness; and (c) to describe those with persistent or recurrent bodily complaints, single or multiple, for which no organic basis can be found. Hypochondriasis in the first sense, as a character trait, is widespread, as the demand for laxatives, tonics, and vitamins demonstrates. It becomes more prominent as age increases and may well be stimulated by the readiness of our profession to prescribe medicaments for any complaint – no matter how trivial.
Hypochondriasis in the second sense, as a symptom, is also common but usually only in a setting of some other psychiatric condition – in an anxiety state (q.v.) or a depression (q.v.), and sometimes in schizophrenia (q.v.) also. In anxiety states hypochondriacal symptoms usually take the form of fears or worries based on one of the somatic manifestations of anxiety, e.g. worry about having a 'weak heart' after experiencing palpitations. In schizophrenia, on the other hand, and also in involutional melancholia, hypochondriasis is usually delusional and often bizarre, e.g. a conviction that the two sides of the brain have been transposed. Depressives are often preoccupied with the possibility of having a serious bodily illness, as they are with the possibility of other calamities, and in severe depression such fears may become delusional.
Hypochondriasis in the third sense is seen mainly in women with prominent personality defects and is very resistant to treatment, probably because the invalid role which the patient's symptoms allow her to adopt produces important benefits, like sympathy, attention and the avoidance of unwelcome obligations.
Psychodynamic theories of hypochondria-

sis generally interpret it in terms of unconscious feelings of badness or guilt. Whatever truth there may be in this it is a fact that unilateral symptoms are referred to the left side of the body far more often than to the right, and it is difficult to resist equating this with the widespread symbolic connotations of left as 'sinister' or bad.
SEE ALSO Psychosomatic disorders and Neurasthenia.

Hypoglycaemia

Attacks of hypoglycaemia have many possible causes. In adults the most important are insulin overdosage, islet-cell tumour and 'functional' hypoglycaemia. Severe hypoglycaemia causes impairment of consciousness, often with inappropriate behaviour, followed by coma and perhaps convulsions. The reaction may on occasions be mistaken for alcoholism. The adrenergic response to hypoglycaemia may cause anxiety and palpitations. All the symptoms occur episodically.

Hypomania

Kraepelin (q.v.) originally distinguished four varieties of mania (q.v.) – hypomania, acute mania, delusional mania, and delirious mania – although he recognized that they represented a gradation in severity, rather than distinct conditions, and that patients often passed from one to another and back again. Hypomania is the only one of the four terms to have remained in common use. It is used to describe a state in which there is a mild elevation of mood with restlessness, distractability, increased energy and sometimes pressure of speech and irritability, but without any prominent flight of ideas or grandiose delusions.

Hypoparathyroidism

Hypocalcaemia is the most important feature of this rare disorder. Clinical features include tetany, convulsions and emotional disturbance – lability, anxiety and depression. Episodes of delirium may occur. Young children with hypoparathyroidism if not adequately treated become mentally retarded, although it is said that the retardation is reversible.
SEE ALSO Endocrine disease.

Hypothalamus

The hypothalamus, lying in the diencephalon, integrates autonomic (q.v.) and endocrine (q.v.) functions. Afferent connections come directly or indirectly from most other parts of the brain and efferents descend to influence autonomic neurones in the spinal cord. The posterior pituitary hormones, e.g. antidiuretic hormone and oxytocin, are produced in the hypothalamus and transported via the nerve trunks to the posterior pituitary. The release of anterior pituitary hormones, such as growth hormone, corticotrophin and the gonadotrophins, is controlled by releasing factors which again appear to originate in the hypothalamus and are transported to the pituitary by the hypothalamic – hypophyseal portal blood vessel system. The hypothalamus is important in the control of food and water intake, cardiovascular functions, body temperature, digestive functions and sexual functions. It organizes the motor and visceral expressions of emotional reactions.

Hypothymic personality

At the opposite end of the mood spectrum to the hyperthymic personality (q.v.) is the 'hypothymic personality'. These individuals have an average mood level below the mean; they are the natural pessimists, morose, despondent, lacking energy, are poor colleagues at work or companions in leisure.

Hypothyroidism

Thyroid hormone deficiency in foetal life and early infancy causes retardation of physical and mental development (see Cretinism). In adults hypothyroidism produces characteristic psychological effects, which are not infrequently the presenting clinical features. Psychological functions generally are slowed and the patient becomes dull, lethargic and forgetful. Emotional disturbance occurs, usually apathy but sometimes depression. Hypothyroidism is sometimes misdiagnosed as depressive illness or as pre-senile dementia. Thyroxine treatment relieves both the psychological and physical symptoms of the illness.

In some hypothyroid patients frank psychoses develop. In these cases thyroxine alone may not relieve the psychiatric disorder, which then needs treatment in its own right (see Myxoedema).

SEE ALSO Endocrine disease.

Hypsarrhythmia

Frequently mistaken as a synonym for infantile spasms (q.v.) (lightning seizures, salaam seizures), the term describes the EEG record which is commonly found in these conditions. The record is a chaotic, disorganized, desynchronized mixture of random spikes and slow waves, which in its fullest form, replaces all normal rhythms. Gradations of severity occur which do not correlate fully with the clinical picture. The EEG may normalize in the course of treatment of the disorder underlying the infantile spasms, but only rarely does normalization of the record and arrest of the spasms lead to normal mental development.

SEE ALSO Epilepsy.

Hysteria

Few conditions in the history of medicine have been so long enduring, so indefinable and so popular with doctors as hysteria. Speculations as to its nature have been endless; it has been called 'the mocking bird of nosology' and each generation of medical men has seen theories of pathogenesis advanced which have delighted the more nimble brains of the profession. Unfortunately little has emerged from all this activity which can be accepted today as evidence for a specific condition called hysteria. In fact neither twin studies, follow-up studies, nor clinical studies support the concept of an entity of hysteria; rather they suggest that hysterical symptoms may appear in any psychiatric condition, especially that of depression, or as a reaction to some unbearable stress.

Hysterical *symptoms* stem from a patient's inability to cope with reality and his attempt to resolve the conflict provoked by this failure by certain aspects of thought or behaviour which, though inconsistent with reality, are not seen in this way by the patient ('dissociation'). The patient's anxiety about his basic conflict is said to be '*converted*' into an hysterical symptom, the symptom usually carrying a '*secondary gain*', e.g. avoidance of the original situation. As an example, whenever a man went to work his neighbour made love to his wife. Unable to face this situation, the patient developed an hysterical paresis of his legs which necessitated him staying at home. Occasionally the patient shows a lack of concern for his disability (belle indifférence) though nowadays the converse is usually the case.

Symptoms may take the form of:

1. *Disorders of memory*. This is not a true and complete memory loss but merely a loss of memory for personal events, which is frequently patchy, and at times of personal identity.
2. *Disorders of consciousness*. The commonest form is a fugue state where often the patient seems to be escaping from an intolerable situation.
3. *Disorders of intellect*, such as pseudodementia or the rare Ganser syndrome.
4. *Disorders of mobility*. Any part of the somatic musculature may be affected by an hysterical paralysis. Tremors, disorders of gait, dysphonia and hysterical convulsions are other manifestations.
5. *Disorders of perception*. This is usually a loss of cutaneous sensation, but hysterical blindness and deafness are not uncommon.

A description of women in the words of men, the term hysterical personality is usually applied to women rather than men. Attention-seeking, lively, flirtatious, shallow, self-centred, dependent, and overreactive emotionally are all character traits which have been linked with the hysterical personality. In fact these personality traits would best be described by the term *histrionic*. Certainly only a minority of patients with hysterical symptoms have this personality.

A history of head injury or organic disease of the central nervous system appears to predispose patients to hysterical symptoms, especially amnesia and fugue states.

As mentioned above, hysterical symptoms

may be precipitated by any severe stress or conflict and probably a capacity to develop an hysterical symptom is latent in all of us. Cultural factors, however, play a part and the incidence is much commoner in primitive societies.

Hysterical symptoms may occur as part of any psychiatric disorder. This is particularly so in depression and a recent study revealed one third of patients with hysterical symptoms to be suffering from an underlying depression.

Treatment is of the underlying cause but over-all the outlook is good for cases with a recent onset. Of these roughly two thirds are symptom free at the end of twelve months. The remaining third have a gloomier outlook and after five years a quarter of the whole group still suffers from symptoms. As the years go by a number of cases diagnosed as suffering from conversion hysteria develop either schizophrenic or manic-depressive psychoses or epilepsy. In summary, hysteria is a diagnosis which should be used with considerable caution and reservation. The exact meaning of whatever terms are used should be so defined as to be easily understood, and consistently applicable to the clinical picture presented by the patient. The ICD classification recognizes under hysterical neurosis two subgroups – dissociative states and conversion phenomena. There is also a coding for hysterical personality disorder. Each is defined in simple understandable terms; not everyone may be satisfied, but attempts should be made to adhere to this international classificatory system.

Hysterical disorders in childhood

Loss of speech, vision, or power in the limbs for non-organic reasons is extremely uncommon in the pre-pubertal child and only slightly more common in early adolescence. The occurrence of such symptoms in childhood is therefore grounds for extremely careful neurological evaluation. Occasionally a child will develop a limp as an imitative or attention-seeking phenomenon for a few days, but this can usually be cured with a mild degree of suggestion and encouragement.

Abdominal pains and headaches in children occur by contrast very commonly in situations when no organic cause can be found. Sometimes clear-cut emotional reasons for the pain are then forthcoming, e.g. concern over a relative with an organic disorder, a problem in school, or tension over parental disharmony, but more commonly neither organic nor emotional reasons can be found for the pain. In this situation the child and parents should be encouraged to allow the pains to interfere as little as possible in the child's life, and the benign prognosis of the symptom should be emphasized.

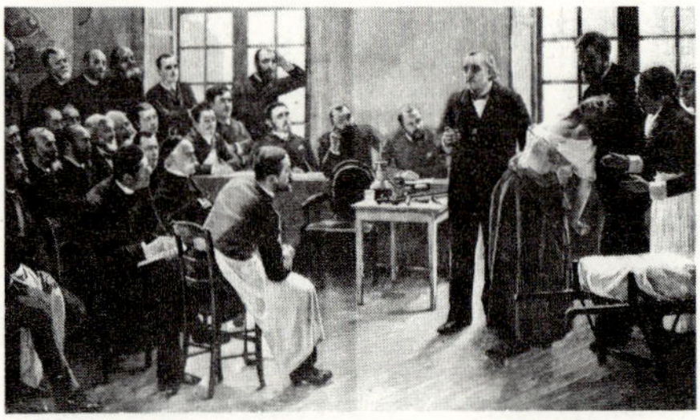

Charcot inducing hysterical fits before an audience

Hysterical fits

Apart from the classical manoeuvres of Charcot, who precipitated seizure-like activity in susceptible persons in front of an audience, fits can only rarely be regarded with safety as having an hysterical basis. Certain individuals may, for a variety of reasons, dissemble or act out the events which they know or imagine represent a major convulsive seizure. Sometimes epileptic patients do so. The absence of neurological signs and the failure to void urine, bite the tongue or damage the person each classically regarded as distinguishing the real from the masquerade, are unreliable. The problem is resolved by experts with great difficulty. 'Hysterical fits' always deserve investigation to exclude an organic cause.

Hysterical pseudo-dementia

Often used synonymously with the Ganser syndrome, the term 'hysterical pseudo-dementia' is an example of psychiatric double talk, seeking to exonerate a patient who simulates amnesia from any responsibility for his performance. The unconscious is involved and the outmoded and imprecise term 'hysteria' used by the doctor, who should instead be competent enough to decide whether or not there is a true dementia. In general this is not a difficult task, provided the psychiatric examination (q.v.) is carried out correctly and that the doctor is able to physically examine his patient and interpret his findings.

SEE ALSO Ganser syndrome and Malingering.

Iatrogenic illness

The influence of medical theory on the handling of the sick individual may result in the production of invalidism, complicating physical disorder, or even the death of the patient. Thus when all heart murmurs were regarded with apprehension, systolic murmurs at the apex led to a cardiac invalidism entirely produced by the doctor. Effort syndrome is rarely seen today and yet was a major cause of invaliding in the first world war. Today iatrogenic illness is less commonly psychogenic and is much more dangerous, being the result of the use of complex diagnostic techniques fraught with possible difficulties and of highly potent pharmaceutical agents. Overtreatment, the complications of treatment, and the injudicious use of drugs are all responsible for the production of iatrogenic illness.

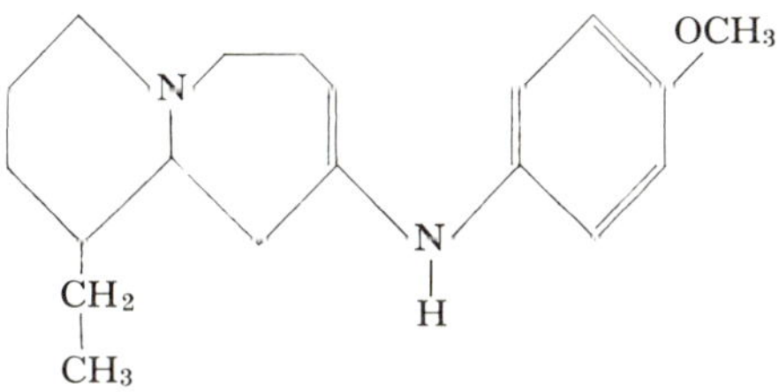

Ibogaine

Ibogaine

Ibogaine is an alkaloid from an African shrub. It is used by natives stalking game to enable them to remain motionless for up to two days yet retain mental alertness. It has been proposed as an anti-depressant but its place in medical practice is not established.

Id

The id is the instinctual reservoir from which drives arise. Controlled by ego and super-ego, a balance is struck in the normal individual between these forces so that the individual is able to adjust to the environment in which he moves.

Ideas

The conscious or subjective counterparts of cognitive processes include percepts (q.v.) – internal representations of the immediate environment; images – internal reconstructions of previous sensory experience; and thoughts (q.v.) which involve conceptual and symbolic processes and have semantic significance. Images and thoughts are both subsumed under the more general term idea.
Pathological ideation occurs in several psychiatric conditions. For example, ideas of influence (q.v.), i.e. of external control, are common in schizophrenia (q.v.) as are autochthonous ideas (q.v.) which appear to have no source, and are unrelated to the current train of thought. Ideas which arise with a subjective sense of compulsion overcoming internal resistance are typical of obsessional states.
SEE ALSO Cognition, Obsessional ideas, and Perception.

Ideas of influence

These are the expression of a subject's feeling that his thought, feeling, or his body is being interfered with by an outside agency. They may arise from passivity feelings (e.g. the feeling that thought is controlled from outside or strength drained away) or from tactile hallucinations. The idea may be expressed in terms suggesting an explanation of its mechanism, e.g. influence by radio or radar. This symptom is characteristically schizophrenic.

Ideas of persecution

The feeling of being singled out, passed over, slighted, being spied on, followed, slandered is the material of ideas and delusions of persecution occurring most characteristically in paranoid states (q.v.). Persecutory feelings also occur in depressive states, but here guilt predominates and instead of resenting the subject believes he deserves what he fears.

Ideas of reference

The essential element in this symptom is correct perception (q.v.) but misinterpretation, through self-consciousness, guilt, or suspicion. Statements, gestures and other indications of opinion are inappropriately applied to oneself as derogatory, disapproving, or persecutory. Thus a newspaper or radio item concerning a murderer may be regarded by the subject as an accusation or a hint of incriminating knowledge; an advertisement for deodorant as a personal insinuation. Self-conscious adolescents may believe that innocent remarks or gestures indicate attention to them or betray contempt, rebuff, or disdain.

Identification

When an individual incorporates or introjects within himself a mental picture of something external, and then thinks, feels, and acts according to the conception of the introject, this is termed identification. The process is largely unconscious and is the mechanism whereby, in early life, a child should come to have an appropriate internal model, e.g. of the same-sexed parent, on which to build and modify. Identification may often be used as a defence mechanism – a sensitive person protects his self-esteem and love by identifying himself with aspects of his frustrating environment. This is the basis for the mechanism of 'identification with the aggressor'.

Idiopathic hypoparathyroidism

This rare disorder, sometimes familial, occurs most often in childhood. Girls are more often affected than boys. In childhood convulsions, vomiting and papilloedema occur as well as tetany. If the hypocalcaemia is not corrected, psychological deterioration may occur, rendering the child mentally subnormal.

Idiopathic spontaneous hypoglycaemia of childhood

Attacks begin in infancy, more often in boys, with convulsions as the main feature. Affected babies are often listless and poor feeders. Repeated attacks of untreated hypoglycaemia in young children is a rare cause of brain damage and consequent subnormality. In the older hypoglycaemic child, psychological support is an essential part of treatment.

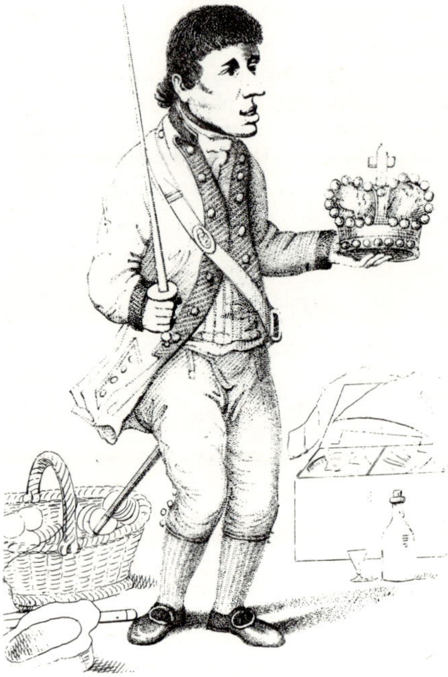

Henry Dinsdale 'Mayor of Garratt' 1821

Idiot

This is an obsolete term (SEE Mental subnormality). Such individuals are now legally regarded as severely subnormal. It became customary to link the designation of idiot with the intelligence quotient, and to class individuals with an IQ under 20 as idiots. Through usage, this association persists, and the term 'idiot-level' is still meaningful in psychological assessment.

Idiot savant

In very rare instances a severely mentally subnormal patient will show an isolated ability of normal or even outstanding quality. Such an individual is known as an idiot-savant. It is possible that a good proportion of such instances have been cases of infantile autism (q.v.) in which islets of ability against a background of apparent subnormality are sometimes observed.

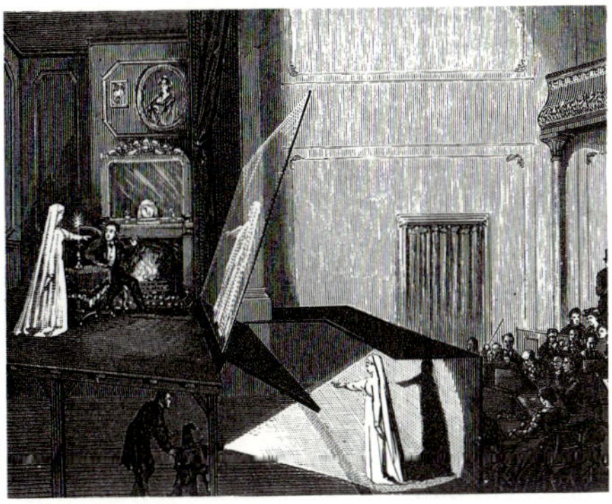

Illusions

An illusion is a perceptual distortion whereby a stimulus is misinterpreted. It may occur under conditions of poor perception (e.g. mistaking a tree for an animal in the dark), or under conditions designed to mislead the senses (optical and theatrical illusions). Illusions may occur and be generated by a mood or expectation (e.g. fear or hope) and occur frequently in mental illness in association with delusions (q.v.).
SEE ALSO Perception.

Imbecile

An obsolete term (SEE Mental subnormality).
Through long custom the term 'imbecile level' is still used to denote a psychological level between IQ 20 and 50.

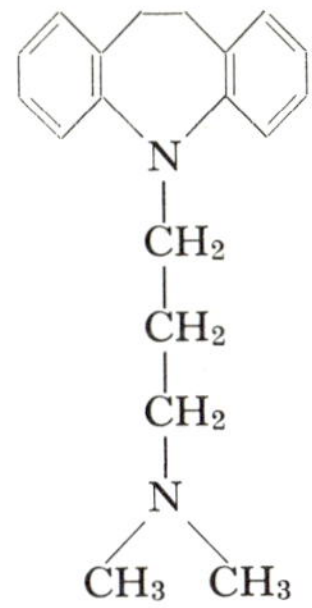

Chemical structure of imipramine, a typical iminodibenzyl compound

Iminodibenzyl derivatives

Iminodibenzyl compounds are tricyclic anti-depressants. Imipramine (q.v.) is the prototype of this group. It is comparatively non-sedative and has the general properties of the tricyclic anti-depressant compounds (q.v.). Desipramine (q.v.) is closely related to imipramine from which it is derived metabolically. It may act fractionally more quickly than its parent compound and has similar actions, although it is claimed to have a lower incidence of side effects. The third member of this group, trimipramine (q.v.) differs from the others in having a sedative action. Smaller doses of these compounds are often used in treating elderly patients because of their greater sensitivity to tricyclic compounds. A further recent addition to the series is clomipramine (q.v.).
Side effects of the group include dry mouth, accommodation difficulties, disturbances of micturition, and hypotension. They are contraindicated in liver damage, circulatory failure, urinary retention, and glaucoma, and should be used with great caution concurrently with or within fourteen days of monoamine oxidase administration.
SEE appendix for details of individual drugs.

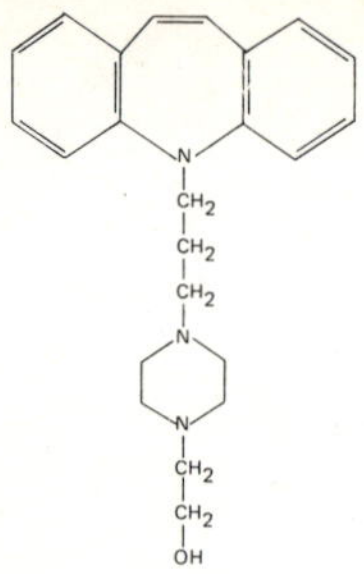

Chemical formula of opipramol, an iminostilbene derivative

Iminostilbene derivatives

One of the iminostilbene derivatives, opipramal (q.v.), is an anti-depressant compound with some sedative effects. A related compound carbamazepine is an effective anticonvulsant in temporal lobe epilepsy and an analgesic.

Imitation

Copying the behaviour of another person. In psychological terms the action of the other person provides the stimulus for a response which is an attempted reproduction of that stimulus. A related process, called modelling (q.v.), does not involve precise copying but the adoption of the general style of behaviour of another. Imitation and modelling are important in social learning (q.v.) generally and particularly in early character (q.v.) and personality (q.v.) development when the same-sex parent usually provides the model.

Implosion

SEE Flooding.

Impotence

Impotence is the inability in the male to obtain or sustain penile erection sufficient to conclude heterosexual coitus satisfactorily. It is distinct from premature ejaculation (q.v.) although both may coexist. Impotence, from first attempts at intercourse (early onset impotence), commonly occurs in the male with an anxious, self-insecure personality. Repetitive attempts at intercourse produce humiliation and anticipatory anxiety. 'Honeymoon' impotence is of this type, and is particularly likely to occur where the wife is sexually timid and inexperienced. Early onset impotence may sometimes be due to an underlying sexual perversion such as latent homosexuality (q.v.).

Impotence, occurring after a period of previous sexual adjustment in middle life (late onset impotence), may be due to boredom and disenchantment with the marital partner, but personality and intramarital tensions are common. Obesity, personal hygiene, menstrual disorders, and vaginal discharges may be remediable contributing factors. Late onset impotence may be symptomatic of some organic disease, particularly diabetes mellitus, pituitary disorder, alcoholism, peripheral arteriosclerotic disease, neurological disorders, and cerebral tumours. Endogenous depressive illnesses may give rise to impotence, whilst some drugs, particularly the anti-depressants themselves, antihypertensive agents, corticosteroids and neuroleptics may induce impotence. Even though at the age of 70 years 50% of the male population is still potent, there is a progressive increase in biological impotence in later life.

Where anxiety plays a major role, as in early onset impotence, joint counselling between the marital partners should be the first step in treatment in order to promote communication and to explore mutual fears and hostile feelings. Simple tranquillizers, such as diazepam 5 mg. nocte, may be useful. If impotence is persistent then a period of complete abstention from intercourse for four to six weeks should be imposed whilst permitting a full range of mutual sexual fore-play. This may be combined with desensitization (behaviour) therapy directed to the patient's anxiety about intercourse and possible failure. Only when there is strong sexual desire with confidence in erectile capacity should intercourse once again be allowed.

Evidence of endogenous depression should be an indication for appropriate anti-depressant treatment. There are no effective aphrodisiac drugs, although amphetamines are thought to have some psychosexual stimulant properties. In the biological impotence of later life systemic testosterone may be tried. Hormone therapy, however, is usually only effective when there is an endocrine disorder present. Where impotence has been present for longer than two years prognosis for recovery is poor. In this type of resistant case the Lowenstein penile splint may be tried. This is a mechanical device devised to allow penetration with the flaccid penis in order to avoid anticipatory anxiety. Claims for its success are offset by aesthetic objections raised by marital partners.

Impotentia ejaculandi

Inability to ejaculate or to experience orgasm in sexual intercourse (impotentia ejaculandi) is much rarer than premature ejaculation (q.v.) but may be so complete as to lead to sterility. It can be due to interference with sympathetic nervous outflow in patients with diabetic neuropathy, tabes dorsalis, following lumbar sympathectomy or as a complication of hypotensive drugs and some phenothiazines and tricyclic anti-depressants. It may occur as an early symptom of Parkinsonism. Psychogenic causes include latent homosexuality and a repressed fear of heterosexual orgasm leading to total orgasmic inhibition; idiopathic cases also occur.

Imprinting

Many young animals learn to recognize the characteristics of their parents early in life. The process involved was first studied in birds, where it is often rapid and relatively irrèversible, and it was regarded as a special form of learning. It is now clear that its peculiarities depend on the context in which it occurs, and that it in fact shares many properties with learning studied in other contexts (e.g. perceptual learning,

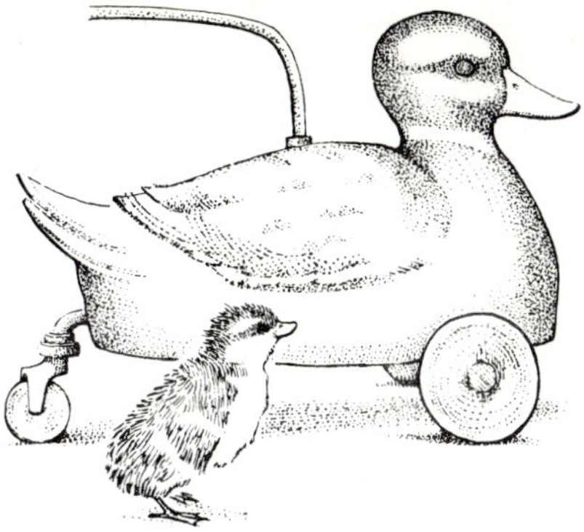

observational learning). However, in so far as the early formation of the parent-offspring bond depends upon it, its importance can hardly be overestimated. Use of the term is often extended to other contexts in which learning is rapid and stable.

Impulse

In its most general sense, a tendency to act without preliminary deliberation or 'act of will' and, therefore, arising suddenly and usually from instinctual sources. Freud (q.v.) used the term particularly with reference to action tendencies directed by the 'id' (q.v.). Impulsive behaviour is associated with emotional arousal and individuals described as 'impulsive' tend to be emotionally labile. Extreme individuals of this type, who appear to be unable to defer emotional gratification, represent one type of psychopathic personality (q.v.) and may indulge in crime. Obsessive-compulsive neurotics (q.v.) experience strong impulses to carry out their compulsions, but may also show equally strong resistance when these are immoral, anti-social or criminal in nature.
SEE ALSO Emotion and Will.

Incest

Sexual intercourse between individuals of opposite sex closely related by blood kinship. The degree of kinship that is regarded as morally and in many communities legally wrong often depends on social custom.

Incest is a very common offence and takes several forms. The most frequent is a father-daughter relationship, more uncommonly a sister-brother relationship, and only very rarely a mother-son relationship. In the latter case one or other or both of the partners is found to be suffering from a serious mental illness. Pre-pubertal sexual play between brothers and sisters is to be considered normal; it is the intensity of the relationship which determines its pathological nature. Father-daughter incest follows several patterns. Most usually there is an unhappy marriage, the husband weak, but with a high sex drive to which the wife does not respond. For comfort the husband seeks out his daughter who may indeed take her mother's place. Another characteristic situation involves the father of a problem family who drinks, and coming home drunk, seduces or even rapes his young daughter. Lastly, there is a true love relationship which develops between father and daughter, who behave as lovers and may run away from home together.

Pregnancy, when it does occur from incestuous relationships, is often carried through for fear of detection, although indications for termination might be manifestly present. The doctor who discovers a case of incest must be particularly cautious in his handling of the situation, for prosecution and imprisonment often produce a total collapse of the family. He should refer the problem to a psychiatrist.

SEE ALSO Sexual disorders and Sexual offences.

Incidence

The occurrence of new cases of a particular condition within a defined population during a particular time period – usually twelve months.

Incontinence in the aged

In advanced dementia (q.v.) there may be true neurogenic loss of bladder control, in which there is a severe continuous incontinence by day and night, and little can be done except to keep the patient dry by regular changing. More often, urinary incontinence in dementia is due to a combination of disorientation and apathy, and is often associated with a loaded rectum. The occurrence of periods of restlessness, due to a full bladder, may make possible a regime of simple toilet training which makes nursing easier. In mild dementia incontinence may respond to treatment with antibiotics for urinary infection, or by surgical or conservative correction of pelvic disorders, and relief of severe constipation and faecal impaction.

Incontinence may for a time occur during emotional crises or depressive psychoses, in which it seems to be a way of expressing resentment, anger, or anxiety.

Although they do not have a large part to play in the treatment of incontinence in the aged, drugs with an atropine-like action, such as propantheline or emepronium bromide, which reduce urinary frequency are worth a trial.

Identity crisis

The development of the sense of what one is, what is one's identity, is interrupted at times by crises, particularly during adolescence, when the feeling of identity is subject to considerable strain. The clash between instinctual feelings and social role obligation may lead to a loss of personal identity – 'Whom am I?', 'What am I?' are typical of the self-questioning that may occur. Resolution of an identity crisis may occur, but is often associated with acute or subacute episodes of mental illness.

Individual psychology

The system of psychodynamics developed by Alfred Adler (q.v.), individual psychology considers human behaviour to be based on feelings of inferiority and the attempts to compensate for them. The importance of sexuality was denied by Adler, who was the first of Freud's disciples to break away. The drive for power, the life-style, and the masculine strivings of women are all based on feelings of inferiority which are partly inherited, partly acquired. The inferiority complex is more popular with laymen than with psychiatrists.

Indole derivatives

A group of tricyclic anti-depressant compounds represented in clinical use by iprindole.

Industrial rehabilitation units

Originally introduced in Britain for the physically handicapped, these units have proved their value for patients with psychiatric disabilities. Advantages may be lost if psychiatric patients constitute more than a small proportion of the intake. The atmosphere of the IRU is as realistic as possible, so that a patient's suitability for open employment can be practically assessed. There is also the encouragement of working in a community where others can be seen overcoming similar handicaps.
SEE ALSO Occupational therapy.

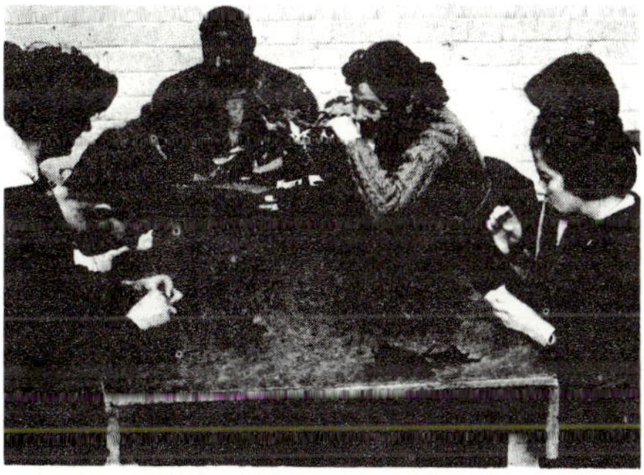

Industrial therapy

In the last twenty years, conventional occupational therapy (which is based mainly on handicrafts) has been largely supplemented and replaced by realistic work processes. Patients are paid on the basis of their performance and the work is usually subcontracted from industrial firms; it is divided into jobs of differing levels of skill. Both inside hospitals and in the community day centres, industrial therapy helps to restore the ability for normal work.
SEE ALSO Industrial rehabilitation units and rehabilitation.

Infanticide

A woman who deliberately causes the death of her child under the age of 12 months is found guilty, in England and certain other countries, of infanticide instead of murder if the jury is satisfied that the balance of her mind was disturbed by the birth and/or by consequent lactation. She is then dealt with as if she had committed manslaughter (q.v.). In practice a verdict of infanticide is brought in wherever possible and courts are lenient with sentencing.
Not all women convicted of infanticide suffer with puerperal psychoses (q.v.); some are psychopathic (q.v.), some are child batterers, some are desperate unmarried mothers (q.v.), and many of the babies are unwanted. Any woman who talks of attacking or destroying her child (whatever its age) is in need of urgent psychiatric advice and may have to be separated from the child to save its life.
SEE ALSO Battered child syndrome, Homicide, Forensic psychiatry, and Murder.

Infantile autism
SEE Autism.

Infantile sexuality

Freud and others have shown that sexuality, used in a wide sense to refer to pleasurable sensations produced by stimulation of various cutaneous (erotogenic) zones is operative long before puberty. There are striking differences from adult sexuality. In infants the body areas concerned are more diffuse, there is a close relationship to excretory functions and there is a sexual colouring to the child's interest in its nearest relatives (the Oedipal situation). The cutaneous areas involved are at first very diffuse, and stimulation of the oral and anal zones, as well as the genital, is connected with infantile pleasure. Fixation at certain phases of this normal process of development is held to be responsible for different neuroses and sexual deviations.

Infantile spasms

(Synonyms: Lightning seizures; Salaam seizures)

This disease consists of periodic spells of jack-knife (whole-body) flexions or extensions and mental retardation. Two thirds of all cases start during the first six months of life and males predominate. The EEG shows chaotic abnormality (hypsarrhythmia), and this term has been used mistakenly as a synonym for the disease. There is a mortality of 15 % and most of the survivors are mentally subnormal. Although the results are disappointing, hospital treatment is advised and some cases have responded to nitrazepam.

Infection, mental symptoms due to

These depend not only on the toxaemia or actual brain lesion, but on the degree of predisposition of the patient, and children and old people are much more likely to develop mental symptoms than middle aged adults. In acute infections confusion and delirium are the characteristic features and no particular infective agent apart perhaps from that causing encephalitis lethargica produces a characteristic picture.
The mental after effects of infection depend on the lowering of the patient's general resistance allowing any underlying predisposition to mental disorder to show itself, depression and emotional lability being the most common.

Inferiority complex

Adler put forward the view that many problems arose as a result of unconscious feelings of inferiority. These might relate to sexual gender, competition for parental love between sibs or a host of situations in which an individual was consistently worsted, made to feel inferior, or was actually inferior. Attempts at compensation, again often unconsciously motivated, might result in aggressive behaviour, sexual over-activity, or a hundred and one different ways of asserting oneself. In addition to psychological inferiority Adler spoke of organ inferiority, a particular organ system failing to develop normally and leaving the individual, for instance, with a 'weak bladder' or a 'weak bowel'. Conflicts might find their expression through such an inferior organ system, e.g. child-parent conflict might be expressed in nocturnal enuresis when nervous control over bladder function has failed to develop completely. Adler recognized, too, that conscious feelings of inferiority were often a powerful motive in the struggle for power, success and mastery.

Information theory

A theory concerned with interpreting communicated messages in mathematical characteristics.

Inhalant addiction

Sniffing of chloroform, ether, nitrous oxide, the synthetic resins and petrol may produce pleasurable psychological effects, and lead to dependence on the substance concerned. Anaesthetists are at risk with regard to chloroform, ether and nitrous oxide. They may conceal their addiction, with unfortunate consequences. Adolescents are the chief users of the other inhalants, petrol in the poorer countries, 'glue' in the more affluent. Serious toxic effects may result from the continued sniffing of these substances – the liver and brain being involved.

Inheritance

A gene is a hypothetical hereditary unit at a specific locus on a chromosome. Characteristics showing continuous variation in a population (with only very small differences from one individual to the next if the individuals are put in rank order) are commonly the result of *polygenic inheritance*, or inheritance through the additive action of many genes of small effect. Often multiple environmental factors add further modification. Intelligence is an example of this kind of characteristic. Characteristics which show sharp segregation in a population may be caused by *single mutant (or altered) genes of major effect*. These may show the familial pat-

terns of Mendelian dominance or recessivity, or may be sex-linked genes. Because the chromosomes are paired, the genes on them are paired. In dominant inheritance, only one of the gene pair need be a mutant for its effect to be shown; in recessive inheritance both genes, however, must be mutants for the full effect to appear. This is a classical view; but in fact there are many intermediate stages of gene function between pure dominance and pure recessivity. Many of the inborn errors of metabolism associated with mental subnormality, such as phenylketonuria (q.v.), galactosaemia (q.v.), maple syrup urine disease (q.v.), gargoylism (q.v.), hepatolenticular degeneration (q.v.), are inherited as recessive traits. Examples of dominant conditions are tuberous sclerosis (q.v.) (epiloia) and neurofibromatosis (q.v.). Sex-linked genes are borne on the part of the X chromosome which has no homologous representation on the shorter Y chromosome. Conditions due to such genes are transmitted familially by unaffected females but are manifest only in males. An example of such a condition is glucose-6-phosphate dehydrogenase deficiency (q.v.). It is assumed that very many genes are involved in the aetiology of conditions in which anomalies of the chromosomes are gross enough to be detected microscopically. Mongolism (q.v.) and other autosomal trisomies are examples of such conditions associated with severe mental subnormality.
SEE ALSO Genetics.

Inherited metabolic defects

Inherited metabolic defects, or inborn errors of metabolism, are very frequently associated with severe mental subnormality. In many the chemical lesion is known, having been identified in a large number of cases as deficiency of a single enzyme, as, for example, in phenylketonuria. In others, though the body chemistry is disordered, the origin is still obscure, as, for example, in Hartnup disease. The great majority of inherited metabolic defects follow an autosomal recessive mode of inheritance. The main disorders are shown in the table.
SEE ALSO Genetics and Autosomes.

Inhibition

The restraint imposed on thoughts, feelings or actions by the unconscious restrictions of instinctual drives. This occurs as a result of the constraints of the 'superego' (q.v.) and the demands of external reality which are opposed to the instinctual drives of the 'id' (q.v.). By this concept anxiety may be experienced in a situation which evokes even symbolic awareness of the forbidden wish. Inhibition of certain feelings, such as anger, are reported to be especially common amongst the sufferers of certain psychosomatic diseases, e.g. bronchial asthma and cholinergic urticaria.

Insanity

A term used frequently in nineteenth-century legislation but now obsolete and being replaced by 'mental disorder' (q.v.) for modern legal practice.
SEE ALSO McNaughton Rules.

Insight

The extent of the patient's understanding of the nature of his condition, the reasons underlying it and the effects it might have on his attitude and behaviour. Loss of insight may be found in a wide range of psychiatric and neurological disturbances – in delusional states, in disturbances of mood, in general paralysis, in disseminated sclerosis, and so on. Insight here is linked with judgement, both being aspects of the highest levels of nervous activity. Quite a different meaning is to be found in the psychotherapeutic situation. Here emotional and intellectual insight must be distinguished, as well as a spurious insight resulting from a desire to please the therapist. Intellectual insight has less therapeutic value than emotional insight – a deeply felt, sudden certainty of the reasons for various emotional disturbances. Many patients improve during psychotherapy without ever gaining insight; in many cases it is wiser to avoid insight-producing procedures.
SEE ALSO Thought.

Insomnia

Insomnia is the complaint of inability to get off to sleep or to remain asleep as personal habit had previously dictated. Needs for sleep (q.v.) vary between individuals. Anxious patients complain that problems flood in as they try to relax and their ruminations prevent sleep. Depressed patients wake to their guilty thoughts in the early hours.

The complaint of insomnia should be seen as a symptom and as far as possible treatment should be directed at the cause. In the absence of physical causes of night waking, thyrotoxicosis, nocturia, etc., it should alert the physician to the possibility of emotional disturbance.

Symptomatically insomnia can sometimes be helped by advising the patient to increase his physical exercise during the day, but for the few hours before bedtime to relax mentally and physically. If a hypnotic is required the benzodiazepines are much safer than barbiturates. Withdrawal of hypnotics should be gradual otherwise the increased REM sleep, frequently accompanied by anxious dreams or nightmares and which may last for several weeks, may convince the patient that he requires hypnotics for ever.

Instinct

1. Instinct or instinctive behaviour implied behaviour that was genetically determined and developed independently of experience. It is now agreed that (a) attempted dichotomies between learned and unlearned behaviour are not useful because learning (q.v.) applies to only some of the effects of experience; (b) attempted dichotomies between behaviour which does and does not depend on experience are not useful because all behaviour involves development within and dependence upon certain environmental conditions; (c) the useful questions about development concern *differences* – does the difference between the behaviour of this animal and that depend on genetic or environmental differences? Once these are answered, questions about how genes or environment produce their effects are fertile.

2. Instinct implied 'driven from within'. This stems from the outmoded energy models of motivation used by Freud, McDougall, Lorenz and others which, though perhaps useful clinically, have little scientific validity. At the behavioural level of explanation such models (a) are often used circularly (e.g. what makes the bird build a nest? – Answer, its nest-building instinct); (b) often imply that different aspects or types of behaviour have a common causal basis when such is not the case; and (c) often imply that behaviour comes to an end only through action, neglecting the roles of goal or consummatory stimuli. Where the term instinct is still used, careful examination of the context is necessary to discern the authors implications.

Insulinoma

Insulin-secreting tumours of the beta cells of the islets of Langerhans are benign adenomas in 90% of cases. The symptoms are those of hypoglycaemia (q.v.) and they are reduced by glucose. The hypoglycaemic attacks are commonest before breakfast, after fasting, and after exercise. Recurrent attacks of unconsciousness, recovering spontaneously, and often without epilepsy and lesser degrees of hypoglycaemia, simply marked by unusual behaviour, may be wrongly diagnosed as hysteria because intercurrent examination will fail to reveal neurological signs, while on occasion, resting blood sugars may be in the low normal range. Fasting, intravenous tolbutamide, and finally insulin assay may suggest the correct diagnosis. Angiography demonstrates a small proportion of tumours, but may be useful in showing multiple tumours. Treatment is by surgical excision.

Insulin therapy

Deep insulin therapy for schizophrenia is of historical interest only. Daily injections of insulin were given to produce periods of hypoglycaemic coma lasting up to forty-five minutes. The coma was interrupted by giving intragastric or intravenous glucose. Treatment was given five days a week over a period of about two or three months, a full course comprising thirty to sixty comas. The treatment demanded a high degree of skill from doctors and nurses and even in the best hands mortality from irreversible coma was a potential danger. Good results were claimed in almost all early cases but the treatment has now been universally abandoned.

Modified insulin therapy has also been largely superseded by antidepressants and tranquillizers, but is occasionally of use in the treatment of patients with chronic anxiety, anorexia, loss of weight, and profound tension and exhaustion. The patient is nursed in bed, at least for the first half of every day. Soluble insulin in increasing doses up to a maximum of about 50 units is given at 8 AM followed at 9 or 9.30 AM by a large breakfast. Sweating, drowsiness and faintness may occur. The patients stay in bed for the rest of the morning, getting up at lunchtime, when they are again encouraged to eat a hearty meal. Weight gain occurs and the patient feels more relaxed and less tense.

Intellectualization

This may be observed as a mental defence mechanism especially in persons with significant schizoid or obsessional personality traits. It is a form of displacement (q.v.) through which painful, but emotionally important impulses are avoided by escaping from the world of emotions into the world of intellectual concepts and words.

Intelligence

In its most general sense, intelligence refers to the all-round efficiency of an individual's cognitive (q.v.) abilities. No single more precise definition has won universal acceptance. Binet, the pioneer of mental testing, considered that intelligence is a combination of intellectual capacities such as judgement (q.v.), reasoning and imagination. Others have described some single more general essential characteristic, e.g. the ability 'to adjust to novel situations', 'to make use of abstract symbols' or 'to perceive relationships'. One of the least unsatisfactory definitions of this nature was proposed by Knight: 'The capacity of relational, constructive thinking directed to the attainment of some end.'

In contrast to these descriptive or analytic definitions, more practical definitions have been proposed by applied psychologists. For them, intelligence is the quality necessary for success in academic, vocational or other situations recognized as intellectually demanding. In a sense, they define intelligence as 'academic aptitude' but, as their tests are designed as good predictors of this type of achievement, they essentially adopt the apparently circular but scientifically sound operational definition by which intelligence is 'what intelligence tests measure'.

Although psychologists, particularly in England speak of general intellectual ability or g, statistical analyses of intelligence test scores indicate a hierarchical structure of abilities with subsidiary group factors of which those representing 'verbal' and 'performance' or 'spatial' ability are the most important. A test such as the Wechsler Adult Intelligence Scale (WAIS) (q.v.) includes two scales, yielding separate scores, one consisting of verbal tests and the other of practical tests involving the manipulation of concrete material such as jig-saws, block designs and the like.

Twenty years ago intelligence was thought of as an innate capacity and the IQ as a more or less stable characteristic of an individual. It is still recognized that genetic factors are important, but it has also become evident that these interact with environmental influences including social-class.

Although definitions of subnormality (q.v.) also refer to social deficiencies, low intelligence is the common element in all types. As a rough guide, subnormals would be expected to have IQs below 75 and the 'severely subnormal' (q.v.) below 50. Of the latter, those scoring between about 20 and 50 represent the imbecile (q.v.) range and those below 20 the idiots (q.v.).

Subnormals are intellectually impaired from birth or early infancy. Brain damage and some forms of psychiatric illness such as schizophrenia (q.v.) may produce intellectual deterioration in later life. This may differentially affect different abilities and the pattern of test scores can be of diagnostic usefulness.

SEE ALSO Psychological tests, Conceptual

thinking, Thought, Thinking, Eugenics, Mental examination, and Brain-damaged child.

Intensive psychotherapy

The more intensive the psychotherapy (q.v.) in terms of length, frequency and number of sessions, the greater the possibility for the patient to develop an emotional insight into his problems through a working transference relationship with his therapist. There is also a greater risk of harm being done to the patient and consequently a greater need for skill in the therapist. Because of these risks intensive psychotherapy should be reserved for patients with disabling symptoms which have failed to respond to more conservative measures and when the prognosis is poor.

Intersex

SEE Pseudo-hermaphroditism.

Intractable headache

SEE Depressive equivalents.

Introjection

As the child's perception of the external world develops, so it has to develop means of dealing with the multifarious impressions streaming into the nervous system whereby it can identify with or reject the objects which are their source. At first the mouth is the chief sensory organ and part objects – the nipple, or the breast, come to symbolize love, warmth and comfort. How this happens is by an active process, that of introjection, whereby the object is incorporated into the developing psyche. As the eye, ear, nose and skin subserve more and more sensory impressions, so these sensory modalities are also used to introject objective perceptions. Introjection is one of the mechanisms contributing to the final identification or otherwise with external objects which produces the individual human being.

Introversion

The turning of instinctual (libidinous) energy inwards upon oneself, the term is especially associated with the work of Jung. With object-love there is need for motor discharge but in introversion satisfaction is obtained in imagined response. There is shown a higher level of conditionability and a higher level of central nervous system arousal in introverted than extraverted subjects. Marked introversion is a feature of some schizophrenic psychoses – especially the 'simplex' subgroup.
SEE ALSO Extraversion.

Involutional melancholia

In the 1920's and 1930's it was widely believed that there was a distinct type of depression – involutional melancholia – which only occurred in middle age. By definition, those developing involutional melancholia had no history of previous depressions and the illness often persisted for several years, and sometimes progressed to a state of dementia.
The characteristics were agitation and bizarre hypochondriacal or nihilistic delusions. Hormone imbalance was regarded as an important cause.
Although the term involutional melancholia is still to be found in the international and other classifications, few people now regard it as a distinct entity. Agitation and nihilistic delusions are not restricted to the depressions of middle age and may occur in people who at other times have retarded depressions or even manic episodes, though the restrictions and increased hypochondriasis and obsessionality which occurs with age may increase their incidence in later life.
The response of involutional patients to ECT and the tricyclic drugs is no different from that of other severe depressions, and genetic studies have made it clear that even the most typical cases do not 'breed true'. Moreover, the classical clinical picture is becoming increasingly rare, probably as a result of earlier and more effective treatment. For all these reasons the term is falling into disuse.
SEE ALSO Geriatric psychiatry.

Irritable bowel syndrome (spastic colon, mucous colitis)

A little understood condition with three main clinical types:
(a) Spastic colon type is commonest, with abdominal pain and episodes of diarrhoea alternating with constipation.
(b) Episodic or chronic painless diarrhoea.
(c) Post prandial pain.
The condition is twice as common in women as men, the onset is in early adult life and rarely comes on for the first time after 50 years of age. In spite of considerable distress the general health remains good. The diagnosis is established by exclusion of organic disease.
The irritable bowel syndrome may occur in patients with normal personalities. In the majority, however, neurotic traits often with a depressive tendency are present and exacerbations of symptoms are often related to stress.
Treatment should include regular supportive interviews, bulk providing medicines and drugs such as diphenoxylate and nebeverine for diarrhoea and pain. A benzodiazepine is helpful in anxious patients and amitriptyline in those with a significant degree of depression.
SEE ALSO Psychosomatic disorders and Ulcerative colitis.

Isolation in the aged

Isolation has to be distinguished from loneliness, although the two often co-exist. Isolation may be defined as a lack of family and social contacts. Loneliness, however, is an explicit or implicit statement about a subjective, internal feeling. Many elderly people who complain of loneliness do in fact have a fair number of contacts, and conversely many who live lives of considerable isolation cope well and make no complaints. The relationship between isolation and psychiatric illness in the elderly is not a simple one.
1. There are the lifelong isolates, usually tough, independent, self-sufficient people, who remain efficient and capable into old age and do not respond to offers of socialization. The extreme types are the eccentric recluses, among whom some are psychotic, who are so reluctant to seek or accept any help that extreme degrees of self-neglect may occur and the prognosis for rehabilitation in the community is very poor.
2. Semi-isolates include those shy and dependent people who have been able to make few friends throughout life. They may become ill when their restricted circle of relatives and close friends are further reduced by death or illness.
3. Lastly, the elderly may become isolated as a result of sensory impairment, poor health, immobility, or bereavement (q.v.) and all these factors may interact to cause illness. This group is perhaps the most likely to benefit from social measures such as visiting, old people's clubs, luncheon clubs and outings.

Isotope scan (gamma scan)

The isotope scan is a plot of the output of gamma radiation over the surface of the head following oral or i.v. administration of a radio isotope. The image is built up by repetitively scanning successive points with a scintillation counter and it is necessary for the subject to be sufficiently cooperative to remain still for about 10 minutes. The technique has been largely superseded by the gamma camera which allows the entire head to be imaged simultaneously without scanning.
Abnormal collections of blood or blood vessels and areas of cerebral oedema take up isotope and produce regions of heightened radio activity in the scan. The technique is chiefly used in investigation of suspected intracranial lesions, notably cerebrovascular accidents, subdural haematomata and tumours.

Jacksonian epilepsy

A type of epilepsy (q.v.) named after Hughlings Jackson, and characterized by local attacks of epilepsy, one sided, and with a characteristic march depending on the anatomical organization of the affected area. Any area may be affected, the most characteristic Jacksonian attack being when the motor cortex is involved. Although originally one sided, the attack may spread to involve both sides, and consciousness may be lost. Jacksonian epilepsy is of great importance in the localization of cerebral lesions.

Jacob-Creutzfeld disease

A miscellaneous group of conditions have been included under this term.
1. Pre-senile dementia occurring together with signs of basal ganglia disorder.
2. Pre-senile dementia occurring together with the signs of motor neurone disease.
3. Pre-senile dementia with no specific features and advancing rapidly to a fatal conclusion.
Recent research suggests that some of the cases in these groups are the result of a slow acting virus; transmission experiments to chimpanzees has produced a condition of subacute spongiform encephalopathy, very similar to the pathological appearance in some of these cases, and in 'Kuru', a tropical disease occurring in New Guinea.

James-Lange theory

It is generally assumed that one has an emotional experience and that this in turn produces the bodily changes associated with it. The James-Lange theory of emotion (1884) claimed that exactly the reverse was true, that the bodily changes came first and the emotional experience is the feeling of those changes as they occur.

Jealousy

Morbid jealousy refers to patients, usually men, whose suspicions or concern about their partner's infidelity are out of all proportion to normal expectations. The

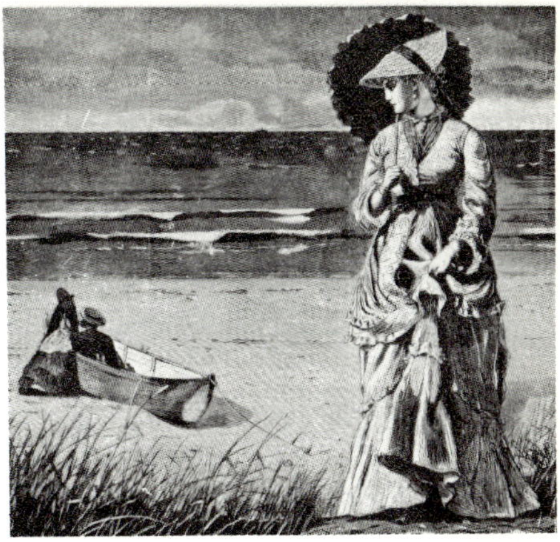

patient may be tormented with thoughts of what really happened in his wife's life, perhaps many years ago during the war, or, more frequently, is concerned about a suspected infidelity currently taking place. In either case the patient searches for evidence to confirm his suspicions by repeated questioning, any variation in the answers being taken as confirmatory evidence. Similarly he may check all his wife's movements during the day, when an unduly long time at the supermarket is held to be significant as are a visit to the hairdresser or the wearing of a new dress. Behind her back her handbag is searched, and her underwear examined for stains. Some patients demand sexual intercourse many times a day in the hope of diminishing the wife's suspected desire for the other man.
Morbid jealousy stems from the patient's underlying personality which shows paranoid traits together with depressive features, frequently related to their feelings of sexual inferiority. Such traits may be exacerbated or may be made manifest by alcoholism.
The disorder runs a protracted course and tends to get progressively worse. Some patients improve markedly with a combination of an antidepressant (preferably an MAOI) and chlorpromazine. In some patients the morbid jealousy progresses to a paranoid delusional state with beliefs that the patient's children are not his own or that his wife is trying to poison him. These latter patients are especially dangerous and there is a definite risk of the patient murdering his wife, often followed by an attempted suicide.

The Jellinek formula

This is a formula developed by Jellinek and used to estimate the prevalence of alcoholism in a population. It is based on reported deaths from cirrhosis.
The formula is

$$A = \frac{PD}{K} R$$

where A = total number of alcoholics alive in a given year,
D = reported number of deaths from cirrhosis in the same year,
P = % of such deaths attributed to alcoholism,
K = % of deaths from cirrhosis among all alcoholics alive with complications in a given year,
R = ratio of all alcoholics to alcoholics with complications (usual value = 4·1).

Jellinek assumed a value for K of 0·694. Though he later discredited its usefulness, many workers have held it to be of value in estimating national alcoholism prevalence rates as it gives at least a minimum figure.
SEE ALSO Alcoholism.

Jensen-Eysenk hypothesis

Jensen's and Eysenk's research supports the view that intelligence is largely genetically determined, probably to about 80%. Jensen suggests that intelligence is the primary determinant of scholastic success and that attempts to compensate for assumed cultural or environmental deprivation are unlikely to be successful.

Judgement

Judgement is a term that lacks precise definition but refers to all cognitive (q.v.) processes in which evaluation or assessment and decision-making are involved, and especially to those by which two or more events or aspects of experience are related to each other. Someone who shows good judgement has the ability to sum up the requirements of a situation and to react in an appropriate manner. Clearly, intellectual ability is important for this but so is relevant experience: highly intelligent adolescents frequently lack judgement, particularly in social situations.
Judgement may be impaired in many mental disorders, particularly the organic brain diseases (q.v.), and in mental subnormality (q.v.). It is assessed during the mental examination (q.v.) from the patient's attitudes to his social, vocational and domestic problems and his plans for the future.

Judicial factor

Otherwise known as curator bonis. This is a term used in Scottish law corresponding to the receiver in England. He is appointed by the court to manage the affairs of a patient who has been compulsorily admitted to a mental hospital or by virtue of mental infirmity is incapable of managing his affairs.

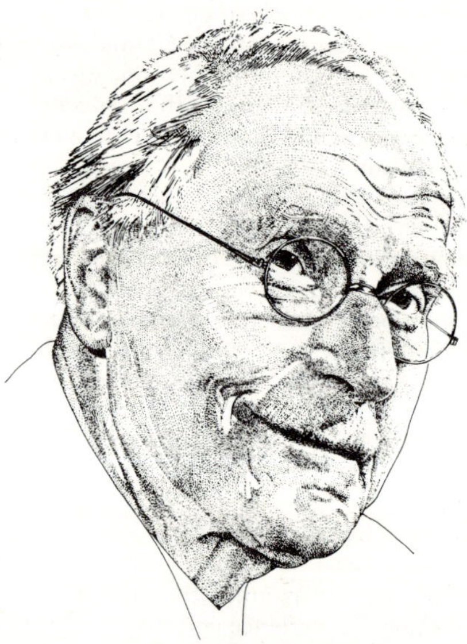

Jung, Carl Gustav (1875–1961)

A pupil of Bleuler (q.v.), Jung also studied under Janet in Paris, his work being very much influenced by these two men. His word-association test and his studies into the thought processes of schizophrenics resulted in a brilliant book, *The Psychology of Dementia Praecox* (1906). He wrote so favourably of Freud's theories, that a mutual interest developed between the two men. Jung organized the First International Psychoanalytical Congress which met in Salzburg in 1908 and became the first President of the International Psychoanalytical Association. Unfortunate disagreements finally led to the secession of Jung and the Zurich group of analysts in 1914 and Jung then began 'to be himself'. An almost endless flow of books and papers was the result, recording Jung's ideas and experiences. He became the leader of the School of Analytical Psychology, received many honours, and has left a permanent mark on the history of psychiatry with such concepts as the collective unconscious, the persona, the complex, introversion and extraversion, the archetype, the shadow, and so on. Jung's early experiences in a mental hospital gave to his work a different direction than that pursued by Freud, who had little, if any, experience of psychosis. Jung's interest in symbols, in magic, and in religion has led many psychiatrists to overlook his lasting contributions to our understanding of the world of the schizophrenic, as well as to the psychology of personality types. Jungian psychology looks forward as well as backwards, and attempts to deal with the totality of man's experience, spiritual as well as psychophysical. The medical model alone is not enough to understand man's problems in their totality and perhaps this may explain why analytic psychology has not met with psychiatry's complete approval of Jung's approach.

Kanner's syndrome
SEE Autism, early infantile.

Karotyping

Chromosomes present in the nuclei of all normal body cells may be classified, numbered and arranged in a systematized order. This process is known as karotyping. The usual arrangement is termed the Denver classification (q.v.).

Katathymic thinking

A thought process in which the emotional aspect is so strong that the logical argument is twisted to fit it. While it is the cause of many prejudiced arguments it is an occasional feature in schizophrenia.

Kayser-Fleischer ring

Is a diagnostic feature of hepatolenticular degeneration (q.v.). It consists of a greenish-yellow pigmented ring on the outer edge of the cornea.

Kempf's syndrome

Attacks of acute agitation, with panic, and escape behaviour occur occasionally in specific relation to a homosexual problem, perhaps the break-up of a relationship, the sudden realization of homosexual love, or the threat of legal proceedings. So acute may be the anxiety that consciousness appears to be clouded, and the diagnosis thus made difficult. Treatment consists of the administration of sedative drugs intravenously or intramuscularly, and when the agitation has been controlled, a common-sense approach to the individual problem presented by the patient. The condition settles quickly; it is akin to the catastrophic reactions.

Kernicterus

Intense bilirubin staining of the basal ganglia in infancy. Usually due to blood group incompatibility (Rh) between mother and infant, rarely drug produced. The clinical picture is variable, but mental defect, spasticity, athetosis, and ataxia may occur. Treatment consists of exchange blood transfusions.

Kinsey's ratings

The late Alfred Kinsey, Professor of Zoology at Indiana State University, in conjunction with Pomeroy and Martin published in 1948 a monumental survey of human sexual behaviour based upon stereotyped interviews of 5300 white males and 5940 white females. Significant numbers of males and females exhibited varying admixtures of heterosexual and homosexual behaviour at different periods of their lives. In order to emphasize the continuity between complete heterosexuality and homosexuality he devised this rating scale.

Kleine-Levin syndrome

A condition of unknown aetiology characterized by attacks of hypersomnia, bulimia, irritability, and uninhibited sexual behaviour, and occurring in young men.

Kleptomania (pathological stealing)
SEE Persistent stealing.

Klinefelter's syndrome
(Synonym: XXY syndrome)

The cardinal features of Klinefelter's syndrome are those of eunuchoidism after puberty in a tall male. They include gynaecomastia, increased excretion of follicle-stimulating hormone and testicular changes producing aspermatogenesis. It occurs in association with an XXY chromosome complement. Mental retardation may occur, but often intelligence is in the normal range. Personality traits include passivity, lack of sexual drive, immaturity, touchiness, paranoid sensitivity, insecurity, apathy, and a poor capacity for work.
SEE ALSO Chromosomal abnormalities.

Klüver-Bucy syndrome

Klüver and Bucy described a characteristic syndrome in monkeys following ablation of major portions of both temporal lobes. The animals showed visual agnosia, loss of fear and rage reactions, bulimia, increased sexual activity and severe memory defect. The uncus and hippocampus appeared to be significant, for these manifestations only occurred if these areas were included in the ablation.

Koro

A culture-bound syndrome occurring in the Chinese. Koro is a state of acute anxiety and panic resulting from the sudden belief that the penis is shrinking, will disappear into the abdomen and that death will then occur. It appears in epidemics, and is an example of anxiety appearing in epidemic form. Treatment consists of reassurance and mild tranquillization, together with appropriate information to the population at risk via the mass media.

Korsakoff psychosis

It is better to speak of the Wernicke/Korsakoff syndrome, for the one develops out of the other; earliest signs of an acute thiamine deficiency manifesting themselves in the signs and symptoms of Wernicke syndrome, viz. confusion, oculo-motor pareses and nystagmus. If the syndrome is inadequately treated, the patient emerges from his acute confusional state over a period of about 4–6 weeks to pass into the amnesic state originally described by Korsakoff. There is a striking memory defect for recent current events, the main difficulty being the inability to retain new material. With appropriate stimuli much material can be retrieved and visual stimuli are more evocative than auditory stimuli. The patient is disorientated in space and time and may or may not confabulate. Confabulation is often a product of the doctor's mode of questioning and is not an essential part of the Korsakoff syndrome. Originally a polyneuropathy was regarded as a necessary part of the syndrome, polyneuropathy, dementia and confabulation being regarded as the key elements in the syndrome. Today it is recognized that there may or may not be polyneuropathy. There is a very characteristic neuropathological appearance – areas of softening with vascular proliferation occurring in the nuclei of the thalamus, brain stem, and cerebellum. Thus, cerebellar signs are frequently to be found on clinical examination. Lesions are bilateral and symmetrical and the mammillary bodies are always affected, a lesion which is specific for the Wernicke/Korsakoff syndrome. Theoretically the Korsakoff syndrome is eminently preventable if adequate thiamine is administered in the early phase of the Wernicke syndrome. Large doses of thiamine (1·0 G. daily by mouth) must be given over a period of approximately 6 to 12 months. Wernicke/Korsakoff syndrome is a clinico-pathological syndrome; the clinical signs and symptoms may be found in a wide variety of disorders such as head injury, cerebral tumour, cerebral abscess, etc., but in these cases the characteristic neuropathological appearance is lacking.

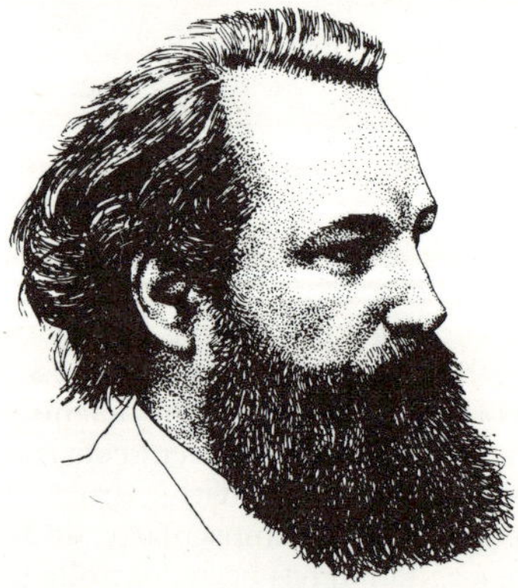

Korsakoff, S. S. (1854–1900)

The friend of Tolstoy, who used to visit Korsakoff's patients and attempt to understand them, Korsakoff was influenced by the work of Charcot (q.v.) and of Maudsley (q.v.). His doctoral dissertation 'On Alcoholic Paralysis' (1887) was concerned with the syndrome later to become eponymously linked with his name. He advocated the non-restraint movement, better conditions for the mentally ill, and classified mental illness mainly according to aetiology SEE ALSO Korsakoff's psychosis.

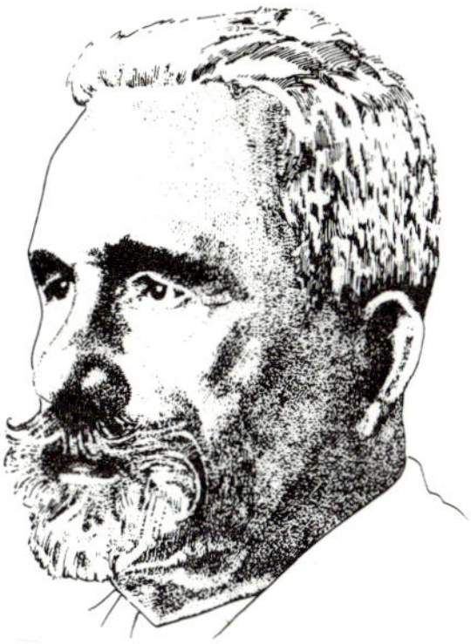

Kraepelin, Emil (1856–1926)

The codifier of psychiatric disorders, Kraepelin trained in neuro-anatomy and physiology. He therefore classified mental illness in accordance with the rules of natural science. Thus he considered that the natural history of the illness, the form it took, its onset and course were all factors to be considered before a diagnosis could be made. He brought order out of relative chaos, separated the manic-depressive illnesses from dementia praecox, and subdivided this condition into three great groups – catatonic, hebephrenic, and paranoid. He further regarded psychiatric illness as exogenous or endogenous. His major work, *Psychiatrie, Ein Lehrbuch für Studierende und Aertze* (1883), went into nine editions. He was Professor of Psychiatry at Heidelberg, moving to Munich in 1903, where he remained until his death. His solid contributions to psychiatry will outlast much of the work of more ephemeral dynamic psychiatrists.

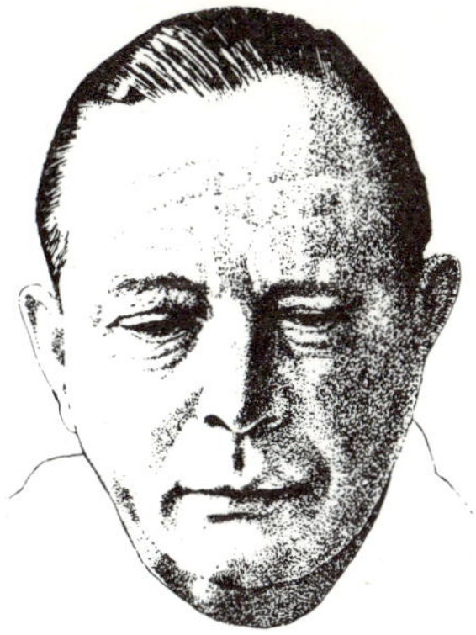

Kretschmer, Ernst (1888–1964)

Perhaps best known for his book *Physique and Character*, published when Kretschmer was only 33. In it he described the alleged relationship between certain mental illnesses and certain types of body build – the pyknic (q.v.) and the asthenic (q.v.), thus beginning a spate of anthropological and scientific work. A man of wide ranging intellect, Kretschmer published books on the sensitive personality, on medical psychology and on psychotherapy, all of them greatly influential on the course of German psychiatry.

Labile

SEE Lability of affect.

Lability of affect

A liability to sudden short-lived changes in mood. In mild form it is characteristic of people with prominent hysterical personality traits and of those suffering from neurotic depressions (q.v.). It may also occur in some mixed manic-depressive states and in these the mood changes are usually unrelated to any obvious environmental stimuli.

Normally, however, the term is reserved for a more dramatic lability seen only in patients with organic cerebral disease, particularly in those with cerebral arteriosclerosis (q.v.). Such patients may be weeping one minute, in a violent rage the next, and rocking with laughter a moment later. Usually these outbursts are provoked by an appropriate but trivial stimulus: floods of tears by the mention of a long-dead relative, uncontrolled rage by some minor inconvenience, and so on. The excessive nature of these responses is often referred to as 'emotional incontinence'. Uncontrolled weeping is generally the most prominent feature. Sometimes it is distressing to the patient but more often the prevailing mood is one of euphoria.

SEE ALSO Brain syndromes.

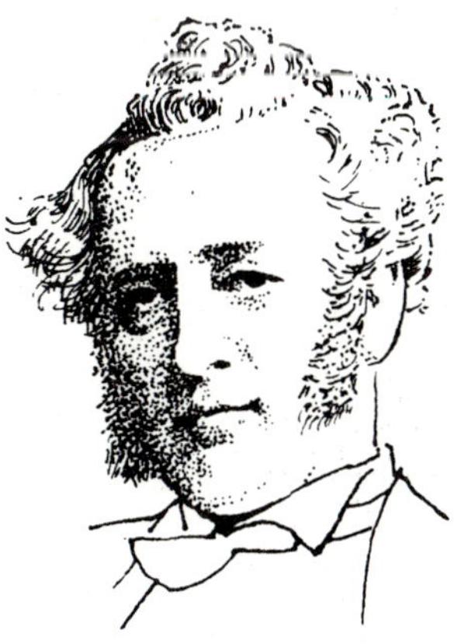

Langdon-Down, John Langdon Haydon (1828–1896)

Combining the medical superintendency of the Earlswood Asylum for Idiots with a post as physician at the London Hospital, he devoted himself to the study of mental deficiency (q.v.). He was the first to describe mongolism (q.v.) in an article in the London Hospital Reports in which he attempted to classify mental deficiency using certain ethnic characteristics. He considered the mongolian type of idiocy was an example of degeneration.

SEE ALSO Mongolism and Down's syndrome.

Language

Social scientists emphasize the communicative function of language. Thus, for the anthropologist Sapir, language is '. . . a purely human and non-instinctive method of communicating ideas, emotions and desires by means of a system of voluntarily produced symbols'. For the psychologist these symbols are also essential mediators of abstract conceptual thinking (q.v.). A word or other symbol conveys a meaning, i.e. it codifies information. This meaning may be 'denotative', indicating or labelling a concrete object or action, or 'connotative', referring to qualities of the object indicated and usually carrying evaluative and attitudinal overtones. Spoken language is based on combinations of a limited number of sound units or phonemes to form a vast number of meaningful units or morphemes which constitute the root words, prefixes and suffixes of a language. Rules concerning the derivation of words and sentences from these morphemes represent the relevant grammar. Advanced human societies develop written as well as oral forms of language. Language functions are controlled from specialized local centres in the cerebral cortex and speech involves complex self-regulatory cybernetic (q.v.) mechanisms. Behaviourists claim that a child acquires language skills from conditioning by and imitation (q.v.) of his parents. However, some modern linguists such as Chomsky propose 'generative' theories and argue for an innate basis for language.

Disorders of language may occur from defects of the underlying neuro-physiological mechanisms as in some organic brain diseases, as a reflection of disordered thinking as in some psychoses, or from a combination of both as is probably true of the dysphasias and dysgraphias associated

with certain types of brain injury. Stuttering is an example of a more subtle dysfunction of language.
SEE ALSO Speech disorders.

Lanugo hair

A fine, downy hair on the back sometimes found in anorexia nervosa.

Latah

A culture-bound syndrome characterized by echopraxia (q.v.), echolalia (q.v.), and startle reactions. It is found in south-east Asia, and bears some resemblance to acute catatonic schizophrenia. It often follows a severe fright.

Lawrence-Moon-Biedl syndrome

This syndrome consists in its full form of retinitis pigmentosa, hypogenitalism, obesity, polydactyly and mental subnormality, usually of severe degree. There is, however, some variability in the form and severity of the clinical signs. It is inherited as an autosomal recessive condition, but the gene is an incomplete recessive, and close relatives of patients may show some of the signs.

Leadership

The ability to lead. Based on the capacity of a person to attract identification (q.v.) from others. This is more likely to occur in times of stress (e.g. war) when people feel inadequate to cope by their own resources.

Lead poisoning

Lead is found in paint (occasionally still on children's toys), ceramic glazes, insecticides, in petrol additives, and in the metal and building industries. Symptoms include a persistent metallic taste, abdominal pain ('lead colic'), vomiting, diarrhoea, the 'lead line' on the gums. Muscle weakness, paralysis of actively used muscles, e.g. at the wrist ('lead palsy'), may be seen with insomnia, irritability, excitement, confusion, convulsions, and coma ('lead encephalopathy'). Diagnosis is by estimation of lead in blood and urine, the findings of microcytic hypochromic anaemia with punctate basophilic stippling of red cells in the blood, coprophorphyrins in the urine and lines of density in X-rays of long bones. Prevention is by industrial protection and the replacement of lead by other compounds in many of its uses. Treatment is by chelating with parenteral sodium calcium edetate or oral penicillamine after withdrawal from exposure.
SEE ALSO Poisons affecting mental state.

Learning

There is no universally acceptable definition of learning. It may be broadly defined as any change in behaviour that occurs as a result of experience, excluding maturational growth processes, and such temporary aberrations as fatigue. Learning is the building of memory engrams (q.v.) in the brain which are used for the interpretation of later environmental experiences.

It is important to distinguish between short-term and long-term memory storage processes. The former decay within a period measured in seconds to hours, are disrupted by mechanical, electroconvulsive and other intense stimuli (e.g. the amnesia of concussion) and may be a necessary stage in the process of long-term memory formation. Short-term memory is needed for the routine of ordinary life, e.g. memorization of a telephone number long enough to dial it. From the short-term memories, certain components are selected for long term storage.

There are three known psychological models for learning procedures. The first, imprinting (q.v.), occurs during the first few hours of the animal's life and is seen in its most marked form in birds. This initial learning procedure forms the basis of attachment to the parent which gives a stable base for subsequent development. The second learning model is the respondent or classical conditioning (q.v.) first studied by Pavlov. In respondent conditioning, the capacity to elicit a particular response is transferred from one stimulus to another. This type of conditioning is probably relevant to some emotional

behaviours, e.g. the way in which fear responses can become conditioned to a formerly neutral situation.
The third learning model is instrumental or operant conditioning (q.v.) associated with the name of Skinner. In operant conditioning, the frequency of a response increases if it is instrumental in achieving a goal, i.e. the animal must itself make an appropriate 'voluntary' response to the stimulus. Operant conditioning can be both negative and positive depending upon whether the goal is a noxious stimulus or the achievement of a reward.
Although it is possible to analyse the learning process under experimental conditions, the natural forms of learning in life are probably more complicated. Thus, for example imitation (in children), experience and trial-and-error, all common natural forms of learning, involve perceptual, respondent and operant conditioning processes.
It is important to remember that there are constraints on learning which are not solely ones of capacity – thus the subject is more likely to respond to some stimuli than others, to make some responses rather than others, and to form some associations rather than others. There are thus differences between species and between individuals of any one species (including man) in the ease with which learning in any one context occurs. Within such limitations, the factors which determine what is learned and which stimuli are associated with which responses is still a matter of dispute.

Left-handedness

The majority of children naturally favour and develop skill with right eye, hand and foot; in them the left cerebral hemisphere is dominant (dextrality). Some children prefer the left eye, hand and foot and a proportion of these have right hemisphere dominance (sinistrality). What proportion of children are left-handed is unclear as many are converted to dextrality by educational means; left-'eyedness' is resistant to such change. The question of whether such conversion of a 'natural' sinistrality leads to learning and speech difficulties is undecided. Left-handedness appears to run in families, but this may be more apparent than real in that some parents may be more willing to tolerate sinistrality. The validity of these correlations between cerebral dominance and laterality is still a matter for discussion; certainly mixed or confused laterality is often associated with behaviour disturbance in children (i.e. hyperkinetic syndrome).

Legal aspects of psychiatry

Most societies have recognized mentally ill persons as requiring different treatment in respect of responsibilities, behaviour and management of their affairs and laws have been enacted to protect other members of the society and the individual himself. These laws differ from one country to another, indeed in a Federal community like the United States of America from one State to another. Each physician and each psychiatrist should therefore become cognizant of the laws which govern in the area in which he practises.
There are, however, in general, three main areas in which the law and psychiatry interact: (a) the care of the mentally disordered; (b) assessment and treatment of offenders; (c) advice to courts on both criminal and civil matters. The care of the mentally disordered is now governed in most developed countries by special laws.
The underlying spirit of all these laws is to provide hospital treatment for the psychiatric patient on the same informal basis as is granted to the physically ill, but with special provisions for those who because of their disorder require compulsory care (q.v.).
Psychiatrists may be required to give evidence to the divorce court, or to the civil court in a case where sanity is in dispute (see Contract) and psychiatrists are needed from time to time to give evidence in regard to testamentary capacity (q.v.) and in regard to compensation claims (q.v.).
The doctor examining an offender has to ask himself three questions: (a) is the client fit to plead? (q.v.); (b) does he have absence or diminution of criminal responsibility (q.v.) by reason of mental disorder? (q.v.); (c) can a medical disposal of any kind be recommended?
In a British court of law and in those of other countries including the United

States of America the doctor, unlike the lawyer, cannot claim immunity from speaking 'the whole truth' – if a court directs that he breaks his professional confidence with a patient then he keeps that confidence in risk of being sent to prison for contempt of court. Lawyers do not exert their power of breaking professional confidence in this way too often. When examining a client for a court report, the examiner's identity should be revealed, the reason for the report given, and the persons to whom it will be disclosed.

A court report should not be too long – only the conclusions and the logical development of these conclusions need be presented. If the client has not yet been found guilty incriminating statements by the accused are legally inadmissible in the court and should not be introduced into the report, i.e. statements such as 'he says he broke into the house because he was frightened' should be avoided. The source of any evidence should be indicated, e.g. if the client gives a relevant family history this should be reported but reported as the client's statement, not as a matter of fact unless it has been checked. Psychodynamic explanations of behaviour are unwelcome, psychiatric diagnoses are welcome. Technical language should be avoided as far as possible. Realistic medical recommendations for disposal or treatment are always welcomed, particularly if the examining doctor has provided the court with a means of implementing the recommendation; a treatment recommendation when no treatment facility is available is not regarded as sensible.

SEE ALSO Contract, Court of protection, Divorce, Forensic psychiatry, and McNaughton Rules.

Leptosomatic

Kretschmer (1936) (q.v.) suggested that bodily height in relation to breadth and depth was related to a person's temperament and his predisposition to mental illness. A tall, thin body build, described as leptosomatic, was associated with a schizothymic personality and with schizophrenic illness.

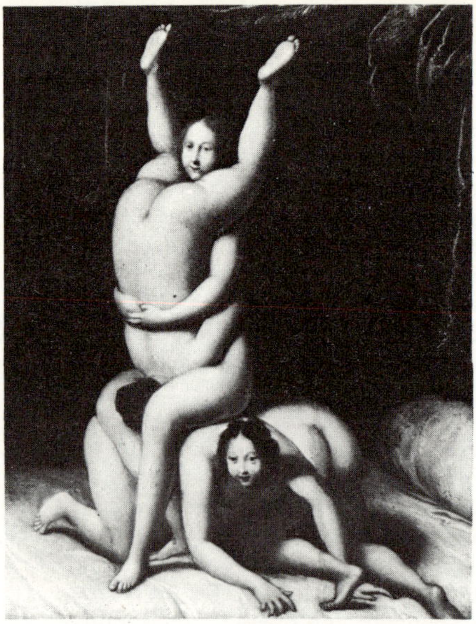

Lesbian

Lesbian is the popular term for a female homosexual (q.v.), derived from the group of habitual female homosexuals who lived in classical times on the Greek island of Lesbos. In its most common form it is limited to mutual physical adulation with emotional attachments and with frigidity in heterosexual coitus. Erotic stimulation, such as inducing orgasm by the rubbing of genitals (tribadism), cunnilingus (q.v.) or the use of an artificial phallus, is much less common than in male homosexuals.

Kinsey rated female homosexuality, as he did in the male, along a continuum. He found that by the age of 30 years, 25% of women had had recognized erotic responses to other women whilst 17% had had actual sexual contact. Exclusive homosexuality, however, is found in only 1% of married and 4% of unmarried women. A number of theories exist explaining Lesbianism; none is entirely satisfactory. Treatment is rarely requested since the condition is socially tolerated; psychiatric symptoms when they do occur are usually reactive to the life situation in which the Lesbian is existing.

Leucotomy

Prefrontal leucotomy was introduced by Egaz Moniz of Lisbon in 1935. The original standard leucotomy consisted of severing the white matter of each frontal lobe as widely as possible. This operation had many undesirable side effects, such as apathy and a high incidence of epilepsy. The beneficial effects of the operation are due to the interruption of the connection between the dorsomedial nuclei of the thalamus and the frontal cortex. Similar therapeutic efficacy can be obtained with a minimum of side effects by cutting the thalamo-frontal bundle (bimedial leucotomy) or by orbital undercutting. Recently stereotactic methods have been used to produce very localized lesions either by coagulation or the introduction of radioactive yttrium.

The main indication for the operation is prolonged and intractable tension and anxiety, particularly in resistant cases of depression and in obsessional neuroses. Nowadays it is rarely performed in schizophrenia. The best results are obtained in patients of good previous personality where drive and activity are prominent features. Since self-control may be lessened the operation is contraindicated in patients with marked psychopathic or hysterical traits.

Although immediate symptomatic improvement usually takes place, thorough rehabilitation is needed particularly in cases of obsessional neurosis to make the patient a fully effective member of society.

Libido

A Freudian term to connote the biologically determined innate drive for sexual pleasure, which he maintained was responsible for the motivation of much adult behaviour. In the infant libidinous energy is concentrated first around the mouth, and thereafter progressively moves to the anus and then to the genitals. Final resolution of the Oedipal conflicts results during the latency period in repression of the libido, which re-emerges at adolescence as the overt sexual drive. Jung used the term libido in the wider philosophical sense of a 'life force'. The direction of the libido, i.e. heterosexual, homosexual or autosexual, is determined by a number of factors, genetic, constitutional, and environmental. The strength of the libido varies in different genetic strains of animals, but in man is much influenced by social conditioning.

Lilliputian hallucinations

Seen most frequently in delirium tremens; the hallucinated objects are reduced in size, so that a herd of elephants or of monsters may be seen by the delirious patient moving over the bed sheets. Rarely, a lesion of the mid-brain will produce vividly coloured, very mobile tiny hallucinatory figures – appearing particularly when falling asleep.

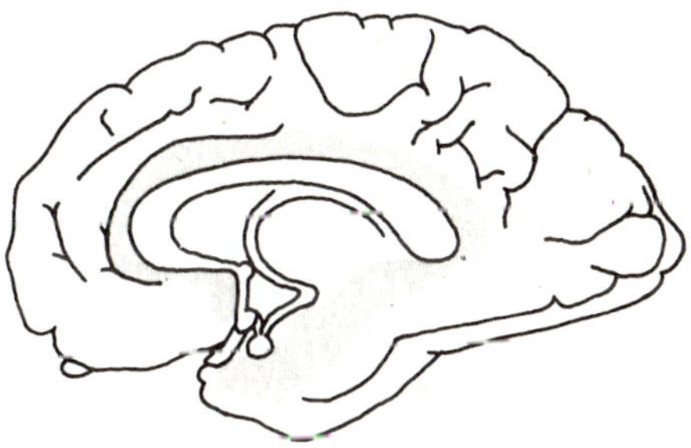

Limbic system

The limbic system is the term applied to the concept of a circle of grey matter lying around the interventricular foramina in the cerebral hemispheres. The main structures are the amygdala (q.v.), hippocampus (q.v.), cingulate and dentate gyri, but many other areas especially in the temporal lobe have been included by one or another author. The input to this system is mainly from the reticular formation (q.v.) and frontal lobes and the output tends to run back to these same structures. The limbic system appears early in phylogenesis and is concerned with emotional experience and expression. In animals, lesions of this lobe result in the Klüver-Bucy syndrome (q.v.) with visual agnosia and overattention to visual stimuli, excessive oral activity, hypersexuality and hyperphagia.

Lipochondrodystrophy

SEE Gargoylism.

Lissencephaly
SEE Agyria.

Lithium carbonate

Lithium salts find their main use in the treatment of manic depressive disorders. They lower mood in manic states and in approximately 75% of patients with endogenous affective illnesses of either unipolar or bipolar type, appear to reduce the amplitude of mood swing and the recurrence of mood disturbance. Some schizo-affective illnesses have also been found to benefit from lithium.
Lithium may exert its effect by partially replacing body sodium, preventing the shift of sodium which accompanies mood swings or by affecting membrane permeability. However, it also has well marked effects of brain amine metabolism, markedly affecting 5-hydroxytryptamine (serotonin) turnover and possibly making 5-hydroxytryptamine physiologically more available within the cell.
As a prophylactic lithium carbonate is given in doses varying between 800 and 1600 mg daily, preferably in a long-acting preparation once or twice daily. A small initial dosage and a very gradual increase is recommended to minimize early side effects. Prophylactic serum levels (0·8–1·2 m.Eq./l.) approximate to levels when side effects (1·5–2·0 m.Eq./l.) and toxic effects (2·0 m.Eq./l.) occur. Regular estimation of serum levels of lithium is recommended. Side effects include fine tremor (often helped by a beta blocking drug such as propranolol), polyuria and occasional diarrhoea and nausea. Toxicity may be suspected if the tremor becomes coarse, the nausea persistent and accompanied by vomiting, and if ataxia, drowsiness or other CNS signs develop. Poisoning is serious and may be fatal with coma and convulsions and is best treated by dialysis. Serum lithium should be estimated fortnightly during the first three months of treatment as a guide to dosage. The aim is to keep the serum levels between 0·8 and 1·2 m.Eq./l., though some patients do well on a lower dose and some resistant patients are only controlled by higher levels. Lithium is metabolized like sodium and potassium and excreted by the kidney. Thus, it is dangerous to give lithium to patients such as those with cardiac or renal failure where the electrolyte balance may be disturbed.
Lithium occasionally causes a colloid goitre and less commonly hypothyroidism, both of which can be controlled by a small daily dose of thyroxine. Six monthly estimation of thyroid function is, therefore, advised, a rising TSH being an early indication of thyroid malfunctioning.
There is evidence that lithium is teratogenic and patients likely to become pregnant should stop lithium at least until after the first trimester of pregnancy.

Lobectomy, anterior temporal

Anterior temporal lobectomy may be carried out for intractable temporal lobe epilepsy. The results are most satisfactory when a structural lesion can be found, e.g. a vascular anomaly or tumour, but even in cases where the damage is hypoxic and presumably more widely spread the operation may be successful, probably by breaking a vicious circle of epileptic activity. Seizures are usually reduced if not eliminated and disturbed behaviour and intellectual performance may both be improved. The operation can only be carried out on one side since bilateral temporal lobectomy profoundly impairs memory. The complications of this operaation include a small upper quadrantic defect in the opposite visual field, transient dysphasia and diplopia and, rarely, hemiparesis. When the ablation is in the dominant hemisphere the subsequent defect of auditory learning may constitute a severe disability.

Lobotomy
SEE Leucotomy.

Locus coeruleus

A pair of minute nuclei lying below the floor of the fourth ventricle. The fine axons spread extensively through the brain and transmit via noradrenaline. It appears to have a part to play in such behavioural states as sleeping, waking and rewarding.

Loneliness and mental breakdown

Social contacts and support are necessary for good mental health, whilst isolation is a factor in many forms of psychiatric disorder. Modern urban living and increasing social mobility lead to greater loneliness, compared with the established patterns of the village or terraced street. In Western societies, loneliness is particularly common after bereavement and in old age because of the breaking up of multi-generation family groups. Suicide rates are related to (*inter alia*) increasing age, widowhood, single and divorced states and residence in large towns – all of which are aspects of loneliness. Attempted suicide – which is a different condition – may have a very high rate in young working-class women, who are emotionally isolated, and in the separated or divorced. It is often difficult to separate the isolation produced by external factors from that due to personality problems. Social clubs may be helpful in combating loneliness.
SEE ALSO Isolation.

Long-acting phenothiazines

Phenothiazines (q.v.) are an effective form of therapy in many patients with schizophrenia and in a large proportion of such patients relapse occurs if therapy is not continued. Unfortunately, psychotic patients are far from reliable over maintenance therapy and in consequence a form of parenteral therapy which can be administered at infrequent intervals by the physician or nurse is desirable. Two esters of the phenothiazine fluphenazine (the enanthoate and the decanoate) the decanoate ester of flupenthixol and fluspirilene suspension, satisfy the requirement and can be administered at intervals of between one week and four weeks depending on the drug and the patient. Although this form of patient management has some advantages, extrapyramidal (q.v.) side effects are often troublesome and this form of therapy is less useful than it would appear to be.

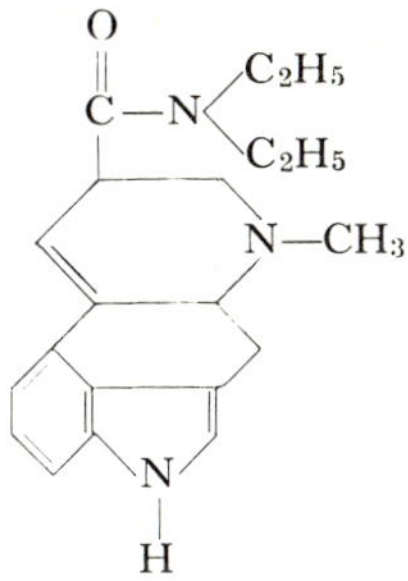

LSD (lysergic acid diethylamide)

LSD 25 is the best-known hallucinogenic drug. It is chemically similar to tryptamine, being a synthetic derivative of lysergic acid. Its hallucinogenic properties were accidentally discovered by Hoffman. It is among the most potent biochemical substances known. It is absorbed via the gastro-intestinal tract. Its most clearly defined action is serotonin antagonism. Tolerance to LSD develops quickly with frequent use and there is cross tolerance with psilocybin (q.v.) and mescaline (q.v.). Physical dependence (q.v.) does not occur though psychological dependence (q.v.) may be extreme. In this the user comes to overvalue the perceptual changes and spurious insights associated with its use and this may have profound effects in altering his way of life. Adverse reactions to LSD occur. They are of three types: *acute reactions* with paranoid excitement and confusion – sometimes ending in aggression or suicide; *severe panic states*, probably not drug related but caused by the subjects fear of the drug-induced changes; *recurrent reactions* – similar to the above can occur up to eighteen months after LSD use. Long-term LSD effects are usually those of severe de-personalization and persistent troublesome visual perceptual disturbances.
The unequivocal evidence of its therapeutic usefulness is as yet not available, though some have found it of value in the treatment of alcoholism.
SEE ALSO Hallucinogenic drugs.

Lying
SEE Pathological lying.

Magical thinking

Magical thinking occurs as part of the normal development of the mind. In childhood, before reality becomes fully accepted omnipotent feelings are associated with ideas that external objects will conform to the child's imperious wishes. Alas, the child has to abandon his magical thinking as a result of the harshness of reality, but during times of stress in later life the individual may return to this earlier, more archaic, and, in some ways, satisfying mode of thinking. Magical thinking is encountered in schizophrenics and in some types of neurosis, particularly obsessional-compulsive neurosis.

Maladjusted homes

Maladjustment, applied to children, means a failure to act in one's own best interests, or with proper regard to the well-being of those around. This can only be judged, however, in relation to the normal, accepted standards of the child's own social group. Within the home, maladjustment may result from the harmful influences of individuals, or from general deprivation or disintegration of the family. Whether a particular child reacts one way or another to such stresses of the environment depends largely on his own temperament. The same disturbed home and parents may produce both maladjusted and normal children at the same time.

Malaria therapy

This great advance in the treatment of cerebral syphilis was introduced by Wagner Jauregg in 1917 in the mistaken belief that GPI was very rare in those countries in which malaria was endemic. The patient was infected with plasmodium vivax (benign tertian malaria) and after about ten rigors the malaria was aborted with quinine. Malaria therapy has been superseded by penicillin but may very occasionally be used in resistant cases of GPI.

Malingering

Although malingering is widespread amongst the working population of many industrially developed countries, doctors have a curious reluctance to believe that 'their' patient could be capable of such ungentlemanly behaviour. Children frequently simulate illness, complaining of sickness, pains in the head or legs, or numerous other symptoms in order to avoid going to school, going to a party and so on. In all cases of malingering there is a desire for gain; many so-called compensation neuroses are nothing more than calculated attempts to deceive the doctor – attempts which unfortunately all too often succeed. The psychiatrist is particularly gullible, having the unconscious to fall back upon whenever he has a need to excuse his own mistakes or his patients' deceptions. The range of simulated illness is immense and its detection demands high clinical skills. The Munchausen syndrome (q.v.) is a notorious example of skilful malingering.

SEE ALSO Compensation neurosis, Criminal responsibility, Ganser syndrome, and Hysterical pseudo-dementia.

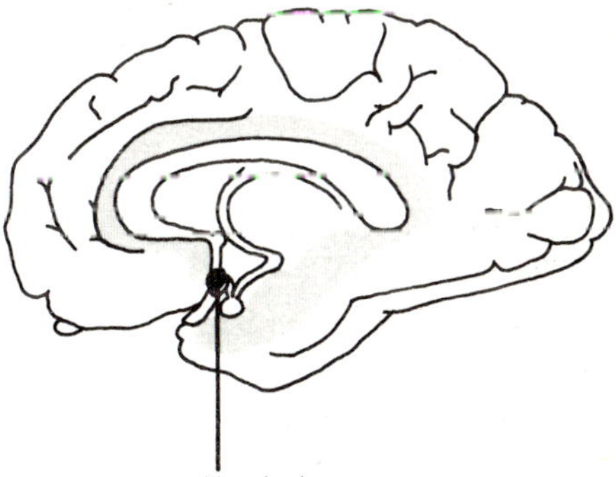

Mammillary bodies

The mammillary bodies are a pair of rounded masses of grey matter lying in the posterior part of the hypothalamus. They receive fibres from the limbic lobe (q.v.) via the fornix (q.v.), and connect with the thalamus via the mammillo-thalamic tract, and with the mid brain via the mammillo-tegmental tract.

Manganese poisoning

Manganese poisoning is most often found in ore grinders and miners, but the metal is used in electric welding, steel, paint, ceramic, linoleum, soap, and dry cell manufacture. Poisoning causes cirrhosis of the liver, neurological manifestations of degeneration of the basal nuclei, and mental symptoms. Prevention is by industrial protection, treatment by chelating with sodium calciumedetate. Exhaustion, weakness, sleep disturbance, emotional lability and psychosis usually recover. The accompanying Parkinsonian syndrome (sometimes with pyramidal and cerebellar signs) most often persists.
SEE ALSO Poisons affecting mental state.

Mania

Mania is one aspect of a manic depressive disorder (bipolar affective disorder). Four main types are recognized: hypomania, acute mania, delirious mania and chronic mania, the first three being simply gradations in severity of the illness. All varieties are characterized by elated and unstable mood, flight of ideas and increased psychomotor activity. In severe cases clouding of consciousness and disorientation may occur and also hallucinations and delusions, but these latter are transitory, occur at the height of the illness, and do not have the ominous significance of the more firmly held delusions or persistent hallucinations which occur in clear consciousness in schizophrenia.

Manic illnesses almost always have a rapid onset measured in days or weeks, are frequently preceded or followed by depression, and in fact depressive features are common in the course of the manic illness itself and in hypomania a lability of mood when elation turns into tears, is often a characteristic feature.

The patient rarely has any insight into his condition and this makes treatment of the milder cases where compulsory hospitalization may not be justified, especially difficult. Disinhibited sexual, excited and perhaps aggressive behaviour may lead to embarrassment, marital distress, or loss of his job. For these reasons a holiday in a non-stimulating environment may be advised when the patient is persuaded to take chlorpromazine or haloperidol while a careful watch is maintained to ensure that he does not swing into a more severe form of the illness.

The more severe forms should always be treated in hospital, frequently under a compulsory order. Chlorpromazine or haloperidol are the drugs of first choice, though ECT is invaluable in the severe forms. Lithium is being increasingly used in the treatment of the manic attack, but it takes 7–10 days to become effective, so that other treatments must be given concomitantly in the initial stages.
SEE ALSO Manic-depressive psychoses.

Mania à potu (pathological intoxication)

This is a rare condition in which drinking relatively small amounts of alcohol is followed by intense psychotic excitement with wildly aggressive and assaultative behaviour. Consciousness is clouded and loosely held delusions are present as are hallucinations. It may last for less than an hour or for a few days. It stops abruptly and is followed by sleep. It usually occurs in persons with severe personality disorders.
SEE ALSO Alcoholism.

Manic-depressive psychosis

Manic-depressive illness (bipolar affective disorder) is the most clearly defined subgroup of the affective disorders, and manifests itself in two distinct and contrasting forms – depression (q.v.) and mania (q.v.). The depressive phase has a number of distinctive characteristics which differentiate it, albeit imperfectly, from other depressions. Often it comes 'out of the blue' without any preceding loss or disappointment. The depression deepens rapidly and sometimes has a 'distinct quality' quite unlike that of ordinary sadness. It does not vary in severity from day to day as neurotic depressions do but may show a distinct diurnal variation, being worst in the early morning and lifting somewhat as the day goes on. Some degree of retardation, affecting both speech and motor activity in general is common and is often accompanied by a distressing inability to concentrate and a loss of interest even in favourite pastimes. Vegetative disturbances may be profound. The patient loses his appetite and his libido and his weight falls rapidly. He also has difficulty sleeping, particularly in the second half of the night. Guilt feelings are common and often centre upon trivial misdemeanours perpetrated long ago. In the majority of cases the depression is sufficiently profound to make the patient feel that life is hardly worth living and as a result suicide is always a serious risk. Characteristically, too, the patient's judgement is impaired. He does not believe he is ill, but attributes his plight to his own weakness or folly, and he may develop delusions centering either on the theme that he is wicked or worthless or on ideas of impending catastrophe.

The manic phase of the illness is in many respects the mirror image of its depressive counterpart. The patient is elated and impervious to disappointments and setbacks. He has far more energy than normal and may stay up half the night, not because he can't sleep but because he has so much to do or doesn't feel tired. He is more sociable and less inhibited than usual and may cause consternation by making obscene remarks or inappropriate sexual advances to casual acquaintances. When remonstrated with his sunny good humour quickly gives way to anger and at times irritability is more conspicuous than elation all along. Nearly always his thinking is speeded up. Plans and ideas flood into his mind and expensive impracticable projects may be embarked upon. At the same time he talks rapidly and incessantly ('pressure of speech') and often loses the ability to maintain a consistent train of thought ('flight of ideas'). His self-esteem is raised and he may develop grandiose delusions – that he is a world-famous poet, or has the solution to the country's economic problems.

Mixed states are also common. Depressions are often preceded or followed by brief episodes of hypomania and the converse is equally true of manic illnesses. Indeed most manic illnesses show depressive features at some stage. Often the elation is punctuated by brief spells of weeping, and suicide is by no means rare. The duration and course of the illness are very variable. Although chronic depressions, and even chronic manias, are well known the majority of illnesses eventually recover completely, with or without treatment, and however many times they recur there is no residual 'defect state' comparable to that of schizophrenia. The average duration of a manic episode is about three to five months compared with six to eight months for a depression, but both are subject to great variation. The commonest age of onset for bipolar illnesses is the second or third decade, but unipolar illness often appears for the first time in middle age or even later. Once a clear cut manic-depressive illness has occurred further episodes are almost inevitable, and tend to get more frequent with increasing age, but again there is much variation from one patient to another.

There is a strong genetic component to manic-depressive illness and several studies have shown that about 15% of the parents, sibs and offspring of manic depressives are similarly afflicted. These figures are probably somewhat inflated through being derived from hospital populations but the risk of the illness being transmitted to a child is unlikely to be much less than one in ten. The mode of transmission is unknown, though the most likely possibilities are either a dominant gene with incomplete penetrance or multifactorial inheritance. Either way it is clear that environmental influences are at least equally important and there is some evidence that the loss of a parent in childhood may be one such factor. Recently it has become clear that there are important differences between bipolar and unipolar illnesses. Both tend to some extent to 'breed true' (the afflicted relatives of bipolar probands tend to have bipolar rather than unipolar illnesses, and vice versa) and the genetic loading is more prominent in the bipolar group. There also tend to be systematic personality differences between the two, those with both manic and depressive illnesses tending to be energetic and extroverted with considerable emotional warmth, and those suffering only from depressions tending to be more anxious and retiring and to have prominent obsessional traits.

Within the last few years important insights have been gained into the physiology and biochemistry of manic-depressive illness. There is evidence that severe

depression of manic-depressive type is often associated with depletion of both catecholamines (noradrenaline and dopamine) and indoleamines (5 hydroxytryptamine) in the hypothalamus and brain stem, and there are indications that there may be a causal relationship between this and the mood change. Thus reserpine causes a similar depletion of brain stem amines and is well known for its liability to precipitate depression; on the other hand both groups of anti-depressant drugs, the tricyclic group and the monoamine oxidase inhibitors raise the levels of physiologically active amines in the brain stem. And finally it is possible that suicides have lower brain stem amine levels than people dying suddenly from other causes. There are also reports, based on whole body balance studies, that the intracellular sodium content is abnormally high in depression, and even more so in mania, and that these abnormalities persist in recovery (SEE Electrolyte distribution in depression and mania).
The treatment of manic depressive illness is relatively straightforward, even if it is not always satisfactory. Most depressions respond either to one of the tricyclic antidepressants or to ECT. Some patients appear to respond selectively to one or the other, but the more severe the depression the more likely is ECT to be necessary. The MAO inhibitors are generally ineffective. Manic illnesses can usually be brought under control with phenothiazines (q.v.) or haloperidol, or more gradually with lithium salts (q.v.). Lithium, however, is most useful in preventing recurrences in patients who have a frequent relapse rate when the drug must be given continuously, the dosage being regulated to produce serum lithium levels of between 0·8 and 1·2 m.eq./l.
SEE ALSO Geriatric psychiatry.

Mannerism

This symptom is a feature of schizophrenia (q.v.) whereby the subject adopts gestures and poses common to normal people but does so inappropriately or in an exaggerated or artificial way. The way of walking may be stilted or eating carried out with unusual movements. Facial expressions and expressive gestures may be affected in this way, as may speech, so that the voice sounds artificially altered or phrases contain meaningless flourishes.

Manslaughter

In English law, this is a lesser form of criminal homicide (q.v.) than murder (q.v.). To convict a person of manslaughter there is no need to prove malice aforethought, e.g. negligence can be sufficient. Convictions for murder can be reduced to manslaughter by means of a successful defence plea of 'diminished responsibility' (q.v.).
The main legal advantage of a manslaughter verdict is that it avoids the mandatory life sentence carried by murder under current English law. Many manslaughter offenders are sentenced to life imprisonment, but fines, probation, or short sentences are also used.
SEE ALSO Infanticide.

MAO inhibitor

SEE Monoamine oxidase inhibitors.

Maple syrup urine disease

This is an inborn error of metabolism in which the amino-acids leucine, isoleucine and valine are excreted in the urine which has a characteristic odour like that of maple syrup. In most cases the symptoms appear in the neonatal period as failure to thrive, feeding difficulties, and usually rapidly progressive neurological deterioration leading to spastic paralysis, convulsions and early death. In some cases patients survive, but are severely mentally subnormal. Success has been claimed for dietary therapy, started early, with a diet low in the branched chain amino-acids. This condition follows an autosomal recessive mode of inheritance.
SEE ALSO Inherited metabolic defects.

Marasmus

This is a chronic state of undernutrition occurring in infancy and resulting in generalized wasting and loss of body fat.

The infant is pale, thin, apathetic and miserable.
Physical causes are usually found, and include chronic infection, congenital abnormalities and underfeeding. Gross emotional deprivation occurring in bad institutions may produce a similar picture in the absence of physical illness, even where adequate amounts of food are available to the child, probably because the child will not eat in these circumstances.

Marchiafava's disease (Marchiafava-Bignami disease)

A rare condition occurring predominantly in Italian males, and characterized by a primary degeneration of the corpus callosum. Convulsions, motor symptoms and signs, together with dementia are found, and there is a history of excessive intake of cheap red wine. The condition may be the result of a toxin, as yet unknown; it is not considered to be a vitamin deficiency disease.

Marfan's syndrome

Marfan's syndrome is characterized by changes in the eye, including coloboma and dislocation of the lens; skeletal changes resulting in a long, narrow head, narrow thorax, long limbs, long spidery fingers and toes (arachnodactyly). Mental subnormality is not a constant feature, but may be present in severe degree. It follows a dominant mode of genetical transmission.

Marihuanha

SEE Cannabis sativa.

Marriage

'A happy marriage perhaps represents the ideal of human relationship – a setting in which each partner, while acknowledging the need of the other, feels free to be what he or she by nature is: a relationship in which instinct as well as intellect can find expression; in which giving and taking are equal; in which each accepts the other, and I confronts Thou.'
In *law* a marriage is regarded as a contract: 'the voluntary union for life of one man and one woman to the exclusion of all others'. Hence the two parties must be legally capable of entering into a contract, and there must be no force, deceit or mistake. This implies that each party should have the mental capacity to marry (i.e. he or she must be able to understand the responsibilities of marriage and be capable of understanding the nature of the contract), should give free consent with proper understanding of the contract, and be capable of consummating the marriage.
The marital relationship could be called the nuclear powerhouse of our society. Mature marriages tend to produce mature individuals who in their turn produce more mature marriages. From these individuals we derive a mature society. In sociological terms each family can be regarded as having its own unique subculture which is passed on to the next generation. On the other hand 'dis-ease' in the marital relationship may cause not only unhappiness but may produce physical symptoms, e.g. the woman with backache which is a defence against sexual activity. Such patients almost invariably go to their own medical practitioner, at least in the first instance, and he needs to understand how illness may be related to marital and social tensions as well as to pathology and biochemistry. Such couples do not usually come for help together. Often a marital problem is uncovered when some physical complaint is related to the patient's life. Given one partner only the doctor must try to avoid the first pitfall, namely collusion against the absent partner. There is a tendency to be seduced into seeing the problem from the wife's or the husband's point of view. Usually indeed the best method of therapy is the joint interview with husband and wife when the doctor's function is:
1. To facilitate communication which has often broken down.
2. To avoid sitting in judgement and apportioning blame.
3. To examine the vicious circle of each blaming the other for the symptoms and to help the couple to realize that no progress can be made until each partner is prepared to examine his or her contribution to the problem.
A particularly difficult situation is that where the couple will present with a ready-

made scapegoat, such as the wife saying it is all the husband's fault and the husband guiltily accepting the blame.
4. The concept of blame must be jettisoned and replaced by the concept of understanding motivation and trying to clarify patterns of interaction.
5. The doctor must resist the temptation to give advice and to make decisions on behalf of the couple.
A simple conceptual framework for the description of relationship involves 'power' and 'identity'. The concept of power is used by political commentators in the description of relationships between nations, and the concepts 'balance of power', 'power vacuum', etc. are used. Furthermore, the business man knows about the power game or the rat race. In every marriage, however, there is also a struggle for power and there is also a certain degree of conflict between the wills of the two partners. For the marriage to remain healthy the power balance should be roughly even.
The other important concept is that of identity. The problem of the adolescent is to achieve identity in his own right and in order to do this there has to be some degree of conflict with the parents. In our society, with the tendency to early marriage, it often happens that adolescents do not achieve full maturation of their identity but exchange dependency on parent to dependency on the spouse. The state of being in love involves a surrender of individual identity with a fusion of selves. After marriage, however, a certain degree of individuality has to reassert itself if only because reality demands different roles for husband and wife. If the partners are mutually dependent so that each is trying to get security from the other then the assertion of separate identity by one becomes a threat to the security of the other. A battle for dominance ensues – whose pattern of behaviour is to take precedence over whose, and this commonly is at the basis of marital conflict.
In fact the relationship between the concepts of identity and power can be stated as follows. The person who is the greatest threat to an individual's identity is the person who has the greatest power over him. For the child that person is the parent for the adult that person is the spouse. Using these concepts the doctor can formulate a therapeutic aim – namely to help the couple to get the power balance right and to help them to accept and to feel less threatened by each other's individuality.
SEE ALSO Divorce and Nullity.

Marriage counselling

This involves advice, guidance and education in preparation for or to overcome difficulties arising during marriage (q.v.). In many industrially developed countries, marriage counselling is organized by voluntary groups but some local authorities provide a 'family advice service' as part of their child care duties.
Counsellors are usually part time, married or widowed (not divorced) who are middle aged and who are selected for suitability. For every marriage problem taken to a marriage guidance counsellor, five reach the probation officer. These marriages, however, are usually at a much more critical stage of discord and are from the lower social classes.

Masculine protest

An Adlerian concept which supposes that the inferiority feelings of women in certain cases find unconscious expression in a number of different activities sharing a common theme – competition with men. Sporting, intellectual, political, or a whole range of activities may be involved.

Masochism

Masochism, first described by the novelist Sacher-Masoch, is the condition whereby the infliction of pain, humiliation and punishment upon the subject are a necessary prerequisite for the attainment of sexual orgasm. Masochism often co-exists with sadism (q.v.) and is thought to be a turning upon the self of aggressive impulses felt towards others, particularly parents. In autosexual masochism such as 'fettering' the individual binds himself in ropes, or garments, such as corsets, or plastic bags in order to achieve orgasm. In homosexual or heterosexual masochism the individual is commonly whipped or humiliated by a member of the same or opposite sex. Many

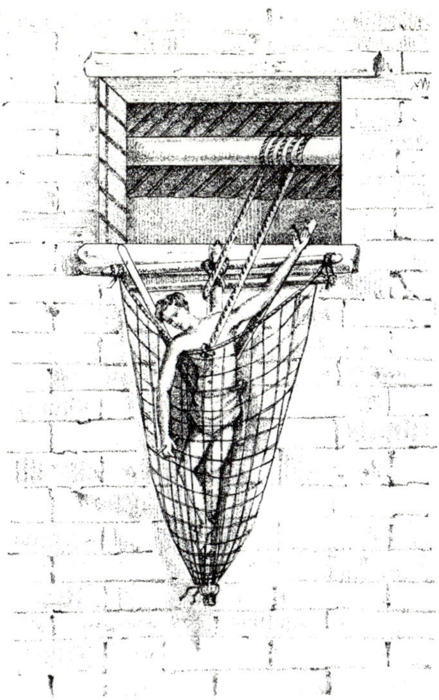

Matthew Lovat, who crucified himself at Venice, July 1805

forms of neurosis, drug addiction, alcoholism, and attempted suicide have a quality of self-punishment involved. This led Freud to view them as forms of masochism in which there was a need for punishment, in order to atone for the guilt of repressed infantile wishes for incestuous sexual impulses towards parents. Moral masochism included the wider social subjugation and punishment seen in some religious practices or experienced in some marital relationships. Treatment is by psychotherapy (q.v.) although in recent years behaviour therapy (q.v.) has claimed some success.
SEE ALSO Sexual disorders.

Masquerading in uniform

Psychopathic behaviour (q.v.) can lead an individual to act out all sorts of phantasies. A posed position in society is one such example. When military personnel are held in high esteem (e.g. during wars) some individuals attempt to deal with their own inferiority feelings by imitating such personnel. Occasionally other people of high prestige value may be mimicked – doctor, clergymen, pop stars etc.
SEE ALSO Lying, Psychopathic disorder, and Phantasy.

Massed practice (or negative practice)

The term includes several treatment methods derived from the learning theory principle that the massed practice (the repeated voluntary performance) of a learned response without reinforcement leads to its extinction. These methods have sometimes been successful with stammering and in cases of tic, disorders which can be regarded as repetitive habits. Treatment entails the subject repeating the problem behaviour as precisely and intensively as possible to the point of exhaustion. This is repeated at least once daily. The point of exhaustion occurring increasingly quickly, until extinction of the response occurs.

Masters and Johnson

Founders of the Reproduction Biology Research Foundation.
Sexual partners are treated both individually and as a couple each with their own therapist. Treatment involves intensive counselling followed by a type of behaviour therapy in practice where the emphasis is on increasing the amount of sexual stimulation. This combination of counselling and behaviour therapy is particularly beneficial in patients whose sexual difficulties stem from anxiety. Desensitization directed to the patients' sexual anxieties can be beneficially combined with a modification of the Masters and Johnson technique.

Masturbation

Masturbation is the deliberate, self-stimulation of the genitals to induce sexual excitement. Self-stimulation of the genital area for the purpose of producing pleasurable sensations can occur from early infancy onwards. The phenomenon is more common in infant girls than infant boys, the baby usually producing a pleasurable sensation by repeated rubbing together of the thighs. A true orgasm can be produced, differing from the orgasm of the sexually mature adult only in the absence of ejaculation. Rarely masturbation may occur to alleviate the itchiness of a nappy rash, or as a result of intestinal infestation.

Masturbation in the older child is very commonly practised both in boys and girls. In itself it is not abnormal and leads to no harmful ill-effects, but if it becomes a compulsive habit (i.e. associated with internal resistance), is accompanied by guilt, shame and depression, or is practised openly, then it is deserving of medical attention. Frequent masturbation in the adolescent, therefore, if practised privately and without mental suffering is of no psychopathological concern. Masturbation practised openly in the older child is usually an attention-seeking phenomenon, and a sign of relative deprivation.

After adolescence, masturbation is carried out to the point of orgasm in about 96% of males and 60% of females. There is no evidence that it has any harmful physical or mental effects. Anxiety and guilt about masturbation, conditioned by religious and moral attitudes during childhood, may, however, lead to anxiety states in adolescence, or to a psychosomatic disorder such as ano-genital pruritus, or pains in the genitals. There is no evidence to support the common idea that masturbation in the female may preclude attainment of orgasm during intercourse in later life.

Rarely, masturbation may be a true perversion when it excludes normal sexual behaviour, as in habitual masturbation, or in anal masturbation where objects are inserted in the rectum for the purpose of inducing orgasm. Masturbation in children is of no pathological significance. If the mother wishes to stop it, she should be advised to fold the nappy in such a way that the thighs are kept apart, but otherwise ignore the child completely when doing it. Habitual and anal forms of masturbation (true autoeroticism) may require treatment of their underlying cause.

SEE ALSO Infantile sexuality.

Matricide

Matricide is almost exclusively a male crime, and indicates serious mental disturbance, usually the result of a schizophrenic illness. At times the killing of the mother may be the only evidence of abnormality, although some coldness of affect, and some lack of interpersonal relations may be detected, both indicating the diagnosis. More uncommonly, a depressive illness may be the setting in which matricide occurs – a long illness of the mother, for instance, may lead to depression in her daughter, and a mercy killing.

SEE ALSO Homicide and Murder.

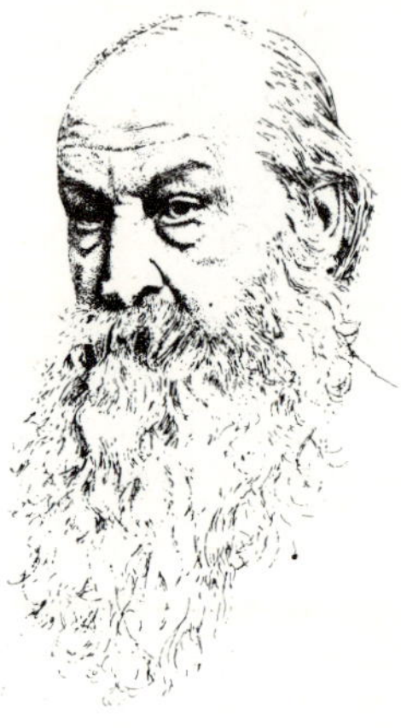

Maudsley, Henry (1835–1918)

Best known as the founder of the Maudsley Hospital, Maudsley had a brilliant career as a student and young doctor. He became the editor of the *Journal of Mental Science*, wrote prolifically and, in a number of books, put forward the view that mental diseases were basically brain diseases. He realized the importance of heredity, and of research into physiology and pathology for the understanding of mental illness.

As a result he offered a large sum of money to the London County Council for the creation of a hospital which would serve a threefold purpose – as a medical school, a research centre, and a clinic with out and in-patient facilities for persons suffering from early mental disorder. Maudsley died in 1918 before the Maudsley Hospital was finally opened.

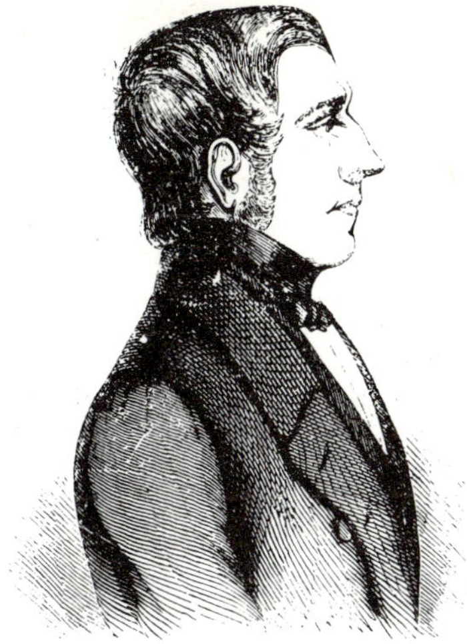

Daniel McNaughton, assassin of Sir Robert Peel's secretary

McNaughton Rules

Rules introduced in the British House of Lords in 1843 to clarify the law following the trial of the deluded McNaughton, who acting in the belief that the Tories were persecuting him, shot and killed the Prime Minister's private secretary (whom he had mistaken for Sir Robert Peel). The defendant was found not guilty, and sent to Bethlem. The ensuing public uproar caused the House of Lords to put certain questions to the judiciary concerning the defence of insanity. The answers became the McNaughton Rules, which lay down that every man is presumed to be sane until the contrary be proved, and that to establish a defence on the ground of insanity it must be clearly proved that at the time of committing the act the accused party was labouring under such a defect of reason, from disease of the mind, as not to know the nature and quality of the act he was doing; or if he did know it, that he did not know that what he was doing was wrong.
The rules are only legally relevant in Great Britain but the principles enshrined have been widely accepted in the legal systems of many countries.
SEE ALSO Criminal responsibility, Diminished responsibility, Forensic psychiatry, and Homicide.

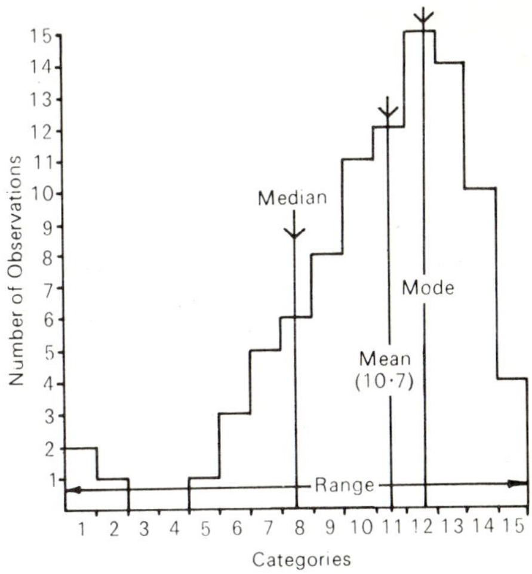

A histogram presentation of the hypothetical data presented in 'Frequency Distribution' – showing range, mean, mode, median. This shows a skew distribution with outlying observations.

Mean, arithmetical

The arithmetic mean is the technical term synonymous with 'average'. It is calculated by adding the individual values of a series and dividing the result by the number of observations.
SEE figure for comparison of Mean, Mode, and Median.

Median

The median is the centre value of a series of observations which are arranged in order (see figure and compare with mean and mode). It is a useful 'average' when the mean is distorted by a large number of outlying observations.

Megalomania

The exaggerations of self-importance and significance comprised under this term occur most characteristically in mania (q.v.) and in paranoid illnesses (q.v.). In the latter the content is more likely to be bizarre and systematized (e.g. being of noble birth or position; the envoy of the Deity). In mania it is more likely to be understandable as an unrestrained, exaggeration of the flattering self-evaluation and self-deception to which most of us are prone (e.g. belief in great talent, perception or wealth).

Megavitamin therapy

During the past few years there has been a vogue for the administration of very high doses of vitamins in psychiatric disorders, particularly schizophrenia. The two vitamins used most commonly have been pyridoxine and ascorbic acid. There is no clear evidence of benefit in the disorder and although such patients may be vitamin deficient from curious eating habits coupled with institutional food, the doses given are well above those required to treat the vitamin deficiency.

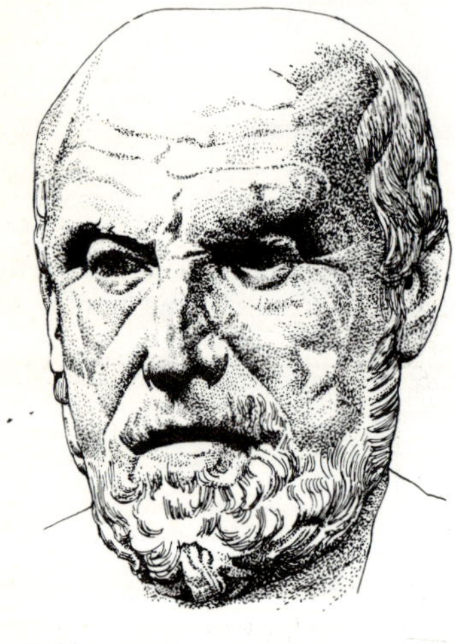

Hippocrates

Melancholia

Melancholia was one of the four types of madness recognized by Hippocrates in the fourth century BC and continued to figure in almost every classification of mental illness for the next 2000 years. But now the term is falling into disuse and being replaced by the more prosaic word depression. When it is used nowadays melancholia should be taken to imply the presence of a severe or psychotic depression. SEE ALSO' Involutional melancholia.

Memory

Memory is the general term denoting the conscious revival, in whole or in part, of past experiences. In another sense, it refers to the specific items of experience revived. The memory process has three phases. The first is the registration (q.v.) phase which requires active attention (q.v.) to be paid to the relevant material and is favoured by conscious attempts at memorization. The possibility of later revival implies that registration modifies the organism in some way by laying down a memory trace or engram (q.v.) which endures throughout the retention phase. Recent research suggests that engrams may be neurobiochemical in nature. The final phase of remembering is studied by tests of recall (q.v.), recognition, reproduction or relearning. Tests of memory span, the number of items, such as digits, an individual can reproduce correctly after one presentation, are frequently employed in the mental examination of patients. Remembering is not an exact process, events as recalled being distorted according to the attitudes and interests of the individual. The Freudian mechanism of repression (q.v.) plays an important part in this distortion.

The American psychologist, Lashley, considered that different parts of the cerebral cortex were equipotential (functionally interchangeable) for functions such as memory, but recent research has shown that bilateral ablation of or damage to the hippocampus (q.v.) has a devastating effect on memory functions.

While hypermnesias (q.v.) are rare in psychiatric disorders, dysmnesias (q.v.) are common, particularly in organic diseases such as senile conditions and Korsakoff's psychosis (q.v.). In these it is likely that the registration phase is more affected than retention and recall. Certain drugs also have specific deleterious effects on memory. In the case of some, e.g. diazepam, this effect is mild and transient and may be useful in alleviating the stress of minor operations.

Memory defects in the aged

Memory defects occur in normal ageing and are invariably present in all dementias (q.v.). Registration, retention and recall of events are all essential to the process of remembering. The mechanisms underlying the first two of these, and thought to be affected by ageing, are difficulty in 'coding' information and defective laying down of short-term memory traces.
Normal forgetfulness, in which parts of past experiences, such as names and dates, cannot be recalled at will on one occasion but may be remembered on another, increases with age and is common among the very aged. The course is generally benign but occasionally dementia develops. In pathological memory defect, associated with dementia, the memory for recent events is most affected, at least in the early stages, but remote memories become affected later. Personality and all mental functions are eventually involved in a global change associated with diffuse degeneration throughout the cortex and elsewhere, but parts of the limbic system seem to be specially important (hippocampal areas, mamillary bodies and adjacent hypothalamus). Circumscribed degenerative or vascular lesions in these areas may give rise to amnestic syndromes with relatively good preservation of other faculties.

Menopause

The menopause means the final cessation of menstruation, but is used synonymously with climacteric. Oestrogen deficiency causes hot flushes and variable atrophy of the genital tract. Emotional disturbance is very common as a reaction to the end of reproductive life and to the physical symptoms of the menopause. Frank anxiety states (q.v.) and depressive illnesses (q.v.) are common at this age, but there is no evidence that they result directly from hormonal changes.
There is no reason why an active sex life should not continue during and after the menopause. Genital atrophy may make intercourse more difficult, but can be relieved by oestrogen treatment.
Menopausal women are helped by explanation and reassurance, but frank psychiatric disorders need appropriate treatment. Oestrogens are indicated only by marked physical features of oestrogen deficiency.
SEE ALSO Climacteric.

Mens rea

A central concept in British law and applied in principle, and sometimes in practice in other countries, roughly meaning 'guilty mind'. It is held that before a person can be found guilty he must have shown some degree of moral turpitude and criminal intent. He must have foreseen and intended the consequences of his act; it must have been carried out wilfully and maliciously knowing it was both legally and morally wrong. In other words pure accidents, however disastrous, are not infringements of the criminal law. Nevertheless there are a few laws of 'absolute liability' which bypass this concept, e.g. some driving laws.
SEE ALSO Criminal responsibility, Diminished responsibility, and McNaughton Rules.

Menstruation

There is a complex relationship between the menstrual cycle and psychological function. Mood disturbance is characteristic of pre-menstrual tension (q.v.) and pre-menstrual aggravation of anxiety or depression is common in neurosis. Many women are less efficient and more accident-prone before and during menstruation. At this time, women are more likely to commit suicide or crimes of violence. In some epileptics fits are more frequent in the pre-menstruum.
Disturbance of the menstrual cycle occurs in many psychiatric disorders: amenorrhoea (q.v.), oligomenorrhoea (q.v.), or menorrhagia (q.v.) may occur. Often menstrual irregularity is secondary to psychological disturbance, but it may itself provoke anxiety.

Mental ages

The results of intelligence tests in children or in adults with mental subnormality are frequently converted into the mental age;

i.e. the life age at where an average child attains that level of intelligence.

Mental deficiency
SEE Mental subnormality.

Mental deterioration

A progressive impairment of mental functions which occurs in organic and some functional psychoses. Intellectual functions are primarily affected and, when the deterioration is general, it is most clearly revealed by a declining IQ from a basic pre-morbid level together with indications of impaired memory functions. As pre-morbid measures of intelligence (q.v.) are rarely available, a number of tests have been designed to yield concurrent measures of present and past intellectual ability. For example, scores on the various subtests on the Wechsler scale (q.v.) decline differentially with age. These 'hold' and 'don't hold' scores may be compared to calculate a rather unsatisfactory 'deterioration index'. The distinction between 'hold' and 'don't hold' is related to that between 'fluid' intelligence, available to apply to new problems, and 'crystallized' intelligence which reflects past learning. An individual's vocabulary is a good indication of his crystallized ability and, in the Babcock-Levy (q.v.) and some other psychological tests of deterioration, the vocabulary score is compared with more vulnerable 'fluid' scores. The danger of this approach is that verbal functions are affected by specific types of brain damage. Other functions which may show specific impairment are those related to memory, speed of mental functioning and spatial functions. A variety of drawing tests have been designed to assess spatial ability, and learning efficiency is often measured by 'paired association' tests in which words become linked in pairs.
During the psychiatrist's examination of mental state, deterioration is assessed from the patient's account of his life, his answers to questions and his performance on a variety of informal tests.
SEE ALSO Mental examination, Memory, and Zangwill's test.

Mental disorder

In the United Kingdom since 1959 this term has begun to replace insanity (q.v.) as a legal term. In the English legal sense mental disorder means 'mental illness', 'arrested or incomplete development of mind', 'psychopathic disorder', and any other disorder or disability of mind. Nowhere in the act is mental illness defined, but it is usually equated with psychosis (q.v.).
Arrested or incomplete development of mind refers to severe subnormality (q.v.) and subnormality (q.v.). Psychopathic disorder is defined elsewhere.

Mental examination
SEE Examination, mental.

Mental Health Acts – Great Britain

The care of the mentally disordered (q.v.) is governed in Great Britain by three separate but very similar Acts of Parliament: for England and Wales, 1959 Act; for Scotland, 1960 Act; for Northern Ireland, 1961 Act. There are no differences in spirit between the three Acts and therefore only that for England and Wales is considered. The aim of this legislation was to sweep away the old system of 'certification' and stigma, and to put the psychiatric patient in the same position as any other sick person, whilst at the same time providing society with some means of compulsory care for those who by way of their sickness are endangering themselves or others. A third principle embodied in the legislation is that the emphasis of psychiatry should be shifted from institutional care to community care.
1959 Act – England and Wales
Part III of the Act lays duties upon the local health authorities to provide mental nursing homes and residential homes.
Part IV embodies a code for compulsory admission to hospital.
Under *Section 25* the nearest relative or the mental welfare officer can apply for a mentally disordered patient to be observed for twenty-eight days. This must be supported by two medical recommendations (one must be a psychiatrist approved by a local health authority). Under *Section 26*

application can be made for a mentally ill or severely subnormal patient (and psychopaths and subnormals under 21 years) to be treated in hospital for up to one year in the first instance. In an emergency under *Section 29* an application for a three day period of observation need only be supported by one medical recommendation (it could be the patient's own practitioner).

Section 33 gives a similar procedure to Section 26 for receiving a patient into guardianship with similar age limitations about psychopaths and subnormals. Any patient under compulsory care or guardianship has the right of appeal to the mental health review tribunal.

Patients under treatment or guardianship can be discharged by the doctors or by the nearest relative (unless the psychiatrist objects, when appeal can be made to a mental health review tribunal).

Mentally disordered persons convicted of a criminal offence can be compulsorily detained under a hospital order (q.v.) made by a court (there are no age restrictions for subnormals and psychopaths). This is under *Section 60* of the act. *Section 65* gives special restrictions so that the patient cannot be discharged in the normal way but only by the Home Secretary. Under *Section 135* a magistrate and a mental welfare officer can commit a patient to a 'place of safety' for three days' observation if the patient is ill-treated, neglected or unable to care for himself.

Mentally disordered persons found in a public place can similarly be committed to a 'place of safety' by a policeman under *Section 136*.

Although the law only applies in England and Wales, the general concepts embodied in it are now widely accepted in many countries.

SEE ALSO Forensic psychiatry and Legal aspects of psychiatry.

Mental mechanisms

SEE Defence mechanisms

Mental retardation

SEE Mental subnormality.

Mental subnormality (deficiency, retardation, amentia)

The term mental subnormality is used to denote deficiency of intellectual function. It is the term used in English law, and has almost completely superseded the previously used terms: mental deficiency or defect in medical practice. Mental retardation is a term commonly used in the United States. Amentia (= without a mind) and oligophrenia (= small mindedness) are synonyms derived from Greek and are little used today.

Two grades of mental subnormality are defined.

Subnormality is 'a state of arrested or incomplete development of mind which includes subnormality of intelligence and requires special care or training but does not amount to severe subnormality'.

Severe subnormality is 'a state of arrested or incomplete development of mind so severe that the patient is incapable of leading an independent life or guarding himself against serious exploitation (or, in the case of a child, that he will be so incapable when adult)'. Severe subnormality corresponds approximately to the formerly used terms, idiocy and imbecility.

There are various criteria by which an individual can be judged to be mentally subnormal. The main psychological criterion is that of the intelligence quotient, which is based on the concept of mental age. This criterion, however, is not without its drawbacks; the IQ is not always constant; the same IQ in different tests may indicate different abilities; the IQ and social performance are not absolutely related. Social criteria depend very much upon the surrounding culture. In communities dependent upon advanced technology more individuals are likely to fail with respect to social competence than in primitive rural communities depending largely on manual labour. Educational criteria are also likely to vary from region to region and culture to culture and cannot be regarded as hard and fast.

Aetiology may be regarded under the two classical headings of genetical and environmental, though in individual cases there is often probably considerable overlap. Environmental causes may operate before birth, for example, maternal infections such as rubella which may produce an embryopathy; at birth, for example, prolonged or difficult labour or any birth trauma causing anoxia severe enough to damage the brain; or after birth, such as meningitis or encephalitis. Genetical factors in aetiology can be listed very roughly as polygenic factors to which milder degrees of mental subnormality are not infrequently attributed; rare major genes (dominant, recessive and sex-linked) which cause specific clinical conditions associated with mental subnormality, usually of severe degree, such as the inherited metabolic defects; and chromosomal abnormalities which can be detected by cytogenetical methods, of which Down's syndrome (mongolism) is the most common example.

As regards social factors in the aetiology of mental subnormality, there is much interplay between heredity and the environment. Many individuals with mild degrees of mental subnormality come into a category described as the 'subcultural' group; their defect is considered as a part of the continuum of normal variation in the population, which is attributed to polygenic inheritance. They are born to parents of somewhat similar intelligence to their own, who tend to belong to or drift towards the lower social classes where poverty leads to nutritional deficiencies and possibly to unchecked infection; these in turn may play their part in the aetiology of mental subnormality.

Enthusiasts have recommended eugenic measures such as sterilization of the mentally subnormal, and such programmes have been carried out in certain states of the USA. Such measures cannot be expected to produce significant results in the prevalence of mental subnormality in the community (see section on Eugenics).

Hope for prevention of mental subnormality in individual families lies in genetical counselling. The antenatal detection of chromosomal abnormalities and certain inherited inborn metabolic errors by amniocentesis is being developed. Improvements in antenatal supervision and obstetrical services may be expected to lead to the birth of fewer mentally subnormal children.

Very few specific forms of treatment exist for conditions associated with mental subnormality. Surgical treatment is limited almost to the insertion of valves for hydrocephalus and the repair of associated defects such as spina bifida. A few dietary treatments exist for inborn metabolic defects such as phenylketonuria and maple syrup urine disease. Most treatment is symptomatic, such as medication for the relief of epilepsy, and physiotherapy and orthopaedic operations for physical deformities of various kinds. Partial deafness should be looked for and, if present, corrected.

In the main treatment is confined to general care and training the child to use his intelligence to its full potential. Patients with an IQ much below average may have to attend special schools for the educationally subnormal (ESN) and perhaps later be supported by a training centre or sheltered workshop. They are slow to learn and have difficulty in adapting to new situations yet are often quite capable of being trained to do work of varying degrees of economic value, especially if the work is of a simple repetitive nature. The extent to which they can lead an independent life depends also on other personality factors. Unfortunately some may be easily led astray and delinquent offences or sexual promiscuity may then necessitate close supervision.

Early diagnosis is important. The earlier the special training the better. Attendance at an ordinary school and perhaps punishment for alleged laziness may result in secondary neurotic symptoms.

The more severe degrees of subnormality are often best cared for in a long-stay hospital, particularly if there are associated neurological disabilities. Hospitalization may also be needed in those cases of milder subnormality where temperament, instability, and social factors etc., make life outside hospital unwise. In these cases, maturation may lead to improvement sufficient to enable discharge in due course.

The following are some factors which should be taken into account when considering institutional care:

1. Degree of retardation and type of defect – e.g. the hyperkinetic and destructive child.

2. Age of child. The guilt of the mother may not be so intense if the child is kept at home for a while. Severely subnormal children become an increasing problem as they get older and heavier.

3. Parental attitudes – e.g. rejection.
4. Effect on siblings – younger sibs may suffer because the mother is over-occupied with the defective child all the time.
5. Effect on the prevention of a further pregnancy. The mother may feel that another child would be too much for her to cope with.
6. Social circumstances – e.g. overcrowding.

SEE ALSO Child psychiatry.

Mental subnormality and inherited syndromes

Recognized inherited syndromes associated with mental subnormality fall mainly into the categories of syndromes inherited as rare Mendelian single major gene defects or chromosome abnormalities. Single major gene defects comprise autosomal recessive defects, autosomal dominant defects and sex-linked defects. The largest group of these, though the individual conditions in it are extremely rare, is the group of autosomal recessive defects; this group includes most of the inherited metabolic defects such as phenylketonuria (q.v.), maple syrup urine disease (q.v.) and galactosaemia (q.v.). Examples of autosomal dominant defects are in the group known as the phakomatoses (q.v.) which include epiloia, neurofibromatosis and von Hippel-Lindau's disease. Examples of sex-linked defects are glucose-6-dehydrogenase deficiency (q.v.) and sex-linked hydrocephalus (q.v.).
Of chromosomal abnormalities, those involving the autosomes are most commonly associated with mental subnormality, which is usually severe. Examples of inherited syndromes associated with autosomal chromosomal abnormalities are mongolism (q.v.) (Down's syndrome), Edward's syndrome (q.v.), Patau's syndrome (q.v.) and the cri-du-chat syndrome (q.v.). Mental subnormality is a less constant concomitant of the sex chromosome abnormalities, and when it is present it is usually of less severe degree. Thus, for example, milder degrees of mental subnormality are found not infrequently amongst patients with Klinefelter's syndrome (q.v.).

SEE ALSO Inherited metabolic defects.

Mental subnormality and physical abnormalities

In populations of severely mentally subnormal patients a very high proportion of individuals show some physical abnormality. The most general of these is shortness of stature which in the majority of cases may be attributed to a concatenation of aetiological factors, both constitutional and environmental. More specific physical defects may also arise from the combined action of multiple factors; but in a number of cases a single major basic cause is implicated, though, again, this is often only a starting point for a chain of events leading to physical malformation. These major causes may be genetical, as in, for example, recessively inherited microcephaly or sex-linked hydrocephalus. On the other hand they may be environmental, such as meningitis which may cause intracranial lesions blocking the flow of cerebrospinal fluid and causing hydrocephalus. Often severe physical malformations such as those seen in cerebral palsy are the end result of primary neurological impairment, which again may be a concomitant of an inherited condition such as familial amaurotic idiocy, or the result of an environmental accident such as birth trauma. Epilepsy, seen in many severely mentally subnormal patients is attributable to physical abnormality of the brain, often neuro-pathologically demonstrable, due to a wide variety of causes both genetical and environmental.

Mental Welfare Officer

This is a statutory office in England under the Mental Health Act. Every local health authority must employ mental welfare officers. They have certain statutory duties, but increasingly they are trained psychiatric social workers (q.v.), involved in the whole range of investigatory and after-care social work in mental health services.

Mercury poisoning

Mercury is still encountered in the manufacture of mirrors, thermometers, in therapeutics and occasionally in suicidal

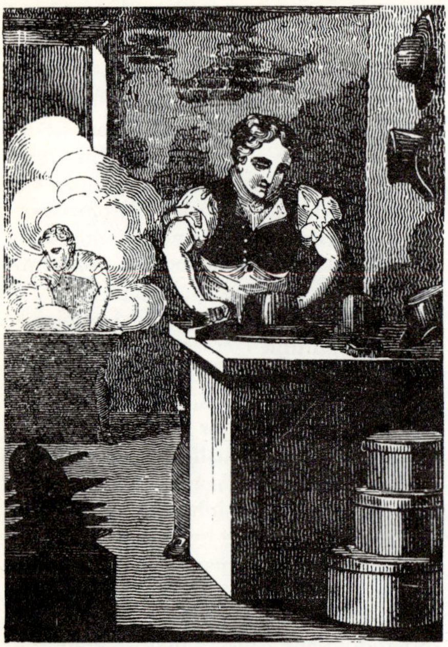

Mercury used in the production of hats

attempts, and was formerly used in the process of felt hat making. The symptoms of chronic poisoning are a metallic taste, gingivitis, salivation, anaemia, colitis, and progressive renal damage. The mental symptoms resemble those of neurasthemia – fatigue, irritability, tremor, poor concentration, depression and insomnia. Their occurrence in hatmakers gave rise to the saying 'as mad as a hatter'.
SEE ALSO Poisons affecting mental state.

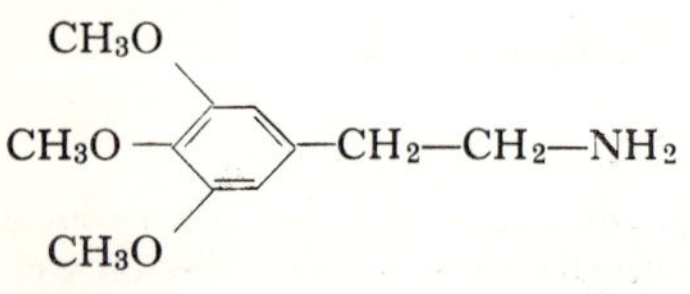

Mescaline

Mescaline is an alkaloid produced by the north Mexican cactus *Lophophora williamsii*. Mescaline depresses the central nervous system and induces psychotic changes similar to those produced by lysergide (q.v.), but is less potent. It is occasionally used in psychiatry, similarly to lysergide, and it is also capable of inducing trance-like states. To produce hallucinations the average dose required is from 400 to 700 mg. by intramuscular injection.
SEE ALSO Hallucinogenic drugs.

Mesial temporal sclerosis

First described as Ammon's horn sclerosis, then as incisural sclerosis, the term mesial temporal sclerosis more accurately describes the lesions of Ammon's horn, the uncus, amygdaloid region, and mesial aspects of the temporal grey matter which are found in certain cases of epilepsy. Mesial temporal sclerosis is associated with epilepsy which has been present since childhood, or infancy. Two factors may be possible causes, birth injury, or infantile convulsions. No explanation of pathogenesis is completely satisfactory; repeated episodes of hypoxia affecting a particularly vulnerable part of the brain is the most likely. Roughly 50% of temporal lobes resected for temporal lobe epilepsy show a mesial temporal sclerosis.

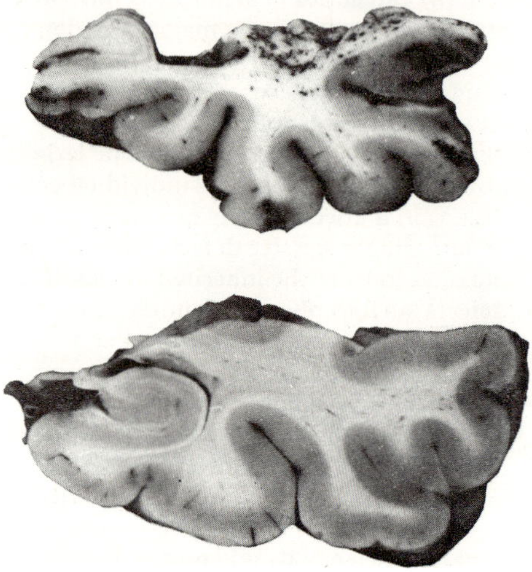

Mesial temporal sclerosis (above)
compared with normal Ammon's horn

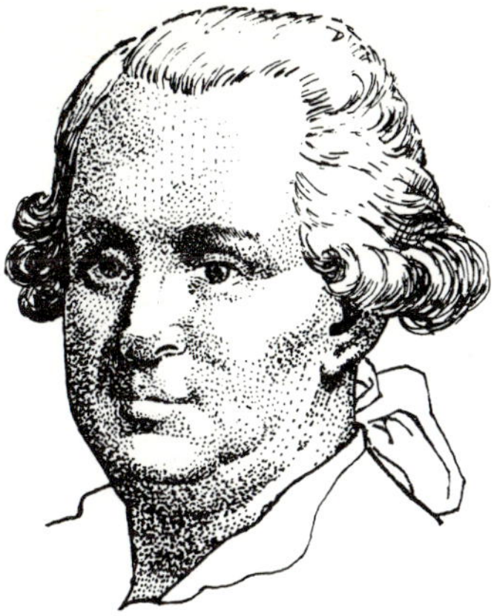

Mesmer, Franz Anton (1734–1815)

Graduating from the University of Vienna in 1766, Mesmer's thesis was concerned with the influences of the planets upon human physiology. After contact with a Jesuit priest, Father Maximilian Hell, who had been experimenting therapeutically with magnets, Mesmer seized on the idea of a cosmic force of great healing power, which could be likened in its properties to magnetism. It soon became evident that magnets were not essential for the force to be transmitted to the patient, for a touch from the healer, or even passes made at a distance could be equally effective. In 1778 Mesmer left Vienna, travelled to Paris at the request of Louis XIV, and soon became a sensation. Mesmer longed for medical recognition, but a Royal Commission on animal magnetism concluded in 1784 that there was no such thing, only 'imagination'. Mesmer was thenceforth a broken man. His work, however, had wide repercussions. Magnetism was taken up, particularly in England and America where it led to the discovery of hypnosis. Dynamic psychiatry, Christian Science, and spiritual healing are all in direct line of succession from animal magnetism.
SEE ALSO Braid, Hypnosis, and Spiritual healing.

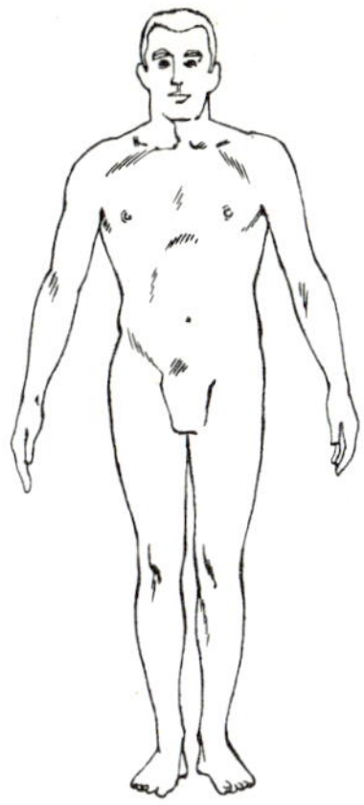

Mesomorph

A mesomorph is an individual displaying features of one of the three main types of body-build in Sheldon's classification of somatotyping. Characteristics include a well-proportioned athletic frame and good musculature.
SEE ALSO Constitution.

Metabolism of the brain

The metabolic reactions of the brain are broadly similar to those elsewhere in the body, but there are reactions found only in the brain and other features have a different emphasis. Protein synthesis follows the usual DNA-RNA pattern and one remarkable feature is the very high level of turnover of brain proteins. Lipids of various kinds compose a large proportion of brain weight and phospholipids like lecithin are of particular importance. The carbohydrate metabolism is based entirely on glucose since the brain has no stores of glycogen. Much of the energy metabolism of brain is expended on maintaining the resting potential of the neurones. Transmitter metabolism is naturally of great importance and the enzymes for their synthesis and destruction are located in the specific neurones. Central transmitters (q.v.) probably include acetylcholine (q.v.), serotonin (q.v.), glutamate (q.v.), GABA (q.v.), glycine (q.v.), catecholamines (q.v.), especially noradrenaline (q.v.) and dopamine (q.v.) and possibly in the cerebellum prostaglandins (q.v.).
The action of many important drugs is exerted on these systems. Also very im-

portant are transport mechanisms for all manner of metabolites across membranes. Particular examples are the reuptake of noradrenaline back into the axon terminals in adrenergic synapses – blocked by antidepressants such as imipramine. Hormones and vitamins also play important roles in brain function and disturbances in their function can lead to psychiatric disorders such as the dementia of pellegra (q.v.) and the psychoses associated with thyroid (q.v.) and adrenal cortical (q.v.) diseases. Brain function is also exquisitely sensitive to oxygen lack, as all high altitude climbers know, and to disturbances in electrolyte balance. Certain compounds such as GABA are found only in the brain. One recent development of great interest has been the suggestion that the laying down of permanent memory depends on ongoing protein synthesis.

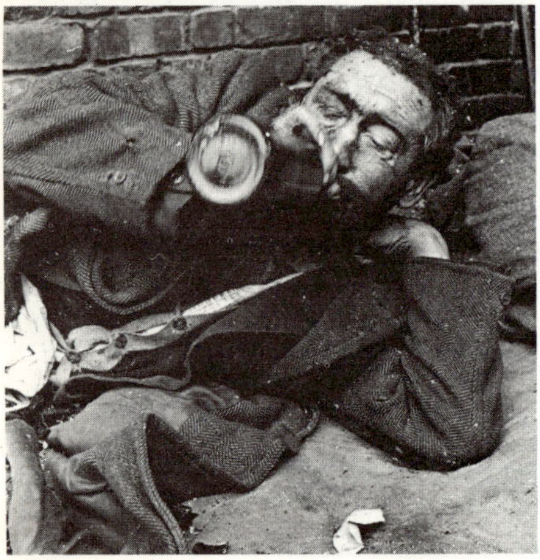

Methylated spirit drinking

The drinking of surgical and methylated spirits is an important aspect of the natural history of alcoholism (q.v.). Drinking crude spirits presents a method of achieving profound intoxication comparatively cheaply. This is in no sense a special form of alcoholism but clearly to be regarded as an economically determined variety since surgical spirits are cheap and strong and can be obtained fairly easily. The drinkers are not a special group except in the sense that their alcohol dependence is so severe and their socio-economic status so low that they can only maintain their intoxication with cheap strong drink. This determines their beverage preference. The spirits are often diluted or mixed with fruit juices etc. Sometimes groups of spirit drinkers congregate in certain areas. the 'typical' crude spirit drinker is likely to be a truly recidivist drinker with a long history of hospital admissions and imprisonment. Methyl alcohol is oxidized to formic acid and formaldehyde and may result in a severe metabolic acidosis. Blindness, delirium, coma and ventilatory or peripheral circulatory failure may occur. Haemodialysis is highly effective in severe cases. As a first-aid measure, the stomach should be washed out if the patient is seen within three hours of ingestion. Ethyl alcohol, by competing with oxidative processes, will inhibit and delay the toxic effects of methyl alcohol.

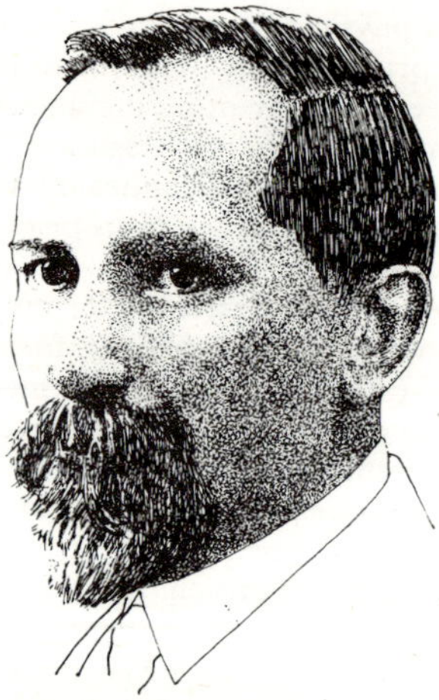

Meyer, Adolf (1866–1950)

Born in Zurich, Meyer emigrated to the United States soon after qualification. He started work as a neuro-pathologist, but influenced by Hughlings Jackson, and by Thomas Huxley, he developed a broad and common-sense approach to the problems of mental illness. His wife became so interested in her husband's work that she began to visit the families of his patients, and became the first American psychiatric social worker. They grasped the broader social implications of mental illness for the patient and his family. Meyer saw each person as a psychobiological whole, responding to life's problems in a manner determined by his genetics, his constitution and his particular social situation. As Professor of Psychiatry at Johns Hopkins, Meyer gathered around him a distinguished group of pupils – Harold Wolff and Aubrey Lewis amongst others. He remained sceptical about psychoanalysis, believing that an integrated approach, a truly psychosomatic approach to medicine, offered the best means of both understanding and of curing the patient. Together with Clifford Beers, an ex-patient, he helped create the mental hygiene movement, which was to lead to the development of preventive psychiatry and of child-guidance clinics.

Microcephaly

The term means 'small-headedness' and is usually taken as a head circumference smaller than three standard deviations below the mean for the age and sex. It is a clinical sign seen in many mentally subnormal patients such as mongolism (Down's syndrome) and phenylketonuria; or genetical microcephaly attributable to a rare autosomal recessive gene; radiogenic microcephaly; 'physiological' microcephaly which is considered to represent one extreme of normal variation; and microcephaly associated with ateleiotic dwarfism or pygmy types.

Microglia

SEE Neuroglia.

Micropsia

Distortions of the size of objects occur in normal subjects during dreams, on waking from sleep, or in 'brown studies'. When these distortions occur in pathological conditions they indicate, in general, a toxic confusional state – deliria, drug intoxications (LSD in particular) or more rarely temporal or occipital lobe epilepsy.

Migraine

(Synonym: Vascular headaches)

Migraine is caused by vasoconstriction followed by dilatation of pain-sensitive cranial branches of the external carotid artery leading to headache, which is usually unilateral at its onset, and associated with irritability, nausea, photophobia and sometimes visual and sensory disturbances, constipation or diarrhoea. The personality of migraine sufferers is characteristically obsessional with high ambition and efficiency, rigidity and reluctance to express hostility openly. At times of conflict these patients become progressively more anxious, frustrated and sometimes resentful. Migraine is sometimes precipitated by emotional stress (q.v.), but there is often a hereditary predisposition, and it occurs five times more frequently among hypertensives than normotensives. It is thought that serotonin (q.v.) or other amines, e.g. tyramine, may also play a part in the production of the syndrome, and reserpine, which depletes it, may precipitate an attack. Methysergide, an antagonist of serotonin, often reduces the frequency of attacks, but is ineffective during one. If the headache is mild, analgesics such as aspirin or codeine phosphate may be effective, but if severe, ergotamine tartrate to produce vasoconstriction may be necessary. The frequency of attacks can also be reduced if situations leading to frustration can be delineated and if possible avoided. SEE ALSO Psychosomatic disorders.

Milieu therapy

The manipulation of the environment for therapeutic purposes, milieu therapy ranges from three meals a day and a comfortable bed, to totally shared activity by all persons in the patients environment. Shorn of its mystique, milieu therapy consists of the kindly efforts of a wide range of individuals to fit a sick person into some niche in the society in which he exists. Group participation, work, and social activities, all are included. SEE ALSO Environmental modification.

Minnesota Multiphasic Personality Inventory (MMPI)

The MMPI is a questionnaire of 550 items in the form of statements with which the subject is required to agree or disagree. Although described as a 'personality' (q.v).

inventory, this test is not concerned with normal dimensions of personality but with pathological tendencies towards hypochondriasis, depression, hysteria, psychopathy, paranoia, psychaesthenia, schizophrenia and hypomania. There are also scales designed to assess 'masculinity-femininity' and to control for lying and more subtle distorting response tendencies. The scales were established and standardized on the basis of responses made by patients of the relevant diagnoses but the direct diagnostic validity is low. Patterns of scale scores or 'profiles', however, have been shown to differentiate neurotics and psychotics from normal subjects and, with skilled interpretation, the test can be a useful screening device.

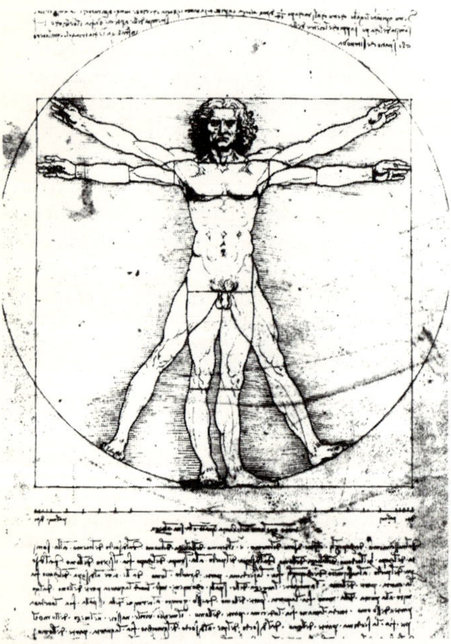

Mirror-writing from the notebooks of Leonardo da Vinci

Mirror writing

A script which runs in the reverse direction to normal with reverse of individual letters. It occurs in normal children and adults, may be learned, and used as a secret mode of writing (e.g. by Leonardo da Vinci in his notebooks). It is also found in states of disturbed consciousness, brain damage, and in dyslexic children. Mirror reading (strephosymbolia) may also occur in dyslexic children.

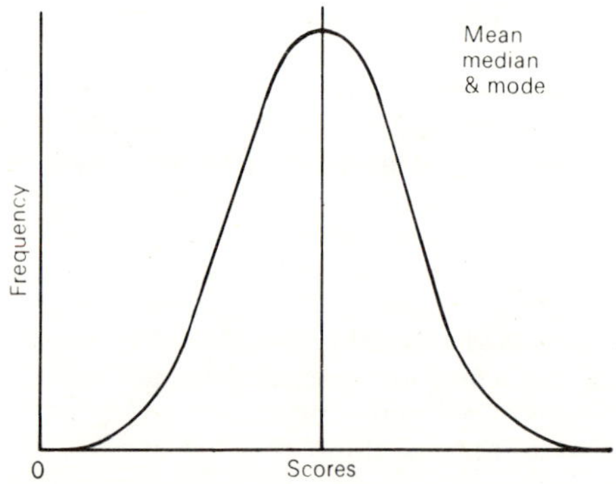

Mean, median & mode in normal distributions.
In normal distributions mean, median & mode coincide

Mode

The mode is the measurement which occurs most frequently in a series of observations (see figure and compare with mean and median). The mode indicates the most frequent occurrence and is particularly valuable when there is a skew frequency distribution.

Modelling

Or imitation. Seeing a therapist enter a phobic situation can induce a patient to do so. It is most used in animal phobias either alone or combined with other techniques such as flooding (q.v.) or desensitization (q.v.).
SEE ALSO Shaping.

Model psychosis

The term 'model psychosis' arises from the observation that small doses of a number of substances (e.g. LSD (q.v.), mescaline (q.v.)) produce an effect resembling schizophrenia. The expectation that this will afford a clue to specific chemical or metabolic abnormalities underlying schizophrenia has not been fulfilled but remains a possibility. It must be borne in mind that emotional and perceptual changes follow intoxication with a wide variety of substances; sometimes sought (e.g. alcohol), sometimes incidental (side effects of drugs) and sometimes accidental (industrial substances); also that, despite a striking superficial resemblance, there are important differences between the effects of hallucinogens (q.v.) and naturally occurring psychoses.

A state resembling psychosis is also produced by depriving the subject of sensory stimulation for a continuous period of more than twenty-four hours (see Sensory deprivation).

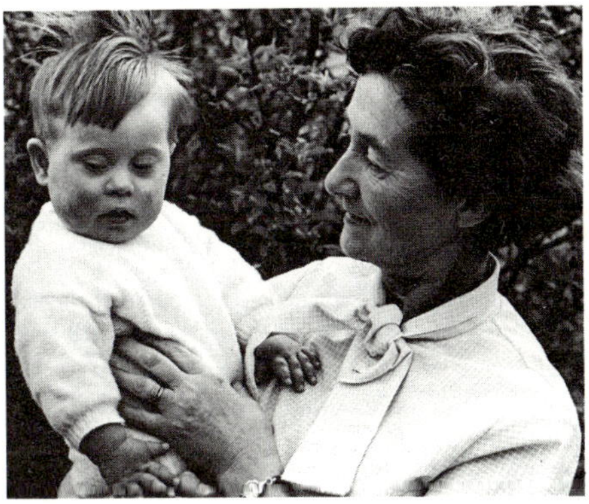

A mongol baby being cared for in a home for mongol babies

Mongolism

(Synonym: Down's syndrome.)

Approximately 97% of mongols have an extra autosomal chromosome of the G group presumed to be a No.21 chromosome trisomy; of the remaining 3% some are mosaics with a mixture of normal and trisomic cells, others have chromosomal translocations in which the extra G group chromosome is fused to another G group chromosome (G/G translocation) or to a D group chromosome (D/G translocation). Parents and relatives of patients with translocation mongolism may be carriers of a balanced translocation, detectable by cytogenetical techniques, which is of importance in genetical counselling because such carriers stand at increased risk for producing mongol offspring.

The incidence of mongolism is about one in every 660 live births. It is recognizable at birth. Clinical features include the typical face; short trunk with deep body-cavities; generalized hypotonia; mottled skin; distinctive dermatoglyphics including single transverse palmar creases in some cases and a plantar furrow on the sole running backwards from the cleft between first and second toes; blepharitis; speckled iris (Brushfield's spots); frequently a congenital heart defect. Mental subnormality is in many cases severe. The highest levels of mental functioning that can be expected in mongols are around IQ 60, but this is unusual, for most function at much lower levels.

Improvement in antibiotics has greatly ameliorated the picture regarding life-expectancy; many mongol's now who have survived the first year of life may hope for a normal or near-normal life-span, though they are exceptionally prone to respiratory infections and pneumonia.

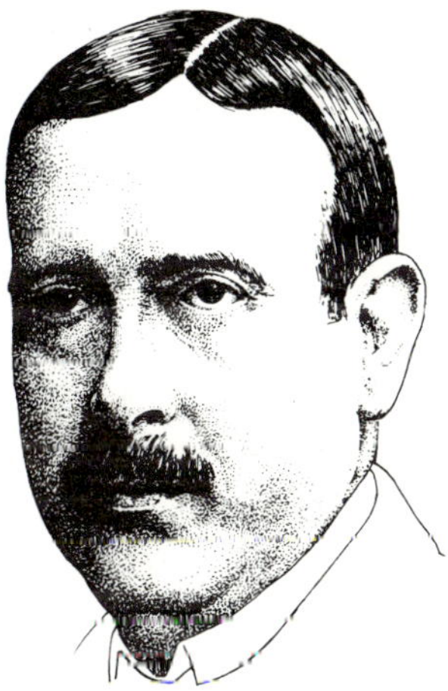

Moniz, Egas (1874–1955)

As Professor of Neurology at Lisbon, Moniz was responsible for two great advances, leucotomy and cerebral angiography. He postulated that by severing the frontothalamic fibres, anxiety would be reduced. His neuro-surgical colleague Almeida Lima, performed the first frontal lobotomy on a psychiatric patient in 1935. Despite the vicissitudes the operation has undergone, neuro-surgical procedures still hold a secure place in the psychiatrists therapeutic armamentarium.

SEE ALSO Leucotomy and Stereotatic operations.

Monoamine oxidase inhibitors (MAOIs)

The euphoriant effects of the MAOIs were noted during their use as anti-tubercle agents. The initial uncontrolled trials induced a wave of enthusiasm. Subsequent more critical evaluations and recognition of the problems of side effects and toxicity have modified this enthusiasm.

As their name indicates these compounds interfere with the action of the enzyme monoamine oxidase (MAO) which is responsible for the degradation of monoamines. Their anti-depressant activity is thought to depend on the inhibition of MAO within the brain, resulting in an increase in the amount of transmitter amines at synaptic junctions.

These compounds are readily absorbed and metabolized, active intermediate compounds may be produced, and most of a single dose is broken down and excreted within a day.

The majority of compounds used clinically are hydrazine derivatives, e.g. iproniazid, nialamide, isocarboxazid, phenelzine and mebenazine. Iproniazid was the prototype of this group but has largely been replaced by the later members because of its toxicity. The other members of the group are therapeutically less active but less toxic than the original iproniazid. Phenelzine and isocarboxazid have probably achieved the widest use.

One non-hydrazine MAOI, tranylcypromine, has anti-depressant use. This compound possesses dual properties resembling both iproniazid and amphetamine to which it has chemical similarity.

The MAOIs have a limited but none the less valuable place in the treatment of depressive illness, particularly when this is associated with anxiety and phobic states. The clinical effect is delayed from five days to three weeks or more from the beginning of treatment.

Autonomic side effects include hypotension, which is rather frequent, blurred vision, dry mouth, constipation, hesitancy of micturition, and delayed ejaculation; they are minor but troublesome. Phenelzine may produce drowsiness, but tranylcypromine because of its stimulant action may produce insomnia. Excitatory states and toxic psychoses have been described.

There are more serious toxic reactions. Many of the MAOIs may cause hypertensive crises due to the liberation of free catecholamines from binding sites, this occurs most frequently with tranylcypromine (one in 200). Hypertensive crises may be precipitated by other drugs, especially sympathomimetic compounds such as amphetamine, ephedrine and phenylephrine. A variety of foods containing pressor amines may initiate a crisis and since cheese was the first of these foods to be identified the reaction has become known as a 'cheese reaction' (q.v.). A rare complication of hydrazine compounds is hepatocellular jaundice.

Most of the MAO inhibitors interact with a wide variety of drugs. They potentiate the action of alcohol, barbiturates and insulin. Dangerous reactions have occurred with various narcotic analgesics. Excitation may occur with anti-Parkinson drugs, and reserpine. Various interactions occur with anti-hypertensive drugs; methyl dopa may cause excitation, ganglion blocking hypotensive drugs may be powerfully potentiated, and guanethidine antagonized. Tricyclic anti-depressants may induce a central excitation which rarely can induce convulsions, coma and death.

Drug interactions are a serious disadvantage of MAOI compounds, but in a psychiatric context the interaction with tricyclic anti-depressant is particularly difficult, since failure of depression to respond to MAOI requires that treatment should be discontinued for three weeks before administering a tricyclic substance. However, certain psychiatrists have shown that a proportion of severe depressions respond best to simultaneous administration of an MAOI and a tricyclic anti-depressant (usually amitriptyline). Such therapy should however always be under the direct control of a psychiatrist.

Monoamines

SEE Amines.

Monosomy X

SEE Turner's syndrome

Mood

The feelings of the person, particularly those experienced internally. The related term affect (q.v.) is used to refer not only to the feelings of the subject but also to the external manifestation of the emotional reaction. Mood swings between wellbeing and 'blueness' are seen in normal people but are exaggerated in the neuroses, particularly manic depressive illness. Experimental evidence suggests that the mood depends on activity in the limbic system (q.v.).

Moral
SEE Responsibility.

Morita therapy

Dr Shoma Morita developed a therapy based on Zen Buddhism (q.v.) and particularly suited to his Japanese patients. Strict discipline imposed from both within and without the patient, intensive work, a repeated denial of illness and of symptoms, the frank recognition of what one really is, all combine to enable the patient to live in the community without complaining. Morita therapy, as well as Zen Buddhism are much used in Japan, largely for neurotic disorders and for those suffering from character disorders.

Moron
SEE Mental subnormality.

Motive

That which moves or induces a person to act in a certain way. Motives are to a considerable extent based on instinctual drives which have been transformed and thereby to some degree concealed.

Motor disturbances

Motor disturbances are very common and varied in mental disorders. Reduction of movement may amount to complete immobility, as in stupor, or the statuesque poses of catalepsy (q.v.). There may be slowness and reduction of movement, as in the retardation of depression (q.v.), where expressive movement and gesture particularly are absent. Increase of movement shows in the rapid, exaggerated and varied movements seen in mania (q.v.) or in the restlessness and more repetitive movements of agitated depression. Abnormality of movement appears as stereotypy (q.v.), mannerisms, and automatic obedience of catalepsy, or in the repetitive rituals of obsessional (q.v.) patients. Limited repetitive movements may occur in tics, tremors, and habit spasms, while many organic illnesses may show motor disturbances (e.g. Huntington's chorea (q.v.)).

Mourning
SEE Bereavement.

Mucous colitis
SEE Irritable bowel syndrome.

Multifactorial inheritance
(Synonym: Polygenic inheritance)

The genetical transmission of a trait through the additive action of many genes of small effect. Traits inherited in this manner show characteristically a continuous distribution throughout the general population, with very small differences in measurement between one individual and the next if placed in rank order. Stature and intelligence are examples of such traits.
SEE ALSO Genetics.

Multiple sclerosis
(Synonym: disseminated sclerosis)

A patchy demyelination and subsequent gliosis, the sclérose en plaques of French neurologists, occurs in certain parts of the central nervous system – in the cerebral white matter, brain stem, cerebellum and spinal cord. Beginning in early adult life, the condition progresses in fits and starts. Retrobulbar neuritis affecting one eye commonly heralds the onset of the disease, whilst transient limb weakness, or sensory symptoms serve to alert the physician to the diagnosis. Nystagmus, dysarthria, intention tremor and ataxic paraplegia are the classical outcome. 85% of patients show some evidence of psychiatric disturbance, the commonest being some degree of intellectual deterioration. This is reported as moderate or severe in 20% of patients and consists particularly of failure to abstract thinking and memory. It may be associated with a mood of euphoria and disorder of judgement, particularly as far as recognition of personal physical limitations is concerned.

Multiple X syndromes

Chromosomal abnormalities associated with duplication or triplication of the X chromosome. Seen in the male as Klinefelter's syndrome (q.v.) or in XXX females (see Trisomy). Mental defect is common but not invariable.

Munchausen syndrome

There is a small group of individuals who repeatedly seek admission to hospital with signs of serious abdominal disorder, for which operation may be considered necessary. Laparotomy reveals no abnormality, the patient is discharged, and later appears at another hospital with similar symptoms. Wandering, repeated laparotomies, psychopathic features of personality, and deliberate production of disability characterize this strange condition, which is ill-understood. Patients rarely come under psychiatric investigation, preferring to move from hospital to hospital in their search for admission to a medical or surgical ward.

Murder

The incidence of murder differs from community to community. In England and Wales about 160 murders are committed a year, whilst in New York alone there are about 5000 homicides each year. In the United Kingdom 25% of murderers commit suicide, in America far fewer. The motives for murder do not greatly differ from country to country, although the relative frequencies of types of murder do – erring wives are much more frequently killed in some Far Eastern countries than in European countries. Jealousy, sexual violence, revenge, gain, self-defence and quarrelling all may lead to murder. It is useful to recognize certain patterns which occur. For instance, the female child victim has most often been killed by a near relative; the middle-aged married woman by a jealous, depressed husband; the whole family by a parent suffering from a depressive illness; the mother by a schizophrenic son. Murders of prostitutes are most commonly carried out by psychopathic individuals, although a true sado-masochistic murder is rare. Morbid jealousy often leads to murder. The psychiatrist may be able to prevent murder taking place if he is familiar with this syndrome.

There is a relationship between murder and certain times of the day and of the year. For instance, the majority of murders occur between 6 p.m. and 1 a.m.; if a murder is committed between 6 and 8 a.m., it is highly likely that it has been carried out by a depressed individual. In the United States it has been shown that killing is particularly common at the weekend or over public holidays. Physical defects and illness are common amongst murderers whether sane or insane.

SEE ALSO Forensic psychiatry, Legal aspects of psychiatry, Homicide, Homicidal threats, and Psychopathic states.

Muscle tone

Voluntary muscles consist of numerous contractile cells arranged in parallel attached either directly, or through a tendon, to the bone. Between these extra fusal muscle fibres lie scattered intrafusal fibres (muscle spindles) which are specialised proprioceptor cells responsible for the controlled muscle contraction of muscle tone which maintains body posture and for the servo mechanism which smooths muscle contraction (see voluntary movement). The muscle spindles are stretch receptors and when the antigravity muscles are stretched feedback impulses probably travelling through the cerebral cortex lead to the contraction of the related main (extrafusal) fibres through the α motor pathway from the anterior horn. The muscle spindle action is itself under γ motor control from the anterior horn. Thus normal muscle tone depends on the integrity of this γ-α loop and on the nervous downflow from brain centres. These include *inter alia* those that cause increased muscle tone in anxiety states and the 'extrapyramidal' downflow that is disturbed with dopamine depleting neuroleptic drugs.

Music therapy

The manipulation of mood by the use of music has been applied to the treatment of mental disorder. Certain pieces of music are selected with regard to their soothing, exciting, fantasy stimulating or other attributes; the patients usually listen in groups. With children percussion groups or more sophisticated musical groups may be formed, the resultant activity being useful in socializing the disturbed child.

Mutism

In catatonic schizophrenia mutism may occur as a negativistic (q.v.) symptom. It may occur in hysteria (q.v.) as an isolated symptom revealed by other evidence of laryngeal function, e.g. coughing. 'Elective mutism' refers to the symptom of childhood where speech is produced in one situation (e.g. home) but not in another (e.g. school).

Myxoedema

Psychological function is disturbed early in myxoedema. Patients become increasingly slow and forgetful, with impairment of concentration and interest. Some patients become apathetic, others morose, irritable and querulous. All of these symptoms improve with thyroxine treatment. Frank psychosis is seen in a proportion of cases, the so-called 'myxoedematous madness'. Some patients present with an organic psychosis: a few with features of dementia, others with subacute delirium. In the latter disorder various psychotic features may occur, but in a setting of impaired consciousness. Other patients present with a functional psychosis. Some are severely depressed, usually with retardation but occasionally with agitation. In other patients a schizophrenia-like illness occurs, with auditory hallucinations and paranoid delusions in a setting of clear consciousness.

The organic psychoses usually clear up with adequate thyroxine treatment. In the functional psychoses response to thyroxine is not so certain and in many cases electroconvulsive treatment and psychotropic drugs are necessary as well.

Naevoid amentia
(Synonym: Sturge-Weber syndrome)

A rare condition in the group of phakomatoses (q.v.). It is associated with mental subnormality, often severe. The most prominent physical manifestation is a facial haemangioma usually unilateral, occasionally extending to the other side of the body. Dilated, tortuous vessels which may become calcified with age are found in the meninges. Epilepsy is common and contralateral hemiplegia is seen. Severely affected patients die early in life, but others have a longer, even normal, life-span. Management depends largely on the degree of mental subnormality; symptomatic treatment of epilepsy and physiotherapeutic regimes for paralysis should be given when called for.

Nail-biting

Most children bite their nails at some point and for the majority the symptom is not a sign of emotional disorder, but a habit that occurs when the child is bored or absorbed, for example in watching television. Some tense and anxious children bite their nails at times of stress and here the management of the problem requires understanding of the more general emotional disorder.
The isolated habit usually remits spontaneously. Certainly, punishment and painting the nails with bitter substances is rarely helpful. In older girls permission to wear transparent nail varnish has been said to act as an incentive to allow the nails to grow, but in general the habit is not worth troubling about.

Narcissism

During psychological development the infant passes through a phase of primary narcissism, when his libido, or mental energy is concerned with his own body, to a stage of secondary narcissism, when his own self-love reflects attitudes of parents and other authority figures. In adult life love objects may be reflections of the individual himself – a narcissistic object choice. Some homosexuals choose partners of this type.

Narco-analysis

A form of treatment used extensively in the war neuroses of the second world war. The usual technique is slow intravenous injection of a short-acting barbiturate such as thiopentone or methohexitone sodium. Intravenous sodium amylobarbitone may also be used. Injection should be slow and in subhypnotic dosage. The subject attains a state of complete relaxation and a feeling of wellbeing and serenity, with a desire to communicate thoughts and a capacity to verbalize easily. Repressed memories, affects and conflicts may be expressed. The technique is particularly successful in relieving hysterical conversion symptoms if there has been a recent, obvious and severe trauma. Psychogenic amnesia may also be relieved – but amnesia of organic origin is likely to be aggravated by this technique and deaths in such patients have been reported.
SEE ALSO Abreaction.

Narcolepsy

An increased tendency to lapse into natural sleep. The sleep is provoked by those circumstances which are normally conducive, such as boredom, relaxation, and monotony as well as by emotion such as sexual excitement. But sleep may supervene in narcoleptics whilst walking, playing cards, eating, and may be not only embarrasing but can interfere with work.

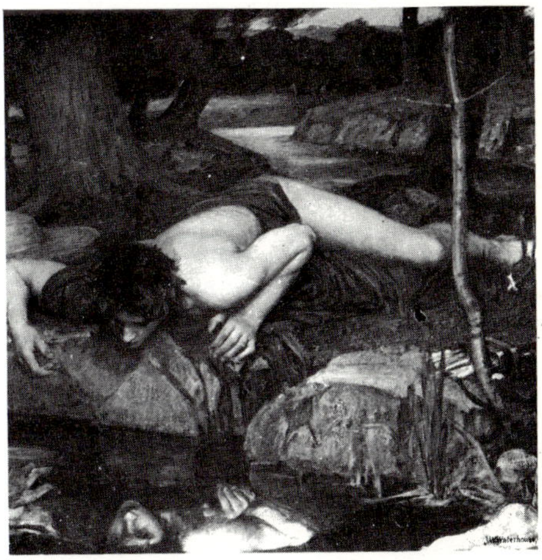

From 'Echo and Narcissus' by J. W. Waterhouse

With the onset of symptoms there may be some weight gain leading to obesity. Neurological examination is negative despite troublesome additional symptoms which may suggest a sinister intracerebral disorder. The symptoms include cataplexy (q.v.), sleep paralysis, and hypnagogic hallucinations (q.v.). The EEG is normal and during the attacks reveals the changes characteristic of sleep though the REM (q.v.) phase is reached unusually rapidly. Treatment with amphetamines (q.v.) has been successful in promoting wakefulness but with the large doses that may be required the danger exists of acute paranoid psychoses supervening.

Narcosis

Continuous narcosis (q.v.) for a period of two to three weeks for conditions such as involutional melancholia has been abandoned in favour of other and more effective methods of treatment. However, modified continuous narcosis for five to seven days is frequently useful as an initial stage in the treatment of reactive states of anxiety and tension particularly if the patient has lost weight. Recently narcosis, combined with ECT and antidepressant drugs, has been suggested as being particularly beneficial in the more resistant types of depressive illnesses.
Some anxious and tense patients find difficulty in recounting their problems, particularly if they have been through some very painful experience. Inducing a state of semi-narcosis in these patients with a drug such as thiopentone will allow them to ventilate their feelings and experiences often with a considerable catharsis and the dependent relationship which this method brings about may also be useful in later therapy if properly managed. A very acute and painful experience, such as was more frequently seen in wartime, may lead to a state of amnesia when interviewing the patient under narcosis may allow the experience to come to consciousness and be relived often with considerable emotional discharge and therapeutic benefit.

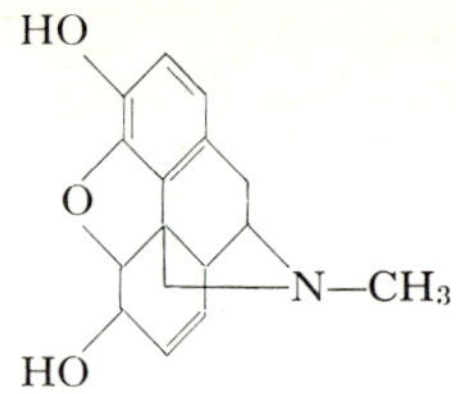

Morphine

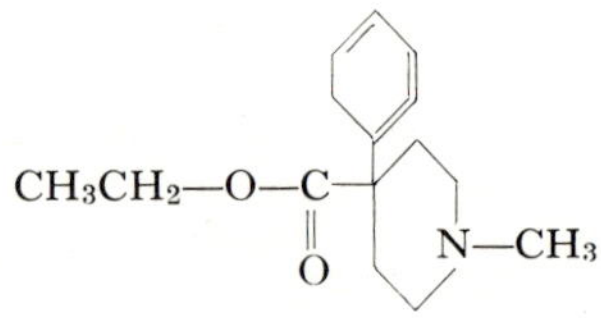

Pethidine

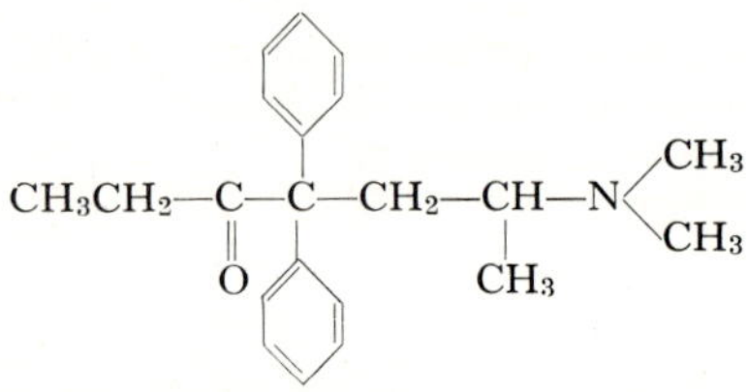

Methadone

The structure of prototype narcotic analgesics

Narcotic analgesics

Full accounts of the properties of these compounds may be found in general pharmacological texts. Psychiatric interest centres on the propensity of these compounds to produce drug dependence (q.v.), and on the treatment of such states. From this point of view all powerful narcotic analgesics may be considered hazardous, although the ease and rapidity with which dependence develops and the severity of withdrawal symptoms show considerable variability. Diamorphine (heroin) is particularly notorious on both counts. However, the prevalence of addiction to a particular compound may reflect other factors such as prescription frequency and availability as well as the inherent properties of that compound.
There are three main groups of narcotic analgesics; morphine and other opium derivatives, methadone and congeners, and pethidine and related compounds (see table). Notwithstanding the enormous amount of work devoted to these compounds, their mechanism of action remains unknown. There are more than twenty

effective narcotic analgesics available today. Despite a considerable degree of chemical diversity, nevertheless they are remarkably similar in their pharmacological actions. The main narcotic action is manifested in analgesia, drowsiness, mood changes and mental clouding; respiratory depression commonly occurs. The mood change induced is usually one of euphoria, and it is this coupled with the ease of drug tolerance development that leads to the major hazard of drug dependence. Cross tolerance occurs and these compounds can partially or wholly substitute for each other in suppressing withdrawal symptoms. Methadone withdrawal produces relatively less discomfort than other compounds, and for this reason the treatment of heroin or morphine addiction commonly begins by changing to an equivalent dose of methadone followed by progressive reduction of the dose.

Similarly the narcotic analgesics show a common spectrum of side effects including nausea, vomiting, drowsiness, dizziness and constipation. A number of psychotropic agents have the property of potentiating the actions of narcotic analgesics; the most important of these are the phenothiazines (q.v.), monoamine oxidase inhibitors (q.v.), and tricyclic antidepressants (q.v.).

Whatever the reason for using narcotic drugs, it is probable that self-administration of drugs and self-induced changes in mood are the critical factors in the development of compulsive abuse. It behoves the physician to remember this when treating patients and indeed should he consider treating himself.

Narcotic antagonists

Simple molecular modification of narcotic analgesic substances has resulted in the production of a series of compounds that are antagonists or partial antagonists of the analgesics. Most narcotic antagonists also possess varying degrees of agonist activity. Nalorphine is the prototype of these compounds, and other important members include levallorphan, naloxone, and cyclazocine.

Narcotic antagonists have the property of preventing or abolishing many of the actions of the narcotic analgesics, and in narcotic addicts will precipitate immediate and severe withdrawal symptoms. Antagonists are used mainly in the treatment of respiratory depression induced by narcotics; they have little place in the treatment of addiction.

The [British] National Association for Mental Health (NAMH)

The NAMH was formed in Britain in 1946, its aims being to foster a wide understanding of the importance of mental health in daily life, in education and in the upbringing of children. Practical steps included the establishment of schools and hostels, the encouragement of research, the provision of information regarding mental health and ill-health, and the establishment and maintenance of professional standards. Associations with similar aims have been established in other countries.

Some of the commoner narcotic analgesics

	Opium alkaloids and related compounds	Methadone congeners	Pethidine congeners
Dependency prone powerful analgesics	Morphine Diacetylmorphine (heroin) Dihydromorphinone Metopon Levorphanol Phenazocine Pentazocine	Methadone Dextromoramide Dipipanone Phenadoxone	Pethidine Alphaprodine Anileridine Pimonidine
Low abuse potential mild analgesics	Codeine Dihydrocodeinone Oxycodone Pholcodine	Dextropropoxyphene	Ethoheptazine

Necromania

Pathological preoccupation with dead bodies.

Necrophilia

A sexual perversion in which sexual gratification is obtained by sexual contact with a dead body. In most cases the individual concerned is suffering from schizophrenia. but there has recently grown up a cult-interest in death amongst certain young people of a psychopathic character which may lead to necrophilic activity.

Negative practice
SEE Massed practice.

Negativism

Negativism occurs most characteristically in catatonic schizophrenia (q.v.) and manifests itself as an opposition to compliance by resistance or by active contrary action. Thus, a subject may refuse to swallow food put into the mouth, or, having remained silent to questions, begin to speak as the interview is terminated.
SEE ALSO Mutism.

Neo-Freudians

A somewhat imprecise term embracing those analysts who follow Freud (q.v.), but who depart in one or other way from classical analytic theory. Jung (q.v.) and Adler (q.v.) founded their own schools of psychoanalysis, and may or may not be regarded as Neo-Freudians; in general the Neo-Freudians are represented by Karen Horney, Erich Fromm, and Harry Stack Sullivan together with their followers. They place greater emphasis on the reaction of the individual to his current environment, the patient-doctor relationship, and to anxiety. There is less emphasis on sexuality and the analysis of early infantile experiences. Books by Karen Horney are useful tools in psychotherapy, for they are well written and can be understood by an educated layman. In particular her book *Self-Analysis* may be used by patients in areas remote from trained psychotherapeutic help.

Neologism

Neologisms are part of the speech disturbance which reflects the disordered thought of schizophrenics (q.v.). They are words of the patient's own making, often condensations of other words and having a special meaning for the patient.

Nephrogenic diabetes insipidus

A sex-linked disorder in which males are affected, with female carriers, showing polyuria from infancy. It often also shows mental subnormality.

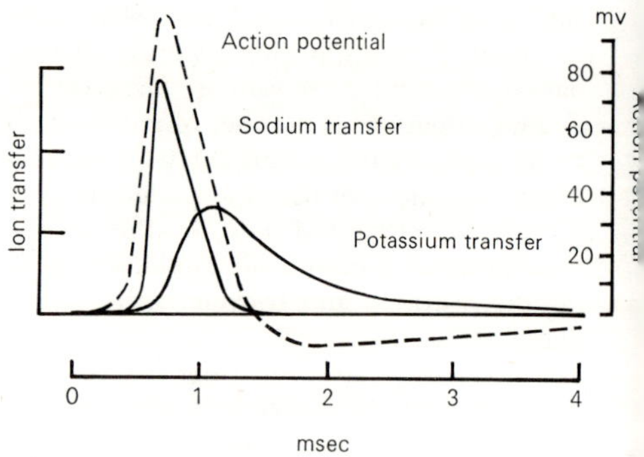

Nerve fibre transmission

Nerve cells transmit messages in the form of brief electrochemical impulses. These travel along the outer membrane of the cell, notably along the membrane of its long principle fibre, the axon. It is possible to obtain an electrical record of impulses in a single nerve fibre by placing an electrode near it. Such measurements have shown that impulses travel along the nerves at velocities of between 0·5 m. and 100 m. per second.
The rate of conduction depends on the diameter of the nerve fibre and on whether it is myelinated. The electrochemical changes which form the basis of the nerve impulses depend on movements of ions (sodium and potassium) across the membrane surrounding the nerve fibre. In myelinated fibres these changes only occur

at the gaps (nodes of Ranvier) in the myelin sheath. The impulse thus achieves a rapid rate by jumping along the nodes (saltatory conduction).

Neurasthenia

First introduced by Beard in 1867, the word neurasthenia was used to describe a condition he believed was caused by exhaustion of the nerve cell. Intense fatigue, feelings of weakness and nervousness characterized the clinical picture, with many psychosomatic complaints. The diagnosis is rarely used today, although occasionally a patient is encountered whose only symptom is persistent fatigue for which no reason can be discovered, and for which no treatment is of any avail. It is easy for the truly neurasthenic patient to be misdiagnosed as a case of depression.
SEE ALSO Hypochondriasis.

Neurilemma
SEE Neurones.

Neurofibromatosis
(Synonym: Von Recklinghausen's disease)

Characterized by skin pigmentation, subcutaneous fibromata, and neurofibromata of peripheral and cranial nerves, the condition is due to an irregularly dominant gene. Malignancy may develop in both skin and nerve tumours, as well as within the brain itself.
SEE ALSO Inherited metabolic defects.

Neuroglia

There are two basic cell elements in the nervous system, the nerve cells (neurones, q.v.) and the neuroglial cells – of which there are several types. The full functions of the neuroglial cells, collectively and individually, are not known though it appears that among the functions is support and nourishment of the neurones. The main neuroglial cells that are distinguished are the ependymal cells (lining the ventricular cavities), the oligodendrocytes (perhaps associated with myelin integrity) the protoplasmic and fibrous astrocytes (the latter showing characteristic attachments to blood vessels) and the microglia (probably showing phagocytic activity). In the absence of adequate knowledge of their function, the main medical importance of these cells is their frequent association with intracranial tumours.

Neurohypophysis

Otherwise termed the posterior pituitary. It is derived from a downgrowth from the diencephalic portion of the embryonic forebrain and hence consists of modified neural cells, the bodies of which lie in nuclei in the hypothalamus and the axons and their terminals in the neurohypophysis. The two hormones which it stores and secretes (antidiuretic hormone or vasopressin and oxytocin) are formed in the cell bodies in the hypothalamus and pass down to the nerve terminals for storage and subsequent secretion under appropriate stimuli. The stimulus for antidiuretic hormone secretion is an increase in osmotic pressure in the plasma passing through the hypothalamus, that for oxytocin is a reflex derived from stimulation of the cervix or suckling of the nipple.

Neuroleptic drugs
(Synonym: Major tranquillizers)

The major tranquillizers or neuroleptic drugs were developed after the successful use of chlorpromazine, the prototype of the series. Several distinct chemical groups now fall within this general category: the phenothiazines (q.v.), the rauwolfia deriva-

Table of the main groups of neuroleptic drugs and representative members.

Phenothiazines	Chlorpromazine Trifluoperazine Fluphenazine
Rauwolfia derivatives	Reserpine
Butyrophenones	Haloperidol Trifluperidol
Thioxanthines	Chlorprothixene Thiothixene

tives (q.v.), the butyrophenones (q.v.), and the thioxanthines (q.v.).
These neuroleptic drugs have many features in common. They calm the patients without producing sleep, they attenuate emotion, diminish the impact of external stimuli and reduce initiative. They also produce a constraint on behavioural disturbance. A number of minor side effects such as drowsiness and hypotension are commonly encountered, but extrapyramidal syndromes are of most importance. Neuroleptic agents are the main stay in drug treatment of psychotic disorders, particularly in the schizophrenias and manic states when they are usually administered in higher doses. They also find a valuable place in controlling symptoms in organic confusional states, in brain syndromes and as adjuvants to antidepressant treatment when there is marked agitation. Neurotic illnesses and anxiety states are customarily treated with minor tranquillizers, but the neuroleptic compounds should be borne in mind as an alternative in refractory cases.

Neurones

Each neurone (nerve cell) possesses a cell body with nucleus, nucleolus and within the cytoplasm the Nissl granules. One single, long, regular fibre, the axon, conducts the impulses from the cell body to its ultimate destination while a large number of short, irregular, branched processes, the dendrites, conduct the impulses to the cell, receiving the transmission from axons of other cells via synapses (q.v.). Axons vary very much in length and in diameter. The diameter of the fibre is mainly determined by the sheath of myelin surrounding the axon. This myelin sheath covers all axons; for some the myelin sheath is very thin and these fibres are by tradition still called 'non-myelinated'; the remaining fibres have a thicker and obvious cover and are termed 'myelinated'. These latter fibres show constrictions of their myelin at intervals termed the nodes of Ranvier. The speed of nerve conduction in thick myelinated fibres is much greater than in thin non-myelinated fibres, the impulse jumping (saltatory conduction) from one node of Ranvier to the next. The speeds vary from about 1 metre per second to 100 metres per second (SEE Nerve fibre transmission). In the peripheral nervous system the nerve fibres have an outer nucleated sheath – the neurilemma. Fibres with this neurilemma sheath can regenerate after section, those without it cannot; hence regeneration is possible in the peripheral nervous system but not within the central nervous system. The axon may give off collateral branches, one or more of which can synapse with its own dendrites or cell body (recurrent collateral). The axon ultimately divides into a number of terminal branches which either form the motor end plates to the muscles or the presynaptic bulbous ending for transmission to another neurone. This general description of neurones applies to most areas of the nervous system though specialization occurs in some sites serving special functions.

Neuroses

SEE Psychoneuroses.

Neuroses in the aged

Although elderly patients with neuroses are only occasionally seen in psychiatric clinics, it has been found that 10–20% of people aged 65 or over have moderately disabling neurotic symptoms. General practitioners are aware, mainly, of their life-long neurotics, but these on the whole suffer less as they grow older. Neurotic illness beginning in later life manifests itself mainly as a depression (q.v.) or anxiety state (q.v.). True psychogenic hysteria is rare, though hysterical symptoms are common in both functional and organic psychoses. At this age neurotic reactions are usually precipitated by physical ill-health, especially cardiac disease. Bereavement (q.v.) loss of income due to retirement (q.v.) and isolation (q.v.) are not in themselves specially frequent causes. Low intelligence and an anxiety-prone insecure personality may be important predisposing factors.

Neurosyphilis, congenital

Whereas but fifty years ago individual neurologists were able to collect series of patients running into hundreds, congenital syphilis is now a rarity and congenital neuro-syphilis correspondingly three times rarer. Convulsions, hydrocephalus, paralysis, optic atrophy, intellectual deficit were seen within weeks or months of birth. In two or three years deafness and interstitial keratitis were observed with a saddle nose and peg teeth, while in the early teens general paralysis or juvenile tabes emerged. A small number of surviving adults with stigmata are still to be seen. SEE ALSO Syphilis.

Neurotic depression

In contrast to endogenous (psychotic) depression, the depressive symptoms are not biologically determined but stem from the patient's neurotic personality. Characteristically such patients have long-standing personality problems, the depressive symptoms come on insidiously and the symptoms show a pattern of reactivity, inadequacy, hysterical or other neurotic features, initial insomnia, hypochondriasis and self-pity. In the USA the term neurotic depression includes reactive (exogenous) depression.
It is better to assess 'how much' of the patient's depression stems from neurotic or endogenous factors rather than to classify it as exclusively one or the other. The more the patient's symptoms stem from neurotic factors the less they are likely to respond to physical methods of treatment such as ECT or tricyclic antidepressant drugs.

Neurotic reaction types

SEE Psychoneuroses.

Neuroticism (N-factor)

In attempting to classify psychiatric disorders, Eysenck has suggested that a medical diagnosis may be appropriate for certain conditions, but that disorders of behaviour acquired through the learning processes must be based on a different classificatory system. He has identified three broad dimensions of personality, psychoticism (*P*-factor), neuroticism (*N*-factor), and extroversion-introversion (*E*-score), On these may be constructed a grouping of the behavioural disorders – the neuroses, some psychoses, and the psychopathies. Tests used to identify these factors include the Eysenck personality inventory (EPI) – formerly called the Maudsley personality inventory (MPI).

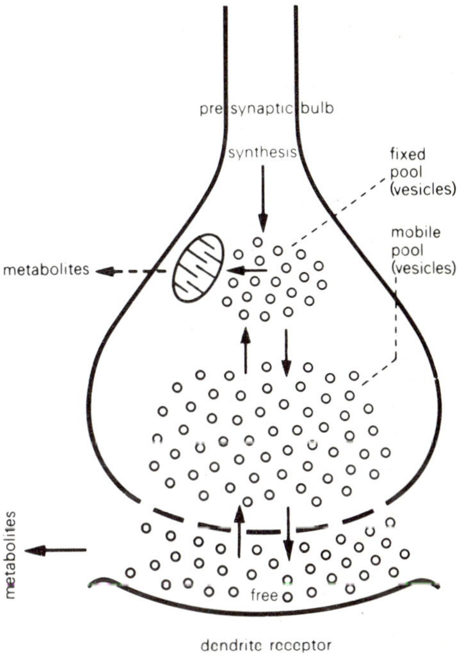

Ideal representation of typical synaptic transmission mechanism

Neuro-transmitters

Transmission of the nerve impulse from one cell to another occurs at the synapse and proceed in one direction only. It passes from the pre-synaptic fibre across the synaptic cleft of about 200Å units and to the post-synaptic membrane of the second neurone. Synaptic transmission results from the release of a small amount of a specific substance through the pre-synaptic membrane. This substance (neuro-transmitter) is contained in minute synaptic vesicles at the end of the axon. The neuro-transmitter reacts with the membrane of the next nerve cell and either excites the cell or inhibits it. In excitation the substance acts to bring the cell into a state in which it is more likely to transmit a further impulse. In inhibition the

substance acts to prevent such activity. The nature of the neuro-transmitters is well known for the peripheral nervous system and consists of acetylcholine and noradrenaline in various synapses. The nature of the neuro-transmitters within the central nervous system is less well established. The substances probably involved are acetylcholine, noradrenaline, dopamine, serotonin (5-hydroxytryptamine) γ-aminobutyric acid (GABA), glycine, and glutamic acid.
SEE ALSO Synapse transmission and Transmission in synapse of brain cells.

New town neuroses

Epidemiological studies do not support the idea that there is any great excess of neurotic or psychotic illness in communities such as the new towns. Those who already have personality problems or poor physical health tend to react unfavourably to the change, whereas the more stable do not.
SEE ALSO Family.

Newer group therapies

Over the last fifteen years, dissatisfaction with the control of psychotherapy by the medically qualified and with its results has led to much experimentation by other professionals, mainly psychologists and educationalists, and by persons interested in their unhappy or disturbed fellow creatures. In 1962 the Esalen Institute was founded in California to enable people to come together and examine themselves in a group setting. Gestalt therapy (increasing immediate awareness), sensory awakening, meditation and encounter techniques were used. Encounter groups had developed out of earlier work by social psychologists, and had been envisaged as a method of education – therapy for normals, education toward greater understanding of self and others and, consequently, greater sensitivity. Many individuals with personality problems, as well as psychiatric patients, have sought help by joining these groups.
Transcendental meditation (TM) is a development of natha yoga – a form of inward contemplation related to autohypnosis. Reciting a Sanskrit word and cutting out external stimuli the meditator practises for 20 minutes twice daily and attains a state of bodily and mental relaxation. The Maharishi, the founder of TM, has developed a theory which is an amalgam of Western science and of Vedic philosophy.
Primal scream therapy is based on the theory that there is a primal pool of pain and that the individual seeks to avoid experiencing the pain by a number of manœuvres. Reliving the pain in a setting of contemplation, isolation or abstinence from psychotropic substances such as alcohol and the medical and non-medical drugs, is a prerequisite to recovery from the tensions and symptoms which are seen as defences against this primal pain. Arthur Janov, who created the Primal Institute in Los Angeles, believes that it is necessary to relive painful emotional experiences in all their original intensity.
Self-help groups – such as Synanon, a residential facility created in the United States for drug addicts, may offer opportunities for a wide range of unhappy or disturbed individuals. Alcoholics Anonymous is the best known of such groups.

Niemann Pick's disease

A hereditary lipoidosis in infancy with irreparably disordered nervous system and hepatosplenomegaly.
SEE ALSO Inherited metabolic defects.

Nightmare

Nightmares are frightening dreams producing a sense of suffocation, and often waking the individual. Occurring at all ages, it is difficult to explain their occurrence. In children nightmares become a problem when recurrent, both parent and child becoming apprehensive as each night approaches. A simple sedative for both is indicated. In adults frightening life experiences may be relived in sleep and thus produce recurrent nightmares, even many years after the event. It is strange how rarely psychiatric patients complain of nightmares.

Night terrors (pavor nocturnus)

Virtually limited to children between the ages of 3 and 9 years, these experiences are reported by parents or attendants. The child's sleep becomes suddenly disturbed and with a groan, shout or scream it claims attention. The child appears to be in a state of terror, it is however inaccessible, will not be comforted and cannot be fully wakened. Finally the child relaxes back into normal sleep. The child is amnesic for the attack and for the dream content, unlike its recollection of a nightmare where the child gives an account of its frightening dream. These attacks should be considered potentially serious symptoms of emotional maladjustment or cerebral dysfunction.

Nihilistic delusions

Nihilistic delusions are most typically encountered in severe agitated depressions – so called involutional melancholia (q.v.). The patient may insist that he has no feelings, that he is dead, that the wife who visits him daily is dead, that the world does not exist, and so on. Similar delusions are encountered in severe retarded depressions and sometimes also in organic or schizophrenic illnesses. They are much less common than in the past, probably because most severe depressions are now effectively treated before such florid symptoms have time to develop.

Nocturnal enuresis

Bed-wetting at night. The significance of this common disorder in children is considered under enuresis.

Nodes of Ranvier
SEE Neurones.

Noradrenaline (norepinephrine)

Noradrenaline is the transmitter of the post-ganglionic adrenergic nerves and also probably in parts of the brain. In the periphery it stimulates mainly α receptors of the sympathetic nervous system, leading

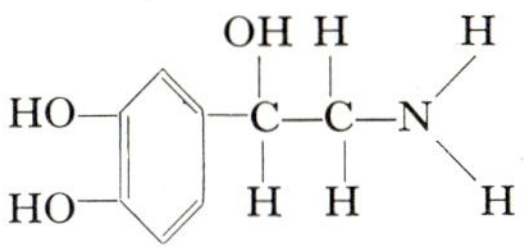

to a rise in blood pressure and increased peripheral vascular resistance. The cerebral blood flow is reduced. In the brain noradrenaline is probably concerned in mechanisms underlying mood, learning reactions and reward signalling systems. At the adrenergic synapse it is stored in 'dense-core' vesicles as a complex with ATP (adenosine triphosphate) and is released by exocytosis. Termination of its action on the receptor depends on reuptake into the pre-synaptic terminal. Drugs like cocaine, amphetamine and imipramine block this reuptake and raise effective levels of free amine at the receptors. This may explain their mood elevating effect. MAOIs (q.v.) also raise mood by raising free brain noradrenaline by blocking the main enzyme – monoamine oxidase which destroys it. Some of these compounds may also release noradrenaline from its stores or act themselves on the noradrenaline receptor. Reserpine acts by disrupting the stores for both catecholamines and serotonin leading to profound falls in the levels of brain and periphery. This may lead to clinical depression.

A second enzyme involved in noradrenaline metabolism is catechol-O-methyltransferase which O-methylates noradrenaline to produce normetadrenaline and vanyl mandelic acid (VMA).

SEE ALSO Amines, Adrenaline, Catecholamines, and Brain monoamines.

Normal curve

Otherwise known as a Poisson or Gaussian curve. It is the curve of frequency of observations which is symmetrical about the mode (which in this case is also the median and mean). It is the typical form of the scatter of measurements in a healthy population.

Nullity and voidability of marriage

In British law, the grounds for nullity of marriage are: (a) invalid ceremony, (b) non-age; (c) consanguinity; (d) bigamy;

(e) insanity at the time of the marriage; and (f) lack of consent. Five further conditions render a marriage voidable (g) impotence at the time of the marriage; (h) wilful refusal to consummate; (i) unsoundness of mind, mental disorder or epilepsy; (j) venereal disease at the time of the marriage, (k) pregnancy by a person other than the husband at the time of the marriage.
For insanity to be a ground of nullity it has to be shown that the respondent was incapable of understanding the nature of the marriage contract and the duties and responsibilities it creates.
SEE ALSO Contract, Divorce, and Marriage.

Nymphomania

Nymphomania is a rare episodic state, of intense sexual excitement in the female directed indiscriminately at any male, but sometimes at the female. In spite of the intense erotic excitement, orgasm is rarely achieved, thus leaving the patient to continue seeking further sexual partners. It can be symptomatic of the heightened excitement of a manic psychosis, acute encephalitis, or drug-induced psychosis, e.g. from amphetamine or LSD, or may be due to a neurological lesion in the temporal lobes (Klüver-Bucy syndrome (q.v.)). It may form the basis of amorous delusions relating to doctors or film stars in some schizophrenics (De Clérambault's syndrome). Nymphomania must be distinguished from hypersexuality, which is a commoner condition manifest in sexual promiscuity and prostitution.
SEE ALSO Sexual appetite and Satyriasis.

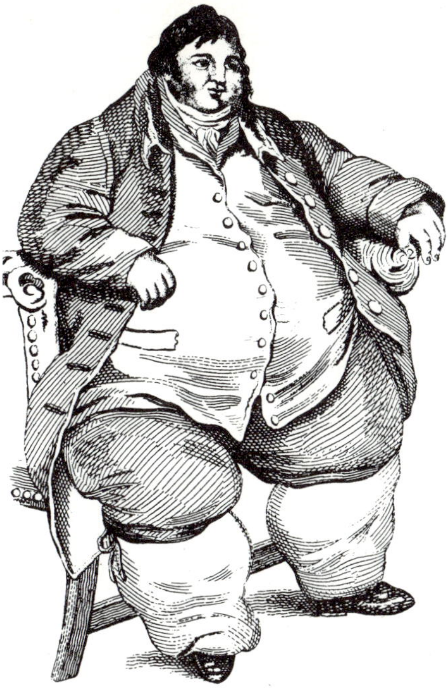

Daniel Lambert of Leicester who weighed 49 stone 12 lbs

Obesity

Obesity is a state of excessive accumulation of adipose tissue resulting from calorie intake which is greater than calorie expenditure. Multiple factors, including genetic, cultural, metabolic, and psychological, are responsible for its development. In its extreme form it tends to be familial and it has been found that monozygotic twins reared apart are closer in body weight than dizygotic twins reared together. The maternal attitude to feeding is an important aetiological influence, especially during the first year of life, and may result in a life-long pattern of overfeeding. Depression, anxiety and loneliness may be associated with a tendency to overeat and if weight gain is rapid, especially in young girls, feelings of guilt accentuate the depression. Appetite-suppressant drugs, especially amphetamines, should be avoided because of the risk of psychological dependence. In some cases psychotherapy is indicated. The long-term prognosis is not good, because there is a tendency for the condition to relapse.

Objective psyche

A term replacing Jung's earlier reference to the 'collective unconscious'. He conceived it as a reservoir or substratum of psychic phenomena existing prior to the conscious mind and functioning together with, or despite, consciousness. The two chief elements of the objective psyche are the 'archetypes' and the complexes which surround them. The archetypes are analogous to instinctual behaviour patterns observed in animal behaviour. In man they express themselves in typically human emotion and behaviour patterns shared in common with all men. The structure of complexes are archetypal – that is, they are based on 'transpersonal' and universal forms of human experience. Thus a 'mother complex' is determined not only by unique, personal experience of the individual mother, but predetermined by a universal, preformed human concept of 'the mother'. The term 'persona' (q.v.) refers to the archetypal drive towards conformity and external reality. The 'animus' (q.v.) and 'anima' (q.v.) are archetypal representations – the former in the repressed male side in the female and vice versa. The 'shadow self' (q.v.) is represented in dreams as another person of the same sex as the dreamer and personifies the dreamers repressed *personal* unconscious qualities.

Obscene telephone calls

The caller is most often a man, who chooses a particular woman as the target for his telephone calls. The content of his talk is usually of a sexual and aggressive nature, and is strangely upsetting to the recipient, who feels threatened and fearful. The calls may be made at all hours; night calls are particularly disturbing. Occasionally a schizophrenic individual may make offensive and abusive telephone calls to a doctor. In such cases the doctor would be well advised to call in the police, it is better to be safe than sorry, for the patient is usually impervious to advice or reason.

Obsessional disorders in childhood

Rituals are common and normal in middle childhood, and are shown for example by unwillingness to step on the cracks between paving stones, stereotyped bedtime habits, etc. Full blown obsessional disorders are rare. When they occur, they can frequently be seen as an attempt to control the behaviour of other members of the family. Parents are usually involved in seemingly endless rituals at meals and bedtime. When the whole of family life is disrupted, as sometimes occurs, admission to a psychiatric unit away from the family can produce a sudden surprising cessation of symptomatology. Milder obsessional disorders may pass unnoticed until late adolescence or early adult life, when they may gradually come to affect the patient's function at work.

Obsessional neurosis

An obsession is a mental experience which is accompanied by a feeling of compulsion which the patient tries to resist and to which he retains insight. Obsessional symptoms may occur in different kinds of mental and nervous illness, e.g. depression, but in an obsessional neurosis they form the kernel of the disorder and its predominant symptoms.

Obsessional neurosis is the least common of the neuroses, constituting only 5% of these disorders. The majority of patients (and relatives) have a premorbid obsessional personality characterized by excessive conscientiousness and adherence to method, order and cleanliness, almost as if the patient has to be sure that things work out correctly and dislike leaving things to chance. Obsessional symptoms come on characteristically between 18–30 years of age. Occasionally the disorder is of a transient or perhaps cyclic nature, but usually, after a sudden onset, the severity increases insidiously over a number of years. The symptoms may take several forms: phobias, ideas and images, ruminations or compulsions.

A phobia (q.v.) is an unreasonable fear associated with a situation, object or idea, e.g. fear of closed spaces, feathers or death.

The patient may be tortured by thoughts or images which intrude into her mind, for instance of a sexual or blasphemous nature. Although the patient denies that she wants to have these thoughts she recognizes that they are indeed her own thoughts and thus can be distinguished from passivity feelings in schizophrenia where the patient insists that the thoughts are not her own but have been put into her head by an external source.

In obsessional ruminations the patient is preoccupied with some topic, for instance 'how old is the world', the question continually obtruding on her mind and causing increasing distress.

Compulsions involve doing things a certain number of times, counting the letters in a word, checking that certain things have been done or not done (folie de doute) or to wash repeatedly in case dirt on her hands might contaminate and harm someone. Occasionally the compulsion might be an aggressive act, for instance an urge to kill her own child. This is often associated with a fear of knives or other dangerous objects. Such aggressive urges are rarely, if ever, carried out.

Obsessional neurosis has to be differentiated from the obsessional symptoms which occur normally, for instance when fatigued and in childhood. Obsessional symptoms in depression are common but are not the predominant symptoms, whereas they are in obsessional neurosis however severe the secondary depression becomes. Rarely the obsessional symptoms may be so bizarre as to suggest a schizophrenic illness.

Treatment should certainly involve explanation and reassurance, for instance that she has a well recognized syndrome, that she will never go mad or give in to her aggressive urges and kill her child. Such reassurance should be continued as a part of supportive psychotherapy. Behaviour therapy may be useful, either of a simple type when the patient is encouraged to omit some of the minor compulsions she carries out, or of a more formal type including reciprocal inhibition, flooding, or varieties of operant conditioning. Anxiety and tension are the main accompaniments of obsessional symptoms and if these can be allayed the patient is better able to resist the symptom. Benzodiazepines are the drugs of

first choice, MAOIs have been recommended especially in the multiple phobias. Tricyclic antidepressants may be useful for secondary depression and some authors suggest that clomipramine may be especially helpful in obsessional disorders. In long-standing patients where the tension and anxiety is marked psychosurgery may be indicated when two-thirds of patients can be expected to have a worthwhile improvement.
SEE ALSO Psychoneuroses, Obsession, Obsessional states.

Obsessional states

Such states, in which an unwanted, but repetitive thought, image, idea, impulse or doubt intrudes imperatively into consciousness, may occur in otherwise normal persons at times of particular stress; or may be associated with physical or psychological illness such as encephalitis, schizophrenia or depression.
Otherwise normal persons who experience such symptoms under stress may have shown a previously obsessional (anankastic) disposition. Such persons tend to be bound by habit, rigid and punctual, worriers over detail, meticulous and conscientious. They may be described as perfectionists by their acquaintances. Emotionally they tend to be controlled and inhibited: indecisiveness in action may be taken as obstinacy or stubbornness. They tend to resist change and to be plagued by feelings of inadequacy and self-doubt.
Such traits occur in many normal persons and, far from leading to an interference with living, are quite consistent with excellent routine work. Such people are dependable, scrupulous and have high ethical values. However, by their nature, their life styles are limited and not expansive, and their social contacts are restricted and conventionalized. Obsessional states occurring secondary to depressive illness may remit as the depression improves, but the obsessionality in persons who have become depressed secondary to obsessional states is less likely to be readily resolved by anti-depressant treatment. Obsessional states occurring in the course of a schizophrenic illness are said to indicate a relatively good outlook with regard to resistance to schizophrenic deterioration.
SEE ALSO Obsessions.

Obsessions

These are contents of consciousness which are associated with a subjective feeling of compulsion together with a desire to resist. They may tend to be recurrent and pathological in that they may substantially interfere with adequate performance and mental activity; or brief and occasional as may occur in normal subjects. Obsessions may take the form of recurrent ideas or images which cannot easily be voluntarily dispelled, or impulses to perform some compulsive act. Recurrent doubtings, ruminations and preoccupations may also occur. Repetitive compulsive acts may take the form of rituals, but strictly speaking a ritual is not, in itself, necessarily accompanied by the desire to resist – which is a hall-mark of the obession. Obessions and compulsions are, however, usually seen in the same person and it is often difficult to decide into which category a particular act fits, i.e. whether there is a desire to resist.
Such phenomena occur particularly in those of obsessional (anakastic) personality in whom traits of orderliness, control, inflexibility and procrastination are marked.

Obsessive compulsive reaction
SEE Obsessional neurosis.

Occupational therapy

Until recently, this has mainly taken the form of handicrafts, such as basket-making, weaving, pottery or toy-making, and such activities have been prominent in the training of occupational therapists.
Occupational therapy is now much more directed towards active rehabilitation, rather than diversion. Shopping, cooking and housecraft are taught to female patients, who are encouraged to make the most of their experience and existing knowledge. For men, the emphasis is on industrial therapy (q.v.), in a realistic work setting, with payment for the results achieved. This has developed mostly out-

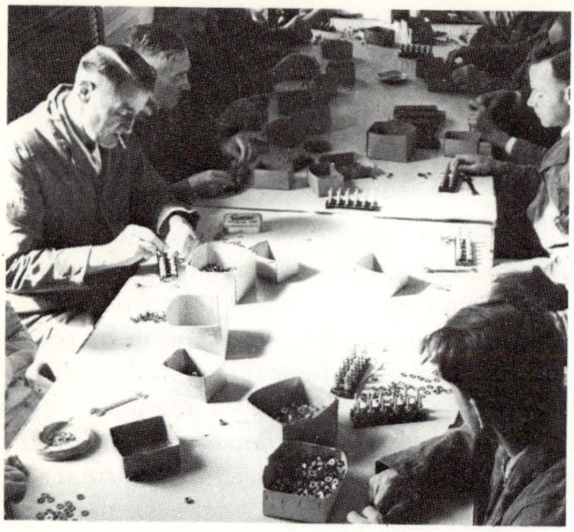

side the professional sphere of occupational therapists, with supervision by psychiatric nurses or specially recruited personnel who have industrial or craft experience. Some psychiatric nurses have accompanied groups of patients into open industry. Although occupational therapy developed mainly in hospitals for the mentally ill and subnormal, it is now active in general hospital psychiatric units, in day hospitals and centres and in services for geriatric and physically disabled patients.

Oculo-cerebro-renal syndrome (Lowe's syndrome)

The oculo-cerebro-renal syndrome is probably transmitted as a sex-linked character. It comprises mental retardation and defects involving the eyes (congenital cataracts and buphthalmos), the kidneys (progressive renal tubular defects) and the central nervous system. The presumed genetical carriers are apparently clinically normal, though in some, renal tubular aminoaciduria has been demonstrated and in others lens opacities have been seen on slit lamp examination.

Oedipus complex

Oedipus, 'The Lame One', who had been abandoned by his parents, in his wanderings came to Thebes at a time when the Theban sphinx – part woman, part bird and part lion – was devastating the city by demanding of each passer-by the answer to the riddle she had learnt from the Muses. Unable to give the answer, one by one the Thebans were carried off and devoured by the sphinx. Oedipus solved the riddle, the sphinx killed herself and Oedipus entered Thebes, killed the King and married the Queen, Jocasta; he himself becoming King of Thebes, not knowing that they were his own parents. His punishment was blinding, madness, and death. This myth became the cornerstone of Freud's theory – the Oedipus complex. The boy's incestuous wishes toward his mother, his hostility to, and envy of, his father and the consequent castration anxiety are phases of normal

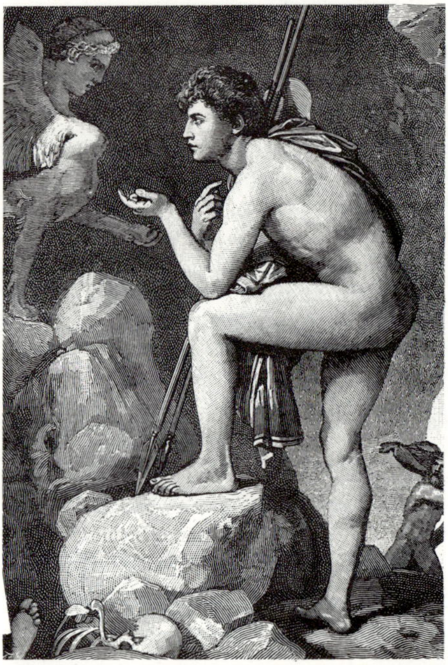

Oedipus and the Sphinx

development. They may be resolved in a variety of ways but failing resolution may give rise to many problems of later adult sexual activity.
SEE ALSO Alloerotic.

Oligodendrocytes

SEE Neuroglia.

Oligophrenia

Defective mental development – synonymous with mental retardation (q.v.).

Oneiroid

Dreamlike. Particularly in those psychotic states where contact with the real environment is lost. In the schizophrenias (q.v.), the immediate surroundings, although they may be misinterpreted and imbued with delusional significance, are recognized and usually accepted. In psychoses of the oneiroid type the patient seems entirely distracted from reality and lives in a dream world of fantastic content. The quality of this experience was captured by Salvador Dali in his dream sequence of the film *Spellbound.*
The experiences are not unlike the paramnesias (q.v.), but in oneiroid states the experiences are extended over weeks rather than seconds or minutes. Catatonic and hebephrenic schizophrenias may show oneiroid phenomena at their onset.

Open door

The change from custodial care, with patients living in closed wards in security conditions, began in the first half of the nineteenth century. It reached its climax about thirty years ago and wards became more or less identical in their security conditions to these in the general hospital. Changes in attitudes to mental illness have been both a cause and a result of the open door policy.

Operant conditioning

Operant conditioning is the learning process which results from the selective reinforcement (rewarding) of certain emitted responses or operants. This reinforcement increases the probability of the same response occurring on subsequent exposure to the same stimulus situation. Conversely, negative reinforcement (punishment) reduces the probability of repetition of the response.
SEE ALSO Conditioned reflex and Conditioned response.

Operant conditioning therapies

Behaviour therapies based upon the operant conditioning theories of B. F. Skinner, in which behaviour is regarded as modifiable by positive and negative reinforcement. Individual treatment programmes are based upon the observable symptoms which require modification and the identity of the reinforcers which may affect them. In general, positive reinforcement is given when desired responses occur and withheld when undesired behaviour is performed. One useful variant is the 'token economy', in which patients on a ward earn tokens by prescribed desirable behaviour, the tokens being used, later if preferred, to 'buy' rewarding activites such as time off the ward and talking to other patients. Shaping (q.v.) is another type of operant therapy.

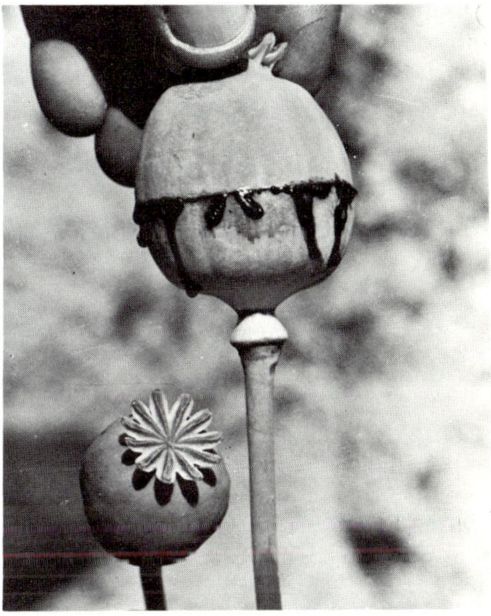

Opium obtained from poppies

Opium alkaloids

Preparations of opium alkaloids obtained from the poppy Papaver somniferum have been used and abused since antiquity. Full accounts of the properties of these compounds may be found in general pharmacological texts. This group of compounds includes a number of natural opium constituents of which morphine is the most important, and also a number of semisynthetic derivatives (see table). The group is therapeutically heterogeneous, and includes powerful and mild analgesics, anti-tussives, anti-diarrhoeal agents, and an emetic.

Examples of natural and semisynthetic opium alkaloids

Natural opium alkaloids	
Phenanthrene	Morphine Codeine Thebaine
Benzylisoquinoline	Papaverine Noscapine
Semisynthetic alkaloids	Diacetylmorphine (heroin) Apomorphine Hydromorphine Oxymorphone Hydrocodone Oxycodone

The powerful analgesics also combine euphoriant activity with readily developing drug tolerance which result in a high liability to drug dependence. Psychiatric interest in these compounds centres on their proclivity to produce drug dependence (q.v.), and on the treatment of such states.
Apomorphine has found a small place in aversion therapy (q.v.), of alcoholism (q.v.), a treatment in which apomorphine-induced vomiting coincides with taking an alcoholic drink.

Oral contraceptives

The Pill has complex effects on psychological state and sexual behaviour. The psychological effects are usually beneficial, since it is such an efficient contraceptive. However, the side effects are well known and suggestible women are more likely to complain of them. The occasional harmful effects are equally well-known and this knowledge sometimes provokes great anxiety.
The Pill often relieves pre-menstrual tension (q.v.) and depression. Yet it makes some women irritable and in 5–7% it causes depression, which is often at its worst pre-menstrually. Depression may become severe and should always be taken seriously. It seems more likely to occur with strongly progestogenic pills and in women with a previous history of pre-menstrual depression or depressive illness. For such women the Pill must be prescribed with caution. But depression can occur in women of previously stable personality.
Usually the Pill benefits sexual life by removing fear of pregnancy. In a small proportion of women, however, it decreases libido and capacity for orgasm. This may be a direct chemical effect since the same effect occurs in experimental animals. But suggestion may sometimes be important, since this side effect is very widely known.

Organic brain syndrome

SEE Organic syndromes.

Organic disease producing mental disorders

General medical disorders
Depression frequently follows influenza, and other virus infections and must be recognized for what it is, rather than attributing it to a lessening continuance of the illness itself. Similar effects may follow any debilitating illness. The significance of other disorders will depend on the patient's circumstances in life and his previous personality. Thus, a relatively minor osteo-arthritis of the hip may render a postman incapable of coping with life and precipitate psychiatric symptoms. Similarly, a patient may be particularly susceptible, psychologically, to physical disorders, either of a general or specific type. This may be due to a hypochondriacal personality, to a specific traumatic medical experience, or particularly in old age, to the increase in social isolation to which physical disability so often leads.

Surgical operations and childbirth
Major psychiatric illnesses are a not uncommon complication of both surgical operations and childbirth, the breakdown tending to come on several days post-operative or post-partum the average being ten to fourteen days. The psychiatric breakdown seems to be unassociated with the type of anaesthetic, sepsis, or other complications, but there is evidence that the incidence can be reduced by measures taken to allay the patient's anxiety about his operation or by proper antenatal preparation. Operations on elderly patients such as for arterial disease or cataract, are likely to cause post-operative mental confusion or paranoid psychoses.

Organic disorders of the central nervous system
Disorders such as dementia, space-occupying lesions, and vitamin deficiency (e.g. vitamin B_{12}) usually present as a typical 'organic' mental state. However, the patient may present with 'functional' symptoms, brought about indirectly by the organic disorder. A brain tumour, by detracting from a patient's efficiency and ability to cope with his work may lead to the formation of neurotic symptoms. Thus a previously stable patient who presents in middle or late age with hysterical or other neurotic symptoms should not be dismissed as an hysteric. Rather, a reason should be sought for the appearance of an hysterical symptom in a previously stable personality.

Organic syndromes

The commonest signs of organic brain reactions are: impairment of memory, disorientation and loss of intellectual ability in the adult, and arrested intellectual development in the infant and child. Special attributes may be specifically impaired by local damage resulting, for example, in loss of speech, spatial ability, etc. The general causes of organic brain reactions are:
1. Trauma – resulting in concussion, laceration, subdural haematoma.
2. Infection (bacterial or viral) – resulting in cerebral abscess, meningitis, general paralysis, encephalitis.
3. Arterial disease – resulting in arteriosclerotic dementia.
4. Degeneration – senile dementia, Alzheimer's disease, Pick's disease.
5. Intoxication – from alcohol, chemical compounds, including gases and drugs, or systemic extracranial infection, e.g. pneumonia.
6. Metabolic – such as liver failure, uraemia alkalosis, acidosis.
7. Hormonal – such as myxoedema, thyrotoxicosis, Cushing's disease, insulinoma.
8. Deficiency disease – Pellagra, vitamin B_{12} deficiency, or anaemia.
9. Anoxia – from anaemia, respiratory or cardiovascular causes, drowning or gassing.
10. Neoplasm – e.g. glioma, meningioma.
11. Congenital and inherited conditions – resulting in foetal damage or birth injury. The former may be due to maternal viral infection during the first trimester. Inherited conditions include the inheritance of metabolic defect, e.g. phenylketonuria and degenerations, e.g. Huntington's chorea.
12. Other causes: collagen diseases, diseases of unknown aetiology, e.g. disseminated sclerosis, idiopathic epilepsy.
For detailed accounts see Individual disorders.

Orgasm

Orgasm is the mental experience accompanying the sexual climax. Four stages are recognizable in its development. During the excitatory phase there is rise in blood pressure, pulse, muscular tension, vasocongestion of pelvic tissues and vaginal lubrication in the female. A plateau phase then occurs until the third phase of orgasmic inevitability is reached when there is rhythmic contraction of the pelvic organs in the female and congestion of the outer third of the vaginal barrel whilst in the male waves of muscular contraction in perineal muscles lead to emission and ejaculation. The resolution phase with decongestion is slow and in about 10% can be followed by repetitive orgasms. There is no evidence of any difference in the quality of the female orgasm produced by clitoral, vaginal or breast stimulation. A constitutional inability to experience orgasm occurs in 1–2% of females (sexual anhedonia) whilst in the male inability to ejaculate and experience orgasm (impotentia ejaculandi (q.v.)) may be due to constitutional factor, drugs, or to repressed, hostile feelings for sexual intercourse. More commonly inability to achieve orgasm is due to inadequate levels of sexual arousal due to lack of sexual attraction for the partner or the underlying conflicts of latent homosexuality. The rare paradoxical association of inability to obtain orgasm in a state of acute sexual excitement occurs in nymphomania (q.v.).
SEE ALSO Sexual drive.

Orientation

Self-awareness in time, in place and in person. Personal orientation, name, age, job, status, is rarely lost though may be

forgotten completely in dementia or briefly after cerebral injury and it may never fully be learned by the severely subnormal. Orientation in time, year, month, time of day is more often disrupted in delirium and in amnesic syndromes. The elderly become confused about place, especially when severely ill and moved to hospital or to relatives. Orientation of time and place may fluctuate or be unstable due to confabulation (q.v.). Left/right disorientation, a difficulty in establishing which side of the body is being pointed to or touched accompanies some cerebral lesions. Loss of orientation suggests organic rather than functional disorder.
Schizophrenics need to establish a double orientation, one in the real and one in the delusional world. Mere delusion is not disorientation.

Orthomolecular psychiatry

Orthomolecular psychiatry, according to Linus Pauling, is the 'achievement and preservation of mental health by varying the concentration in the human body of substances that are normally present, such as vitamins'. In schizophrenia this involves the use of vitamins (megavitamin therapy) and minerals, the control of diet, especially the intake of sucrose and, during the initial acute phase, the use of conventional treatments such as phenothiazine drugs.
It is certain that vitamin deficiency can cause mental symptoms and that some, rare, patients may need a very high intake of certain vitamins to maintain health. There is no evidence to suggest that schizophrenics fall into these groups. However, megavitamin therapy might act in a different way and it has been suggested by Osmond and Hoffer that nicotinamide might be beneficial as a methyl group acceptor and thus prevent the formation of psychotogenic methylated compounds. After initial encouraging reports this suggestion has not been confirmed.
Regardless of the theoretical basis for the theory there is no good evidence, for instance double blind studies, to suggest that orthomolecular treatment of schizophrenia is beneficial.

Orthopsychiatry

An approach to the study and treatment of human behaviour where the emphasis is on prevention of morbidity and the promotion of healthy emotional development especially in children and adolescents.

Overactivity

Increased activity may have psychiatric significance in a number of contexts. A fairly sudden onset accompanied by optimism, expansiveness, impulsiveness and a decreased need for sleep is typical of manic illnesses. Patients with dementing processes, particularly Alzheimer's disease (q.v.), sometimes show a characteristic purposeless overactivity (q.v.) – packing and unpacking a suitcase, or repeatedly polishing the same piece of furniture – but usually their impairment of memory and increasing incompetence are equally obvious. There is, of course, an element of aimless overactivity in agitation (q.v.), but it is clearly secondary to the patient's feelings of tension and apprehension.
SEE ALO Motor disturbances, Akathisia, Hyperkinesis.

Overdetermination

Individual or neurotic symptoms, as well as dream events, are believed by psychoanalysts to have many determining causes. Thus one particular symbol in a dream (q.v.) may represent a number of determinate problems, conflicts or events, and is thus overdetermined.

Overinclusion

Overinclusive thinking is one aspect of thought disorder in acute schizophrenia. There is an inability to preserve conceptual boundaries, so that ideas only distantly related to a particular concept become included in that concept. The 'woolliness' of schizophrenic thought is a result of this type of thought disorder.

Overprotection

The 'overprotected child' is allowed to do little for himself, is treated in a manner suitable for a younger age, and is exposed to an excess of physical contact with his mother. This pattern of childhood upbringing arises in a variety of ways. The mother may be overreacting to her own guilt about not wanting the child; a habit of overprotection may have been kept up from a time when the child was unduly fragile or physically ill; the mother who had a deprived childhood herself may identify herself with her child and overcompensate for her own deprivation. Such behaviour frequently leads to delay in maturation and emancipation on the child's part (e.g. school phobia (q.v.)), protracted dependence on the mother and 'spoiled child' behaviour.

Oxycephaly
SEE Acrocephaly.

Pachygyria

A developmental defect possibly of genetic origin in which only a few large convolutions are present on the cerebral cortex. There is a severe mental defect in such patients.

Paedophilia

Paedophilia is the abnormal sexual attraction, usually in the male, for children of the same or opposite sex. It may manifest itself in attempts to induce the child to look at or masturbate the male penis, to touch the female's genitals or in more severe cases to attempts at actual intercourse per vaginam or per anum. The child is seldom a total stranger to the offender. In the psychopathic or brain-damaged male frustration of sexual arousal may lead to overwhelming aggression with physical assault upon the child and may culminate in murder. The condition commonly begins in adolescence as an expression of frustrated childhood desires to be loved by a parent. It is intensified by accompanying personality disorder which then prevents normal sexual contacts. Late onset paedophilia may be symptomatic of progressive organic cerebral disease such as cerebral arteriosclerosis. Homosexual paedophilia has a high rate of recidivism (up to 28%). In heterosexual paedophilia the risk of repetition is only up to 13%.
SEE ALSO Sexual offences.

Pain
SEE Gate theory of pain.

Pain asymbolia

The patient, though perceiving pain, shows an abnormal lack of emotional response to it. This is due to lesions in the left parietal lobe.

Palilalia

The repetition of words or short phrases with increasing speed and diminishing audibility, palilalia is most frequently observed in post-encephalitic Parkinsonism but also occurs in cases of Pick's disease.

Panic attack

This refers to the occurrence of acute, overwhelming dread. The panic attack is distinguished from the anxiety state by the accompanying explosion of autonomic activity with dizziness, palpitations, pallor, sweating, tremulousness, urge to vomit, micturate or defaecate. The onset is usually fairly abrupt and the attacks are usually self-limiting, although they may last from a few minutes to some hours. During this period controlled mentation is impossible and the subject may rush around aimlessly. Depersonalization and derealization are likely to occur. The attack leaves the patient feeling weak and exhausted. Panic may be quickly controlled by the intravenous injection of a short-acting barbiturate, usually administered in sub-hypnotic doses, e.g. methohexitone or thiopentone sodium. Oral administration of sodium amylobarbitone or quinalbarbitone may be given at the same time to prolong the effect after the shorter action has worn off, but these medications should only be used in an emergency and not continued thereafter. Investigation of the cause should proceed before further treatment is initiated.
SEE ALSO Psychiatric emergencies and Kempf's syndrome.

Paradoxical sleep

The stage of sleep in which rapid eye movements (REM) occur with loss of muscle tone and sometimes twitching of the limbs. During this phase subjects can only be woken with difficulty. Paradoxical sleep in the human adult is cyclical and makes up 20–25% of the normal night. This is the period of sleep during which dreaming occurs and it forms an essential component of the sleep process. Sleep deprivation leads to an increase in the percentage of paradoxical sleep during the recovery phase and this proportion is also changed by hypnotics and stimulants.

Paraesthesiae

Abnormal sensations, e.g. burning sensations, tingling, numbness, 'pins and needles', usually maximal in the limb extremities and attributable to dysfunction of the peripheral nerves or the central nervous system. In pellagra the patient complains of bilateral burning sensations affecting the extremities, the mouth, tongue and epigastrium. Hysterical paraesthesiae are usually described as numbness or tingling; respiratory alkalosis resulting from overbreathing may provide an intermediate mechanism. Tactile hallucinations have been reported as a hypnagogic phenomenon (q.v.).

Paramnesia

Paramnesia, or falsification of memory, occurs most characteristically in the dysmnesic (disordered memory) syndrome. Here gaps in the subjects recall may be filled by a fabricated account of previous events (confabulation (q.v.)).
A deluded subject may falsify memories to conform with the sense of his delusions, e.g. a belief in royal status may produce the memory of a coronation.
'Déjà vu' (q.v.) refers to the feeling of having previously undergone a contemporary experience, or a feeling of familiarity with surroundings, which have not been known previously.

Paranoid reactions

Paranoid reactions are the exaggerated response to disappointing or humiliating circumstances displayed by certain sensitive individuals and by many otherwise normal people in special circumstances. The mechanism of projection (q.v.) is operative here; they are displayed normally where individuals feel mistakenly that they are the centre of attention, being talked about, or that some embarrassing private matter is being referred to. Such a reaction is readily understandable by the subject and easily dispelled. It becomes morbid where it persists and carries conviction. Abnormal personality (shyness, inferiority feeling, excessive self-esteem), special disabilities (deafness, sexual deviation, disfigurements) and special circumstances (imprisonment, national alienation) form the soil in which this growth proliferates. In so far as the reaction can be understood in the light of the circumstances and personality of the subject, it is differentiated from psychosis. Acute forms may occur in response to massive or accumulated stress. The prognosis for these reactions is good as they usually respond to removal of the precipitating causes; their liability to recur in many cases is obvious, however.

Paranoid schizophrenia

Paranoid is the most clearly differentiated of the subtypes of schizophrenia (q.v.) and the least variable in character. Its onset is usually insidious and occurs often after the age of 30. It is characterized by the development of clearly formulated, persistent delusions, mostly of a persecutory content. The delusions are often widespread but interconnected. Sometimes, however, 'encapsulated', single delusions occur which seem not to affect the rest of the subject's ideation. Grandiose delusions often occur which interconnect with the persecutory feelings, through a feeling that the subject's status is ignored or envied with resultant slights or animosity. Hallucinations may occur which share and expand the content of the delusions. Both emotion and behaviour may be affected by the delusions showing depression, anger, resentment, resignation or apathy. Serious antisocial acts are infrequently the result of acting on the delusional beliefs, more often these acts are merely a nuisance (complaining to the police, writing to royalty, ministers and other prominent persons) or the subject appears eccentric. Remissions occur but in at least half of the cases delusional belief, oddity of behaviour or social disability remains. Prognosis and treatment are similar to those of other forms of schizophrenia.

Paranoid states

Kraepelin (q.v.) (1856–1926, the father of modern psychiatric nosology) described paranoia as the development of systematized permanent, mainly persecutory, delusions (q.v.) in a setting of otherwise un-

disturbed thought and consciousness.
The term 'paranoid states' embraces those conditions in which the paranoia symptom complex occurs; characteristically paranoia, paraphrenia and paranoid schizophrenia (q.v.). In all of them suspicion and resentment arise from the conviction that the environment is changed; innocent matters are taken as a direct attack on the patient who believes he is not estimated at his true value. Associated with this last sentiment are grandiose delusions.
Thus 'paranoid states' covers the broad range of disorders from paranoid schizophrenia (q.v.) in which thought and personality are poorly preserved, through paraphrenia with hallucinations but minimal personality deterioration, to the suspicions of a paranoid personality.
Freud (q.v.) suggested that paranoia originated in the subject's attempt at adjustment to incestuous homosexual desires. As a result, homosexuality has uncritically appeared in psychiatric mythology as a cause of paranoia, a view not upheld by clinical evidence as a comprehensive explanation.
Paranoid schizophrenia (q.v.) has a later onset than other types of schizophrenia (q.v.) and is usually insidious. It is possible that it owes its distinctive features to this; that the more mature and stable personality is less disintegrated assimilating the alien experiences of the schizophrenic process.

Paraphrenia

Schizophrenia arising for the first time after the age of 60 years. The majority of patients have a more or less organized delusional system, usually with hallucinations, and in a setting of a well preserved personality and intellect.

Pareidolia

An illusion in which visual images are given a fantastic interpretation.

Paresis

Weakness of muscles of organic origin or an incomplete paralysis. The term is sometimes used as an abbreviation for general paralysis of the insane (q.v.).

Parietal lobe syndrome

The mental symptoms secondary to damage to the parietal lobes, e.g. from cerebrovascular disease, neoplasm, and as a part of Alzheimer's presenile dementia. The characteristic feature is an inability of the patient to comprehend and make use of sensory perceptions. Often the most striking feature is an impairment of spatial relationships. The relatives state that the patient easily gets lost, even in his own house. This defect can be demonstrated in his inability to construct designs (constructional apraxia). Dressing apraxia is usually due to a lesion of the right parietal lobe. Tactile agnosia (astereognosis) is associated with lesions in the post-central convolution and visual agnosia with lesions in the occipito-parietal region. Disturbances of body image (supramarginal gyrus) and even an unawareness of the opposite side of the body (autotopagnosia) may occur. Comprehension and expression of speech may be disturbed and in lesions of the angular gyrus a combination of finger agnosia, acalculia, agraphia and right-left disorientation may be present (Gershmann's syndrome).

Parkinsonism

In 1817 James Parkinson described in a masterly fashion the disease that was later given his eponym. This consists clinically of the classical triad of akinesia, tremor and rigidity together with other features such as festinant gait, drooling of saliva and sometimes oculogyric crises.
It was subsequently shown that there are several different causes for the disorder and the current tendency is therefore to refer to the group as Parkinson's syndrome or Parkinsonism or, less appropriately, the extrapyramidal syndrome (q.v.).
Although there are many causes for the disease the constant physiological abnormality is an imbalance in the cholinergic and dopaminergic antagonistic components of the basal ganglia (q.v.). In the

classical form of the disease this is due to degeneration of the dopaminergic nigro-striatal path with predominance of the cholinergic pathway. Improvement can be effected for several years in about 60% of such patients by the administration of levodopa, preferably with a peripherally acting decarboxylase inhibitor. This enables high concentrations of levodopa to cross the blood brain barrier to be subsequently converted into dopamine within the corpus striatum. The alternative though usually less effective therapy, is to block the cholinergic activity with a centrally acting anticholinergic, e.g. orphenadrine.
Parkinsonism is also seen as a troublesome side effect with reserpine (q.v.) and related compounds, with the phenothiazines (q.v.) and with the butyrophenones (q.v.). Many physicians believe that the administration of any of these groups at a dosage level which produces a consistent antipsychotic effect is almost certain to produce some clinical signs of Parkinsonism. Even if this is not quite true the difference in the two levels is small. This iatrogenic disorder appears to be due to dopamine depletion but it does not respond to levodopa administration and should be kept under control with an anticholinergic drug if the causative drug cannot be withdrawn due to relapse in the psychosis.

Partial monosomy 5 disease
SEE Cri-du-chat syndrome.

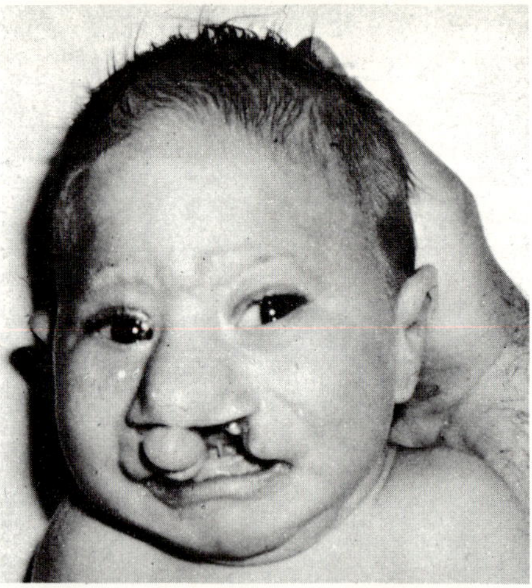

Patau's syndrome (Trisomy D)

The syndrome associated with trisomy of an autosomal chromosome in the D group (see Denver system) comprises severe mental retardation and gross physical malformations: death in early infancy is to be expected. The multiple physical defects involve the face, head, hands, feet, heart and abdominal viscera. Specific defects in the central nervous system include absent olfactory tracts and trigones and a fusion of the frontal lobes. As in mongolism and other autosomal syndromes the appearance of the signs is very variable, and any combination may be seen in an individual case.

Pathological lying (pseudologia phantastica)

Lying is either (a) normal or (b) pathological. Normal lying (also called defensive lying) occurs in everyone from time to time when under attack or stress, and is a mechanism for avoiding painful consequences. Pathological lying (pseudologia phantastica) occurs without obvious stress and usually in patients with psychopathic disorders (q.v.). Fantastic stories are told usually of a boastful or grandiose nature without being as incorrigible and egocentric as delusions (q.v.); sometimes both storyteller and listener can be aware of their fantastic nature and aware of the other's awareness. They occur quite frequently as a substitute for a harsh repressive reality (e.g. in recidivists (q.v.)).

The condition has to be differentiated from Korsakoff's syndrome (q.v.) where memory loss for recent events is coupled with confabulation.
SEE ALSO Hysterical pseudo-dementia.

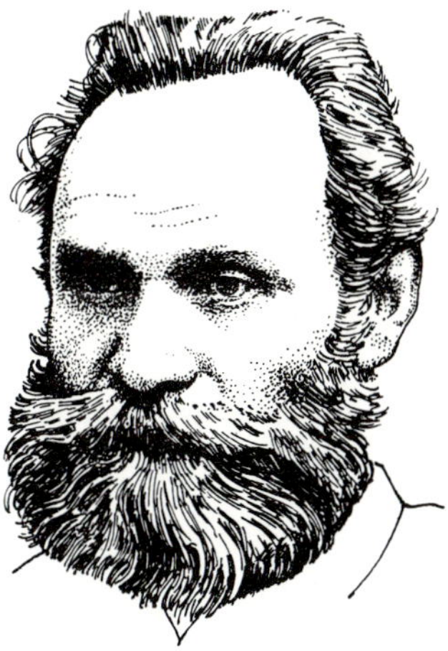

Pavlov, Ivan Petrovich (1849–1936)

The son of a poor priest, Pavlov had to struggle against poverty to complete his medical training. In 1890 he was appointed Professor of Pharmacology at the Military Medical Academy in St Petersburg, and five years later became Professor of Physiology. His *Work of the Digestive Glands* (1897) led to the Nobel Prize. His decisive methodological advance was in the use of the chronic as opposed to the acute experiment. His great surgical skill enabled him to create fistulas in the stomachs, salivary and pancreatic glands of dogs and thus to study the function of these organs in otherwise healthy animals. He studied, by objective physiological techniques, the behaviour of his animals, and discovered the conditioned reflex (q.v.).
Pavlov, late in life, became interested in psychiatric illness and applied his theoretical construct of nervous activity to the understanding of mental disorder. He believed that inhibitory processes in cortical and subcortical areas, normally protected neural structures, but when excessive could be pathological. Harassed in his early formative years by the Czarist authorities, he was generously treated by the Soviet Government. The discovery of the conditioned reflex has been important in the development of psychology, particularly in the field of learning.
SEE ALSO Behaviour therapy and Learning.

Pavor nocturnus
SEE Night terrors.

Pellagra

Pellagra, from the Italian 'pelle agra' or rough skin, is a nutritional disease which in underdeveloped areas is associated with the intake of white maize and in richer countries is usually secondary to alcoholism. Deficiency of nicotinamide, its precursor tryptophan, and other vitamins of the B-complex, or malabsorption result in a triad of skin (a persistent erythema, later scaly brown pigmentation), alimentary (bright red glossitis and diarrhoea) and neuro-psychiatric lesions. The neurological lesions resemble those of subacute combined degeneration (q.v.). The psychiatric state is in the earlier stages a neurasthenic syndrome, but later delirium and persistent organic confusional and confabulatory states are seen.
SEE ALSO Vitamins and Brain syndromes.

Penis envy

Penis envy has a central role in the Freudian theory of female sexuality. On realizing that she lacks a penis, the little girl turns away from her mother in anger and resentment, towards her father. He will give her a penis in the form of a child – an addition to her body. Thus the female Oedipal complex (Electra complex) comes into being. Penis envy underlies many neurotic and personality problems – for instance in lesbianism, masochism, and the girl's masculine strivings and identifications. It is, however, only one aspect of the powerful role in human development played by the twin emotions of envy and jealousy – emotions connected with every stage of growth.

Peptic ulcer

Emotional factors such as sustained anxiety or frustration can lead to increased hydrochloric acid secretion and susceptibility to peptic ulceration. The general management is facilitated by a good doctor-patient relationship, the reduction of stress, rest in bed if necessary, sedation as required and the avoidance of emotional conflicts.
SEE ALSO Psychosomatic disorders.

Perception

The process of recognizing or knowing objects or events from stimuli impinging upon and exciting the sense receptors. Sensation refers to the elementary subjective qualities of sensory experience, perception is concerned with the meaningful interpretation of this sensory information in terms of an objective external environment or, via the interoceptors, of the perceiving individual's own physical self. The latter type of perception leads to the development of a stable body-image (q.v.). Certain aspects of perceptual functioning have an innate basis but learning (q.v.) is also important. Perception can be surprisingly accurate as demonstrated in the perceptual constancies, the stability of external objects in respect of size, shape, colour, etc., despite variations in the viewing conditions. Sometimes, however, perceptions may be distortions of reality, either from the patterning of stimulation as in the illusions (q.v.), or from the needs, motives, attitudes and mood of the observer. Perceptual defence (q.v.) is a term descriptive of a tendency to fail to perceive stimuli of an anxiety-provoking nature. More severe distortions of perception occur in many psychiatric conditions. These may be 'functional' in nature or have an organic basis. Hallucinations (q.v.) perceptual experiences in the absence of appropriate stimulation, represent the extreme of perceptual distortion.
SEE ALSO Apperception, Brain-damaged child, Gestalt, Hypochondriasis, and Perceptual deprivation.

Perceptual deprivation

A condition in which the patterning (and, therefore, information content) of sensory stimulation is drastically reduced. Often confused with sensory deprivation (q.v.), a reduction in the level of sensory input. The wearing of dark glasses is a form of sensory deprivation, translucent glasses impose visual perceptual deprivation. Prolonged exposure to either condition has adverse emotional effects, impairs cognition (q.v.), and may produce a confused state in which hallucinations (q.v.) may occur. It has been suggested that analogous effects underlie certain psychotic phenomena. There is also evidence that lack of varied perceptual stimulation in infancy adversely affects intellectual development.
SEE ALSO Perception.

Periodic catatonia
SEE Catatonia.

Pernicious anaemia
(Synonym: Addison's anaemia)

Even minor changes in the blood picture may be associated with significant nervous and mental symptoms in pernicious anaemia due to malabsorption of cobalamin (q.v.) (vitamin B_{12}). Paradoxically also, while folic acid may improve the anaemia it may precipitate signs in the central nervous system. Degeneration of the spinal cord and peripheral nerves gives the clinical picture known as subacute combined degeneration. Mental changes of depression or of a paranoid or neurasthenic type are often encountered, and an organic picture with confusion may be seen.
SEE ALSO Anaemia and Cobalamin.

Persecutory states in the elderly

These may be idiopathic or associated with affective disorder or organic disease.
1. *Symptomatic paranoid states*, often with hallucinosis, are common in acute confusional states (q.v.). The patient is usually suffering from an acute physical illness or recovering from an operation. Nursing procedures may be misinterpreted with accusations of poisoning and maltreatment; food and drugs may be refused, and

behaviour be resistant or frankly hostile. The degree of clouding of consciousness is variable but perplexity is often marked. Every effort should be made after removal of an old person to hospital to keep him in touch with his environment, to allay his fears and to promote confidence in his attendants. Phenothiazine drugs (e.g. chlorpromazine 50–100 mg. orally or intramuscularly followed by 50 mg. t.d.s. orally) are generally very effective once the psychosis has developed. ECT may bring to an end delusional states which persist after the confusion has cleared.
Persecutory ideas, of simple, transient kind, but sometimes persistent and more organized, may also arise during the course of dementing illnesses. Defects of hearing or vision may contribute. In affective disorders delusions of wickedness and punishment secondary to the change in mood are quite common in old people, and require treatment in hospital, usually with ECT.
2. Persistent delusions of paranoid type (usually persecutory, but sometimes erotic, hypochondriacal or grandiose) occurring in clear consciousness are characteristic of late paraphrenia (a late form of schizophrenia). Hallucinations of hearing are conspicuous, and of taste and smell common. The mood which may be fearful, depressed or indignant at first, later becomes shallow, incongruous and euphoric. The personality tends to remain well preserved, but insight is totally lacking and the patient may call for police protection, abuse or assault her neighbours, barricade herself in her room or commit suicide. Physical health, memory and intellect are good but hearing defects are rather frequent. Women predominate. The premorbid personality is often eccentric, and there may be a family history of schizophrenia.
Adequate and indefinitely prolonged medication with phenothiazine drugs is essential to control the psychotic features. Dosage should be as low as possible (e.g. trifluoperazine 2–5 mg. t.d.s.) and anti-Parkinsonian drugs given if necessary (orphenadrine 50–100 mg. t.d.s.). The long-acting preparation, fluphenazine decanoate, 12·5 mg. intramuscularly every two to three weeks, is suitable for robust but not for frail patients. Failure to persist usually leads to relapse. A relative or social worker should be involved, and attendance at a day hospital permits socialization and effective supervision.

Perseveration

Perseveration is the involuntary persistence of a word or phrase and its obtrusion into subsequent responses. It may be demonstrated by presenting a series of objects for naming or may be observed in the patient's spontaneous speech. It is a type of aphasic disturbance, and is found in organic cerebral reactions and dementias.

Persona

A term from Jungian psychology implying the personality mask or façade which is presented to the outside world.

Personality

The unique, dynamic and integrated organization of relatively stable and predictable qualities of behaviour (q.v.), expression and thought which are characteristic of an individual and constitute the social stimulus to which others respond. Thus, personality is perhaps the most inclusive term in psychology. Apart from all other personal characteristics it includes qualities of temperament (q.v.), character (q.v.), and intellect (q.v.).
Various attempts have been made to classify individuals into personality types. Notable among these was Jung's (q.v.) description of introverts (q.v.) and extraverts (q.v.) according to the inward or outward direction of their interests. It is now recognized, that such 'types' represent extremes of continuous dimensions. Thus extraversion is now regarded as a higher level of organization of unidimensional traits such as sociability, activity, impulsivity and dominance. The importance of organization in personality is demonstrated by conditions of multiple personality in which relatively independent systems develop of which one is usually dominant. There are various theories of personality development, ranging from the behavioristic to the Freudian. Most stress the importance of social learning during infancy. Personality disorders represent various

forms of social maladjustment which may isolate the individual, e.g. the obsessional, paranoid or schizoid, or place him in conflict with society as in the sociopathic and psychopathic disorders. Personality disintegration frequently accompanies intellectual deterioration in chronic organic and functional psychoses.
A variety of psychological tests (q.v.) and techniques have been devised for the assessment of personality. These include the objectively scored self-report 'Inventories' or questionnaires such as the Minnesota Multiphasic Personality Inventory (q.v.) and the projective techniques, such as the Rorschach (q.v.) and thematic apperception tests (q.v.), which are based on the subject's interpretations of ambiguous stimuli. Less formal personality assessment, based on the patient's history and his responses during interview, is an important aspect of the mental examination.
SEE ALSO Perseveration, Cyclothymic personality, Child psychiatry, Depersonalization, Mental deterioration, Conflict, and Delinquency.

Personality disorders

As there are over fifty different definitions of personality it is important to remember that in general the psychiatrist regards personality as the motivational and temperamental qualities of an individual. These qualities vary in much the same way as height, body weight, or intelligence. It is in terms of these normal variations that disorders of personality can best be conceived. There are many frank and clear-cut abnormalities of personality, which include the passive-aggressive, the schizoid (q.v.), the paranoid (q.v.), the cyclothymic (q.v.), the emotionally unstable, the compulsive (q.v.) and the hysterical (q.v.). These deviant types may exist in society perfectly satisfactorily, both personally and socially. It is only when society suffers from the consequences of the abnormalities that we speak of psychopathic (q.v.) or sociopathic personalities – terms which are often used incorrectly and all too imprecisely as synonyms for personality disorder. Personality disorder is a feature of the psychopathic personality, but it is the behaviour of the individual in a social situation which determines the appropriateness or otherwise of the term psychopathic.

Persuasion

Persuasion as a psychotherapeutic technique was developed by Freud. By means of discussion, argument, and the use of the physician's knowledge the patient is persuaded, indeed convinced, that his symptoms are no more than figments of his imagination, harmful to himself and to others. To practise this method the physician relies on his superior knowledge, and on his dominance of the patient.
SEE ALSO Psychotherapy.

Perversion

A perversion is a morbid craving for a form of sexual behaviour which is fixed and excludes normal heterosexual intercourse. Much deviant sexuality is, however, incidental to normal sexual behaviour. As a result, it is now considered that the term perversion should be abandoned, and that sexual deviation should be used to express the continuum of sexual behaviour which exists from the most minor form of deviation to the most bizarre and exclusive forms.
SEE ALSO Sexual disorders.

Petit mal

A form of epileptic attack starting during childhood, and only rarely starting after puberty, petit mal is characterized by sudden, transitory losses of consciousness, or 'absences'. They last for five to ten seconds, and may be accompanied by small muscular twitches about the face and in the upper limbs. There is no warning and the absence may pass unnoticed by those around the child, for he does not fall and resumes whatever activity he is engaged in, possibly after slightly shaking his head as though to re-orient himself. The attack is accompanied by an outburst of bilaterally symmetrical 3 cycles per second spike and slow wave activity in the EEG, the origin of which is considered to be in the diencephalon.
A number of variants exist, either in the

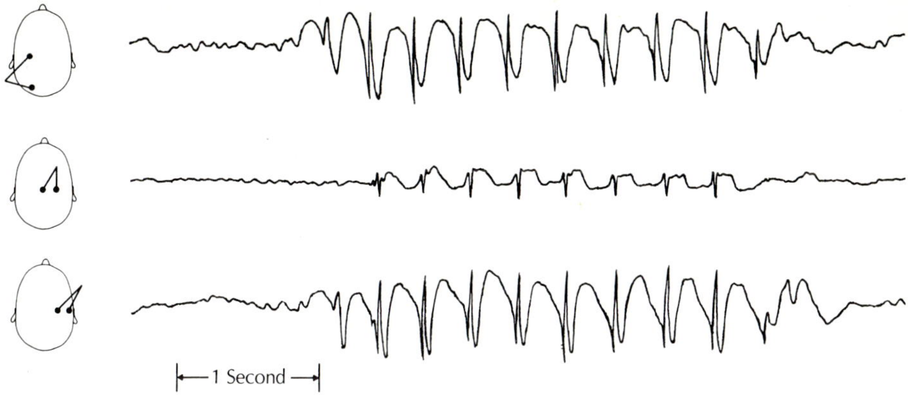

EEG in case of petit mal showing 3 c/second burst of bilaterally synchronous alternating spikes and waves. The amplitude varies with the electrode

time or frequency of the attack. When the attack lasts longer than five to ten seconds more complex motor activities may be noticed, such as lip smacking, or chewing movements, and there is an accentuation of clonic movements. One attack may follow another so rapidly as to produce a petit mal status, in which the child may become confused, or show automatic behaviour. At other times the only clear cut abnormality is to be found in the EEG, the child showing no outward evidence of change of consciousness.

The cause of petit mal is unknown; genetic factors are considered to play some part in the aetiology of the condition. The course is usually benign, and good control may be obtained with ethosuximide or troxidone.

Petrol sniffing

Uncommon in the United Kingdom, petrol sniffing is more common in the United States amongst youngsters who inhale volatile solvents such as benzene etc. Typically the petrol sniffer or 'huffer' inhales fumes from car petrol tanks or from lawn mowers; cigarette lighter liquid fuel may also be used. Rapid intoxication occurs, with dysarthria, ataxia and confusion. Since the vapour is highly concentrated coma and death may easily occur. SEE ALSO Addiction. As with other addictions, the response to treatment is uncertain.

PGR (psychogalvanic response)

SEE Skin conductance level.

Phakomatoses

The phakomatoses are a group of genetical conditions not infrequently associated with severe mental subnormality in which the main pathological involvement is in the skin and central nervous system. They are so called on account of the presence of nerve tumours of the retina in many cases (phakomata) which are benign nerve tumours and whose name is derived from the Greek for lentil. The phakomatoses include tuberous sclerosis (q.v.) and the Sturge-Weber syndrome (q.v.), both of which are commonly associated with severe mental subnormality.

Phantasy

(The alternative spelling is Fantasy)

In psychiatry this is the equivalent to day dreaming (q.v.). Freud also postulated a type of night dream which does not undergo the type of additions or alterations by the mechanisms of distortion, condensation or symbolization which occur in ordinary dreams. These he termed the 'phantasies of sleep'. The driving force behind fantasy is regarded as an unsatisfied unconscious wish or striving – it is able to give the illusion that wishes and aspirations have been fulfilled. Phantasy, and the inner world of reveries and contemplation, may be more satisfying to the introverted personality than the outside world of action and external reality.

Phantom limb

Following amputation, or interruption of sensory pathways, the illusion that a part is still present may persist, and in the limbs gives rise to the phenomenon of the phantom limb. The phantom usually shrinks and disappears into the stump, only to re-occur in periods of psychological stress or physical disturbance. The phantom limb may be painless or painful, and it is when the pain persists and does not respond to treatment that the psychiatrist is consulted. At times neuro-surgical intervention such as tractotomy, or even leucotomy, may become necessary. Suicide may result from intractable pain in a phantom limb.

Phenomenology

The scientific description of symptoms and signs and the recognition of similarities between patients from which it is hoped to deduce causes.
Recently there has been a reaction away from phenomenology towards a study of the individual person. However, a study of the phenomenological aspects of a patient's disorder remains of fundamental importance, if not for understanding the patient at least for understanding the illness from which he is suffering and the difficulties he may have in coping with his symptoms.

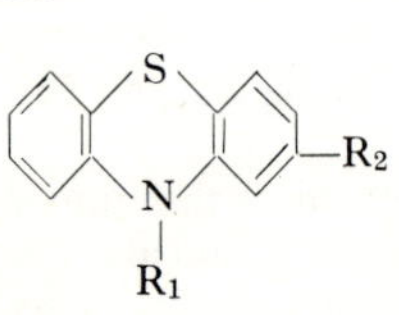

Phenothiazine nucleus

Phenothiazines

The phenothiazines have had an enormous impact in psychiatry and the beginning of modern psychopharmacology was the development in 1952 of chlorpromazine, the prototype of the series.
These compounds are all based on the phenothiazine nucleus (see illustration). Three subgroups exist with small differences in properties according to the nature of the side chain in the 10 position. The aliphatic side chain, which includes chlorpromazine and promazine, tends to have sedative effects and prominent postural hypotension but relatively little extrapyramidal disturbance. The piperazine group, including trifluoperazine, perphenazine and fluphenazine, shows comparatively little sedative or hypotensive effect and these compounds are chosen when activation is required; extrapyramidal effects are pronounced. The third group has a piperidine side chain and falls roughly midway between the amino and piperazine groups. The main members are thioridazine and pericyazine. A related group of drugs is the azaphenothiazine derivatives, of which prothipendyl has been studied clinically.
The phenothiazines block metabolic pathways at a number of different sites and have a general inhibiting effect on catecholamine metabolism.
They are absorbed promptly from the gastrointestinal tract and effects appear within an hour. The rate of excretion varies within the group but complete elimination after discontinuing the drug often takes several weeks.
The main psychiatric effect is that of tranquillizing and the use of phenothiazines in the treatment of the schizophrenias depends upon this action. With a reduction of intensity of disturbed affect, specific psychotic symptoms such as delusions and hallucinations fade, thinking becomes more orderly and emotion more appropriate. Symptomatic restraint can be dramatic, behavioural disturbance is constrained and psychomotor hyperactivity and mania are controlled, but often at high dosage; aggression is modified; agitation and anxiety are settled.
Phenothiazines are most widely used for treating the schizophrenias and manic-depressive psychoses. But they find a valuable place in organic brain syndromes including confusional states, epilepsy, dementia and Huntington's chorea. In general, acute disturbance calls for a sedative phenothiazine and parenteral administration may be needed in a crisis. When rehabilitation is being attempted the use of an activating phenothiazine minimizes interference with initiative and

activity. Psychiatric patients are unreliable pill takers, and depot fluphenazine enanthate and decanoate is valuable for maintenance therapy. Intramuscular injections are given at intervals varying between one and four weeks.

Agitated depression may be treated by a combination of a phenothiazine with an anti-depressant. In neurotic illness the phenothiazines are used in smaller doses, often in addition to minor tranquillizers.

The commonest side effect is the appearance of Parkinsonism when higher doses are used and anti-Parkinsonism drugs can be given prophylactically with advantage. Other extrapyramidal syndromes (q.v.) include akathisia (q.v.), dystonic reactions, oculogyric crises and torticollis (q.v.).

Toxic confusional states appear in about 1% of patients and may include a vivid hallucinosis in the elderly. Jaundice of an intrahepatic obstructive type is due to an allergic response and occurs after two to four weeks in between 0·1% and 4% of patients according to the compound used. Agranulocytosis is fortunately rare. Both these effects call for prompt cessation of treatment. The phenothiazines are epileptogenic and grand mal convulsions are occasionally precipitated; reduction in dosage is usually all that is required. Especially with long continued high doses of chlorpromazine and thioridazine unexpected death may occur, possibly due to a quinidine-like effect on the heart. Photosensitivity can be a real problem, but can be avoided by using ultraviolet barrier cream on the exposed surfaces.

Other unusual side effects include amenorrhoea, lactation, diuresis, diabetes mellitus exacerbations, keratoconjunctivitis, pigmentary retinopathy, hypotension, tachycardia, weight gain, blurred vision, dry mouth, impotence, skin rashes and pruritus. Most of these have a nuisance value but it will usually be possible to continue therapy.

Phenylketonuria

Phenylketonuria is an autosomal recessive inherited defect of aminoacid metabolism due to a deficiency of the enzyme phenylalanine hydroxylase. The incidence has been quoted variously from about one in 25,000 births to one in 10,000 births. High levels of phenylalanine are found in the body fluids, and the biochemical diagnosis rests on the phenylalanine level in the serum; screening tests of urine by the addition of ferric chloride or use of Phenistix strips which give a colour reaction due to presence of phenylpyruvic acid are insufficient on their own.

Clinical features include dilution of hair, skin and eye colour, reduction in head size, hyperreflexia, hyperkinesis, epilepsy in childhood in a number of cases and infantile eczema. Mental subnormality is nearly always of severe degree, but in a very few exceptional sporadic cases intellectual function has been within normal limits. Genetical carriers (heterozygotes) for phenylketonuria are apparently clinically normal although the carrier state can be detected by biochemical means.

Some measure of success has been claimed for dietary treatment. This should be started as soon as the condition is diagnosed shortly after birth. It consists of giving a diet low in phenylalanine, and should be biochemically controlled so that the phenylalanine levels in the body are regularly checked. The age at which the diet may be discontinued is controversial, but between the ages of 4 and 6 years has been suggested. Homozygous patients should be put back on their diet during pregnancy.

SEE ALSO Inherited metabolic defects.

Phenylpyruvic oligophrenia

SEE Phenylketonuria.

Phobias

A phobia is the experience of a persistent excessive fear when in contact with an object or situation which is not a significant source of danger. The patient's anxiety increases the closer she approaches the situation and diminishes as the feared situation recedes. Phobias have three main components:

(a) the subjective experience of fear or anxiety which accompanies contact with the feared object,

(b) physiological changes associated with such anxiety, and

(c) behavioural tendencies to avoid or escape from it.

Some truly phobic subjects therefore experience fear very rarely because they avoid contact with objects or situations which make them anxious.
Phobias are of three main types: agoraphobia (q.v.) and claustrophobia (q.v.), specific phobias (q.v.) and social phobias (q.v.). Fears of illness and obsessive symptoms with pronounced phobic qualities including fears of killing, stabbing or cutting are included in a fourth miscellaneous 'group'. As a general rule, specific phobias such as for spiders, cats or dogs are associated with a normal personality, they are 'learned' phenomena, and when the patient is removed from the situation she is symptom free. Such specific phobias are resistant to drugs and psychotherapy but respond well to behaviour therapy, either desensitization or flooding. The agoraphobic/claustrophobic syndrome is a multiple phobia; the patient frequently has personality difficulties and anxiety symptoms, though diminished, are often present even when the patient is removed from the feared situation. Psychotherapy and drugs both of the benzodiazepine and antidepressant groups are the mainstays of treatment. Behaviour therapy is often helpful in association with psychotherapy and may also be used to desensitize the patient to some more fundamental fear which has been uncovered by psychotherapy. Social phobias and many of the miscellaneous phobias may be treated in similar ways. Phobias may occur without other psychiatric symptoms or in association with other psychiatric syndromes. Primary depressive illnesses are often accompanied by mild phobic symptoms, especially of the agoraphobic variety but may present as phobias, the underlying depression being masked. When phobias exist with other problems the management is of the prepotent or primary disorder.

Phobic anxiety

SEE Anxiety neuroses, Phobia, and Anxiety.

Physical dependence

In the World Health Organisation definition of dependence a distinction is made between physical and psychological dependence (q.v.). This, though somewhat arbitrary, has practical uses. Physical dependence implies a real physical need in the patient to continue taking the drug to avoid physically determined abstinence symptoms. These differ between the different drugs, but include such symptoms as confusion and convulsions. Many regard physical dependence as having greater medical significance than psychological dependence.
SEE ALSO Addiction.

Physical treatments, special methods of

Just as one should never prescribe 'penicillin for pyrexia' a doctor should not prescribe a drug or other physical treatment for a psychiatric symptom without a full assessment of the patient and the cause of the symptomatology. On the basis of this information he should then plan his treatment. Only in this way can the doctor determine what he expects from and how long the physical remedies should be continued, and how they might best be combined with general social and psychotherapeutic procedures.
The greater the endogenous component of the illness, be it depression, mania or schizophrenia, the more effective the physical treatments designed to alter such a biochemical disturbance. Thus in a typical endogenous depression, antidepressant drugs or ECT are likely to result in cure, other treatments playing a relatively small part. Where personality or reactive factors are marked, however, the anti-depressant drugs might only be expected to result in partial improvement, though perhaps sufficient to enable the patient to face up to and, perhaps with psychotherapeutic help, eventually overcome her difficulties. In such a case the anti-depressant may have to be continued for one or two years until such time as the patient has adjusted to her problems. Such 'maintenance' type of treatment is common in patients with schizophrenia and in certain cases, especially when the illness is not fully controlled, may have to be continued indefinitely as relapse may lead to a permanent deterioration of their mental health.
In neurotic patients in particular, physical

treatments are aimed at symptom relief rather than being directed at a specific biochemical disorder. Patients with a neurotic personality develop neurotic symptoms when they are unable to cope with some stress either single or cumulative. Ill-health, insomnia, or loss of weight can add to the patient's difficulty in facing life and easily lead to a vicious circle of increasing symptoms causing greater inadequacy and hence more symptoms. In such a patient physical measures designed to relieve symptoms may not only help the patient to face up to her problems but to get back to work and develop her social and other interests, factors which in themselves help to stabilize her personality. To this end hypnotics, tranquillizers, and at times sleep therapy, modified insulin, or narco-analysis may be used. It is important to remember, however, that these drugs are intended to help the patient *do* something. Patients given tranquillizers simply to relieve symptoms and without any help to alter the underlying problem may easily become dependent on them. In some patients on the other hand personality or reactive factors are so intractable that the doctor may intentionally have to continue such symptom relief indefinitely rather than allow the patient to lose what social capacities she has.

Physiological basis of mental disorders

SEE Biochemical and neurophysiological background to mental disease.

Physique

Kretschmer (q.v.) led the way in modern psychiatry in the search for correlation between psychological variables and physique. He associated the pyknic build (stocky stature, broad face, thick neck, large visceral cavities, slender extremities and slight shoulder girdle, and a tendency to accumulate subcutaneous fat on the trunk) with a cyclothymic temperament and affective psychoses. On the other hand, he associated the leptosomatic build (tall stature, narrow trunk, long limbs, paucity of subcutaneous fat) with schizoid temperament and schizophrenic breakdown. Later workers in this field included Sheldon, who developed another typology, and Rees and Eysenck.

SEE ALSO Somatotypes and Constitution.

Piaget, Jean (1896–)

The Swiss psychologist and philosopher known for his studies of child development, of language, and of intelligence. Piaget's theory of intelligence is an epigenetic one – intelligence develops in response to and as a consequence of stimuli from the environment. Thus he regards the child as progressing through four stages of intellectual development. First the sensorimotor – occurring in the first two years of life as a relatively blind exploratory behaviour. This is followed by a phase of preoperational representation – the acquiring and storing of information and its coding ready for stage three, concrete operations, when testing out is performed in a simple, concrete manner. Finally, the fourth stage of formal operations sees the mind fully developed – abstract concepts now coming into action. Piaget's work on cognition has been pursued over a period of fifty years and is, perhaps, the most important contribution to the subject.

Pica

Pica (derived from the latin, pica – a magpie) involves the indiscriminate picking-up and ingestion of inappropriate material. This occurs as a phase in normal development, in the second six months of life, but it occurs as a pathological entity up to the age of puberty. The child is often mentally retarded and from a disturbed family. Iron deficiency anaemia may be found, most probably as a secondary phenomenon. The most serious complication is lead encephalopathy, sometimes producing an organic confusional state. Treatment involves dealing with the disturbing family influences and this may mean admission of the child to hospital. Estimation of lead levels may indicate the need to treat lead poisoning with chelating agents.

Pick's disease

Lobar atrophy, particularly of frontal and temporal lobes, distinguishes this pre-senile dementia from the generalized cerebral atrophy of Alzheimer's disease (q.v.). Beginning in the pre-senium (50–60), focal signs such as apraxia, aphasia, and agraphia precede the development of generalized memory disturbance. Women are more commonly affected than men. Neuropathologically the changes are confined to the affected areas, and consist of a ballooning of nerve cells, shrinking of white matter and neuroglial changes. Differential diagnosis from Alzheimer's disease is not easy and cortical biopsy may be the only method of establishing the diagnosis. Prognosis is poor – death occurring rather more rapidly than in Alzheimer disease. No specific treatment is available.

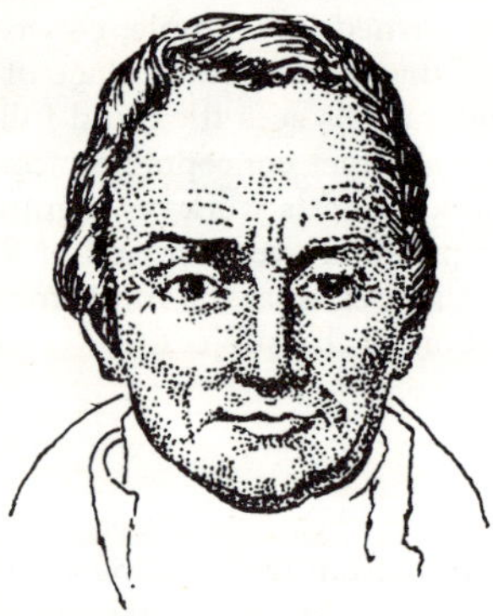

Pinel, Philippe (1754–1826)

Popularly known for his work in freeing the lunatics in the Bicêtre from their chains, Pinel has become one of the myth heroes of psychiatry. The son of a physician, he was much influenced by English and Scottish medicine, and he was interested in the classification of mental illness, and in the moral management of the insane. He paid particular attention to the psychosocial aspects of insanity, exposed as he had been to the turmoil of the French Revolution and of the Napoleonic era. His famous book the *Traité Médico – Philosophique Sur L'Aliénation Mentale, ou La Manie* (1801), is one of the classics of psychiatry.

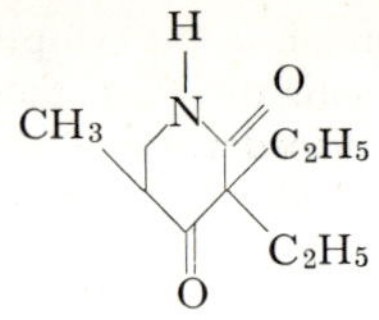

Piperidinedione derivatives

Glutethimide and methyprylon are piperidinedione derivatives, used as hypnotics. These compounds closely resemble the barbiturates in potency and adverse effects, and tolerance and dependence may develop.
The ill-fated thalidomide was structurally related to glutethimide, but its metabolic fate in the body was different; glutethimide has not been shown to possess teratogenic activity.

Placebos, placebo reactor

A placebo is a tablet or capsule or other vehicle containing only inert ingredients and no active drugs. Placebos are frequently used as controls (q.v.) in blind controlled clinical trials (q.v.) and are matched in appearance to the active drug. They are also used to test response to therapy, and to reduce drug dosage in addicts.
The placebo reactor is an individual who responds, positively or negatively to placebo administration. Various personality features are associated with specific types of reaction to placebos. Placebos should not be administered therapeutically without considerable thought: deception in medical practice is dangerous.

Play therapy

In cases where a child too young or too inhibited to communicate verbally is thought to have developed an internal mental conflict amenable to psychological methods of treatment, techniques of play therapy have been devised to deal with the situation.
The psychotherapist (who may be a medically qualified psychiatrist or a lay therapist) usually has a standard set of play equipment with which to confront the child. Commonly, this will consist of a sand tray,

a set of containers, a low basin with cold running water, a doll's house and a set of toy soldiers. Paints, crayons, plasticine and paper are provided. The child may be taken into the room with the therapist and invited to play without any further explanation, or, depending on the age of the child, the therapist may say that some children who are upset and have difficulties find it helpful to play or paint a picture. The role of the therapist depends largely on his or her personality and theoretical orientation. Some therapists are virtually silent while the child plays, whereas others make interpretations (comment on the child's behaviour according to their understanding of it) very freely. The focus of the therapist's interpretations may be on the way the child is playing in relation to his feelings about his parents, or about the therapist himself. Interpretations about the possible symbolic significance of the child's play may also be made.

Although the value of play therapy as an effective treatment technique is not established, it is certainly possible to obtain valuable diagnostic insight into the way a child is thinking by placing him in this sort of play situation. It is probable also that, at the very least, a child can learn in this way to explain himself imaginatively in the presence of a skilled and sympathetic observer. Greater claims than this are at present unjustifiable.

SEE ALSO Child psychiatry.

Pleasure principle

Instinctual life, according to Freud, is governed by the pleasure-pain principle, the immediate attainment and fulfilment of pleasure, and the avoidance of pain of any sort. The workings of the id are governed by this principle, but controls exerted by the ego and super-ego may lead to modifications of instinctual demands – as, for instance, with fantasy fulfilment instead of reality fulfilment. Thanatos, or the death instinct, was a later development of Freud's thinking on the pleasure-pain problem.

Poison pen letters

The persecution of an individual by anonymously written letters may produce much mental anguish in the recipient and his or her family. The contents of the letters usually refer to alleged infidelities, or dishonesties, and often reveal a close knowledge of the person to whom the letter is addressed. So much so that at times the recipient must become the suspect letter writer. Threats of a terrifying nature may be made against family members; at times whole groups of persons may be persecuted by such letters. Doctors are common targets. The letters should not be lightly regarded, each one should be read, and the police should be informed, particularly when threats of violence are made. A paranoid schizophrenia which is not overtly manifested may underlie this poison pen activity, which may be the only sign of the schizophrenic illness.

Poisons affecting mental state

Exposure to poisons can occur in industry, agriculture, in therapeutics and in the home. Poisoning may be the result of accident, negligence, addiction, suicide or homicide. Acute poisoning is often suggested by gastrointestinal, hepatic or renal symptomatology, with the rapid onset of excitement, delirium, convulsions and coma. Chronic poisoning involving the central nervous system most often follows an insidious course with apathy, loss of concentration, impairment of memory, irritability, insomnia and, terminally, excitement, convulsions or coma. The specific poison may be identified clinically by the history of contact, for example with heavy metals or industrial solvents, and by any special features – the punctate basophilia and hypochromic anaemia, the coproporphyrinuria and the wrist drop of lead (q.v.); the pigmentation, exfoliative dermatitis and foot drop of arsenic; the alopecia of thallium, the cherry-red cyanosis of carbon monoxide (q.v.); the breath odour of bitter almonds of cyanide. The variety of substances for which addiction may develop – 'glue', petrol, arsenic, anaesthetics, as well as drugs – and the development of new toxic substances – e.g. paraquat – should be borne in mind.

SEE ALSO Suicide, Addiction, and Drugs.

Polyphagia

Excessive eating, which apart from those in whom overeating and obesity is the central problem, often occurs in women with mild neurotic depressions, and as a common reaction to unhappiness. It also occurs in short bouts in some young women with anorexia nervosa (q.v.).

Pornography

The description of the habits, lives, patrons and practices of prostitutes, in literature and in art, pornography may be regarded as an acceptable facet of a civilized society. However, in certain circumstances these descriptions may overstep the bounds of what is acceptable in a particular society and so become obscene – that is, offensive to the senses, to modesty and decency.

Porphyria

Porphyria is inherited by an autosomal dominant gene with incomplete penetrance so that a proportion of those bearing the gene do not suffer clinical symptoms, although they have an abnormality of porphyrin metabolism which can be demonstrated biochemically. There are at least five distinct types of porphyria, of which the most important are acute intermittent porphyria (Swedish type) and porphyria variagata (South African type).

In the Swedish type, which is the most common type in Britain, the symptoms appear episodically with hypotension, acute headache, vomiting, abdominal pain polyuria and neurological signs which take the form mainly of a motor neuropathy. Psychiatric symptoms consist of confusional states in which the patient becomes noisy and behaves as if hallucinated. Porphyria is rarely seen in childhood and the onset is usually in the third decade.

Its relationship to drugs is important since attacks may be precipitated by barbiturates, sulphonals, sulphonamides, allyl isopropyl-acetylurea and aminopyrine.

It is particularly important to avoid the use of barbiturates for psychiatric symptoms during an attack; these may produce paralysis and lead to death by respiratory failure.

SEE ALSO Inherited metabolic defects.

Portal systemic encephalopathy

In cirrhosis of the liver a high portal vein pressure may allow blood flow between portal and systemic veins. Ammonia and other substances normally detoxicated by the liver enter the systemic circulation and neuro-psychiatric phenomena are observed. Confusion, lethargy, altered awareness, and finally coma are seen with a characteristic flapping tremor and other extrapyramidal signs. The condition is exacerbated by a high protein diet, infection and intestinal haemorrhage. Selective drugs should be avoided. The EEG reflects the altered state of awareness. Restricted protein, sterilization of the gut with neomycin (1–2·5 g. daily), purgation, and colectomy have been reported as successful treatment.

Positive conditioning

In operant conditioning (q.v.) the learned process results from the selective reinforcement of certain responses. These may take the form of rewards (positive conditioning) or punishments (negative conditioning).

SEE ALSO Conditioned reflex and Behaviour therapy.

Positive conditioning therapy

'Positive conditioning' implies using conditioning methods to establish new (operant) responses which are incompatible with the existing response to the stimulus and leads to its elimination. The treatment of nocturnal enuresis offers a good example of this; classical (Pavlovian) conditioning does not explain this treatment satisfactorily. The bell and pad is effective and often used. A pad is placed under the sheet on which the patient lies and is so arranged that when it is wet a bell rings and wakes the patient, inhibiting micturition.

The strengthening of assertion behaviour to counter anxiety in certain social situations is another example.

Possession

Demoniacal possession was, for centuries, regarded as the cause of insanity, the devil needing to be exorcized and driven out before recovery could take place. Today, states of possession by an alien spirit are rare in the Western world, but not uncommon in the Negro, particularly in the Caribbean area, and in West Africa and Nigeria. The ideas prevalent in a particular culture modify the presentation of mental illness, so that ideas of possession are, in general, non-specific and may occur in conditions as different as simulated insanity, culturally determined trance states and schizophrenia.

Post-infective depression

Depressive symptoms, of variable severity and duration, are a not uncommon sequel to many physical illnesses. The patient feels despondent and is easily moved to tears; he feels weak and has no energy; he sleeps badly and complains that he cannot concentrate; and sometimes he has paranoid or histrionic outbursts quite alien to his normal personality. Such symptoms are perhaps understandable in the aftermath of a long and serious illness but they are equally common after many relatively mild illnesses like glandular fever, infective hepatitis, brucellosis and, particularly, influenza. Usually the symptoms are neurotic in character and predominantly neurasthenic but sometimes deep depressions with endogenous symptoms like retardation are seen. The roles of organic and psychological factors in the aetiology of these post-infective states are ill-understood.

In cases where the depression is severe tricyclic drugs or even ECT may be necessary, and effective.

SEE ALSO Infection, mental symptoms due to.

Post-operative psychoses

Post-operative psychoses occur in one out of 1600 operations, the incidence depending on the site of the operation, the patient's age, nutrition, and general condition. Common operations followed by psychiatric disturbance are those performed for cataract, peptic ulcer, and cardiac disease. Confusional states are common, as are depressive and paranoid reactions. The risk may be diminished by preoperative discussion and explanatory attention to the patient's general condition and specific attention, e.g. in eye operations regarding the temporary blindness. Treatment will depend on the diagnosis, but particular care must be taken not to over-sedate the patient.

SEE ALSO Organic disease producing mental disorders.

Post-partum disorders

Emotional disturbance in the early puerperium is so common that it must be regarded as normal. After the first two or three days many women undergo a brief episode of depression and tearfulness – the so-called fourth day blues. To the primipara, and to her husband, this sudden change of mood is likely to be unexpected and even alarming, so that reassurance about its ephemeral nature is needed.

General emotional lability with over-reaction to emotional stimuli is also very common during the first days after childbirth. Both types of emotional disturbance may be partly of hormonal origin, since very large changes in the circulating levels of steroid hormones occur during and shortly after delivery. But personality and environmental factors are also important.

Frank psychiatric illness is at least four times as common in the puerperium as in pregnancy, with a peak incidence in the first month after delivery. It is convenient to discuss neurotic and psychotic illness separately, although the distinction may not always be readily made in an individual patient.

Neurotic symptoms may appear shortly after delivery or may be delayed for several weeks. Puerperal neurotic disorders do not differ in form from neurotic disorders generally. The commonest syndromes are states of anxiety (including phobic anxiety) and of 'reactive' depression, but obsessional and hysterical symptoms may also be seen. Understandably anxiety about the baby is very common.

Puerperal neurosis is commoner in primiparae and in patients who have had similar symptoms during pregnancy. It is rare for neurotic symptoms to appear for the first time after childbirth; there is usually a history of previous neurotic symptoms or

of personality vulnerability and there is often a family history of neurosis. Childbirth and its consequences act as both a physical and a mental stress, liable to provoke neurotic symptoms in susceptible personalities.
The treatment is the same as for neurotic illness generally, with particular attention being paid to the patient's relationship with her baby. Other members of the family, particularly the husband, may also need help. It is important in the early stages to ensure that depressed or tense patients get sufficient sleep, since sleeplessness can exacerbate tension and establish a vicious circle. Many untreated patients do improve after a few weeks or months, but some become chronic neurotics, so that early diagnosis and treatment are important. Furthermore, puerperal neurosis may cause family and marital discord, which in turn may perpetuate the neurosis.
In puerperal psychoses (q.v.) psychosocial precipitants are less obvious. The onset is often acute, within a few days of delivery. The prognosis in treated cases is good, although there is a risk of suicide and infanticide. Treatment is no different from that of the same psychoses occcurring outside of the puerperium. It is important that the patient should continue looking after her baby as much as she is able. When in-patient treatment is necessary, as in cases of schizophrenia or severe depression, patient and baby should both be admitted.

Post-partum psychosis

SEE Puerperal psychosis and Post-partum disorders.

Post-traumatic dementia

SEE Head injury and Mental sequelae.

Post-traumatic syndrome

The post-traumatic syndrome is characterized by symptoms of anxiety, depression, attacks of giddiness, irritability, and poor concentration and the absence of any signs of physical abnormality. It is not necessarily associated with head injury, but may occur following any frightening injury. The term post-concussional syndrome should be reserved for those cases where a head injury has led to momentary loss of consciousness, then followed by the previously mentioned symptoms. In the majority of cases of concussion no sequelae occur, but when they do, they are not necessarily a sign of psychiatric disturbance, but rather, many consider, a result of a disturbance in the haemodynamics of the cerebral circulation. They usually disappear over the course of twelve months at the most. The more severe the head injury in general the less likelihood the occurrence of 'post-concussional' symptoms; it is striking how uncomplaining are the severely head-injured patients.
The problem posed by the post-traumatic syndrome is almost invariably of a medico-legal nature. It is unusual to see this syndrome unless some form of compensation is involved. This naturally poses the question of just how much the symptoms are produced or prolonged deliberately for the purpose of financial gain. In the absence of any abnormal physical signs, and the lack of adequate follow-up statistics, it remains a matter of opinion as to how much the patient may be malingering.
In general the following factors may prove helpful in assessing the situation: the financial situation of the patient, who may receive enough financial benefit from Social Security to make work unattractive, the legal handling of the case, the treating doctor's attitude, the character of the patient, and his financial expectations.
There is no reason why a man should not return to work within three months of a medically trivial injury – certainly twelve months is the maximum period to be allowed for recovery. Doctors too often forget that human beings may be greedy, envious, grasping, or dishonest, and possess a remarkable tendency to deceive themselves and others regarding their motives. On this view the majority of cases of the post-traumatic and post-concussional syndromes are situationally determined, the situation being the desire for financial reward. None the less, care must be taken to exclude a depressive or anxiety reaction precipitated by the traumatic experience, so that adequate treatment may be given.

Pregnancy, psychological aspects of

In normal pregnancy mild anxiety and other transient mood disturbances are common in the first trimester; the second trimester is characteristically marked by tranquillity and wellbeing, but anxieties tend to reappear as term approaches. Typical fears are of death during labour or of the birth of a malformed child. While steroid hormones no doubt influence emotional state during pregnancy, psychosocial factors are important, in particular the pregnant woman's relationship with her husband and with her own mother. Food craving and fads during pregnancy are common and are thought to have a physiological basis. The role of maternal stress on the development of the foetus is controversial, some evidence suggests that it is not to be ignored.

Prejudice

A preconceived opinion or bias, usually unfavourable. It is an aspect of displacement (q.v.) and projection (q.v.) whereby one's own disclaimed and objectionable character traits, attitudes or desires are projected outwards and attributed to others.

Premature ejaculation

Premature ejaculation is persistent, precipitate ejaculation in the male before, or immediately after, penetration of the female introitus: sexual potency is normal. About three quarters of normal males ejaculate within two minutes of penetration. Some males, particularly those of neurotic personality, are unable to control sexual excitability and delay orgasm long enough to bring satisfaction to the partner. Treatment consists in the female partner repetitively stimulating the penis extravaginally to pre-orgasmic levels of excitability, and then allowing detumescence to occur. This activity is continued until an erection is maintained for periods of up to twenty minutes without ejaculation. When anticipatory anxiety to coitus is a significant factor anxiolytic drugs may be useful.

Premenstrual tension

This term refers to a group of symptoms that occur in the days immediately preceding menstruation. The disorder varies in severity from a mild discomfort to a disabling burden, and in duration from a day to a week or more. In general more severe symptoms tend to last longer.
The main features are (a) mood change: tension and irritability, but sometimes also depression. The mood is often variable with a tendency to worsen as menstruation approaches; and (b) physical symptoms: general physical discomfort, a bloated feeling, painful breast swelling, sometimes weight gain.
In its mild form this is a very common disorder. More severe symptoms are more likely in women with neurotic personalities. Hormonal factors are also important. An imbalance between progesterone and oestrogen secretion, with a relative deficiency of progesterone, has been postulated. There is now good evidence that the psychological symptoms are improved by an oral contraceptive or by a progestogen such as norethisterone. Physical symptoms respond better to a diuretic. This suggests that at least two physical mechanisms are involved.

Prescriptions for addicts

Each country has its own specific legislation governing the prescription of drugs of dependence to known addicts. The United Kingdom law places upon the doctor the legal obligation to notify to the Chief Medical Officer of the Home Office Drugs Department the names and other details of any patient whom the doctor sees in a professional relationship who is diagnosed as being addicted to any of the drugs covered by the Act.
Under the current regulations for the United Kingdom, heroin and cocaine may only be prescribed to addicts by specially licensed doctors, but there is no bar on their customary medical use as analgesics for other patients.

Pre-senile dementia

Under this term are included idiopathic degenerative diseases of the nervous system that give rise to dementia (q.v.) between the ages of 40 and 60. The main conditions are Pick's disease (q.v.), Alzheimer's disease (q.v.) and Jacob-Creuzfeldt's disease (q.v.), and a group of dementias without special features, none of which, however, is strictly confined to this period. Huntington's chorea (q.v.) which often begins before 40, is not usually included. There are also secondary dementias due to syphilis, cerebro-vascular disease, cerebral tumour, myxoedema, alcoholism and chronic neurological disorders such as subacute combined degeneration of the cord.

Priapism

A painful chronic erection, priapism is sometimes regarded as a psychosomatic manifestation, but, in fact, is always a manifestation of some underlying illness, either local or general, such as thrombosis of the corpora cavernosa, leukaemia, or Hodgkin's disease.

Primal scene

The experience of parental sexual intercourse during childhood is usually repressed, but may appear in fantasies, more or less distorted. In some individuals this primal scene may have powerful effects on future sexual development. The child may interpret his parents' behaviour in a variety of ways, as an example of terrifying male-female struggle, or of masculine aggression and violence, or of mother's betrayal of the child's love for her. Sexual behaviour in the presence of children varies widely from culture to culture – in parts of Polynesia it is accepted by adults and children as perfectly normal. The primal scene has probably less significance than was originally postulated by Freud.

Primary gain

There are two types of gain which result from neurotic symptoms – primary and secondary. Primary gain consists of relief, by symptom production, of the anxiety and distress produced by the basic conflict and is unconscious; secondary gain consists of those conscious benefits obtained as the result of neurotic symptoms – attention from the entourage, financial gain, avoidance of unpleasant situations. Secondary gain is often imputed to psychiatric patients, usually unjustifiably. The doctor should be most careful before regarding his patient's behaviour as dictated by secondary gain.

Prison medical service

Arrangements for medical care show marked variations from one country to another. In England and Wales a specialized medical service has been established within the Home Office to provide medical care for prisoners. Most of our large prisons have at least one full-time medical officer. Apart from providing general medical services, prison medical officers provide a medical report service to the courts and psychiatric clinics are increasingly being established within prisons. Some of these prison medical officers also hold specialist hospital psychiatric appointments.
SEE ALSO Forensic psychiatry, Psychiatric prisons, and Special hospitals.

Prison psychoses

A psychotic breakdown which only occurs within a prison setting, the clinical picture is usually that of a paranoid illness, although depressive, and even delirious, features may occur. The special strains imposed by imprisonment, with all its social and personal consequences for the prisoner, affect the form of the illness. Although sometimes regarded as simulated insanity, it is wise to treat psychotic symptoms arising in prison with caution – otherwise the unexpected suicide, or an impulsive attack on a warder under the influence of delusions may take place. Psychopaths are more liable than normal individuals to develop psychiatric illnesses, and doctors should take particular care that his judgement should not be affected by the fact that a man is labelled a psychopath.

SEE ALSO Ganser syndrome and Hysterical pseudo-dementia.

Probation and after-care

Under United Kingdom legislation, a probation order may be made on an offender aged 17 or more years in lieu of sentence. The order requires him to be under the supervision of a probation officer for one to three years, and if he breaks the terms and conditions of his order he is liable to be punished for both the breach of probation and the original offence. The aim of probation is to re-establish an offender within the community and to avoid institutionalization. Usually the probationer has to agree to be of good behaviour and to keep in close contact with his supervising officer. Sometimes other conditions are included in the order, e.g. residence at an approved probation hostel, or in- or out-patient medical treatment. A probation order can only be made with the consent of the offender.

On leaving prison in the United Kingdom, all medium and long-term prisoners may opt for voluntary aftercare (i.e. supervision and assistance from a probation officer). Parole has recently been introduced in the United Kingdom as a method of enforcing after-care, a prisoner who has served one-third of his sentence (a minimum of twelve months' imprisonment having been served) being eligible for consideration. The parole licence may contain certain provisions, such as conditions of residence, work, etc., to which the parolee must adhere, or else be liable to revocation of the licence.

Problem families

In problem families, multiple difficulties have clustered together to such an extent that the family fails to conform to the minimum demands of society. An inability of one or both parents to cope with the complexities of life in an industrial society or an active rejection of conventional standards and a turning to crime and delinquency are frequently encountered. The parents are unemployed – except irregularly – and the children stay away from school, sometimes from lack of proper clothing (at a time when almost all schoolchildren are now adequately clothed), or when the older children are kept at home by an inadequate mother to look after younger children. More important is a failure to understand or identify with the aims of the educational system; this tends to become hostility when there are official attempts to enforce regular school attendance. When adolescent, the children often become active truants, which leads to delinquency. Uncontrolled fertility is one of the commonest problems, particularly as the mothers are often unco-operative in antenatal care. Efficient contraception is virtually unknown, except where a domiciliary family planning service is available, and pregnancies may continue until one or other partner consents to sterilization. With each additional child, the family may sink deeper into rent and hire purchase arrears and eventually suffer eviction. Possibly as a result of the outside hostility they tend to arouse, problem families often have a strong internal loyalty, at least until the older children grow up.

Projection

An important mental mechanism, projection consists of the attribution to others of undesirable personal feelings and attitudes. In pathological conditions paranoid delusions are based on the projection of hostile and aggressive feelings.

Prolactin

A hormone secreted by the anterior pituitary gland. It is one of the hormones necessary to prime the breast for lactation and secretion is raised during pregnancy. It is also important in the control of gonadal function, an increase in circulatory prolactin is accompanied by impaired gonadal function which may result in impotence and oligospermia in men and amenorrhoea or abnormal and anovular menstrual cycles in women.

Prolactin secretion from the pituitary gland is controlled by a prolactin inhibitory factor from the hypothalamus which is probably controlled by dopaminergic neurons. Dopamine antagonists such as the phenothiazines or butyrophenones will cause a marked rise in circulating prolactin with consequent side effects. High levels of prolactin have been found in mania but this may only represent abnormal hypothalamic feedback mechanisms in this disease.

Promiscuity

Promiscuity is indiscriminate sexual relationships between partners who have no emotional bondage. In the female delinquent, promiscuity can be a form of 'acting out' behaviour and the counterpart of criminal behaviour in the male, and is often an expression of aggression and rebellion to parental authority through the flaunting of accepted social standards. Females with hysterical personality disorders are often promiscuous and use seduction of the male as a manipulating technique to obtain emotional indulgence. Promiscuity may be symptomatic of manic states and diffuse brain damage when hypersexuality results. Promiscuity, due to weakening of the normal social inhibitions, may become a serious problem in chronic schizophrenic and subnormal females living in the community. Sterilization may be necessary to avoid recurrent pregnancy. Promiscuity in the male is less socially disapproved of than in the female. Male promiscuity is sometimes a manifestation of latent homosexuality (Don Juanism) where the successful seduction, particularly of married women, is not only a reassurance against impotence but an aggressive act towards other males.

Property of mentally ill patients

This is managed in England by the Court of Protection (q.v.) who appoints a receiver (curator bonis, judicial factor (q.v.)). An equivalent system exists in several other countries.

Propf schizophrenic

Schizophrenic syndromes occur in the mentally subnormal, often as rather acute, but transient attacks of florid mental disturbance. German psychiatrists regarded the schizophrenia as grafted onto the subnormality. However, childhood schizophrenia itself may be a cause of defect, so that the psychosis may be part of a continuing process. Whatever the theory may be, in practice the prognosis is good, and response to ECT is often gratifying.

Prospective inquiry

In a prospective inquiry the characteristics of a group are known and the subsequent development of disease is noted in an attempt to define aetiology. A typical example was the recent study of smoking habits and subsequent mortality in doctors. The differences between this and a retrospective inquiry (q.v.) should be noted.

Prostaglandins

A large group of substances, related to and biologically synthesized from the unsaturated fatty acids. They are widely distributed in animal tissues though few physiological activities have been confirmed. Among possible physiological roles is an action in synaptic transmission at adrenergic sites.

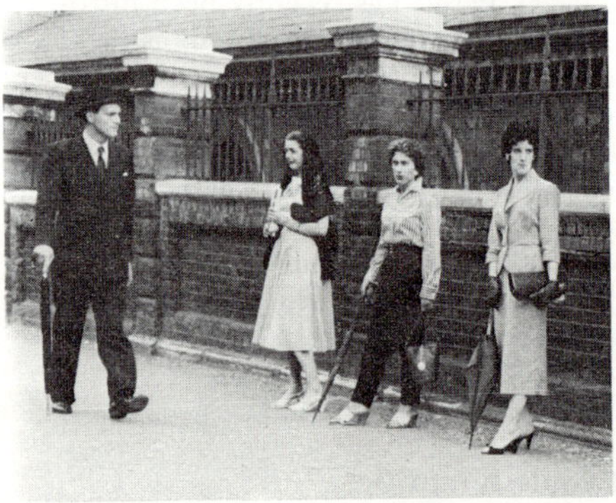

Prostitution

Prostitution is the promiscuous bartering of sexual favours by females or males for financial gain. The emotional relationship between the prostitute and client is usually one of mutual contempt. Prostitution now occurs mainly in sexually disorganized urban communities and is associated with other forms of social pathology such as drug addiction, criminality and alcoholism. Female prostitutes have varying degrees of personality disorder and intellectual endowment. Some are homosexuals who manifest their hostility to the male by degrading him through involvement in an asocial relationship, although in the actual heterosexual coitus they are often frigid. Male prostitutes for elderly females (gigolos) are often partial homosexuals.

Pseudo-cyesis

In this uncommon disorder a woman, usually nulliparous, becomes convinced that she is pregnant and develops symptoms and signs that mimic pregnancy. The symptoms include amenorrhoea, morning sickness and reports of quickening. Abdominal swelling and breast enlargement occur. While many features of pseudocyesis can be reproduced voluntarily, in some cases there is a hormonal disturbance, with a persisting corpus luteum.

In most patients there is an intense desire for pregnancy. The condition must be distinguished from the occasional delusion of pregnancy expressed by a schizophrenic patient, and from the deliberate fraud, aimed at blackmail or notoriety.

Pseudo-hermaphroditism

Is more common in the male where the genetic constitution is 44–XY. There is testicular feminization due to the enzymic failure of the somatic cells to respond to the masculinizing action of androgen. The external genital organs are rudimentary at birth and the child is reared as a female until adolescence when masculinization makes the mistake evident. The sex may then have to be re-assigned.

Pseudo-neurotic schizophrenia

A condition first described in 1949, in which an apparently neurotic condition progresses to a schizophrenic illness. Anxiety is prominent and pervades all aspects of the patient's life and the neurotic manifestations are usually varied with obsessions, hysterical symptoms, somatic manifestations of anxiety such as vomiting and palpitations, and a variety of sexual abnormalities. The symptoms are severe and the disturbance of behaviour and personality is more pervasive than is usual in neurosis. Short-lived psychotic episodes with clear cut schizophrenic symptoms may be distributed throughout the illness and gradually become more pronounced. The diagnosis is made more commonly in the United States than in Europe.

Pseudo-reminiscence

A general term indicating the pathological 'remembering' of events not experienced by the patient. There are three subcategories: (a) confabulation (q.v.) which occurs in organic states; (b) pseudo-logica phantastica; (c) retrospective falsification (q.v.) which can occur in organic, psychopathic, or psychotic states.
SEE ALSO Pathological lying.

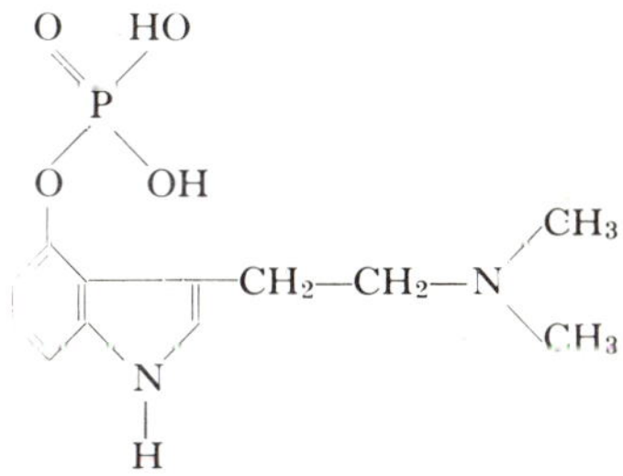

Psilocybin

Psilocybin is a hallucinogenic substance chemically similar to tryptamine. It is the

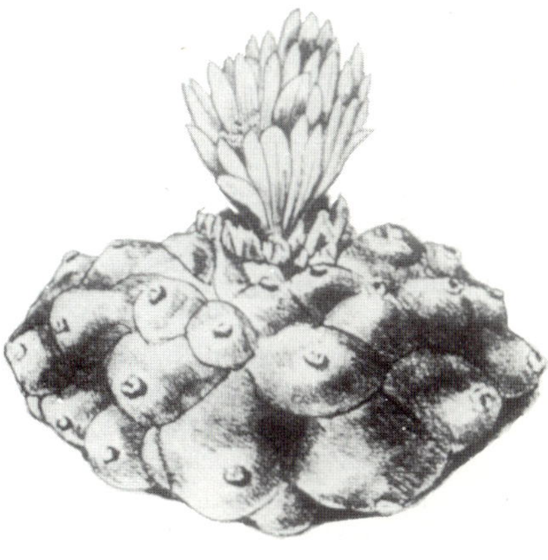

Psilocybe mexicana

active principle in the sacred Mexican mushroom known as 'teonanacatl' or Psilocybe mexicana. It has been used, taken by mouth in the setting of tribal religious observance. In recent years, particularly in the United States, psilocybin has become a popular hallucinogenic drug, mainly because of its effects on perception and the feelings of cosmic revelation associated with its use.
SEE ALSO Hallucinogenic drugs and LSD.

Psychedelic

Synonymous with hallucinogenic (q.v.), and psychotomimetic (q.v.). Applied to drugs and based upon the concept that they are mind expanding.

Psychiatric prisons

A distinct overlap occurs between the offending and the mentally disordered populations. As a result a need exists for special psychiatric facilities within the penal system. Psychiatric prisons have been pioneered in Scandinavia (notably Herstedvester and Horsens prisons in Denmark). Britain has one such prison at Grendon Underwood. The prison has a doctor as its governor, and is run on therapeutic community lines, with a special emphasis on group psychotherapy. All other forms of psychiatric treatment are also available within the prison. An offender cannot be sentenced to Grendon – the decision to treat him there is made by the Prison Medical Service (q.v.). The prisoner can refuse to accept. His sentence is in no way affected by admission to Grendon. Some other countries have introduced an equivalent system.
SEE ALSO Forensic psychiatry and Special hospitals.

Psychoactive drugs

Psychoactive drugs are substances which act directly or indirectly on the central nervous system and affect mental and emotional processes; psychotropic and psychopharmacological are alternative terms. The main types of psychoactive drugs used today are the major tranquillizers, the anxiolytic compounds, and the anti-depressants. Some psychostimulants and psychotomimetic agents are particularly liable to abuse. Description of psychoactive agents will be found under the appropriate headings.

Psychoanalysis

Strictly speaking this only refers to those techniques evolved from the work and theories of Sigmund Freud. In Freudian theory the 'ego' (q.v.) is the whole of the psychic faculties of the person and the function of the ego is to test and to relate to external reality. It is experienced by the individual as the unique 'me' or 'self'. It is constantly under pressure from the unacceptable instinctual demands of the 'id' (q.v.) which are in conflict with the requirements of external reality and the 'superego' (q.v.) or conscience, which is broadly determined by the mental acceptances of parental attitudes, morals and restrictions on behaviour. Mental defence mechanisms, e.g. repression (q.v.), dissociation (q.v.), projection (q.v.), etc., serve to protect the ego from being overwhelmed. Free association (q.v.) is the tool of psychoanalysis. The patient contracts not to censor any thought or feeling in therapy, however apparently trivial or meaningless to him. Interpretations are made by the analyst on the basis of this material, relating past experiences to present behaviour.
Patients are selected as suitable for psychoanalysis on the basis of ego strength, i.e. the ability of the ego (self) to survive interpretation of defences without disintegration; on the age of the patient, level of intelligence, ability to make symbolic and insightful connections – and the availability of time and money. Motivation for change is also of vital importance in assessment, as 'resistance' virtually always occurs at some time in treatment. This may take the form of 'forgetting' appointment times, late arrival, or inability to use interpretations profitably.
Treatment is terminated when more appropriate, adaptive defence mechanisms have been adopted and the patient is free of neurotic symptomatology. Analysis of children involves play therapy and observation in a permissive atmosphere to

gain insight into underlying emotional attitudes and conflicts.

The psychoanalytic view – an introduction to

The psychoanalytical school was originally based upon the ideas of mid- to late nineteenth-century psychologists, but the main development of these ideas, their practical application and their subsequent defence were due to Sigmund Freud (1865–1939) and his followers.

Regions of the mind. The mind consists of three distinct regions: the conscious, the subconscious and the unconscious. Beyond the threshold of consciousness is the subconscious region; its contents are immediately accessible to a conscious wish or a relevant stimulus. Thus the subconscious region is that portion which stores the myriad of readily available memories. There is a memory store deeper in the mind which is termed the unconscious. Therein are stored the instinctual drives, repressed urges, painful emotional memories and unresolved conflicts. They are inaccessible to conscious scrutiny by virtue of an active force which Freud termed 'the censor'. The censor may be overwhelmed by a massive upsurge of ideas of great power from the unconscious – as in the psychoses. Alternatively, these ideas could appear in a disguised form as dreams. Dream theory and dream interpretation thus became an integral part of Freudian psychoanalytical theory.

The personality structure. Freud described three components of the personality: (1) The id (q.v.) consisted of the instinctual and pleasure-seeking drives for food, sex and aggression. It is amoral, entirely self-centred and demanding. It is entirely unconscious.

(2) The ego (q.v.) is largely conscious, even though it has to react with the unconscious regions of the mind. It is the fundamental personality of the individual which has moral standards, uses logic and matches the demands of the unconscious with the needs of the individual in the environment. This principle of balance between the two is termed the reality principle (q.v.) and depends upon assessment of the environment via the sensory processes which form a vital part of the ego. It is thus constantly involved in establishing the compromises of life's reality.

(3) The superego (q.v.) is a differentiated part of the ego corresponding to the conscience. It is largely unconscious but contains the moral restrictions and ideals of the person. The superego is derived from the assimilation of the moral standards of peers, and particularly parents. When the person carries out actions derived from the id which are contrary to the principles contained in the superego, the pain of guilt is felt. By the use of guilt the superego attempts to keep the person within his bounds of moral restrictions.

Personality developments. The most important factors which influence personality are at work during the first seven years of life. After this the personality is largely developed. An essential force in this development is the libido. In its broadest sense, libido as used by Freud can be defined as 'desire' or 'craving'. It is the motivating instinctual force which is the basis of desire and achievement drives throughout life. Freud spoke of these first seven years as the period of 'psychosexual development', using the word 'sexual' in the sense of pleasure. The stages of development he described were each related to a different erogenous zone of the body.

In the first year of life the oral zone was connected with pleasurable and painful sensations, with attachment to, and dependence on, the mother. The infant's whole well-being depends upon the quality of maternal care; as indeed does his future love and relationships with women! Biting as an outlet for aggression comes with the growth of teeth and the mother may be the object of this type of aggression if she fails to satisfy the demands of the infant. In the next stage, which occurs between the ages of 2 and 3, the excretory apparatus becomes the focus of interest. This anal phase of development sees the beginning of conflict over toilet training. A good child is one who is clean, regular in his excretory habits, obedient and submissive. Rebellion may be quickly suppressed by the parent and the seeds laid for future obsessional neurosis. The third or 'phallic phase' lasts from 3 to 7 years of age when the erogenous zone moves to the genitals. The child, for the first time, distinguishes the difference between the sexes. The boy forms an attachment for the mother (the Oedipus situation) and hostility for the father. The association of guilt over the Oedipus situation and recognition of the female lack of a penis leads to a 'castration anxiety'. In girls, a 'penis envy' occurs with father affection (the Electra situation) and hostility to the mother. Out of the healthy resolution of Oedipal and Electra situations are developed the normal feminine and masculine attitudes and ideals. Unresolved Oedipal and Electra complexes are regarded as the basis for a wide variety of psychoneurotic, psychotic and personality problems. If the child undergoes profound emotional trauma at any stage, maturation ceases and he may regress to a previous period of emotional satisfaction where he becomes fixated – for example at the oral or anal phases. The latency period then supervenes and lasts until puberty. The child is concerned with the acquisi- of social skills and with adjusting to extra-familial groups. With the onset of puberty the child starts his move into the adult world, painfully going through a series of real experiences as compared with what were previously mainly fantasy experiences, and emerging in the end as an adult person.

Psycho-biological psychiatry

Theories of psychiatry are usually sharply divided between the psychological and the physical. Adolf Meyer considered that illness could only be understood by taking into account the psychological, biological and environmental situation of the individual. The doctor must manipulate the social, medical and psychological environments of the sick person, whose sickness is seen as a reaction to a number of factors. The type of personality will colour the manifestations of illness, mental or physical so that, particularly in mental illness, it is important to distinguish between what is the reaction of a certain personality to certain external circumstances, and what is a truly endogenous illness. British psychiatry is, in general, based on psychobiological theory.

Psychodrama

Primarily a form of group psychotherapy (q.v.) which involves a structured, directed and dramatized acting out (q.v.) of the patient's personal and emotional problems as well as his immediate group interaction problems. It has been used in schizophrenia in which further understanding and interpretation of the patient's illness is attempted, based on the concept of faulty communication in schizophrenia associated with projection of feelings and experiences onto others in the group. Neurotics with motor disturbances, such as stammering or tics have been treated in this way. In homosexuals, psychodrama is used as a reconditioning-behavioural technique.
Psychodrama is based on the principle that action and dramatic psychotherapy allows greater depth of awareness than is available by verbal means. Spontaneity, rather than insight, is the goal. The acting subject (patient) is called the protagonist. The therapist leads the production in accordance with clues provided by the patient about his basic anxieties, conflicts and frustrations. Auxiliary egos are provided by other members of the group who act out the roles directed by the therapist in order to intensify the impact or clarify the meaning of the transference situation. SEE ALSO Psychotherapy.

Psychogenesis of organic disease
SEE Psychosomatic disorders.

Psychological changes in normal and abnormal ageing

1. *Intellectual changes.* Normal ageing is accompanied by reduction in speed of response, in some impairment of memory (q.v.), in perceiving new relations and learning new material, and in the capacity for abstract thought. Scientific originality lessens, though artistic creativity may persist to an advanced age. There is a falling off of performance on cognitive tests, e.g. the Weschler Adult Intelligence Scale (q.v.), so that IQs must be standardized for age. However, there is much individual variation in the rate of decline so that differences tend to become accentuated.

Moreover, abilities do not all decline equally, and psychological tests may cover a wide range of skills. Well-established ('crystalline') knowledge, e.g. vocabulary, is usually preserved, while the power to solve new problems ('fluid' ability) declines. Non-verbal tests, which involve sensori-motor abilities, tend to show more decline than verbal tests.

Clinically, the question often arises whether an old person's mental decline is or is not excessive for his age, since if it is, further investigation may be indicated. Psychological tests may reveal that the present IQ (age corrected) is incompatible with the patient's educational standing and occupational history, which will suggest that his decline is pathological. The IQ derived from the verbal part of the test is often used to give an estimate of the previous intellectual capacity, and the difference between this and the non-verbal IQ then regarded as an 'index of deterioration'. However, this and similar indices are not of great clinical value, since considerable verbal-performance discrepancy may exist at any age. Moreover verbal abilities themselves eventually decline if the disease progresses. Lesions in the dominant hemisphere may cause dysphasias. Repeated testing will be more revealing than single tests.

Test performance is also reduced in the presence of anxiety, depression or a psychotic illness. The best discrimination between supposedly 'organic' and 'non-organic' patients is obtained by tests which measure the ability to learn new material, e.g. the new word learning or paired associate learning tests, which correctly classify about 75% of patients according to clinical diagnosis. When there is clinical doubt, however, the tests themselves are often equivocal.

Simple clinical methods will betray gross cerebral disease or dysfunction. The patient's orientation in time and space, and for persons, and his memory for past and recent personal and general events are explored, and he is given simple tests of memory (name and address), mental arithmetic and concentration. Disorientation and loss of memory for recent events are characteristic of all severe organic states, but in dementia (q.v.) the errors are global and persistent, in acute confusional states (q.v.) patchy and fluctuating, and in amnesic syndromes other mental functions are relatively intact. Suitable tests may bring out features indicating involvement of the frontal, temporal or parietal lobes, or of the dominant or non-dominant hemisphere. The degree of dementia and its progress may be roughly quantified by asking the relatives or attendants to rate the patient's usual behaviour on a simple scale, on items such as the ability to dress, feed and keep himself clean, to perform simple tasks, to deal with money, and to orientate himself in and outside the house.

2. *Personality*. In many ways the personality remains stable in middle and old age. Some changes occur, however. Extroversion decreases, intraversion increases. Interests become less outward looking, more concerned with the immediate family and with the somatic changes in the person's own body. Attitudes become more rigid, opinions and habits more fixed. These changes affect neurotic traits and personality deviations. It is rare for psychopathic behaviour to persist into old age and even severe psychopaths become less antisocial. Neurotic 'acting-out' and manipulative behaviour of hysterical type tends to be replaced by verbal complaining. On the other hand anxious, depressive and obsessional traits become more marked. Sexual drive decreases, but individuals with a strong libido in youth, a habit of regular intercourse and a surviving partner may be sexually active into the eighth decade. Sexual aberrations are not uncommon (q.v.) but extramarital intercourse is uncommon.

It has been said that people come to resemble each other as they grow older. Existing evidence suggests the opposite: personality traits become exaggerated in the aged, who are 'themselves only more so', sometimes to the point of eccentricity. However, differences in the social roles of men and women become less marked. Me may take on housekeeping and child care while women become more aggressive and assertive, as exemplified in the stereotype of the elderly 'virago'.

There are various patterns of *adjustment* to ageing, which in themselves are neither good nor bad. It is often assumed that the greater the activity and involvement of old people, the better their adjustment to ageing. While this may often be true, a

frantic kind of overactivity may be 'counterphobic', i.e. a defence against neurotic breakdown, and suggests an unstable adjustment. A different pattern has been described as 'disengagement': there is a withdrawal from social ties and an increased self-absorption.
An important aspect is the attitude towards death. This is something which is seldom discussed by the aged, who often deny that it concerns them. Intense fears of death, and also strong wishes for it, are undoubtedly present in some of the abnormal affective states of the aged, and may reflect ambivalences which are rarely voiced by the normal elderly person. Acceptance of death without despair may be the main task of the personality in adjusting to old age.

Psychological dependence

A distinction is made between psychological dependence and physical dependence on drugs (q.v.) in the World Health Organisation terminology. Psychological dependence covers not only subjective pleasure from taking the drug, but also the emotional drives that lead the patient to persist in its use. These include the relief of feelings of distress, anxiety, etc. For the main drugs of dependence the situation is fairly clear, but it is often difficult to be certain whether psychological dependence is present with some of the psychotropic drugs used in patients. Such patients have anxiety and depression as the main pre-treatment symptoms. Thus removal of therapy may lead to the return of these symptoms and indeed may precipitate added anxiety as a result of the prospect of return to an unpleasant pre-treatment state. This has been confused by some physicians with psychological dependence. SEE ALSO Addiction.

Psychological tests

A psychological test is a formal assessment procedure, scored qualitatively or quantitatively and designed to ascertain the presence, absence or degree of a particular psychological characteristic or set of characteristics. Test procedures are frequently used for intellectual (q.v.) and personality (q.v.) assessment.
Intelligence tests consist of series of intellectual tasks or items, selected on an empirical basis, graded in difficulty and standardized by testing a representative sample of the relevant population to provide norms against which an individual's score may be assessed. The tester also requires statistical information concerning the reliability and validity of the test. Reliability is usually assessed by measuring the consistency of test scores on different occasions or with different testers. Validity, the degree to which a test measures what it purports to measure, may be assessed by correlating test scores with an external criterion measure such as marks in an examination. Group tests, e.g. Raven's 'progressive matrices' (q.v.), can be administered to a number of individuals simultaneously. The more time-consuming individual tests can only be administered to one person at a time by a skilled tester. Of these, a modern revision of the original Binet-Simon test (q.v.) is still widely used with children. The Wechsler Adult Intelligence Scale (WAIS) (q.v.) is the most popular test for adults. Children's test scores are frequently converted into *mental ages* (MA) (q.v.) based on the average scores achieved by children at each age level. Relative brightness is assessed by relating the mental age to the chronological age (CA) to calculate the intelligence quotient (IQ) (q.v.). Thus

$IQ = \frac{MA}{CA} \times 100$ and the expected IQ is 100.

However, an individual's mental age does not improve after adolescence. For this reason and because of a number of technical difficulties of a statistical nature the IQ, calculated in this way, is an unsatisfactory score especially when testing adults IQs derived from most modern tests are really 'standard' or 'deviation' scores. Percentiles provide another convenient measure.
Personality tests are mainly of two types: personality inventories (q.v.) and projective techniques (q.v.). A personality inventory is a self-report questionnaire, the subject being required to agree or disagree with or answer 'yes' or 'no' (or 'don't know') to a series of statements or questions. Scoring is objective, and the tests are standardized in similar ways to intelligence tests. Various biases affect res-

ponses to questionnaires and, despite ingenious devices to control these, the reliability and validity of a typical personality inventory is considerably less than those of most intelligence tests.

Projective techniques, such as the Rorschach (q.v.), ink blot test and the thematic apperception test (q.v.) involve the presentation of vague, unstructured or ambiguous stimuli to the subject. His responses are therefore largely determined by personal factors and are thought to reveal his characteristic modes of perception of and response to his environment. These techniques lack the objectivity of other types of psychological tests and require very expert interpretation. Even then, their validity is a matter of great dispute.

The main current psychological tests are shown in the following table.

SEE ALSO Mental deterioration and Mental subnormality.

Table of psychological tests*

Test	Type	Assesses	Age of Patient	Output	Administration
Bayley Scales of Infant Development	Infant development	Cognitive function and motor development	1–30 months	Performance on various tests measuring cognitive and motor development	Individual
Bender Visual-Motor Gestalt Test	Projective visual-motor development	Organic brain damage; also used for personality conflicts and ego function	5–adult	Patient copies visual designs	Individual
Benton Visual Retention Test	Objective performance	Organic brain damage	Adult	Patient reproduces visual designs from memory	Individual
Cattell Infant Intelligence Scale	Infant development	Yields mental age scores and IQ's	1–18 months	Performance on developmental tasks	Individual
Draw-A-Person Draw-A-Family House-Tree	Projective	Personality and intellectual performance	2–adult	Unstructured free-hand drawings	Individual
Eisenson Aphasia Examination	Laryngeal ability	Aphasia in organic brain damage	Adolescents and Adults	Profile of laryngeal function ratings	Individual
Eysenck Personality Inventory	Paper and pencil personality inventory	Personality structure	14 years +	Extroversion, neuroticism lie-scale score	Individual or group
Frostig (Marianne) Developmental Test of Visual Perception	Visual perception	Basic perceptuo-motor development	4–8 years	Structured drawings on disposable answer sheet	Individual or group
Gesell Developmental Schedules	Preschool development	Cognitive, motor, language and social development	1–60 months	Performance on developmental tasks	Individual
Illinois Test of Psycholinguistic Ability (ITPA)	Language ability	Psycholinguistic function in young children	2–10 years	Performance on 12 sub-tests measuring various dimensions of language functioning	Individual
Mill Hill Vocabulary Scale	Intelligence	Verbal ability	4½–60 years	Word definition	Individual or group

contd.

* Modified from a similar table in ***A Psychiatric Glossary,*** 4th edn., Amer. Psychiatric Ass. 1975.

Table of psychological tests—*contd.*

Test	Type	Assesses	Age of Patient	Output	Administration
Minnesota Multiphasic Personality Inventory (MMPI)	Paper and pencil personality inventory	Personality profile in psychiatric diagnostic terms	Adolescent–adult	Personality profile reflecting nine dimensions of personality Diagnosis based upon actuarial prediction	Group
Raven's Progressive Matrices	Intelligence	Inductive reasoning, persistence	8–65 years	Performance on visual problem solving items	Individual or group
Rorschach	Projective	Personality structure and pathology	3–adult	Patient's associations to inkblots	Individual
Stanford-Binet	Intelligence	Intellectual functioning	2–adult	Performance on problem solving and developmental tasks	Individual
Thematic Apperception Test (TAT) Child's Apperception Test (CAT)	Projective	Personality structure and pathology	Adult – TAT Child – CAT	Patient makes up stories after viewing stimulus pictures	Individual
Vineland Social Maturity Scale	Social maturity	Profile of concordance with development expectancy in 8 areas	0–25+ years	Performance on developmental tasks measuring various dimensions of social functioning	Interview parent, guardian or nurse
Wechsler Adult Intelligence Scale (WAIS)	Intelligence	Level of and changes in intellectual functioning	16–adult	Performance on 10 sub-tests measuring various dimensions of intellectual functioning	Individual
Wechsler Intelligence Scale for Children (WISC)	Intelligence	Level of and changes in intellectual functioning	5–15 years	Performance on 10 sub-tests measuring various dimensions of intellectual functioning	Individual
Wechsler Preschool and Primary Scale of Intelligence (WPPSI)	Intelligence	Level of and changes in intellectual functioning	4–6½ years	Performance on 10 sub-tests measuring various dimensions of intellectual functioning	Individual

Psychology – Schools of

SEE Schools of Psychology.

Psychomotor retardation

A term describing the slowing of mental functioning and of motor activity seen in manic-depressive depressions (q.v.). The patient rarely speaks spontaneously and his normal gestures and associated bodily movements are lost. In mild cases retardation can be so inconspicuous that it is only detected in retrospect, but sometimes the slowing and restriction are so extreme that they verge on stupor. In the past agitation and retardation were generally regarded as alternatives but this is

not so; the two can co-exist and fluctuate independently. The physiological basis of retardation is complex. What the observer perceives as slowing is experienced by the patient as difficulty, and physiological indices like the metabolic rate and the electromyogram make it clear that retarded patients are in a state of arousal rather than of inactivity. The main importance of the symptom is that its presence suggests that the depression is endogenous in type and that it is likely to respond to ECT.
The phrase 'mental retardation' (q.v.) has quite a different meaning, being a synonym for mental deficiency. Usually which sense is intended is clear from the context, but the double meaning is particularly unfortunate as the retardation of depression is not infrequently misinterpreted as stupidity.
SEE ALSO Motor disturbances.

Psychomotor seizures

A clinical description of epileptic fits characterized by a warning (aura) and a period of disturbed behaviour often followed by other seizure phenomena. Auras are difficult to elicit, the disturbed behaviour may be brief, the whole phenomenon unnoticeably transitory or else overwhelmed, in descriptive accounts, by the major convulsions which often ensue. In a psychomotor seizure there will be impairment of consciousness from dazedness to unconsciousness, motor behaviour from fiddling with the dress to orienting reactions, signs of autonomic dysfunction and often speech disturbances. Complex automatisms (q.v.) may occur. Subjective components in addition to auras (q.v.), include disturbances of emotion, perceptual illusions, and paramnesias.
Most psychomotor seizures are focal temporal lobe epilepsies (q.v.). However, lesions of the insula, inferior orbital cortex and the whole limbic system in general may provoke them. Static lesions of the temporal lobe are associated with chronic epilepsies, but psychomotor seizures may be symptomatic of advancing cerebral lesions. Temporal lobe tumours provoke anxiety and well-formed sensory experiences in addition to crude sensations from autonomic disturbances. Midline tumours contiguous to the limbic system may cause psychomotor seizures, memory disturbances and other symptoms more usually referable to the temporal lobe. There is no characteristic EEG, but it may show a focus in areas known to be conducive to the production of psychomotor seizures. Treatment is difficult, especially where there is automatic behaviour, but anticonvulsant treatment usually reduces the frequency of all attacks especially generalized seizures which supervene. Management includes consideration of the mental and behavioural disturbances with which these epilepsies are associated.
SEE ALSO Epilepsy.

Psychoneuroses

(Synonyms: Neuroses and Neurotic reaction types)

The psychoneuroses may be distinguished from the psychoses by the facts that emotional experience and behaviour is quantitatively, rather than qualitatively, different from normal, insight is usually present and relation to, and sense of, reality unimpaired. Personality deterioration, disorders of concrete thinking and loss of contact with reality do not occur as in the psychoses; nor does disorientation or confusion, as in the organic mental states. They are reactions in which anxiety, generated by the conflict between the subject and internal or external stresses, are typically defended against by such mechanisms as repression, conversion/dissociation, displacement, phobic avoidance and/or repetitive thoughts and acts. The subgroups include: anxiety reaction, dissociative (hysterical) reaction, phobic reaction, obsessive-compulsive reaction and psychoneurotic depressive reaction.
Freud's ideas on aetiology are based on fixation at certain levels of psychological development, e.g. oral, anal, phallic; the type of neurotic reaction being determined by the predominant mental defence mechanisms used, e.g. fixation at the anal level in obsessional neurotics with denial, projection and displacement as important mental mechanisms in symptom formation.
Pavlovian concepts are centred on the idea of neuroses as learnt behaviour patterns reinforced by continuing stress and anxiety avoidance behaviour, but capable

of extinction by appropriate behaviour therapy techniques. Neither theoretical framework is inconsistent with present evidence for an inherited predisposition to specific neurotic reactions, these reactions being precipitated by *personally significant* stress.

Prevalence of neurotic ill-health is high – some 15% of the population being significantly incapacitated by such symptoms.

In childhood certain habits, such as tics, stammers, enuresis, sleep-walking, etc., may indicate emotional maladjustment but specific phobias vary in their significance. Fear of the dark, loud noises, strangers are so common as to be almost universal. Persistent school refusal or phobia requires particular investigation into personal and family dynamics.

Certain neuroses have special characteristics. Compensation neurosis is unlikely to respond fully to treatment until the claim is settled one way or the other. Depersonalization most often occurs in a setting of phobic anxiety or in the young adult of rigid, obsessional disposition with depressive and anxiety features.

In general prognosis depends on constitutional liability to breakdown under stress, the severity of the stress itself, the ability to manipulate the environment satisfactorily and early treatment – appropriate to the specific neurotic reaction type and personality.

Treatment includes psychotherapy of appropriate type, the use of tranquillo-sedative or anti-depressant medication if necessary, behaviour therapy, social and environmental manipulation. Rarely prefrontal leucotomy is indicated in patients with severe, intractable and incapacitating tension.

Psychopathic disorders (psychopathic personality and psychopathic states)

This has been defined legally as a 'persistent disorder or disability of mind (whether or not including subnormality of intelligence) which results in abnormally aggressive or seriously irresponsible conduct on the part of the patient, and requires or is susceptible to medical treatment'. This definition has a large social component but other clinical features are implied in the term psychopath. Firstly, a failure of emotional learning (sometimes, but inadvisedly, called immaturity), in particular a failure to learn how to give and take love: in consequence an inability to form stable or satisfactory interpersonal relationships. Secondly, a failure to develop a normal conscience (or superego), i.e. guilt and remorse may be absent or pathological. Marked impulsivity of behaviour, emotional overreactiveness to stress, and an increased likelihood of EEG abnormalities are also described. Antisocial behaviour (q.v.) is a common consequence and many prisoner recidivists (q.v.) are psychopaths although not every psychopath falls foul of the law. It is less common in women. Psychotic episodes are not unknown complications (see Prison psychoses).

The aetiology is unclear. The disorder runs in families, probably due to a small genetic component and a large faulty training component. Most psychopaths come from emotionally unsatisfactory backgrounds where they suffered cruelty, deprivation of affection, rejection or wildly inconsistent handling as a child.

Such disorders usually start in childhood, but by no means all children with behaviour disorders (q.v.) will become psychopaths. It is wise to defer diagnosis at least until early adult life. Occasionally the disorder can follow severe brain damage.

Treatment for adult psychopaths is in general ineffective, although several methods of institutional therapy are in use at the special hospitals (q.v.), at psychiatric prisons (q.v.), and other selected centres.

Psychotherapy seeks to help the patient form satisfactory relationships, whilst attempting to avoid the particular stresses which precipitate his crimes and outbursts of impulsive or antisocial behaviour.

Psychopaths are encountered less frequently in later than in early adult life, partly because the condition tends to improve with time, and partly because it carries a high mortality via self-neglect, accident, suicide, and other forms of violence.

SEE ALSO Forensic psychiatry, Child psychiatry, and Behaviour disorders in childhood.

Psychopharmacology

Psychopharmacology can be defined as the study of drugs which predominantly affect psychological processes and behaviour. It includes consideration of drug action on both normal and abnormal processes within the higher functions of the central nervous system. The development of psychopharmacology is essentially a modern phenomenon, but its roots go back to antiquity and originate in the ingenuity shown by primitive man in discovering in nature powerful agents which affect the mind.

A number of terms have been coined to express concepts of various types of activity. The general terms psychotropic and psychoactive designate substances acting directly or indirectly on the central nervous system and affecting mental and emotional processes; psychotropic, psychoactive and psychopharmacological are synonymous terms.

More specific names have been used to emphasize the principal actions of the various categories of psychotropic compounds. The tranquillizers (q.v.) are basically inhibitory in action, and produce calmness without impairment of consciousness. They include both the major tranquillizers or neuroleptic (q.v.) agents; the minor tranquillizers or anxiolytic (q.v.) compounds; hypnotic or sleep-inducing drugs; and narcotic analgesics. Antidepressant or thymoleptic (q.v.) drugs have an indirect stimulant action on the central nervous system and elevate depressed mood, whereas those drugs acting directly are called psychostimulants. There remains a group of compounds which have disorganizing effects on mental function. The term hallucinogenic highlights the ability to produce hallucinatory experience, psychotomimetic the relationship of the symptoms to the psychoses.

A more detailed consideration of classification will be found under Classification of psychotropic drugs.

Psychosis

The term psychosis refers to mental illness which is severe, produces conspicuously disordered behaviour, cannot be understood as an extension or exaggeration of ordinary experience and whose subject is without insight. The term may be used if any of these elements is present and is antonymous to the term 'psychoneurosis' (q.v.) in which they are not prominent. In fact the term is not a useful one and there would be no loss to psychiatry if the term was discarded. Some schizophrenics have good insight into their condition and are able to live and work in the community, while some hysterics have no insight and have to be hospitalized. Similarly endogenous depressions may be mild and neurotic depressions severe with repeated serious suicidal behaviour.

SEE ALSO Geriatric psychiatry.

Psychosis in childhood

The criteria by which psychosis is recognized in early childhood are necessarily different from those used in adulthood. For example, it is not easy in the young child to decide whether there is a lack of contact with reality or whether insight is lacking. By convention, however, the term psychosis is used to refer to types of severe mental disorder of infancy in which the child fails to develop or loses any capacity for social relationships despite other evidence of intellectual adequacy. Childhood autism (q.v.) is the most common form of psychosis in infancy and early childhood. It may be apparent from birth or there may be a period of normal development lasting anything up to two and a half years, followed by regression.

Dementia in childhood is rare, and is always a consequence of organic disease of the brain. Any child whose mental functioning shows clear evidence of deterioration (as opposed to failure to progress) is likely to be suffering from organic brain disease. Cerebral tumour, hypsarrhythmia, cerebral lipoidoses, metachromatic leucodystrophy and subacute sclerosing panencephalitides constitute most organic pathology in this age-group.

The functional psychoses, manic-depressive psychosis and schizophrenia, occur only rarely before puberty. With the onset of adolescence, however, the functional psychoses present more commonly, and by the time late adolescence is reached, the peak age for the appearance of premonit-

ory symptoms of schizophrenia has been achieved.
SEE ALSO Child psychiatry.

Psychosomatic disorders

A heterogenous group of illnesses in which psychosocial events can be shown to have a direct relationship to the production of the symptoms and signs of an otherwise apparently physical disorder. They include bronchial asthma, peptic ulcer, some forms of hypertension, of coronary thrombosis. skin conditions, such as eczema, psoriasis and urticaria, a wide range of sexual disturbances, such as impotence, premature ejaculation, menorrhagia, amenorrhoea and so on. In all these conditions the relationship between emotion and physical disturbance is such that physicians cannot avoid recognizing the connection, and as a result this somewhat spurious term came into use. Today it is better to speak of the psychosomatic approach to medicine, that is, the concurrent physical and mental examination of the sick person. Illness in general, of whatever type, is conceived as a reaction by the organism to a variety of changing events both in the external and internal environments. The capacity to react to changing circumstances determines whether the organism remains healthy, falls ill, recovers or dies. All illness is psychosomatic, physical and psychological changes being part of the total response of the organism. The genetical make-up of the individual is of great importance – a relatively weak stimulus from the external environment producing marked changes in the suitably predisposed individual, whilst in others of a different genetical make-up the same stimulus would produce no effect. Illness is considered to be multifactorially determined; for instance in bronchial asthma an attack will often only result when a number of allergic, emotional and infective factors combine to, as it were, trigger off the attack. The form of the illness is dictated by stock, genetic and constitutional factors reacting to a particular environment. Thus under difficult life conditions the illnesses European soldiers develop in tropical countries are different from those experienced in subarctic Siberia.
For the clinician this theoretical approach is important, for it enables him to understand the changes that are going on in his patient's body, as well as in his psychosocial environment. A three-part question should be posed – Why does this particular individual fall ill in this particular way at this particular time? On an understanding of the answers the physician will be aided in formulating a comprehensive diagnosis, therapy and prognosis. The psychosomatic approach to medicine takes into account both mental and physical factors in illness; it has no commitment to either psychological or physical methods of treatment, or to any particular school of psychology.

Psychostimulants

Psychostimulants are drugs which exert a direct stimulant effect on the central nervous system to produce alertness and a general facilitation of psychological processes. A distinction is thus drawn between psychostimulants and convulsants. The main established groups of compounds are the amphetamines (q.v.), other sympathomimetic drugs (q.v.), and xanthines, of which caffeine (q.v.) is the most potent stimulant. In recent years an increasing and heterogenous collection of psychostimulants have been introduced, particularly in the USA. The following compounds are included in this group: methylphenidate, fencamfamine, pipradol, cyprolidol, deanol, pyrovalerone, trioxazine, and centrophenoxine. These compounds have not yet been available for long enough to achieve a firm basis of clinical experience, but they are likely to have similar drawbacks to the amphetamines.
The value of psychostimulants in psychoneurosis, depressive illness, and schizophrenic apathy is controversial to say the least, but when such highly dubious diagnostic categories as chronic nervous exhaustion, neurasthenia, and chronic fatigue are considered then their value is extremely doubtful. Certainly psychostimulants do not form the basis of treatment of clearly defined psychiatric illness, but are more likely to be used as a measure of desperation in the face of unremitting illness and a persistently complaining patient. Indiscriminate use of psycho-

stimulants in psychiatric practice should be avoided.

There are several organic conditions where amphetamines are of established value, and it may be useful to have alternative compounds available. Post-encephalitic Parkinsonism, epilepsy, narcolepsy, and hyperkinesis in children fall within this category.

Psychosurgery

Egas Moniz introduced the standard operation of leucotomy in 1935. This was found to relieve intolerable states of tension and anxiety by interrupting the connections between the frontal cortex and the dorsomedial nuclei of the thalamus. The original operation has been modified repeatedly to attain therapeutic efficacy with the minimum of side effects. The most popular operations are bimedial leucotomy and orbital undercutting; other procedures consist of 'blind' rostral leucotomy, the implantation of radioactive yttrium in the frontal connections, stereotactic thalamotomy and cingulectomy.

The operation is indicated in patients suffering from intractable tension, with a stable and driving personality. Immediate symptomatic relief is often obtained, and thorough rehabilitative measures add to the successful outcome. The operation may decrease the patient's self-control, and although rarely of significance in stable personalities, this is undesirable in patients with unstable and psychopathic traits.

Psychotherapy

This refers to the method of treating illness based on the use of psychological rather than physical techniques. It varies in complexity from the simplest supportive psychotherapy, aimed at aiding the patient to overcome immediate difficulties by guidance, environmental manipulation (q.v.), reassurance (q.v.), persuasion (q.v.), cathartic techniques leading to abreaction (q.v.), to the more complex psychoanalytically orientated psychotherapies, such as psychoanalysis (q.v.) based on the work of Freud, whose object is a reorientation of the patient's personality by interpretation of its defences. Behaviour therapies (q.v.), such as desensitization (q.v.) in phobic states, aversion therapy (q.v.) in alcoholism and sexual deviations and operant or 'positive' conditioning (q.v.) as used in childhood autism, are included. Hypnosis (q.v.) may sometimes be used as a technique for obtaining relaxation in desensitization procedures or suggestion in supportive therapies.

In children play therapy (q.v.) techniques utilizing objects representing emotionally important figures, such as the parents, may be used to help analysis of underlying conflicts, and a permissive environment in the therapeutic play room helps to demonstrate important emotional attitudes, especially in the restricted, overdominated child.

The doctor-patient relationship is of vital importance. In supportive techniques deliberate use of the patient's faith and good will in the physicians omniscience and personal interest is fostered.

In more formal analytic therapies, the transference (q.v.) situation is allowed to develop more spontaneously – reflecting the patient's projection onto the therapist of feelings of love or hate which are analysed according to their earlier, original appropriate source. Any psychotherapy may be undertaken individually or in a group, the latter usually comprising about eight patients with the therapist.

Existential analysis stresses the importance of the patients own personal experience of his existence and significance in his environment.

Psychotic depression

SEE Depression.

Psychotic parents

Severe mental disorders in parents inpinge on the life of their children in a number of different ways. The effect of puerperal psychosis depends on its form, its duration, and its impact on mothering capacity. If the mother makes a complete recovery within the first six months of life and is thereafter capable of looking after her child, the effect on the child's life may be negligible. Parental schizophrenia and manic-depressive psychosis obviously present severe stresses to a child's emo-

tional life, and the effect they have will depend largely on the amount the child is exposed to morbid behaviour. It is perhaps surprising that the rate of childhood psychiatric disorder is lower in the children of psychotics than in the children of parents with neurosis or personality disorders. The explanation of this finding probably lies in the overriding importance of harmonious family relationships in normal child development. The parent with a personality disorder is more likely to show disturbance in marital and parental relationships.
SEE ALSO Child psychiatry.

Psychotomimetic drugs

Psychotomimetic drugs are characterized by their ability to induce disturbance of mood, thought and perception in doses sufficiently small to avoid peripheral effects of any magnitude. These compounds are of no general therapeutic value although they have had some rather special use in psychiatry for abreactive purposes and to facilitate psychotherapy; their effectiveness is equivocal. The main general interest lies in their propensity for abuse.

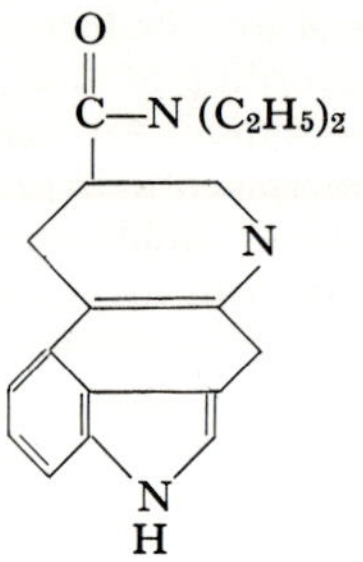

Lysergide

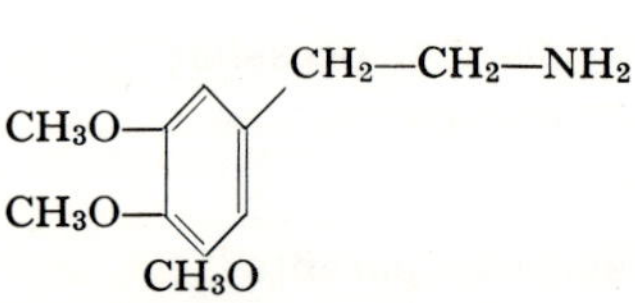

Mescaline

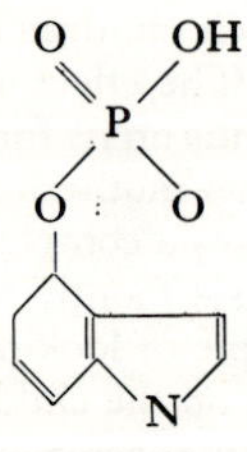

Psilocybin

Some hallucinogenic drugs

The three most important compounds are lysergic acid diethylamide (LSD), psilocybin and mescaline, but there are many others. Lysergide is a synthetic product related to the ergot alkaloids and it is the most potent and most extensively used member of the group. Psilocybin and mescaline were originally both natural products used for religious rites by the indigenous natives of Mexico; the former is obtained from the Mexican mushroom, and the latter is the active ingredient of peyote, the dried tops of the Mexican cactus peyotl.
The effects of these compounds show a striking similarity, and what differences occur may be related to personality factors rather than specific drug effects. Mild somatic symptoms are common and include gastrointestinal disturbance, headache, dizziness, and autonomic symptoms. The commonest affective change is intense anxiety, and this frequently wears off to be superseded by euphoria or hypomania often alternating dangerously with profound depression. Paranoid ideas may lead to aggressive behaviour. Cognitive changes include indecision, distractability and a looser less-discriminative stream of thought. Introspection is typically increased and associated mystical experience is common but often disappointing. The most striking response is perceptual disturbance which is usually visual or tactile; at first the experiences are illusory but not uncommonly develop into hallucinations. Colour, texture, shape, perspective, and time become disconcertingly variable and are frequently accompanied by distortion of the body image. Synaesthesia is a common and interesting phenomenon in which the distinction between the sensory modalities is lost; for example a sound may be associated with an experience of colour or smell.
The concept of drug-induced model psychosis was developed, based on the resemblance between the subjective results of taking psychotomimetic drugs and the experiences described in psychotic illness, but there are recognizable qualitative differences.
Psychotomimetic substances have danger-

ous adverse effects. Psychological dependence rapidly predisposes the indulgent to drug abuse. But more serious is the precipitation of irreversible psychotic illness; this disastrous occurrence was epitomized by a patient with florid schizophrenic symptoms when he described how he had at first taken trips with LSD, but now he could manage trips without it. Prolonged states of anxiety and depression occur, and suicide is becoming increasingly recognized as a consequence of psychotomimetic indulgence.
A number of tranquillizers interfere with the effects of psychotomimetic drugs, and chlorpromazine is the most reliable in this respect.

Psychotropic drugs

Psychotropic drugs are substances which act directly or indirectly on the central nervous system to affect mental and emotional processes. Alternative terms are psychoactive (q.v.) and psychopharmacological.
For classification and cross reference SEE Classification of psychotropic drugs.

Puberty

Adolescence is notoriously a time of emotional turmoil. Changes in endocrine function contribute to this turmoil in various ways. They are, of course, responsible for the physical changes of puberty: these changes are particularly disturbing if they occur either much earlier or much later than in the child's peers. Hormonal changes are also basically responsible for the awakening of adult sexuality. This inevitably requires considerable psychological adjustment and may cause persistent emotional disturbance if previous psychological development has been abnormal.
SEE ALSO Adolescence.

Puerperal psychoses

Acute organic psychoses in the early puerperium are now rare, because of advances in obstetrics. Functional psychoses are notably commoner in the early puerperium than in pregnancy. Both depression and schizophrenia occur, mania is rare. The aetiology is unknown, but hormonal changes may act as precipitants.
Puerperal psychoses differ from psychoses occurring at other times only in that they are more liable to begin acutely and in a setting of transient clouding of consciousness. In the early stages both schizophrenic and affective features may be evident.
The prognosis with treatment is generally good. Milder cases of depression may be treated at home, but schizophrenia and severe depression are best treated in hospital, because of the risk of suicide and infanticide. Both mother and baby should be admitted, if possible. Most patients needing admission respond well to electroconvulsive treatment, supplemented by appropriate drugs. Careful follow-up is essential.
SEE ALSO Post-partum disorders.

Punch drunk
(Synonym: Boxer's encephalopathy)

The syndrome applied to pugilists who have sustained repeated brain traumata. The severity of the syndrome varies from a mild clumsiness of speech and movement to ataxia, dysarthria, Parkinsonism and intellectual deterioration. Excessive aggression and rage reactions may occur. Pathological changes in the brain include lesions of the septum pellucidum, scarring of the cerebellar cortex especially on the inferior surface of the lateral lobes, degeneration of the substantia nigra and neurofibrillary changes in the medial temporal grey matter.

Pyknolepsy

A form of epilepsy in children characterized by very frequent attacks of petit mal.

Pyromania

A morbid compulsion to set fire (see Arson).

Quasi-psychotic states
SEE Ganser syndrome.

Questionnaires

Many enquiries are now undertaken by questionnaires, presented by an interviewer or answered by the respondent without guidance. Usually the respondent answers questions about himself by marking the appropriate alternative on a sheet of questions, e.g. Can you usually go to sleep easily at night? Yes/No/?
Advántages of using a questionnaire are ease of administration and objectivity of scoring. The objective scoring categories allow the formation of norms with consequent ability to compare individuals in numerical terms. By using an established questionnaire investigators gain access to a useful pool of accumulated information. Questionnaires have been constructed for many purposes and activities: smoking behaviour, voting intention, job interests, personality characteristics, medical symptoms.
The major disadvantage, if self-report information is to be accepted as typical behaviour, is honesty. The respondent may deliberately distort his answer if gain may accrue, or unintentionally distort his answer if his view of himself is inaccurate.
In using established questionnaires care should be taken that the available norms are appropriate for the intended respondent. In constructing and using a new questionnaire, expert help should be sought on the preparation of questions and the analysis of pilot data before the final version is composed.

Random sampling numbers

A table of random sampling numbers is used when a perfect random sample of a population is required. Other apparently haphazard procedures may be influenced by bias.

Range

The range is the variation which exists between the highest and the lowest observation in a series. While this gives an indication of the extent and variability of observations in a series, other methods of indication are preferable – see, for example, Standard deviation. The range as a means of measurement gives no indication of the frequency of individual observations, and a particularly distorted picture of the series when there are outlying single observations.

Rape

Sexual intercourse with a woman against her will, whether affected by force, fraud, or intimidation, is a crime of men under the age of 25. There are a number of common situations in which rape occurs, such as after a party, when alcohol has been used excessively, or when gangs of youths forcibly abduct a girl on the way home from a dance and commit multiple rapes. The dangerous rapist is the man who, suffering from intense hostility or resentment towards women, waylays his victim and violently assaults her physically before raping her. The crime may be repeated until the offender is apprehended, a veritable reign of terror occurring in a particular vicinity. Rapists of this sort are particularly dangerous, being usually cold and brutal individuals whose violence verges on sadism. Attempts are often made to throw blame on the woman involved for leading the man on, and whilst there are girls who suddenly become frightened during sexual activity, and panic, in fact this situation is no excuse for forcible intercourse. Treatment is not recommended, and the doctor should exercise considerable caution when dealing with the psychiatric aspects of rape.
SEE ALSO Sado-masochism.

Rationalization

The ego has the task of adjusting the individual to reality, to recognize things for what they are, not for what they seem to be, so that survival can be based on an appropriate adjustment to the environment. It is difficult to reconcile these functions with the narcissistic and instinctual demands of the individual, the self-esteem that is a derivative of narcissism. Rationalization is a process, partly conscious and partly unconscious, whereby failures or mistakes are excused, both to the self and to others, thus preserving self-esteem.

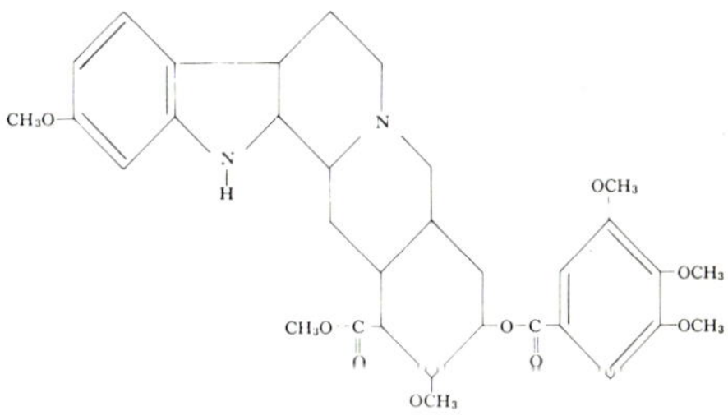

Reserpine, a Rauwolfia alkaloid

Rauwolfia alkaloids

Rauwolfia alkaloids are the active compounds from Rauwolfia serpentina. The principal alkaloid reserpine was widely prescribed both as an antihypertensive and a psychotropic agent in the 1950's. Reserpine depletes stored amines (q.v.) in both the central and peripheral nervous systems. Central amine depletion is the basis of its psychotropic activity and there is a characteristic delay in the appearance of clinical effects. The actions and side effects of reserpine show a broad similarity to those of phenothiazine compounds, but depression reaching psychotic severity was a particular disadvantage.
The advent of more effective drugs has largely displaced reserpine from clinical practice. They have limited use in certain severely disturbed psychotic patients and in Huntington's chorea.

Raven's progressive matrices

An intelligence test in which the subject chooses, from several alternatives, the appropriate part to complete an abstract design which is presented to him. The designs become progressively more complex. It is a test of non-verbal intelligence, is easy to administer, and is a useful tool for use with large populations.
SEE ALSO Psychological tests.

Reaction-formation

An unconscious defence mechanism whereby the person develops attitudes and patterns of behaviour which are directly opposite to the underlying impulses.

Reactive depression

The antonym of endogenous (psychotic) depression, reactive depressions are the result of environmental events such as the loss of a loved person or cherished possession. In a truly reactive depression the content and degree of the patient's depressive thoughts must be entirely explicable in terms of the experience, the condition would not have arisen without this experience, and the symptoms disappear on removal of the cause. In fact pure reactive depressions are uncommon and in nearly every case there is evidence of a constitutional factor and very often psychogenic factors as well. In any particular patient the problem should be how much is the depression due to endogenous, reactive and psychogenic factors, rather than either/or.
In many countries, including the USA, the term has gone into disuse, reactions to both external and internal stresses and conflicts being included under the term 'depressive neurosis'.

Reality-principle

In psychoanalytical theory the pleasure principle (q.v.) which represents the instinctive gratification wish is modified by the demands of the external world – the reality-principle.

Reassurance

Reassurance depends on the acceptance by the patient of the superior knowledge of the doctor, an acceptance which is determined by both conscious and unconscious factors. Reassurance may be both verbal and non-verbal, the mere presence of the doctor being sufficient to comfort the sick person, and to allay his anxieties. The universal need for security and dependence during illness experience provides the setting in which the doctor exerts his capacity for reassurance, which must include explanation of the symptom production.

Recall

The process of returning a memory to consciousness. The term is used in psychiatry to refer to the recollection of facts or events in the immediate past.

Receiver

An official appointed in the English legal system to manage the property and affairs (not the persons) of patients who by reason of mental disorder (q.v.) are unable to do so themselves. He acts on the patient's behalf and may be regarded as the statutory agent of the patient.
SEE ALSO Curator bonis, Testamentary capacity, Forensic psychiatry, and Judicial factor.

Receptors in the sympathetic nervous system

Two different peripheral receptors for catecholamines (adrenaline and noradrenaline) exist in the sympathetic nervous system. These are termed the α and β receptors. The α receptors are associated with contraction of smooth muscle and respond more to noradrenaline than do the β receptors. These latter receptors relax smooth muscle when stimulated by catecholamines. The β receptors have been subdivided recently into β_1 and β_2 receptors.

Recidivists

A minority of law breakers who persist in offending. The majority of offenders are young men who commit one or at the most two crimes. Most recidivists are psychopaths, with poor work records, a family history of criminality, increased alcohol intake, and disturbed interpersonal relationships. Whatever method of control is tried, whether probation, prison, or parole, the recidivist does not learn by experience, and continues to re-offend, thus causing endless social and personal disturbance.
SEE ALSO Forensic psychiatry.

Reciprocal inhibition

This is a term used in learning theories and the behaviour therapy techniques derived therefrom for the treatment of neurotic symptoms – usually phobic. It is firmly based on animal experimentation. It is found that if a psychological and physical state is produced that is mutually opposite to that found in the pathological state (i.e. a state of relaxation (q.v.)) it is possible to undertake graded retraining to eventual extinction of the undesirable response. For example, relaxation induced either by practice and suggestion or the use of short-acting intravenous barbiturates enables a phobic patient to work through a hierarchy related to his phobic object or situation – from the least frightening idea associated with it up to the most fearful. The patient is desensitized gradually, step by step in his own self-constructed hierarchy. Monosymptomatic phobic states, e.g. dog phobia and impotence (gynophobia), respond best in general. Remission rate has been reported as high as 80–90% in some series.
SEE ALSO Behaviour therapy.

Re-employment

Return to employment is one of the most important aspects of rehabilitation (q.v.) although with serious psychiatric illness impaired levels of skill and responsibility may result. In such cases in Britain the Disablement Resettlement Officer in collaboration with social workers either from the hospital or community, may be of assistance. Attendance at one of the industrial rehabilitation units (q.v.) or a training centre is often helpful. If the patient cannot return to open industry, it may be possible to obtain a place for him in one of the special factories which have been established in some communities.

Reference, ideas of
SEE Ideas of reference.

Registration

The term applied to the initial phase of the memory (q.v.) process. Items to be remembered have first to receive selective attention (q.v.) within the perceptual field. Modern research suggests that they then pass initially into a short-term storage system before some are transferred to long-term memory. Tests of memory-span are concerned with this short-term or immediate memory.
SEE ALSO Mental examination, Perception, and Retention.

Regression

Faced with unsatisfying or anxiety arousing situations, a return to an earlier, happier stage of mental life, a regression, is a commonplace experience. In general, during mental development, the individual advances a little, retreats a little, and masters his new goals little by little. Regression may be used to avoid the solution of the problem – the individual remaining obstinately fixed at a certain, to the individual, satisfying developmental stage. Earlier patterns of behaviour come into action once more, but are unsuitable for the current situation. To advance means danger, to remain fixated at a previous stage of development is a compromise between instinctual demands and fear of their consequences. The patient suffers and many of his symptoms can only be understood if the degree and stage of his regression can be recognized by the therapist.

Rehabilitation

Rehabilitation is the process of being restored to functioning as a fairly normal person, in two main respects – work and social living. In the case of psychiatric patients, it is required mainly for schizophrenics and for those who have had brain injury or surgery. The process should normally begin in hospital, through occupational and industrial therapy, and through increasing independence in the patient's daily life, There are also psychiatrically disabled persons living in their own homes who need the industrial therapy units and therapeutic social clubs on a daily basis. The supervision of a social worker is vital in this process, as well as the over-all medical direction of psychiatrist and general practitioner.

Rejection

Survey evidence confirms the clinical impression that it is very common for mothers to experience dismay and disappointment on finding that they have conceived. However, assuming the pregnancy goes to term, it is unusual for maternal feeling not to be aroused by the movements of the infant *in utero*, and later by the sight of the infant and its response to affection.

Deep-seated rejecting attitudes persist, especially in parents suffering from personality disorders. However, sometimes the dislike of one particular child is an isolated psychopathological phenomenon occasionally persisting as an aftermath of puerperal depression. It need hardly be stated that as parental warmth is the single most necessary ingredient for healthy child personality development, so parental rejection is potent in the production of child psychiatric disorder.

Rejection of the aged patient

Community care of the aged patient places an increasing burden on the family, and when this becomes intolerable rejection may occur. Burdens that sooner or later become unacceptable include faecal smearing, persisting urinary incontinence, violence and abuse, disturbances at night and severe restriction on the family's social life or earning power.

If admission to hospital is delayed too long, then a stage will be reached when whatever help, support or temporary relief is offered after discharge, children will refuse to accept the care of their parents again in spite of strong guilt feelings and moral pressure from others.

If difficulties in interpersonal relationships have existed for some time and care of the aged relative is mainly motivated by guilt, a sense of duty or social propriety, rejection will occur at an earlier stage. Prodromal signs of rejection may include inexplicable 'emergency' calls to visit the patient, dissatisfaction with every attempt to assist in management, complaints and criticisms about the treatment or those giving it, and an increasing number of 'mistakes' with administration of drugs or in keeping hospital appointments. An overprotective attitude towards the patient may also be significant.

An awareness of the possibility of rejection, the prompt offer of temporary relief, and good channels of communication to reduce the family's sense of isolation, may help to prolong effective home care.

Relaxation

A state of repose in which voluntary skeletal musculature is inactive and muscle tone reduced, associated with mental calmness. Repeated training may be necessary to attain this state which is used in behaviour therapy (q.v.) techniques such as that of reciprocal inhibition (q.v.) for the treatment of certain phobias. The subject is placed in his most comfortable prone position so that muscle work against gravity is eliminated. Suggestion (q.v.) in hypnosis is aimed to produce this state as a prerequisite of trance. Short-acting intravenous barbiturates can be used to obtain reliable and immediate relaxation.

Relaxation therapy

Training in deep muscular relaxation forms part of most techniques of systematic desensitization, but can also be useful alone, particularly when patients are anxious and therefore preoccupied and unable to cope, and hence more anxious, caught in a kind of vicious spiral. In one simple technique the subject sits comfortably and is asked to concentrate on the words of the therapist, who repeats a series of phrases in a quiet, rhythmical and monotonous voice – 'let your toes (emphasized) – pause – relax, let the soles (emphasized) of you feet – relax', and so on to include the whole body.

Remand homes

Remand homes are now being replaced by a co-ordinated system of community homes (q.v.).

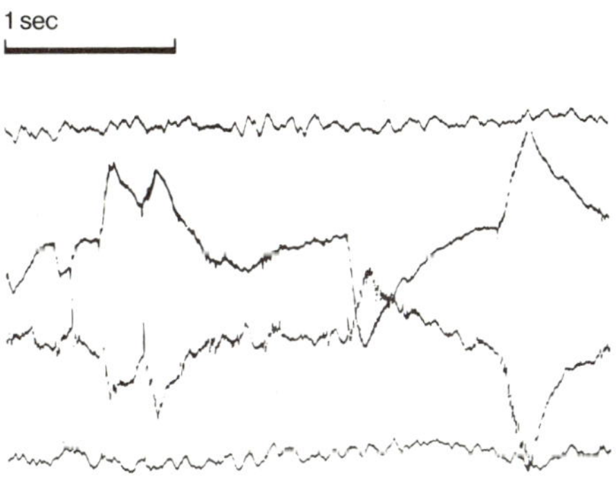

A portion of the electro-encephalogram in REM sleep

REM sleep

Rapid eye movements (REM) are one of the features of paradoxical sleep (q.v.). REM may occur in short bursts of as many as fifty rapid movements from side to side. This phase of sleep is cyclical and makes up 20–25% of sleep in the normal human. It is at present suggested that the REM sleep phase corresponds to brain repair.

Repetition-compulsion

The repetition of patterns of behaviour which serve no useful or pleasurable purpose is frequently observed amongst human beings. It appears that there is a powerful instinctually derived compulsion in some individuals producing this non-goal directed activity. The condition is seen in many types of neurosis and character disorder; it is as if the same gramophone record is switched on in various life situations, playing the same tune, and leading to the same dissatisfactions.

Repression

This is the active, but unconscious, mental mechanism by which ideas or impulses that are unacceptable to consciousness are ejected from it and are held from entering awareness. Such material is not ordinarily subject to voluntary conscious recall. Anxiety is the force which brings about repression and anxiety is experienced if there is the threat of the repressed material entering consciousness. Repression is the foremost defence mechanism especially against the demands of the sexual drives. Freud postulated that repression of sexual desires may give rise to a paranoid reaction by the secondary mechanisms of projection and reaction formation. In this instance the impulse is not only projected onto others so that subjective ideas and wishes are attributed to another, but their sexual nature is converted into hatred by reaction formation so that the subject experiences feelings of hostility or persecution from others. Depression may occur if aggressive feelings have been repressed. Subsequent real or phantasied loss results in introjection of the damaged object and identification with it.
SEE ALSO Displacement.

Respiratory disease

Emotional factors affect the respiratory system, notably in asthma (q.v.) and the hyperventilation syndrome (q.v.). In respiratory failure, clouding of consciousness or delirium may occur and bronchial carcinoma (q.v.), which is either non-metastatic or with cerebral secondaries, may give rise to psychiatric symptoms.
SEE ALSO Psychosomatic disorders.

Responsibility

In British law an individual is deemed responsible for his actions (both civil and criminal) in the sense that he is legally accountable for them, unless he or his attorney can show that he is under the

appropriate age of responsibility for that particular action or did not have the necessary 'intent' at the time of his action. The concept of intent is a legal one.
SEE ALSO Criminal responsibility and Diminished responsibility.

Retardation
SEE Psychomotor retardation, Mental retardation, and Mental subnormality

Retention

The term applied to the intermediate phase of the memory (q.v.) process, intervening between registration (q.v.) and recall (q.v.). Items to be memorized are transferred from the short-term storage of immediate memory by a process involving the consolidation of an enduring memory-trace or engram (q.v.), possibly of a biochemical nature, within the central nervous system. Retention can only be assessed indirectly by tests of recall.
SEE ALSO Attention and Mental Examination.

Reticular formation

The reticular formation is the diffuse central core of the neuraxis extending from the bulbar region to the medial thalamus. There are few well-defined nuclei or tracts but many small subcentres which influence most input to and output from higher centres. The ascending reticular formation initiates and sustains activity of these higher centres by activating the thalamus and cortex. It is thus involved in the mediation of consciousness (q.v.) and alertness and in the direction of attention (q.v.). It also modifies sensory inputs, and modulates transmission along many nerve tracts. On the effector side, the reticular formation influences spinal mechanisms and exerts control over many visceral functions, linking together voluntary and involuntary components of the response of the body.

Retirement

Retirement is considered as a major stress for men, because there is loss of status and income as well as lack of occupation.
Retirement is a phenomenon of Western industrialized societies and the special problems of learning new skills and retraining increase the difficulties of the older employee. Sheltered work shops, although of help in some cases, do not, with the increasing complexity of industry, seem to be viable on any major scale.
There is little actual evidence to show that retirement by itself is a major psychological stress. More men retire from work with physical or psychiatric ill-health than because of age limits. Furthermore, some men would like to retire but for the economic problem.
In general, retirement appears to be acceptable to the bulk of working-class men (whose jobs may be unattractive and physically demanding), but their constant presence in the household sometimes aggravates marital disharmony.

Retrograde amnesia
SEE Amnesia.

Retrospective falsification

Unconscious distortion or falsification of past experiences to bring them into line with current emotional requirements.

Retrospective inquiry

A retrospective inquiry is one made after the event. It begins with a person or group of people with an illness, and seeks to determine possible causes from the histories. A typical example is the search for the source of a typhoid outbreak. The differences between this type of study and a prospective inquiry (q.v.) should be noted.
Retrospective studies in psychiatry may be very unreliable unless the data are confirmed by contemporary records, e.g. hospital records, etc.

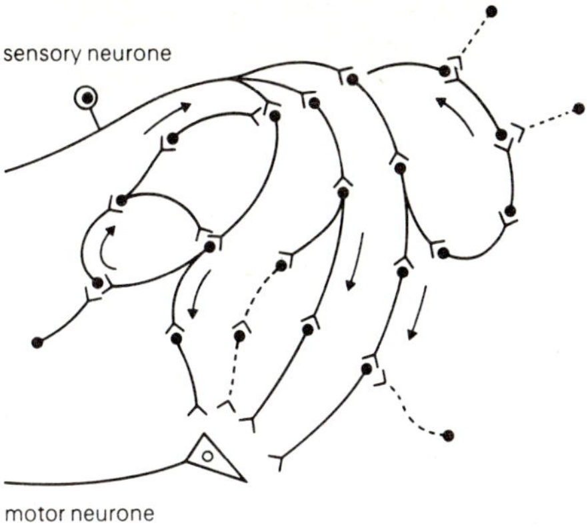

Reverberating circuits

Current theory suggests that important functional units in the central nervous system, particularly at higher levels are the reverberating circuits. A nerve cell discharges through a large number of synapses into other nerve cells either exerting a facilitatory or inhibitory effect which is summated with the other impulses reaching the second (receptor) cell. This nerve cell in its turn, and if the summation is above the excitatory threshhold, fires onto many more. Reverberating circuits are established when neurones ultimately fire back on the original cell (see diagram). During its passage the nerve impulse may be reduced by inhibition or potentiated by spatial or temporal summation of facilitatory impulses. More complex reverberating circuits are postulated by which interrelated brain areas can interact. Modification of reverberating circuit patterns have been used as the basis of theories of memory, learning and behaviour patterns.

Rhesus incompatibility

The rhesus factor is a complex genetically determined blood group factor classifiable as positive or negative. Antibodies may be developed in a rhesus negative mother's blood in pregnancy if the foetus is rhesus positive. The risk is small in a first pregnancy of this kind unless the mother has been previously transfused with rhesus positive blood, but increases progressively with each subsequent pregnancy. The maternal antibodies may lead to excessive breakdown of haemoglobin in the infant, and in the neonatal period the child may be severely jaundiced. Lesions may result in the brain (kernicterus (q.v.)), especially the basal ganglia, and elsewhere throughout the central nervous system, leading to choreoathetoid palsy, deafness and mental subnormality.

Rheumatoid arthritis

A generalized systemic disease with a predilection for peripheral joints, which become swollen and painful. The aetiology is unknown and relapses and remissions may occur without apparent cause, although emotional factors have been implicated. In some patients increase in anger or anxiety is associated with exacerbations of joint pain. The serious invalidism itself at times leads to psychiatric disturbance. SEE ALSO Psychosomatic disorders.

Ritual

The term ritual is used in quite different ways in different disciplines. Anthropologists often use 'ritual' to refer to moderately complex ceremonies, traditional in a given society, and involving anything from one to many hundreds of individuals. They also use the term to refer to individually specific stereotyped patterns of behaviour, often with religious or mystical significance. Descriptively similar patterns of movement are also referred to as ritual by psychiatrists, with often an implication of conflict and of behavioural pathology. Finally ethologists refer to species-characteristic movements, which have become specialized in evolution for a signal function, as 'ritualized'. Clearly there is much room for misunderstanding here, and no assumptions about a common basis for such divergent phenomena are justified.

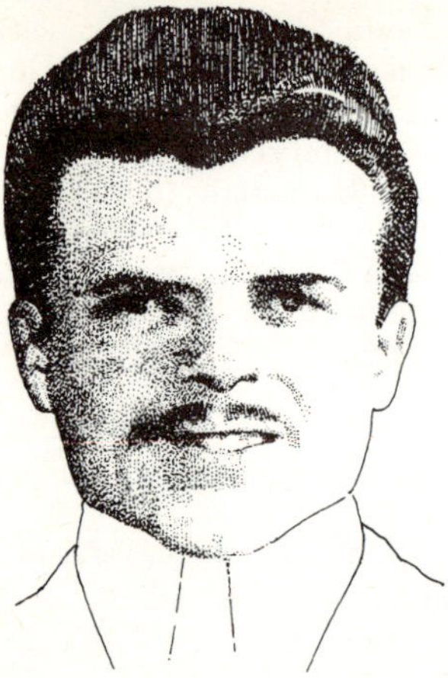

Rorschach, Hermann (1884–1922)

One of Bleuler's pupils, Rorschach experimented with ink blots and, after fourteen years' work, published his findings in a book entitled *Psychodiagnostik* (1921). Bleuler and Jung had introduced him to psychoanalysis, and in keeping with the Zurich's school interest in the individual's inner life, Rorschach developed the projective test named after him. The sensory stimulus provided by the ink blot serves to arouse thoughts and phantasies which may be compared in a variety of individuals and a variety of conditions.

Rorschach test (Ink blot test)

The Roschach ink blot test is one of the most popular projective techniques for the assessment of personality (q.v.). It consists of a series of ten cards, each bearing a complex, bilaterally symmetrical ink blot. Some cards are monochromatic, others include colours. The subject is asked to tell the examiner 'what he sees on the card' and is encouraged to make as many responses as possible, either to the whole blots or to parts. Scoring and interpretation, which is complicated, takes into account such factors as the content of the responses, their locations on the cards, the use made of colour, form and shading, and the extent to which movement is introduced. Advocates claim much for this technique and argue that it reveals unconscious as well as conscious aspects of personality. Attempts at objective validation, however, have proved disappointing. There is more empirical support for the validity of certain specific pathological signs associated with conditions such as brain damage and schizophrenia (q.v.). SEE ALSO Psychological tests.

Rubella

Maternal rubella is a cause of embryopathy. It has been estimated that for every hundred mothers who have had rubella in the first twelve weeks of pregnancy, there will be about seventy infants surviving without serious congenital defects, though about ten of these may have some degree of deafness. The main deleterious effects of maternal rubella on the foetus are deafness, congenital heart defects, cataracts and other ophthalmological defects, and mental subnormality. SEE ALSO Embryopathy.

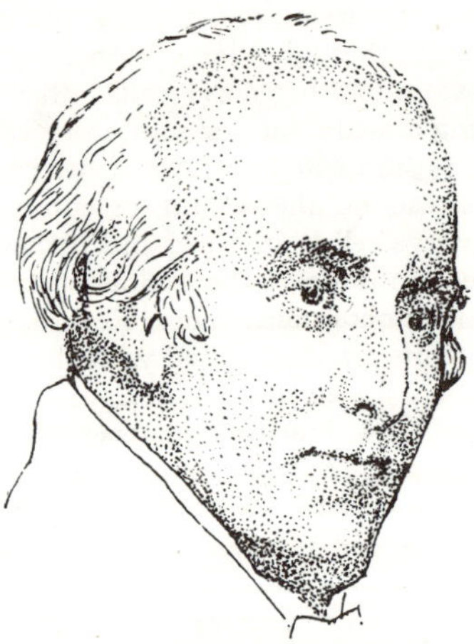

Rush, Benjamin (1745–1813)

Physician to the Pennsylvania Hospital, Rush wrote the first American text-book of psychiatry, *Medical Inquiries and Observations upon the Diseases of the Mind* (1812), and is generally regarded as the father of North American psychiatry. He graduated from Edinburgh and was greatly influenced by William Cullen, the Professor of Medicine. He was one of the signatories of the Declaration of Independence. He believed mental illness was essentially due to excessive irritability of cerebral blood vessels, and used blood letting and other methods to diminish the amount of blood in the brain.

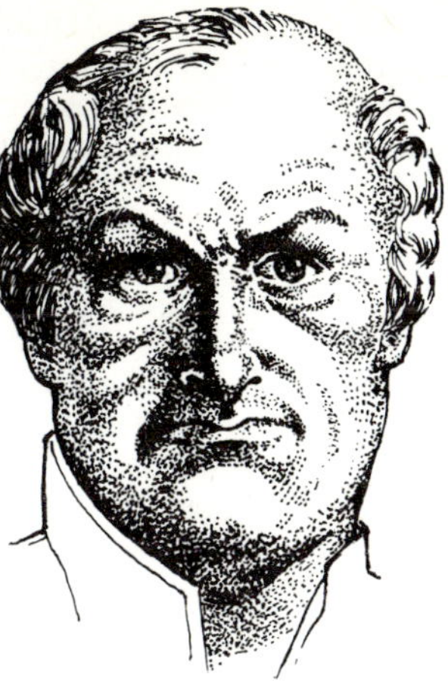

Marquis de Sade

Sadism

Sadism is the sexual perversion named after the Marquis de Sade whose obscene novels are based upon sexual lust and cruelty. It is the exclusive attainment of sexual orgasm through the infliction of pain and cruelty upon another individual, male or female, or upon an animal (bestosexual sadism). It mainly occurs in males who are often otherwise impotent. Rudimentary sadistic impulses commonly emerge in the biting and scratching of normal pre-coital sexual arousal. Sadistic fantasies are common and are often sublimated in pornographic literature. True sadism varies from the whipping or beating of prostitutes who cater for this perversion to physical assaults of rape, buggery or lust murder with mutilation of the corpse. At other times the sadist may subject himself to masochistic (q.v.) stimulation. Sadistic fantasies often date back to childhood and are associated with acts of cruelty for non-sexual pleasure against animals or other children. Treatment is unsatisfactory; the convicted sadistic criminal requires supervision in a security hospital. In some countries chemical or surgical castration (q.v.) is offered to the patient. SEE ALSO Sado-masochism and Sexual disorders.

Sado-masochism

Sadism (q.v.) and masochism (q.v.) were formerly regarded as two distinct perversions, but are commonly thought now as parts of the same complex with each varying in degree. Current ideas suggest that a certain degree of sado-masochism is a normal attribute of most people.

Salivary secretion

Saliva can be collected and its volume measured by means of a suction cup over the opening of the parotid duct or by absorbent dental rolls in the floor of the mouth. Depressed patients have diminished salivary flow which returns to normal as the illness remits. Psychotropic drugs with anti-cholinergic side effects have also been assessed with this technique, although the assessment may be more representative of the side effect than the therapeutic activity.

Samaritans

A voluntary organization, originally started under church auspices and now covering many urban centres in several industrially developed countries. Its main object is the prevention of suicide, but this has extended to cover 'crisis intervention' for many kinds of acute personal stress situations. The staff consists of volunteers, who work under the supervision of professional staff and have a careful training to exclude any who may be attracted to the work because of their own personal problems. Clients usually approach the Samaritans first by telephone and are then encouraged to make a personal visit; further volunteer support may be arranged, or they may be referred for medical treatment.
SEE ALSO Suicide.

Satyriasis

Satyriasis is a rare pathological intensification of the sexual drive in the male which leads to unrestrained and indiscriminate sexual activity. The individuals are often of subnormal intelligence, with a degree of brain damage, particularly in the temporal lobes. Acute satyriasis may be a manifestation of a manic psychosis, amphetamine or alcohol intoxication, an acute schizophrenic illness or rarely it may be the presenting symptom of an acute encephalitis. It is occasionally found in otherwise apparently normal individuals. SEE ALSO Nymphomania.

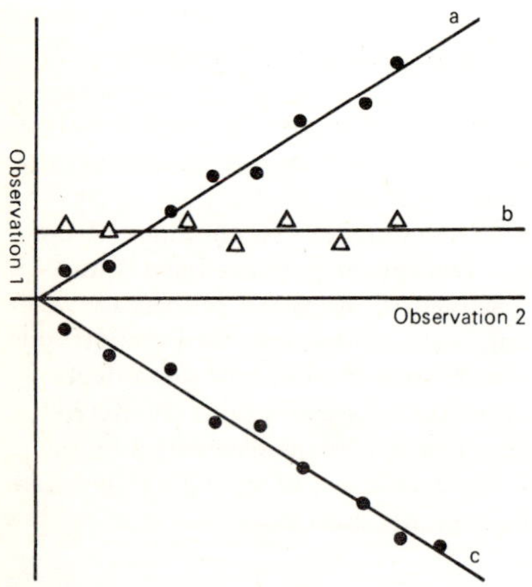

Scatter diagram showing for 3 different conditions the relationship between 2 sets of observations and the equivalent correlation curve

Scatter diagram

A scatter diagram is a graph upon which each observation is shown as a point. The position of the point is determined by the values of the observations used for the ordinate and abscissa of the graph. The scatter diagram is a useful visual representation of the correlation between two different characteristics. The correlation coefficient (q.v.) can be shown as a line on the same graph and the regression coefficient (q.v.) calculated.

Schilder's disease

SEE Diffuse sclerosis.

Schizo-affective disorder

This term refers to clinical states in which elements usually associated with depressive illness and schizophrenia (q.v.) appear simultaneously, making correct diagnostic assignment doubtful.
The occurrence in a considerable number of depressive illnesses of ideas of reference (q.v.), bizarre hypochondriacal delusions, doubts about the subject's sex, suspicion, ideas of persecution (q.v.), etc. should not lead to the application of the term schizo-affective. The course of such illnesses is that of other depressive states and they do not merit a separate label: nor do schizophrenic illnesses in which a depressive picture appears, as, for instance, it does fairly frequently in the paranoid type. Periodicity, that is recurrent illness with full remission between attacks, favours a diagnosis of affective illness but does occur uncommonly in schizophrenia. The most important practical decisions depending on diagnosis relate to treatment or prognosis. Depressive symptomatology is likely to respond to anti-depressive treatment, even in a schizophrenic illness. The schizophrenic symptoms, noted above, occurring in the course of a depressive illness are more likely to respond to anti-depressive than anti-schizophrenic treatment, however. It is not wise to give both types of treatment in all cases of doubt, because it is not then possible to know the agent responsible for the favourable or unfavourable change that occurs. This knowledge is valuable in treating recurrent illness and it is therefore worth treating thoroughly with each treatment separately and carefully noting the result.

Schizoid constitution

This is the term used for those handicapped personalities of the shut in, shy, seclusive type, who tend to be emotionally withdrawn or cold. It is often associated with an asthenic type of body build. Different varieties can be distinguished; the 'backward' type, lacking ambition, absent minded, and often playing truant; the 'precocious' type, the bookish, prudish, 'model' child; the 'neurotic' variety, selfish, deceitful, and with many minor ailments; the 'asocial' seclusive, daydreaming, and the 'juvenile' type which never seems to grow up.
About one-third of schizophrenics show such pre-morbid characteristics and they occur much more frequently in the blood relatives of schizophrenics than in the general population.

Schizophrenia

Schizophrenia is the term used for a group of illnesses whose aetiology is unknown, having characteristic mental symptoms leading to fragmentation of personality. The patient undergoes experiences which are unfamiliar and cannot be understood as exaggerations or prolongations of familiar sensations. Thought, emotion, drive and movement may be disordered. The illness often recurs, each recurrence increasing a chronic disability until a plateau is reached. The final result, oddity, social incapacity or chronic invalidism requiring prolonged hospitalization, may be modified by treatment and its social effects mitigated by professional guidance.

Early adult life is the most frequent period of onset but the illness begins often in adolescence and sometimes at later periods of life. A characteristic insidious onset is often preceded by introversion, subdued behaviour or suspicious secretiveness (schizoid personality). Males are a little more frequently affected than females and single subjects more than married.

First admission rates for schizophrenics are about fifteen per 100,000 of the whole population in Britain. About 80% of the patients under 65 who have been continuously in hospital for two years or more are schizophrenics.

Genetic studies show that if one of a pair of monozygotic twins has a severe form of schizophrenia the other twin will also have the disease in about 70% of cases. Among dizygotic twins of the same sex the figure is 15%. Milder cases have a lower concordancy rate. This is the strongest evidence of a genetic basis for schizophrenia but there is no satisfactory theory of the mode of inheritance. It is probable that schizophrenia occurs more frequently in people of tall, lean or muscular build than in those of tubby (pyknic) habitus, and also that before the onset of their illness many schizophrenics show a 'schizoid' personality, i.e. they are shy, reticent, unsociable, oversensitive or eccentric.

The association of the onset of schizophrenia with the epochs of life has stimulated energetic investigation of endocrine factors. It has produced no unequivocal evidence of endocrine gland disorder as a cause of the disease, although minor anomalies are frequent, many secondary to the disorder.

Many biochemical anomalies have been reported in schizophrenia, the majority are either unconfirmed or considered secondary to the abnormal regimen imposed by the disease. In periodic catatonia, however, the mental changes coincided with nitrogen retention and the remissions with greater excretion. This finding has been confirmed and provides a rationale for the treatment of periodic catatonia (an uncommon condition) with thyroxin.

Only two facts are known for certain about schizophrenic metabolism: (a) L-methionine (20 g./day) induces an acute psychotic reaction in about 40% of chronic schizophrenic patients; and (b) schizophrenics are abnormally resistant to histamine (e.g. intradermal injection). Since most psychotomimetic drugs, such as LSD and mescaline, are methylated derivatives of the brain transmitters dopamine and serotonin, and since methionine is the source of the methyl groups in these reactions, the hypothesis has been put forward that schizophrenia is associated with a weak enzyme system concerned in these transmethylation reactions so that toxic levels of some potent psychotogen, such as dimethyltryptamine, builds up in the brain. This fits the histamine data since histamine is normally metabolized by methylation. This hypothesis is currently directing research in a number of centres.

In both content and course schizophrenia is variable giving rise to 'types' which are not sufficiently distinctive, however, to command agreement among psychiatrists. They are not based upon aetiology nor are there objective tests to distinguish them, thus they rest on prominent clinical features.

The most widely accepted classification is that of Kraepelin into the four categories: (a) paranoid (q.v.), in which persecutory delusions with coherent thought are prominent; (b) catatonic (q.v.), characterized by alternating periods of stupor, and excitement; (c) hebephrenic (q.v.) showing capricious, fatuous emotion and thought; (d) simple (q.v.), where there is an insidious development of social inadequacy and eccentricity. The schizophrenic clinical picture may be coloured by symptoms of other psychiatric syndromes, as in schizo-affective type (q.v.) where depressive or, less frequently, manic features are prominent and as in pseudo-neurotic type (q.v.) where neurotic symptoms and behaviour dominate. During severe stress such as battle or shipwreck, a schizophrenic picture may appear abruptly and subside as the stress is removed. This phenomenon is described as a schizophrenic episode which may occasionally appear in more mundane circumstances.

Schizophrenia is characterized by a change of personality with inco-ordinated thought, emotion and impulses occurring in a setting of clear consciousness, memory and orientation.

Thought disorder is a characteristic feature. Normal association of ideas is lost, and illogical or bizarre sequences occur. The patient may feel that his thoughts are controlled and ideas are put into his mind (feelings of influence) and explain this in terms of external influences, such as radar or telepathy. He may feel that his stream of thought is suddenly cut off (thought blocking) and show this by an abrupt cessation of his flow of speech. There is considerable variety in these manifestations and an accumulation of descriptive terms, some translations of original German phrases, bear witness to attempts to pinpoint particular features; thus 'incoherence' and 'neologism' explain themselves and are summated as 'verbigeration'; 'autism' indicates the patient's immersion in private fantasies and day-dreams; 'negativism' his resistance to being disturbed from them.

Delusions (q.v.), false beliefs unassailable by fact or reason, occur frequently. Their content is varied and may be persecutory, grandiose, hypochondriacal, nihilistic, etc. They may be disconnected or systematized, fleeting or fixed. The patient may believe that announcements on the radio or in the newspaper are about him (ideas of reference (q.v.)) or that his body is affected by external agencies (passivity feelings). Primary delusions arise *per se* (autochthonous ideas (q.v.)); secondary delusions are the patient's attempts to account for his strange sensations and may seem clear and logical if the primary premises are granted.

Incongruity is the most characteristic disorder of emotion; the patient may greet bereavement with laughter or indifference; he may giggle as serious aspects of his future are discussed. Some emotions may be expressed with great intensity, but more frequently the emotions are 'flattened' or 'blunted' so that there is a lack of understandable expression of affection, enthusiasm or dislike.

Hallucinations (q.v.), disorders of perception, may occur in any sensory modality, but hearing is by far the most common in the form of 'voices' which may address the patient, discuss him or publicize his private affairs. They may be attributed to a particular person or agency, but more commonly the patient is at a loss to account for them.

The schizophrenic's speech and writing indicate his thought disorder. Talk may be reduced in amount (mutism (q v.)) or continuous and difficult to interrupt; it shows peculiarities of manner and content. One idea or phase may be repeatedly used and appear out of context (perseveration (q.v.)); the questions or final words of the interviewer may be repeated (echolalia (q.v.)). The manner of speaking may appear affected or stilted; words are sometimes coined by the patient (neologizing (q.v.)).

In the patient's actions and bearing stiffness and oddness may be seen early. Preoccupation may be manifested by inexplicable changes of emotional expression and gesture, or by ignoring the address of others. Grimacing, odd posture, mannerisms of gesture, twitchings and rituals may occur and sudden impulsive actions appear. All movement is sometimes greatly reduced, as in catatonic stupor, and the patient may adopt fixed postures for long periods. The patient may resist or do the opposite of what is requested (negativism (q.v.)) or show undue compliance (automatic obedience (q.v.)) in rare cases to the extent of imitating another's actions (echopraxia (q.v.)). These gross behavioural disorders in schizophrenics appear to have diminished greatly during the past two decades as psychiatric hospitals have allowed more freedom, encouraged occupation and otherwise fostered a more normal life.

The course of schizophrenia somewhat resembles that of pulmonary tuberculosis before the advent of effective pharmacotherapy. Always a serious illness, an acute phase may be followed by quiescence, with some damage to psychic life which successive attacks aggravate. During an acute phase patients are admitted to hospital in all but the most affluent families. About a third of cases will run a chronic course with serious disability; a further third an episodic course free of florid symptoms during remissions. In the last third improvement, quick or slow, will occur to a level of stability which is maintained for a long period.

The prognosis is worse in those patients where the onset is early or insidious, and in those showing schizoid traits before the onset of the illness. The married and those with parents alive have a much better prospect of living outside hospital.

The principles of treatment can be compared to those for poliomyelitis; protective and conserving during the acute attack; stimulating and rehabilitative during convalescence. It is at this stage that the services of a psychiatric social worker should be introduced and can render invaluable service.

During the acute stage of the illness phenothiazines have a controlling and ameliorative effect on symptoms. Chlorpromazine is the longest established and 300 mg. daily is the average dose, which varies widely. The piperazine type of phenothiazines, such as trifluoperazine, are thought by some to have advantages in certain patients, such as the apathetic ones, and the butyrophenones are also a useful alternative. Chronic schizophrenics in hospital become more accessible to socializing and stimulating influences by prolonged administration of phenothiazines. Phenothiazines have largely superseded the use of ECT in schizophrenia, though the latter is still used by many psychiatrists, in conjunction with the phenothiazines, particularly in acute cases and in those with an affective component. The acute side effects and toxic results of prolonged administration of phenothiazines constitute a serious disadvantage of their use. The damage or loss inherent in particular treatments must always be weighed against the advantage hoped for; this consideration usually rules out the use of leucotomy in schizophrenia.

The nature of the schizophrenic illness and frequently the patient's previous personality tend to result in his becoming emotionally shut off and isolated to other people. The regime of a good psychiatric hospital is aimed at countering this, and occupational therapy, social activities, industrial units, and the constant endeavours of the individual nurses are aimed at resocializing the patient, developing his outside interests and contacts, and trying to prevent his withdrawal and occupation with morbid thoughts, hallucinations, etc. The phenothiazines moreover enable the patient to be discharged from hospital much earlier than previously so that he is able to maintain his normal social contacts and interests. However, due to lack of insight into their condition many outpatients cannot be relied on to take their medication regularly and this is a major cause of relapse. Long-acting depot preparations of intramuscular fluphenazine or flupenthixol have been introduced to overcome this problem and in some areas re-admission rates have been halved by using this one simple measure.

Psychoanalysis and insight psychotherapy are, with rare exceptions, contra-indicated. However, psychotherapy aimed at understanding the patient's present difficulties with a view to discussing them and helping him with them on a friendly basis, can often be very beneficial. This benefit is probably due to the relationship he develops with his doctor who helps him to get his feet on the ground and face his difficulties but at the same time offers help and friendship which again counter a tendency to introversion. It is surprising the relationship that can be developed with even an advanced schizophrenic patient and controlled trials have convincingly demonstrated the benefit to patients of this simple method when compared to the more formal type of psychotherapy. The family to which the patient is discharged is important. The possible role of parents in contributing to the aetiology of schizophrenia by the effect of allusive thinking and a generally irrational family life is very controversial and has not been confirmed. However, there is strong evidence that patients returning to a home with either a critical or over-protective atmosphere have a high relapse rate. This is especially so when there is in addition a high face-to-face contact, for instance the patient being unemployed and staying at home all day. In extreme cases the patient is better living in a hostel apart from the family. In milder instances therapy with the family and measures taken to lessen face-to-face contact may suffice.

SEE ALSO Psychosis.

School phobia

Fear of going to school occurs commonly and normally in children on initial school entry or earlier if the child goes to nursery school. Usually this fear passes in the first few hours and it rarely lasts more than a few weeks. Established school phobia or refusal to go to school because of anxiety is a much rarer phenomenon.

The condition must be sharply distinguished from truancy (q.v.) in which the child attempts to cover up his unwillingness to go to school and shows little or no anxiety. The child with school phobia is usually quiet and well-behaved, of average or above average intelligence, and with few or no learning problems. Commonly there is an unduly close mother-child relationship with the father taking an unassertive uninvolved role in the household.

Immediate predisposing factors may include an episode of bullying at school, an altercation with a teacher, or illness in a parent. Commonly the anxiety occurs at the beginning of a school term or year and at change to secondary school. The child may show very circumscribed symptoms of anxiety so that he can play out quite happily in the evenings, though terrified of going to school in the morning. More rarely the anxiety occurs as but one symptom of a depressive or schizophrenic illness.

If no underlying illness is diagnosed and the problem appears to have arisen in the context of an overclose mother-child relationship, treatment should initially involve rapid return to school before a habit of non-attendance is established. This will always be easier if the father can be involved to take the child to school. These 'first-aid' measures should be accompanied by discussion with the parents about the way the problem has developed. If these measures fail, then psychiatric referral is indicated.

SEE ALSO Child psychiatry.

Schools of psychology

While the principles of psychology are as old as civilization yet as an independent science psychology is one of the youngest. From the Graeco-Roman era until the latter part of the nineteenth century, psychology existed as an integral and essential division of philosophy. Both Plato and Aristotle were concerned with aspects of psychology and the Pythagorean school had accurately postulated that the seat of the mind could be found in the brain. Hippocrates, in addition to his important studies in inherited factors and predispositions to mental illness, taught on the disorders of cerebral function and their role in mental illness and insanity.

As with so much in medicine philosophy influenced, overshadowed, and even retarded, all psychological thought to the seventeenth century. However the British seventeenth-century philosophers Hobbes and Locke, who favoured the concept of association in explaining learning and remembering, initiated a gradual emergence of the first, if poorly defined, school of psychology, the associationist school.

The associationist school maintained its ascendancy in psychological thought throughout the eighteenth and greater part of the nineteenth centuries. But by the latter part of the nineteenth century, many found the associationist's methods which relied on subjective introspection outdated.

Wilhelm Wundt in 1879 who set up the first psychological laboratory at Leipzig, founding the new science of experimental psychology, required in his laboratory factual, objective data measured by experiment. Wundt's theories, which stressed the synthesis of conscious experience from sensations and feelings, were further developed by the structural school of psychology born in Germany and in the United States of America, most notably by E. B. Titchener (1867–1927). However, much of the basic doctrine of this school was superseded by the newer theories of the schools of psychology that were emerging.

The school of psychoanalysis founded by Sigmund Freud in Vienna in 1900 rejected the views of the existing schools of psychology and advanced the highly controversial theories of unconscious motivation. Central to these new theories was the role of the dynamic unconscious mind in both healthy mental activity and in the occurrence of mental illness.

Freud's associates, Carl Jung (q.v.) and

Alfred Adler (q.v.) later each formed his own particular school; Jung, the school of analytical psychology and Adler the school of individual psychology.
The gestalt school introduced another new approach to psychological theory. Founded in Germany in 1912 by Max Wertheimer, Wolfgang Köhler and Kurt Koffka, it stressed the importance of '*Gestalten*' or 'wholes'. The prime interest of the gestalt school lay in problems of perception. Learning, memory, behaviour and social psychology, among other special interests, were studied extensively according to gestalt principles.
J. B. Watson founded the behaviourist school in America in 1912, which thought of psychological phenomena as simple physiological functions and sought to explain behaviour by stimulus-response reflex units. The mechanistic theory of mental processes has provoked much criticism from present-day psychologists but behaviour therapy of modern psychiatry is based on the clinical application of selected principles of the behaviourist school.

Sclerosis, disseminated

SEE Disseminated sclerosis.

Scoptophilia

(Synonym Voyeurism)

A desire to observe the genitalia or secondary sexual characteristics of individuals of the same or more usually the opposite sex. It is normal in children, who like to observe each others genitalia, a form of natural curiosity. In adults it may persist as a perversion, the 'peeping Tom' or the man who uses binoculars to observe courting couples being stereotypes of this perversion. The widespread visual interest in nudity may also be regarded as scoptophiliac activity.

Screen memory

The distorted recollection of a significant event, the screen memory has developed as a defence against the painful recall of what actually occurred. The unconscious processes of distortion, falsification, symbolization and repression are all involved in producing the screen memory.

Sedatives

Originally the term sedative was used to designate those properties of a drug which produce quietness and drowsiness short of sleep, usually associated with anxiolytic activity. The only difference between sedative and hypnotic effects is one of degree and is a function of dose; pharmacological consideration of sedative compounds as a separate entity is artificial, and most modern texts do not distinguish between the two terms. Rather is the distinction drawn on grounds of clinical usage, reflected in the dosage. Similarly there is a blurred boundary between sedative and anxiolytic compounds.
SEE ALSO Hypnotics.

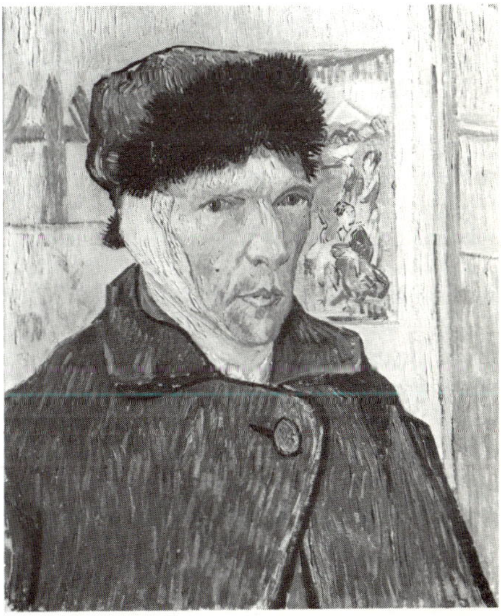

Self portrait with severed ear, by Van Gogh

Self-mutilation

The commonest type of self-mutilation, and the least severe, is the wrist slashing which occurs in adolescents or immature young people, either to attract attention, relieve tension, or as a contagious phenomenon. More rarely self-mutilation is of a serious nature, the individual cutting off his penis, or testes, or even amputating a limb – and perhaps bleeding to death in the process. Such episodes occur in schizophrenics, more uncommonly in depressives with sexual problems, but at times the diagnosis may present difficulties, the behaviour itself being the only sure sign of any mental disturbances. The famous case of Van Gogh's ear illustrates how complex such behaviour may be. Repeated episodes of this very disturbing and serious self-mutilation may lead to great difficulties in management.

In times of war self-mutilation may serve to remove the soldier from the front line. Gunshot wounds of the hand and feet are particularly suspect.

Senile dementia (Chronic brain syndrome, senile type)

This is an insidious and steadily progressing dementia (q.v.) usually beginning after the age of 70–75, and increasing in frequency with age. Roughly 10% of the over 80's are affected. The predominance of females is at least partly due to their longer survival.

The first sign is generally a failure of memory for recent events, followed by a gradual decline in all mental faculties with disorganization of personality and deterioration of habits. The diagnosis may become obvious when a relative falls ill, or when an episode of confusion due to intercurrent illness, a fit, an episode of wandering, the onset of incontinence or dangerously negligent behaviour demand attention. For a time, especially in younger patients, relatively limited defects of parietal lobe type may be recognizable, but eventually the dementia becomes global with incoherence of speech, total disorientation and failure in the simplest tasks.

Apathy or mild euphoria is usual, but some patients become suspicious, aggressive or callous. Persecutory ideas (q.v.) are usually transient, occasionally persistent. Visual hallucinations suggest some clouding of consciousness or a visual defect.

The duration of life is about five years from the onset of definite changes. The cause of death is usually intercurrent infection, myocardial failure or inanition.

The brain shows a variable degree of generalized atrophy with, microscopically, a diffuse loss of neurones, most marked in the cortex, and shrinkage of the remaining cells. The characteristic changes consist of senile (argentophil) plaques throughout the cortex, and Alzheimer's neuro-fibrillary tangles which are most numerous in nerve cells of the hippocampal area. Granulovacuolar degeneration is the rarest cellular change. Vascular lesions may be present but are not characteristic of senile dementia.

Claims for specific remedies are unconfirmed. Management consists of symptomatic treatment, supervisory care and nursing. Relief of intercurrent ill-health, such as urinary or chest infection, silent infarcts, malnutrition, anaemia or heart failure, may bring about a dramatic improvement in behaviour by removing the element of confusion. Restlessness may be due to faecal impaction. In females a ring pessary and in males a condom urinal minimizes the effects of incontinence when regular toiletting has failed. Anxiety, depression or agitation can be relieved by anti-depressant or phenothiazine drugs, starting with small doses because of hypotension. Non-barbiturates such as oxazepam flurazapam, or dichloralphenazone are useful, and excessive sedation must be avoided.

Sensation

The term sensation refers to the primary input to the cerebral cortex of information concerning the animal's internal and external environment. This sensory input is derived from appropriate receptors in the body surface and in key positions within the tissues and organs. While the receptors within the body (interoceptors) all measure changes in the local internal environment, the exteroceptors on the body surface may measure local changes (e.g. sensation of heat, touch, etc.) or via the special senses (e.g. sight, hearing) changes in the distant environment.

The sensory receptors may all be termed transducers because they convert the input energy into a different form, namely the ionic changes that constitute the nerve impulse (q.v.).

Sensation depends on these impulses reaching the contralateral cerebral cortex. With the exception of the sensation of smell they all relay in the thalamus, or its

associated geniculate bodies. The general body surface sensations are arranged topically in the post-central gyrus; vision in the calcarine fissure and neighbouring areas of the occipital cortex; hearing in the middle third of the superior temporal gyrus and smell and taste around the region of the uncus or upper operculum of the Sylvian fissure.
Sensation, which is solely concerned with the reception of the information in the cerebral cortex, must be distinguished from perception (q.v.), which implies the meaningful interpretation of the information.

Sensitivity group
SEE Newer group therapies.

Sensorium
SEE Consciousness.

Sensory aphasia
SEE Aphasia.

Sensory deprivation
SEE Deprivation, sensory.

Sensory disturbances in hysteria

Sensory disturbances in hysteria are produced either by the doctor's suggestions, or by the patient's own ideas as to what kind of sensory disturbances the doctor expects to find. They include every possible type of manifestation from analgesia to hyperalgesia, in every possible area of the body. Neurologists are particularly good at producing hysterical disturbances of sensation; psychiatrists in failing to understand their real origins.

Separation anxiety

Anxiety is common in childhood and separation from the mother, for instance when the child first goes to school or is hospitalized, will normally result in anxiety, usually with some regression and clinging behaviour. A tendency to separation anxiety is much greater if the child has previously been emotionally deprived or if the mother herself is over-anxious and over-protective. In such cases a true school phobia may develop and recur at puberty when the child changes to a new school. Such children frequently show neurotic anxiety in adult life.
The child's personality may be permanently injured by prolonged separation from the mother, for instance if it has to be looked after in an understaffed institution. Such injury, however, can be largely prevented if the child's emotional needs are cared for by a familiar relative or other mother-surrogate.

Serotonin
(Synonym: 5-hydroxy tryptamine – 5HT)

Serotonin is a neuronal transmitter in peripheral and central systems. In the brain, serotonin systems are thought to be concerned in the control of perception, mood, sleep, thinking and behaviour. The hallucinogenic drugs such as LSD and mescaline are specific blockers of central serotonin synapses and many of them are close chemical relatives of serotonin. Rauwolfia alkaloids deplete brain serotonin levels.
Serotonin may also be involved in migraine, the therapeutic agent methysergide being a potent blocker of 5HT. Brain serotonin mechanisms are also concerned in hypothalamic mechanisms regulating pituitary function in oestrus, ovulation and ACTH secretion. Serotonin is also believed to be a synaptic transmitter in the hindbrain (Raphe) area concerned with the sleep mechanism.
SEE ALSO Biochemical and neurophysiological background to mental disease.

Severe subnormality

Severe subnormality is defined in British legal terms as 'a state of arrested or incomplete development of mind which includes subnormality of intelligence and is of such a nature or degree that the patient is incapable of living an independent life or of guarding himself against serious exploitation, or will be so incapable when of an age to do so'. This allows latitude of interpretation from

the point of view of measurable psychological scores, but if severe subnormality is taken to correspond to the now obsolete statutory terms of idiot and imbecile, then it can be taken to cover an intelligence range of approximately IQ 50 and below. As regards aetiology, a greater proportion of severely mentally subnormal patients as compared with more mildly affected patients owe their intellectual deficit to single major factors, such as a single rare deleterious gene of major effect or environmental accident such as birth trauma. Thus severe mental subnormality is not infrequently accompanied by physical deformities and conditions such as paralysis and epilepsy. Few syndromes associated with severe mental subnormality are recognized at birth, unless there are marked physical signs such as in severe microcephaly, or in mongolism or other syndromes associated with autosomal chromosome abnormalities. A very few, such as phenylketonuria, may be diagnosed in the neonatal period by screening tests. In the majority of patients, severe mental subnormality is first suspected through signs of delayed development, such as retardation in reaching the developmental milestones. Prospects of treatment in the conventional sense of this term are limited mainly to symptomatic alleviation, such as the control of epilepsy by anti-convulsants. Prognosis as regards life expectancy varies from individual to individual and often depends on the type of pathological lesion present.
SEE ALSO Mental subnormality.

Sex-linked inheritance

Sex-linked recessive disorders are rare, occur only in males, and hereditary transmission can be assumed to take place through unaffected females. The abnormal gene is presumed to be carried on the X chromosome, masked by the other normal X chromosome in the carrier female but unmasked in the affected male. Rare sex-linked conditions associated with mental subnormality include the oculocerebrorenal syndrome (q.v.), Hunter's syndrome (q.v.), and at least some cases of congenital hydrocephalus (q.v.). Some cases of the Duchenne form of pseudo-hypertrophic muscular dystrophy and nephrogenic diabetes insipidus show mental subnormality. In some sex-linked conditions, for example glucose-6-phosphate dehydrogenase deficiency (q.v.), the female carrier can be detected biochemically.
Recent reports suggest that some cases of mania (bipolar affective disorder) may be due to a dominant gene localized on the X chromosome. In these families, as one would expect, female cases outnumber males by 2 to 1, and fathers cannot transmit the disorder to their sons. In some families the disorder has been linked with an X-chromosome marker such as protan or deutan colour blindness.

Sexual aberrations in the elderly

Libido and potency decline in the aged, but indecent exposure, genital play with children, and occasionally sexual assaults on them constitute 12% of the offences for which old people are prosecuted. Factors contributing are personal predisposition, lack of normal outlets, or, in a minority, disinhibition due to dementia (q.v.). Impotence of recent onset may be due to depression, and flirtatious or overtly erotic behaviour may occur in hypomania. Treatment may include antidepressants, sedation, and encouragement of social and recreational interests.

Sexual appetite, abnormal

Sexual appetite is the episodic craving for sexual excitement relieved by orgasm. It is a direct manifestation of the sexual instinct and is normally distributed in the population. Individuals at the extremes of the continuum have abnormal sexual appetite. At one end are those with little or no sexual appetite (sexual anhedonia) who may present with frigidity (q.v.) or impotence (q.v.). At the other extreme are those with excessive sexual appetites who require two or three orgasms per day for satisfaction (hypersexuals).
Satyriasis (q.v.) and nyphomania (q.v.) are pathological intensifications of sexual appetite due to brain damage, subnormality, drug intoxication or psychopathy.

Sexual assaults on children

Sexual assaults on children of both sexes give rise to much ill-feeling towards the offender, who at times is lucky to escape with a severe thrashing. In prison the punishment from fellow prisoners is often such that the offender voluntarily requests to be isolated from them. It is therefore surprising how little physical or mental damage has been shown to result from sexual assaults on both boys and girls. Several common and relatively harmless situations occur in which sexual assault is committed, *viz.* an elderly retired man attracts a group of 5–12-year old girls into his house, bribes them with sweets or money, and indulges in sex play with them; a backward youth may mix with much younger children, one of whom may enter into a sexual relationship with him; uncles, nephews and other family members may abuse their relationship to interfere with a small girl or boy. The dangerous forms of sexual assault are committed by paedophiliacs (q.v.), men who can only relate sexually to children. The activity tends to be repetitive and stereotyped, and not susceptible to punishment or to psychiatric treatment. Chemical castration may be indicated in the form of hormone implants. The rare but brutal child murders are nearly always committed by paedophiliacs.

SEE ALSO Forensic psychiatry.

Sexual disorders

Probably only a minority of patients with sexual disorders ask a doctor for help. This may be because the patient does not want to be different, as is the case with most homosexuals; in others the patient may feel guilty and hope that with time he may overcome the problem himself. In many cases the patient is married, a good husband and father and a respected member of his community, his sexual deviation being conducted in secret, often at times of stress, for instance when his wife is pregnant and he feels a lack of affection or consideration. In other cases the patient has controlled an underlying urge all his life only to be arrested when his inhibitions have failed either through drink, an affective disorder or in the early states of a dementing illness.

A psychiatric opinion may be requested if the patient has been arrested for lewd or libidinous behaviour. A decision must be reached as to whether the offence was committed during the course of some form of mental disorder or whether it arose *sui generis*. In the former, the patient will need hospital treatment. Similarly in cases of a neurotic nature with obsessive compulsive symptoms, the court may sanction probation providing the patient co-operates in medical supervision and treatment. Mitigating factors may also be mentioned, but the doctor should be scrupulous in ascertaining all the facts to assist the court to come to a fair decision.

Sexual deviations are forms of self-fulfilling sexual behaviour which do not lead to normal heterosexual coitus. They can be further classified as: (a) aberration of the sexual object, such as homosexuality (q.v.), fetishism (q.v.), and bestiality (q.v.); and (b) aberration of the aim, as in scoptophilia (q.v.), exhibitionism (q.v.) and transvestitism (q.v.). Little is known as to the aetiology of these disorders. Psychodynamically they can be considered as due to retardation or deviation in the course of normal sexual maturation. Factors such as a dominant, overprotective mother and a weak or violent father are said to lead to a lack of identification with the parents of the same sex, an unresolved Oedipus complex and hence lack of emotional sexual development. On the other hand genetical studies and anthropometric measurements point to a physical and possibly chromosomal aetiology in at least some cases of homosexuality.

Sexual dysfunction are those conditions such as impotence (q.v.), premature ejaculation (q.v.), dyspareunia (q.v.), and frigidity (q.v.) when the sexual object and aim are normal but the patient cannot carry them out to their own or their partner's satisfaction. These disorders are dealt with separately, but in most cases they all have one thing in common in that the patient is afraid and with repeated failures their guilt, despair and anxiety is increased. This vicious circle is as true of conscious and superficial sources of guilt and anxiety as it is of deeper psychological complexes. Certainly the practitioner can nearly always offer help of great value to many of these patients in whom the guilt and anxiety are reasonably superficial, perhaps with simple behaviour therapy later on.

Shadow

The shadow is the 'dark' side of the individual, the primitive instinctual part of the collective unconscious. It is one of the three main archetypes – the other two being the anima and animus – and has much significance in Jungian psychology.

Shaping

A behaviour therapy based on operant conditioning (q.v.) principles. The patient is systematically instructed to do that which he fears and is rewarded by the therapist with praise when he succeeds and with no response if he fails. Shaping differs from modelling (q.v.) in that the therapist does not set the patient an example by doing the feared act himself. Like modelling, shaping may significantly aid phobic and obsessive symptoms and may be helpful in behaviour disorders secondary to schizophrenia and childhood autism.

Sheldon
SEE Constitution.

Shock treatment
SEE Electroconvulsive therapy.

Shoplifting

An offence which leads to enormous financial loss, particularly by multiple stores. The great majority of shoplifters are dishonest, but otherwise normal individuals working either alone or in gangs; the professional shoplifter is usually a working class woman, who has no scruples in involving children or relatives in her activities. More recently gangs of both men and women have moved in on the rich pickings to be obtained so comparatively easily by shoplifting.
It is only in a minority of cases that the psychiatrist needs to be involved, although attempts may be made to involve him by both professionals and by amateurs of high social standing who have been caught unexpectedly. Particular caution must be exercised regarding the idea of depression in these women, for this is the commonest psychiatric symptom presented by the offender. It may well be reactive in nature, although husband and relatives may indulge in some retrospective falsification. Of women who find their way to prison, a most unrepresentative sample of shoplifters, 13% have drinking problems, a quarter are professionals, and the rest present a variety of psychiatric disturbances. Senile dementia is occasionally encountered in both sexes, a real forgetfulness being responsible for the offence. Male, non-professional shoplifting is almost entirely confined to the theft of books, and merits psychiatric examination. SEE ALSO Forensic psychiatry and Legal aspects of psychiatry.

Sibling rivalry

Siblings are just as liable to experience the whole gamut of emotions towards each other as toward others outside the family. Rivalry for the affection of the mother, father, other sibs, or other family members will depend on the particular composition of the family group. The key figure in the Western family is the mother, and in general it is for her affections that siblings compete. In some cases conscious or unconscious sibling rivalry may persist throughout life, and colour relationships with individuals outside the family circle.

Side effects
SEE under Individual drugs in appendix or Drug groups in main sections.

'Significance'

Statistical analyses are designed to determine the degree of chance between two groups of observations being related. This degree of probability is expressed as a percentage. A difference is said to be 'significant' if the probability is less than 5%, i.e. there is less than one chance in twenty that this could have occurred by chance. While this is an accepted term a more accurate representation of the 'significance' of differences is expressed by giving the probability as a value, e.g. 0·01 > 0·001, i.e. it lies between one in 100 and one in 1000.

Simple schizophrenia

This subgroup of schizophrenia (q.v.) is the least clearly delineated and most difficult to diagnose. Its main features are its insidious onset and lack of florid clinical symptoms. The onset is in late adolescence and is betrayed by odd conduct, neglect of responsibilities, poor social contact, unreasonableness and intolerance. On clinical examination little abnormal may appear except a facile attitude to previous social deficiences. Relatives, however, will be aware of callous indifference or nagging, querulous tyranny replacing previous affection. According to social circumstances and degree of support from relatives there will be a drift into eccentricity or social degradation, such as alcoholism or prostitution. It is believed that the majority of simple schizophrenics are not admitted to psychiatric hospitals but add to the ranks of petty criminals, tramps and other social misfits.

Skin conductance level and response (SCL and SCR)

These terms are superseding the formerly used but confusing 'electrical skin resistance (ESR) and 'psychogalvanic response (PGR)'. The palmar skin's conductance of a small electric current varies with the activity of the sweat-glands. Human palmar and plantar glands are not usually concerned in thermoregulation, but are activated by any alerting stimulus, physical or psychic. Some degree of activity, which is controlled by sympathetic nerves, is normally present throughout the waking day and reflects the level of arousal. Activity declines with age, in the pre-menstrum and in depressive illness, whilst it is high in thyrotoxicosis and in psychological states of hyper-arousal whatever the accompanying emotion.
Individual variation among the healthy (including those whose only complaint is of hyperhidrosis) is so great as to make measurement of skin conductance *level* of little diagnostic value, although repeated observations may help assessment of a patient's progress. Skin conductance *responses* provide more useful information. For example, the morbidly anxious exhibit more 'spontaneous' (psychic) SCRs than do non-anxious subjects, and do not habituate to a repeated simple stimulus such as a tone signal. Diminution of SCRs toward a phobic object may be measured during various forms of therapy.

Skin disorders

Different reactions of the skin such as pallor, sweating or blushing may be produced by emotional states such as anxiety, excitement, embarrassment or anger. Many dermatological disorders have a complex aetiology with allergy and psychological factors playing prominent roles. In times of stress it is not uncommon for dermatitis, urticaria, pruritus ani, or vulvae, or acne to appear, or for there to be an exacerbation of a pre-existing skin condition. A constitutional predisposition may be present, for example in infantile eczema, but more commonly psychopathology such as repressed hostility or sexual conflicts may be uncovered. Conscious or subconscious motives may result in self-inflicted lesions – dermatitis artifacta.
SEE ALSO Psychosomatic disorders.

Skinner, Burrhus Frederic (1904–)

An American psychologist who has undertaken extensive research in the field of operant conditioning (cf. Pavlov's (q.v.) work on classical conditioning). Upon this research are based many of the procedures of behaviour therapy.

Sleep

This is a physiological state of unresponsiveness and greatly reduced mobility which occurs regularly each twenty-four hours. The normal amount of time spent in sleep varies from twelve to twenty hours per day in neonates to five to eight hours in adults.

The two major classes of sleep are rapid eye movement (REM) or paradoxical sleep and non-rapid eye movement (NREM) or orthodox sleep and this latter may be subdivided into four stages depending on the depth.

REM sleep is associated with 4–10 c/s rhythm in the EEG for periods of twenty minutes four to five times a night, taking up approximately 20–25 % of sleeping time. This is the time when dreaming (q.v.) occurs, the more 'active' the dream, the more rapid are the eye movements. Penile erection is another associated phenomenon. It has been suggested that REM sleep is the time during which brain regeneration takes place and that it is particularly associated with protein synthesis in the brain. Thus it is associated with increased brain blood flow, is greatest in amount in neonates and after a drug overdose or brain injury, and is diminished in subnormality and old age.

Orthodox sleep may be related to somatic restitution, is enhanced by physical exercise and is accompanied by a high concentration of growth hormones.

The mechanism of sleep production is uncertain. There is evidence that a balance exists between a sleep system and a wake system, both of which are located in the mid brain area, the wake system predominantly in the reticular formation (q.v.). A sleep-wake balance, which determines the degree of attention or sedation, depends not only on the inherent rhythm of these mutually antagonistic systems, but also on nervous impulses which reach them. The impulses come from peripheral receptors and from higher centres including those for the emotions. A natural sleep occurs when the predominance of factors stimulating the sleep system raises its outflow to a level which inhibits the cortical arousal reaction from the reticular formation. Changes in the concentration of serotonin (5-hydroxytryptamine) in the Raphe system of cells in the hind brain has also been found and may play a role in the sleep mechanism.

Sleep deprivation

Prolonged sleep loss impairs attention and the performance of skilled tasks. If maintained, a proportion of individuals develop hallucinations (q.v.) and transient psychotic manifestations of a paranoid type (q.v.). Recovery from abnormal mental states is complete after sleep has been taken, but skills may still be impaired for some time. Deliberate deprivation of sleep as part of a technique of 'brainwashing' aims at disrupting vigilance and the sense of reality. Sleep after deprivation contains abnormally distributed REM periods. Some evidence suggests that REM sleep is associated with brain repair.
SEE ALSO Sleep and Dreams.

Sleep paralysis

Total inability to move the body while in a state of relative mental alertness on awakening from sleep, lasting only seconds. Frequently associated with narcolepsy (q.v.).

Sleep therapy

In the past continuous narcosis (q.v.) (sleep therapy) for two to three weeks at a time was widely used for patients with involutional melancholia and agitated schizophrenia. These conditions are nowadays far better treated by other means. Modified continuous narcosis is still used as an initial form of treatment in severe anxiety states, particularly those of long duration.

Sleep therapy is now used for states of anxiety and tension secondary to some stress. In times of acute stress insomnia is common and considerable improvement in the patient's condition will result from eight to ten hours' sleep per night. This is best achieved by combining a hypnotic such as sodium amylobarbitone with a tranquillizer such as nitrazepam, or flurazepam, given half an hour before the patient is ready to go to bed. Later the patient may sleep with a benzodiazepine alone, leaving the barbiturate by her bedside relaxing with the confidence that she can take it if sleep is delayed.
SEE ALSO Narcosis.

Sleep walking

SEE Somnambulism.

Social class

Social class is usually measured through the occupation of the family breadwinner and on this basis, the whole population is divided into five classes, from higher professional (I) to unskilled labouring (V). In the USA it has been found that the kind of treatment a psychiatric patient receives depends more on this social class rating than on his diagnosis – richer patients get psychotherapy and poorer patients get physical or custodial treatment. Recent social changes, though, in Britain and similar countries have made it less likely than in the past that lower social class will be associated with a cluster of unfavourable circumstances, such as poverty, malnutrition, overcrowding and poor medical care. In any case, there is no simple relationship between any particular social class and particular forms of psychiatric disorder. Compared with the general population, schizophrenia is found to be much more common at the lower end of the socio-economic scale. However, this does not mean that the illness results from poor social conditions, but rather that there has been a 'downward drift' of the patients, who become capable of only low-level jobs. Depression and neurosis, on the other hand, do not show this kind of relationship to occupation because they do not often cause the same kind of personality damage and disability.

Socialization

Socialization is the process of becoming involved in membership of a wider society, through the establishment or re-establishment of personal and group relationships. It begins in infancy, and is an important aspect of child development, involving learning conformity to certain rules of the social group. Maldevelopment or failure of this part of mental life may be an expression or cause of severe emotional disturbance.
SEE ALSO Social therapy.

Social phobia

Anxiety in the presence of other people. Subjectively the patient is afraid of what other people might think of him. The patient states that he fears people might find him boring or gauche, alternatively he fears he might make a fool of himself in a public situation (e.g. public speaking). These fears may be accentuated by the somatic response to the anxiety (e.g. blushing, stammering, vomiting).
The social phobias are in many ways intermediate between agoraphobia (q.v.) and the specific phobias (q.v.). There may be accompanying general anxiety or depression, and multiple fears of many social situations, or the social phobia may be an isolated problem restricted to a specific activity. The fear may only occur during an activity which is witnessed by a particular class of person, such as strangers (xenophobia) or authority figures or may be more widespread and related to the number and proximity of observers (anthropophobia). A common feature is a strict parental upbringing, particularly concerning attitudes to sex; the age of onset is similar to agoraphobia which is also commonly associated with sexual anxieties. This group of phobias is clinically less homogeneous than either agoraphobia or the specific phobias, but patients may respond well to behaviour therapy (q.v.) methods, including desensitization, modelling, shaping, flooding and assertive training.

Social security

A wide term covering most of the statutory schemes for financial aid in those countries in which the community assumes responsibility for citizens who are unable to support themselves. For most benefit schemes there are two conditions: (a) a minimum number of contributions must have been paid; and (b) a specified number of contributions must have been paid or credited within a given period. *Sickness benefit* is provided for a defined period, *unless* the illness can be said to have been caused by misconduct, or there is a failure to obtain treatment, or the patient works. Paid-up contributors are also usually entitled to *unemployment*

benefit unless they lose their job through misconduct or leave voluntarily.
Many of the chronically sick will fail to qualify for these schemes. Provision may be made for them via *supplementary benefits* – a non-contributory scheme.

Social worker

A member of the mental health team in the United Kingdom, the social worker obtains reports on home and family, as a background to clinical examination, keeps open the communications between a patient in hospital and his relatives, and provides supervision and support after discharge.
SEE ALSO Rehabilitation.

Sociopath
SEE Psychopathic disorders.

Sodomy

Sodomy is anal intercourse with another male, with a female or with an animal, and is a felony under the laws of most countries. In the United Kingdom, homosexual behaviour in private between consenting adults (i.e. men aged 21 or over) is no longer an offence; but sodomy, offending against public decency or victimising children can be punishable by imprisonment. Anal intercourse between marital partners could be similarly dealt with but is more commonly a plea for divorce on grounds of mental cruelty. Medical proof of the offence relies upon demonstration of local anal injury or recovery of spermatozoa from the rectum.
SEE ALSO Sexual disorders.

Somatotypes
SEE Constitution and Physique.

Somnambulism (Sleep walking)

Certain children, particularly those suffering night terrors (q.v.), rise and wander with slow deliberate tread whilst apparently asleep. Usually objects and dangers are avoided, which suggests a

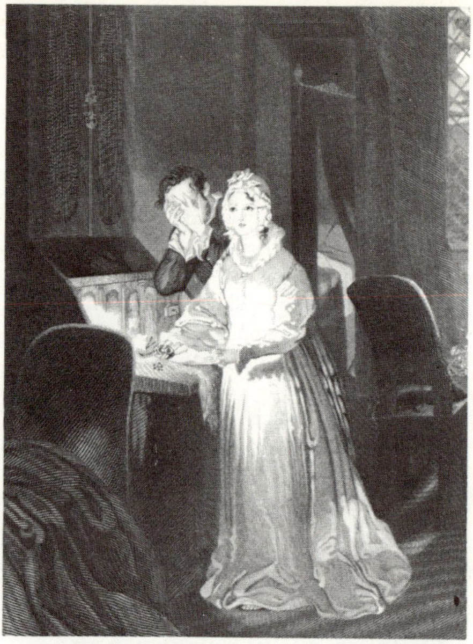

dissociative state rather than sleep. In the absence of electrophysiological evidence this cannot be determined. When offered as a presenting complaint it may suggest unhappiness, tension or familial discord. Usually, apart from taking some sensible precautions such as seeing that the child cannot fall down the stairs, somnambulism may be disregarded. At times, however, crimes are alleged to have been committed in a somnambulistic state, and such a defence may even succeed on occasions.
SEE ALSO Automatism.

Somnolence

Where not clearly attributable to errors of regime (overeating, alcohol, drugs) and in the absence of narcolepsy (q.v.) and the rare Kleine-Levin syndrome (q.v.) of periodic overeating and sleepiness, somnolence should be judged a serious symptom. Many cerebral tumours, raising intracranial pressure, lead to hypersomnia and this tendency increases where the tumours are located around the hypothalamus. Not surprisingly, disturbances of appetite, thirst, and behaviour which themselves might seem to be causal of the hypersomnia are often associated symptoms.
Encephalitis and the encephalopathies of metabolic disorders (uraemic, hepatic)

should be considered. Boredom and carbon dioxide retention in a stuffy room should, however, be borne in mind.

Spastic colon

SEE Irritable bowel syndrome.

Special hospitals

A term applied in the United Kingdom to hospitals which are especially set aside for the care of dangerous patients in all categories of mental disorder. In England there are three special hospitals (Broadmoor, Rampton, and Moss Side) and in Scotland one (Carstairs State Mental Hospital). Not all patients in these hospitals are compulsory detainees but the hospitals are security institutions with specially trained nursing staff and the majority of patients are under hospital orders (q.v.) from a court.
SEE ALSO Forensic psychiatry, Legal aspects of psychiatry, and Psychiatric prisons.

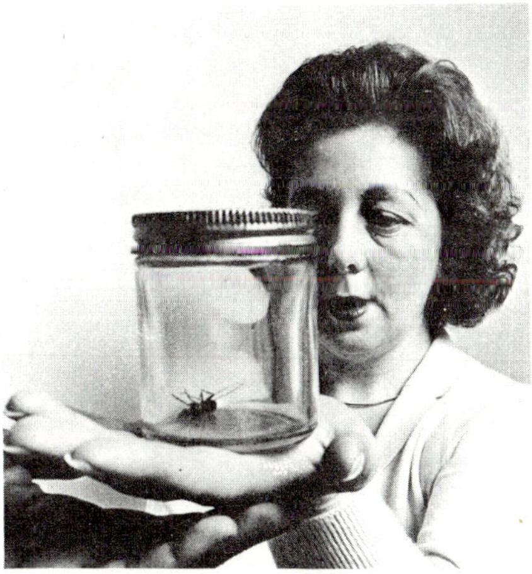

Specific phobias

A fear of a particular object or locus. Specific phobias include fears of animals, commonly cats (ailurophobia), spiders (arachnophobia), dogs (cynophobia), mice (murophobia), snakes and wasps, and fears of heights (acrophobia), thunder and/or lightning, and darkness.
Such fears are widespread before puberty in both sexes, but rarely persist to a disabling degree. Patients with specific phobias represent a small percentage of the phobias seen by psychiatrists. The fear sometimes originates in a traumatic experience in early life involving the object, although frequently the onset is beyond recall. Most such patients are adult women with a history of uninterrupted fear of a specific object since early childhood, and are usually otherwise well-adjusted people without other neurotic symptoms. This may explain why specific phobias in adult patients often respond well to behaviour therapy techniques. Desensitization (q.v.) is comfortable and a proven method, while flooding (q.v.) may be more effective, though more unpleasant, and may work when desensitization has failed.

Speech disorders

The word 'language' is used to describe our means of communication (including gesture and mime). 'Speech' is the expressive or spoken part of language. Speech disorders in childhood can be divided into defects of voicing and articulation, and central disorders of language. Articulatory disorders include disabilities due to structural abnormalities of the mouth, palate and tongue, and disorders due to abnormalities of the neuro-muscular mechanisms subserving these structures (e.g. dysarthria, bulbar palsy). Some articulatory disorders such as stammering, arise in the absence of either structural or neuro-muscular defects.
Central disorders of language may be due to mental retardation, deafness, childhood autism, developmental aphasia, or emotional factors producing so-called elective mutism. In differential diagnosis between these disorders, it is important to note the quality of vocalization used by the child, the use of gestures, the general behaviour of the child especially the relationship with parents and other children, and the child's hearing ability. An assessment along these lines is indicated in any child who is not using single words by the age of 2 or uttering two-to-three-word sentences by the age of 3. Treatment of speech disorders depends on

the underlying condition from which the child is suffering.
SEE ALSO Child development.

Spiritual healing

Of the non-medical psychotherapies, spiritual healing and faith healing are perhaps the most popular, appealing to individuals of all classes, beliefs and intelligence. Their cardinal feature is a belief in some power above man, and in the power of Faith. Little distinction is made between mental and physical illness, so that a case of leukaemia may be legitimately treated by practitioners of these techniques. There are no sicknesses, only sick persons. Prayer, belief, the laying-on of hands, and unction are all used, by the individual or a group. Much comfort may be given to a mortally sick person and for the chronic neurotic spiritual healing may offer more solace than does medical science. Priests and doctors have mutually complementary roles and much present-day unhappiness masquerading as mental illness is the province of the priest rather than the doctor.

Split brain

Section of the corpus callosum, hippocampal commissure, the anterior commissure and the massa intermedia of the thalamus is very occasionally carried out for the relief of intractable epilepsy. The operation functionally separates the two cerebral hemispheres and the effects are academically very interesting. Personality, temperament and intelligence are unimpaired and the patient behaves normally where both hemispheres are allowed to operate freely as in normal circumstances. However, when special conditions prevent one hemisphere from knowing what stimuli are being received by the other, striking deficits emerge. Thus a patient can indicate with his left hand a point stimulated on the left limbs; he cannot indicate this either verbally or with his right hand. Similar experiments with speech, calculation, vision, emotion, consciousness indicate not only the dominance of one hemisphere (contralateral to the dominant eye and hand), but significant differences in the activities of the two hemispheres.
SEE Cerebral cortex.

Stammering

Stammering is synonymous with stuttering, and involves an interruption in the normal rhythm of speech, because of an involuntary repetition, prolongation or cessation of sound.
It occurs in about 1–2% of British schoolchildren and is between two and four times more common in boys than in girls. There is some evidence that boys who stammer are somewhat less bright than those in the general population. There is no association with social class or, as is often stated, with left-handedness or ambidexterity. There is a strong suggestion that parents of stammering children are unusually ambitious and perfectionist. However, most stammerers have little or no evidence of psychiatric disorder and in most cases it is unhelpful to regard this condition as a form of psychoneurosis. Stammering is a disorder of childhood and over 50% of sufferers begin to stammer before the age of 5 years. About 50% of stammering remits either naturally or with treatment. In general, the milder the condition the better the prognosis. Treatment of the mono-symptomatic stammerer lies within the province of the speech therapist to whom a large number of individual and group techniques of treatment are available.
SEE ALSO Speech disorders.

Standard deviation

The statistical expression of a group of observations must give not only the average ('mean' (q.v.)) but also the extent of the scatter about the average. One means of expressing this is the 'range' (q.v.) but this gives a distorted view if there are outlying figures. A better statistical calculation which expresses the variation is the 'standard deviation' – SD. In a 'normal curve' (q.v.) the 95% range of the observations is covered by the mean ± 2 SDs.

Standard error

The standard error (of the mean, of a percentage or of a difference) shows the variation in the figure quoted which might be expected by chance in samples drawn randomly from a population.
SEE ALSO Standard error of the mean.

Standard error of the mean

In order to measure an accurate mean (q.v.) the whole population should be measured. The smaller the random sample selected for study, the greater the chance that the observed mean will not tally exactly with the true mean. The standard error of the mean, calculated from the standard deviation (q.v.) and the number of observations made, gives the calculated estimate of the error.

Stanford-Binet test

A test of intelligence for children consisting of questions arranged in mental ages corresponding to the ages of children who could pass them. The results of the test are expressed as mental age from which one can calculate the intelligence quotient (IQ)

$$\text{IQ} = \frac{\text{Mental age}}{\text{Chronological age}} \times 100.$$

The Stanford-Binet test is deficient in questions for the higher mental age group and is heavily loaded with tests of educational achievement.

Startle reaction

This term has been applied to several different phenomena: in babies subjected to noise or sudden movement the startle reaction (moro response) comprises extension of limbs and trunk; in normal adults exposed to sudden noise the startle response is characterized by dilatation of pupils, extension of spine, sweating of palms and increase in pulse rate: paradoxically patients with anxiety neurosis show less response because they are already in 'top gear' physiologically speaking.

Statistics

The science of determining and comparing probabilities. When used in relation to the biological sciences it is normally concerned with the probability of a particular outcome of a disease, experimental procedure or therapy. This may be extended to the determination of the probability that a defined therapeutic procedure has influenced the normal course of an outcome of a disease. Several techniques are available for such therapeutic comparisons. These include the chisquare (q.v.) and Student's (q.v.) tests.
SEE ALSO Mean, mode, median.

Status epilepticus

Serial epileptic fits without recovery of consciousness; a serious disorder and a medical emergency. Seizure activity continuing unabated for more than fifteen minutes should be treated as status epilepticus. Apparent immobility and profound unconsciousness without 'lightening' after an obvious seizure should suggest that the seizure is continuing. Death may result from cerebral anoxia, cardiac, or renal failure.
The therapy of choice is diazepam 10 mg, i.v., the dose being repeated every fifteen minutes until control is obtained, up to a maximum of 50–60 mg. in one to two hours. For petit mal status ethosuximide may be given in doses of 250 mg, by mouth every four hours. It is advisable after the petit mal status has ceased to give hydantoin sod. 50 mg. t.d.s.
SEE ALSO Epilepsy.

Stealing

In general the doctor will be well advised to limit his intervention to those cases of stealing which present some bizarre or unusual feature, which involve children, or take certain forms, e.g. shoplifting, stealing female undergarments from clothes lines, or repetitive theft of a particular object. Aggression, greed, envy and malice are the common emotional substrates for stealing; in children it may represent a means of obtaining attention. A knowledge of human nature, rather

than of psychiatry, is necessary when considering the innumerable forms of theft, the majority being motivated by a simple desire for easy money.
SEE ALSO Childhood behaviour disorders and Shoplifting.

Stereotactic operations

Stereotactic surgery is a method of producing accurate lesions in certain areas of the nervous system where nuclear structures and fibre tracts are concentrated. The tremor of Parkinsonism and involuntary movements in certain other conditions can be alleviated by thalamotomy and intractable pain controlled by stereotactic cervical tractotomy.
In psychiatric disorders stereotactic surgery has been applied to the amygdala (q.v.), the thalamic nuclei and the substantia innominata. The reduction of emotional disturbance such as aggression, tension or depression with preservation of all other mental function is the objective of such operations. Electrocoagulation or the implantation of seeds of yttrium ^{90}Y in the relevant areas depends on accurate placement of the instruments, a matter demanding a high degree of technical skill.

Stereotypy

Mechanical repetition of an action or group of actions, or words, or the maintenance of a posture for long periods when fatigue would normally induce relaxation. Stereotypy is a catatonic symptom showing in a local manifestation the characteristic catatonic features of both immobility and excitability.

Sterilization

In the United States, twenty-six states have statutes which provide for the compulsory sterilization of the mentally disabled. There is no evidence to show that sterilization for eugenic (q.v.) reasons is justifiable. In Britain the law is not entirely clear. The Brock Report in 1934 recommended that voluntary sterilization should be legalized in the case of a mentally disabled person, a person who suffers from or is believed to be the carrier of a grave physical disability, a person who is believed to be likely to transmit mental disorder. These proposals were never embodied in the law, and it is still technically possible for a surgeon to be charged with an offence against the person if he carries out a sterilization. However, it is a relatively common procedure, and criminal proceedings are extremely unlikely if the consent of both the husband and the wife is obtained.
The majority of sterilization operations are carried out not for eugenic reasons, but on women who are unable effectively to rear children either because of a physical or mental disability, or because of a large family or impoverished social circumstances. In some of these cases a psychiatric report may be required.
SEE ALSO Abortion Act.

Stigmata

The term is used in two different ways: (a) in nineteenth-century European psychiatry when the theory of degeneration required anatomical and physiological stigmata as confirmation of degeneracy; (b) as marks resembling the wounds of Christ, self-produced, and found in both neurotic and psychotic individuals.

Stimulants, central nervous
SEE Psychostimulants.

Strephasymbolia

Difficulty, in children, in learning to read. These children are unable to distinguish between similar letters, such as 'p' and 'q', or 'n' and 'u'. It is a result of mixed motor dominance of right and left hemispheres.

Stress

Psychological stress is any stimulus which is sufficiently intense to produce an emotional response, either because there is a threat to the individual's self-esteem or peace of mind, or because there is a need for a special effort. The 'stress reaction', which is the response of the individual to a noxious stimulus, takes the form of a psychological, physiological or biochemical response, or some combination of these. One behavioural response is that of 'fight' or 'flight' seen in marked form in the traumatic war neuroses, where overwhelming stress leads to the defensive posture of loss of function, e.g. hysterical blindness or paralysis. Different personality structures deal with stress in characteristic ways; an anxiety-prone patient will run from a crowded shop when claustrophobic, a histrionic personality may develop an amnesia, and an obsessional may indulge in rituals; all these reactions are defences against anxiety. The psychological and biochemical responses to stress are not under conscious control and may lead to psychosomatic disorders (q.v.), for example bronchial constriction in asthma, or high gastric acidity leading to peptic ulceration.

Students, emotional problems

About 5% of all students have psychiatric disorders causing serious distress and handicaps, whilst at least twice as many have less serious conditions which need skilled psychiatric help. 14% of the students who begin university fail to graduate and emotional disorder is responsible for a high proportion of these 'drop-outs'. Those who break down are more likely to be female than male, to have graduate parents, to be reading arts rather than sciences and to come from overseas (a particularly vulnerable group). Common problems are depression, which may be connected with loss of the security of life at home, phobic fear of examinations, difficulties over personal relationships and unwise experiments with drugs. Almost all universities and colleges now have a medical service, though many still lack special psychiatric facilities. Counselling (perhaps combined with medication) will relieve most of the less serious conditions, but some cases of depression or of schizophrenia will need intensive treatment as in-patients. Students in some cases may be allowed to take their examinations under special medical supervision whilst patients in a psychiatric hospital.

Students 't' test

The 't' test was first described by G. S. Gosset writing under the pseudonym 'Student' – hence the name. It is used to determine whether there is a significant (q.v.) difference between samples when the number in each is small (usually thirty or less). Since this is a common situation in clinical trials it is a widely used test.

Stupor

Stupor is characterized by immobility and lack of response to stimuli without loss of consciousness. The subject may be mute, completely immobile, and may retain urine and faeces. In milder degree it may be difficult to gain the subject's attention, whose speech and movement are limited and slow. Despite the apparent withdrawal, stuporose subjects may demonstrate on recovery that they have been aware of events around them.

Stupor is one phase of catatonic schizophrenia (q.v.); it also occurs in profound degrees of retarded depression (q.v.). Modern physical treatments have made both types less common.

Stupor may occur in organic conditions – following head injury, or associated with tumours of the third ventricle. Akinetic mutism may be easily confused with a stupor occurring in a functional psychosis.

Sturge-Weber syndrome
SEE Naevoid Amentia

Stuttering
SEE Stammering.

Subdural haematoma

A subdural haematoma is an encapsulated collection of blood between the dura and arachnoid mater, usually frontal or parietal and commonly bilateral. Trauma is the most frequent cause, but those most subject to it are often least able to recall it – seniles and alcoholics. Headache, drowsiness and confusion markedly fluctuate in degree. Arteriography and ventriculography show displacement of vessels or ventricles. The EEG shows an area of diminished amplitude of fast activity with adjacent slow wave activity. Lumbar puncture may show paradoxically low fluid pressure and xanthochromia. Final diagnosis is by exploration and treatment is by surgical evacuation.

Sublimation

The word sublimation like many other psychoanalytical terms, has passed into the vernacular and is usually used to mean the substitution of a socially acceptable form of behaviour for an unfulfilled emotion. The disappointed lover who goes off to shoot big game, instead of disposing of his rival, is a banal example of the common meaning of the word. Technically, however, sublimation is an unconsciously determined substitute activity for an infantile (usually sexual) impulse.

Subnormality
SEE Mental subnormality.

Substantia gelatinosa
SEE Gate theory of pain.

Substitution

An unconscious defence mechanism by which an unacceptable or unattainable goal is replaced by one which is more acceptable or attainable. Compare with displacement (q.v.).

Suggestibility

Suggestion is the process whereby one person induces another by verbal or other non-coercive communications, to accept ideas he presents in an uncritical manner or to behave according to his wishes or example. Suggestibility is a personality trait representing the degree to which an individual is open to suggestion or, as used psychiatrically, indicates a more extreme state of this nature as exhibited during hypnosis and in a number of pathological conditions. In Hull's body-sway test of suggestibility, the blindfold subject stands with his feet together and is told repeatedly that he is falling forward. The extent to which his body sways to and fro in these circumstances is an indication of his suggestibility. Suggestibility is increased in some forms of psychoneurosis (q.v.), especially conversion hysteria (q.v.), some brain conditions, and in schizophrenia (q.v.) in which, however, negativism (q.v.) or negative suggestibility may also occur. The automatic obedience (q.v.), echolalia (q.v.), echopraxia (q.v.), and flexibilitas cerea (q.v.) shown by catatonic patients are all phenomena related to suggestion.
SEE ALSO Conation, Consciousness, Folie à deux and Personality.

Suggestion

This is the process of influencing an individual so that he shows uncritical acceptance of an idea or belief. Suggestion plays a large part in the induction of hypnosis and in the degree of success encountered by the therapist with his persuasive comments to the patient. Psychoanalytic method was born out of, and has evolved from, hypnotic techniques. Prestige-suggestion is a form of psychotherapy. It does not attempt to deal with unconscious motivation for behaviour, but relies on the patient's submission to, and identification with, the omnipotent therapist. The patient gives up his symptoms as part of his obedience to the doctor.
Persons of hysterical disposition are often found to be unusually suggestible. The 'body-sway' test, in which it is suggested to a steady, erect subject with closed eyes that he is beginning to sway from side to side, gives some indication of his degree of suggestibility.

Suicide

In most industrial countries suicide ranks as one of the ten commonest causes of death and, with the virtual elimination of deaths from inanition and exhaustion, it is almost the only psychiatric cause. In young men the mortality from suicide is second only to that from traffic accidents, and amongst university students suicide accounts for a third of all deaths. Contrary to popular belief, and in sharp contrast to attempted suicide, the suicide rate in both Britain and the USA is much the same now as it was at the beginning of the century. It rose in 1930 at the time of the depression and fell in both world wars, but is now steady again at about 1:10,000 population per year.

The epidemiology of suicide has been studied extensively and many facts are well established. It is twice as common in men as in women. It is rare in childhood and becomes steadily more common as age increases. In women the rate is highest in the sixth decade, but in men it continues to rise to the eighth and ninth decades. There is a diurnal fluctuation with a peak after midnight and an annual fluctuation with a peak in the spring and early summer. Catholic communities consistently have lower suicide rates than Protestant ones; probably only part of this difference is due to the reluctance of Catholics to record unexpected deaths as suicide. Urban areas have higher suicide rates than rural ones, but within big cities like London there are large and persistent differences between one area and another. Surprisingly, areas of poverty and poor housing often have quite low suicide rates; the highest rates are found in areas with a changing population and a high proportion of lodging houses and people living alone. The key factor is probably social isolation, for those who are widowed or single consistently have higher suicide rates than those who are married, and widows with children have lower rates than those without. The lack of relationship with poverty is emphasized by the fact that suicide is commoner in upper social classes than in manual workers and is particularly common in doctors and dentists, probably in part because of their ready access to lethal drugs.

Methods of committing suicide vary considerably from country to country and from one generation to another. In the British Isles barbiturate overdosage currently the commonest methods, but overdosage with other hypnotics and assorted psychotropic drugs is increasing steadily. Violent methods (hanging, shooting, stabbing, etc.) have become steadily less common, since the beginning of the century and are largely restricted to men.

About 50% of all suicides are suffering from depressive illnesses (q.v.) and for that reason alone the risk of suicide must be taken seriously in all depressions. However, the risk is much greater in psychotic or endogenous depressions than in neurotic or reactive illnesses; at least 15% of manic depressives eventually die by their own hand. The other group of patients most at risk are alcoholics (q.v.), whose suicide rate is fifty times higher than that of the general population. Indeed, in Britain alcoholics are far more likely to die from suicide than from cirrhosis or any of the other physical complications of alcoholism. Perhaps a quarter of all suicides have personality disorders of one sort or another, often in combination with depression or alcoholism or both. A small proportion, under 10%, are psychiatrically normal; that is, they have no history of psychiatric illness and appeared normal to their friends and relatives up to the moment of their death. Physical illness is present in a high proportion of elderly suicides. This applies particularly to cancer (and to the fear of it) and Parkinsonism.

The motives and states of mind which lead up to suicide can be inferred with some confidence from these facts. Depression and the pessimism, guilt and feelings of hopelessness that accompany it are obviously very important, but probably more important still are feelings of being useless and unwanted and of having no one to live for. It is probably thoughts of this nature which are responsible for the high suicide rate of the elderly and those living alone, and the low suicide rate of young married women in spite of their high incidence of depression.

The prevention of suicide depends upon accurate recognition of potential suicides. All those with depressive illnesses are at risk and for this reason depressives (and alcoholics) should always be asked whether they feel that life is not worth living or are entertaining thoughts of killing themselves. The physician's assessment of the risk of suicide is often the most important factor in determining whether or not the patient is admitted to hospital and will be strongly influenced by the patient's age and sex, whether he is living alone and whether he is drinking, as well as by the severity of his illness. The lay belief that those who talk of suicide do not kill themselves is fallacious. In fact, up to 70% of suicides communicate suicidal ideas beforehand, often to several different people, and about 40% state definitely that they intend to kill themselves. Unfortunately these hints or threats are often ignored, or else have continued for so long that alarm and concern have given way to complacency, or even irritation, by the time the tragedy occurs. Up to now suicide prevention measures have not been strikingly effective. Neither the introduction of ECT nor that of the anti-depressive drugs was followed by a convincing fall in the suicide rate, in spite of the undoubted efficacy of these drugs in the treatment of depressions. Indeed some patients who are too retarded in severe depression to pursue their suicidal intent, commit suicide during the recovery phase. Perhaps of greater significance is the fact that neither drugs nor ECT prevents the recurrence of the depression; the patient's symptoms are indeed relieved but they recur a year or two later and he kills himself then, often before coming under medical care. It is a sobering fact, however, that over 50% of suicides were either currently, or at least recently, attending a doctor, and often a psychiatrist. One of the problems is that a high proportion of suicides are impulsive. The patient may have been depressed and thinking intermittently of suicide for many months but is only impelled to act by some 'last straw' which in itself is trivial. The day and night telephone service provided in many cities by the Samaritans (q.v.) or other organizations seems a logical answer to the problem, though so far there is no clear evidence of falling suicide rates in cities with such services. Major wars are consistently accompanied by a sharp fall in the suicide rate and there is intriguing evidence in the USA that prolonged newspaper strikes are accompanied by a sharp fall in the number of female suicides, but it is difficult to derive practicable medical solutions from either of these findings.

Superego

That part of the mental apparatus concerned with personal and social standards of acceptable behaviour. The maturing child patterns itself, both consciously and unconsciously, on the behaviour and mores of the individuals amongst whom it grows up. By processes of identification and introjection these standards of right behaviour become incorporated into the mind. Conflicts may arise between the instinctual demands of the individual and the super-ego. Then the ego may have to decide just how much instinctual gratification may be allowed in relation to the strength of the super-ego. It is as a result of such conflicts that anxiety, depression, and obsessive-compulsive symptoms may arise.

Super females

SEE Trisomy.

Super males

SEE Trisomy.

Supervision order

In Britain juveniles, by means of either care or criminal proceedings in a juvenile court can be placed under a supervision order. The supervising authority will usually be the local children's department although some young persons (aged 14–17) will be eligible for supervision by a probation officer in special circumstances. It can contain 'provisions' or rules to which the supervised person has to adhere, e.g. it can designate where he must live. As with probation (q.v.) in the adult, the court can add, if it wishes, a requirement of medical treatment if recommended by a psychiatrist. Equivalent systems for juvenile offenders exist in some other countries.

Supportive psychotherapy

The objects of this treatment are to strengthen existing mental defences, elaborate more effective mechanisms to maintain control and restore an adaptive

equilibrium. The techniques used include guidance, environmental manipulation (q.v.), externalization of interests, reassurance (q.v.), persuasion (q.v.), catharsis (q.v.), desensitization (q.v.), and group therapy (q.v.).
The object is to deal with the present problems in the life of the patient. It is invaluable in the milder neurotic reactions resulting from modifiable environmental stress.
SEE ALSO Psychotherapy.

Sydenham's chorea

A disorder characterized by rapid, involuntary, non-repetitive, purposeless movements. Aetiologically it is probably related in some way to collagen disorders as in about 75% of cases there is a previous history of rheumatic fever. It occurs mainly in young girls aged 10–15 years, who have often suffered a haemolytic streptococcal infection a few weeks previously. The treatment is symptomatic, involving no more than the temporary use of a tranquillizing agent such as chlorpromazine. Recovery is complete. The only psychiatric significance of the condition is that it is said to occur most commonly in tense anxious girls. In addition, in the differential diagnosis, it is important to exclude Huntington's chorea and tics of organic or psychogenic origin.

Symbolization

The process of expressing psychic disorder in terms dissimilar from, but standing for, the underlying disorder itself. The symbol may be ideational, affective or somatic. It is an unconscious process built up on association and similarity whereby one object comes to stand for another object, through some quality which the two have in common. The resemblance is usually so slight that the conscious mind overlooks it. As such it may be used as a mental defence mechanism to protect the conscious mind from awareness of unacceptable impulses or ideas by merely substituting a covert, yet linked idea in its place. Dreams are believed to be rich in symbolization, the significance of which may be interpreted during analysis through free association of ideas to the symbol.
Symbolization is a very characteristic feature of schizophrenic behaviour, ideation and speech. He acts like 'a dreamer awake' and the symbolization often gives the illness its bizarre quality.

Sympathin
SEE Adrenaline

Sympathomimetic drugs

In general the effects of the sympathomimetic drugs resemble the response of stimulation of adrenergic nerves, but individual drugs differ in the details and intensity, of their actions. Sympathomimetic agents have both excitatory and inhibitory actions on peripheral structures according to the predominance of α or β receptors (q.v.), they have a cardiac excitatory effect, metabolic actions of glycogenolysis and liberation of free fatty acids, and an excitatory effect on the central nervous system which with some drugs may increase wakefulness and reduce appetite. It is those effects on the central nervous system which are of interest in psychiatry.
The catecholamines adrenaline, noradrenaline, and isoprenaline have essentially peripheral actions. The amphetamines (q.v.) have important psychostimulant properties and are considered separately. Ephedrine has central actions that resemble but are less pronounced than those of the amphetamines, which have therefore superseded ephedrine.
Phenmetrazine like the amphetamines has been used as an anorectic agent, but has similar problems of wakefulness and drug dependence. In contrast to other amphetamines, fenfluramine does not produce wakefulness and therefore may be of special value in the treatment of obesity accompanying psychiatric disorder.

Symptomatology

Psychiatric symptoms arise from three causes:
1. **Environmental factors.**
2. **Personality factors.**

3. Genetical factors and organic disorders of the central nervous system.

1. *Environmental factors.* These are usually self-evident. Thus a psychiatric disorder precipitated by a sad event, such as a bereavement, tends to be coloured by depressive symptoms related to the loss of the loved one. In a more subtle way, the menopausal woman, whose children have left home, may feel useless and rejected, and make excessive demands for her husband's attention.

2. *Personality factors.* These are usually the predominant factors in determining how the psychiatric disorder manifests itself. Thus, if an anxious man is unable to cope with life for one reason or another, his symptoms will be those of anxiety and the form they take will depend on other personality traits, resulting in free-floating (q.v.), phobic (q.v.), or hypochondriacal (q.v.) types of anxiety. Again, patients with an hysterical personality tend to develop hysterical symptoms. In the same context, some people are constitutionally predisposed to a particular psychosomatic disorder (q.v.). In such persons and particularly when physiogenic factors are involved, psychogenic stress acting through the autonomic nervous system, may produce an exacerbation of the psychosomatic symptoms.

3. *Genetical factors and organic disorders of the central nervous system.* If a genetical predisposition results in the development of a specific illness, such as mania (q.v.), depression (q.v.) or schizophrenia (q.v.), the symptoms are fundamentally those of the illness concerned. Similarly, organic disorders of the central nervous system result in characteristic 'organic' symptoms of disorientation, memory loss, emotional lability, etc.

However, none of these factors acts alone and the manner in which a genetically determined illness presents will depend to a considerable degree on precipitating factors and the patient's underlying personality. Thus, a depressive illness precipitated by the death of her child may result either in the patient blaming herself or, depending on paranoid traits in her personality, believing that the neighbours are talking about her and accusing her of causing the child's death by her neglect. Lastly, a genetically determined, though mild, depressive illness or an early dementia might result in a precariously adjusted patient being unable to cope with life and consequent on this develop neurotic symptoms which may predominate and mask the underlying depressive or organic disorder.

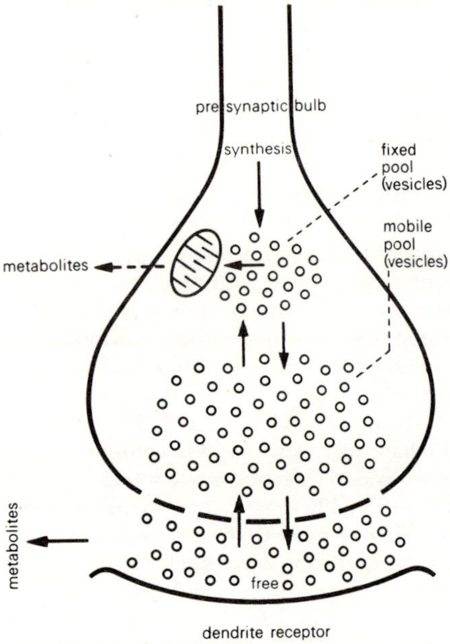

'Ideal representation' of typical synaptic transmission mechanism

Synapse – transmission in

The term synapse refers to the area between two neurones where transmission of the nerve impulse occurs. The pre-synaptic structure is usually a swelling, the 'bouton terminal' at the end of axon branches. Synapses can be axo-somatic, axo-dendritic or axo-axonic according to their site on the post-synaptic neurone. Transmission across the synaptic cleft is always in one direction and is mediated by a specific chemical substance, the neuro-transmitter. This is stored in pre-synaptic vesicles in the boutons terminaux. When the membrane potential of a neurone is reduced to a certain critical level a nerve action potential is triggered which sweeps along the axon by means of permeability changes to sodium and potassium ions. When the impulse arrives at the axon terminal the neuro-transmitter in the pre-

synaptic vesicles is released into the synaptic cleft and diffuses across to its specific receptor sites on the post-synaptic neurone. At the post-synaptic site it initiates an ionic permeability change which is a characteristic of both the transmitter substance and the particular receptor. At some synapses the effect is to produce an excitatory depolarization and an impulse spreads along the next neurone; at others an inhibitory membrane-stabilizing or hyperpolarization effect occurs.
In these circumstances the passage of other impulses in that nerve will be inhibited.
A nerve cell acts by means of the same transmitter at all of its synapses.
In the peripheral nervous system there are two known transmitters. Acetylcholine is synthesized by the enzyme choline acetylase in the nerve. After release excess acetylcholine is broken down by acetylcholinesterase. The other peripheral transmitter is noradrenaline which is synthesized from phenylalanine and tyrosine via dopa and dopamine.
SEE ALSO Transmission in synapses in brain cells.

Synesthesia

(Synonym: Secondary sensation)

These are sensations which accompany those in a different modality; for example, some people experience a sensation of colour when they hear a particular musical note being played.

Syphilis

Despite a rise in the incidence of venereal disease in recent years the number of new cases of syphilis reported in Britain has remained stable at about 1300 per annum – roughly 4·5 per 100,000 population for males and 1 per 100,000 for females. Rates in the United States as a whole are roughly double this, and experience in different areas in this country will vary widely because of the social factors involved in the spread of venereal disease. Congenital syphilis (once a significant cause of subnormality) is now extremely rare because of the routine investigation of and treatment available for pregnant women.
That the central nervous system is involved in about 30% of cases within a few months of primary infection is demonstrated even in the absence of clinical signs by increased mononuclear cells and globulin with possibly a positive Wasserman or similar reaction in the cerebro-spinal fluid.
In tertiary neuro-syphilis Lange's colloidal gold test yields either a 'paretic' curve (e.g. 5542210000) or a 'luetic' curve (1355421000).
The central nervous system is affected secondarily in meningovascular syphilis when vascular and perivascular inflammation leads to impairment of the blood supply and patchy necrosis with surrounding fibrotic reaction (gumma). The brain and spinal cord may, however, be invaded directly by spirochaetes and general paralysis of the insane (GPI) (q.v.), tabes dorsalis, or combinations of these conditions result. Early tabes may be mistaken for hysteria because of crises or lightning pains in the absence of local findings. In cerebral syphilis headache, anxiety, apathy, impairment of memory and intellect are seen with various neurological signs. Convulsions beginning in adults, third nerve palsy, optic atrophy, and hemiplegia in a young normotensive subject should all rouse a suspicion of neuro-syphilis. The Argyll-Robertson pupil (failure to react to light but retention of the reaction to accommodation) is a common neurological sign.
SEE ALSO Infections, mental symptoms due to.

Systematic desensitization

Systematic desensitization (or simply desensitization) is one of the behaviour therapy techniques, and is particularly useful in phobic states when anxiety is associated with particular objects or situations. Theoretically one can hypothesize that in psychological terms the patient has 'learned' a maladaptive response to a particular stimulus. In physiological terms one could visualize it as a result of 'conditioning'. Whichever way one looks at it, the aim of desensitization is to substitute a response, such as relaxation, which is antagonistic to that of anxiety (reciprocal inhibition) and in such a way cause 'unlearning' or deconditioning of the phobia.

In desensitization, a detailed account is obtained of characteristics of the stimulus which influence the intensity of the evoked anxiety; the phobic anxiety experienced in a spider phobia for example, might depend upon mobility and proximity of spiders, and their number. Patient and therapist together construct a 'hierarchy', a sequence of ten to twenty different problem situations from that which evokes minimal anxiety to the most anxiety-provoking one. Starting at the bottom of the hierarchy the doctor helps the patient to imagine as vividly as possible the situation which would make him mildly anxious and apposes this with relaxation so that the patient imagines the situation but remains symptom free. The relaxation can be induced by teaching deep muscle relaxation or by the intravenous injection of about 1 ml. of a $2\frac{1}{2}\%$ solution of methohexitone sodium, which provides quick relaxation which rapidly wears off. The procedure is repeated in sessions of fifteen to thirty minutes until the most anxiety-provoking items have been visualized without anxiety. This procedure is 'desensitization in imagination' and is rarely completed in less than ten sessions. It is often claimed that successful imaginal desensitization leads without further treatment to changed behaviour in the corresponding real-life situations. Desensitization can, however, be adapted to real situations, the subject being encouraged, while in a relaxed state, to approach the problem situation gradually and repeatedly, stopping on each trial when anxiety occurs.

At the same time as desensitization is being carried out the patient is taught to behave in a manner incompatible with his previous anxiety and this can be done in the five to ten minutes required for the patient to recover sufficiently to return to the waiting room. Thus, if the patient's anxiety is interpersonal and he feels self-conscious and embarrassed in the presence of people of superior intellectual, social, financial, or physical status, then assertive responses are used and he is trained to express his feelings (in a socially acceptable way) instead of repressing them. Again, this is the time for simple psychotherapy and possible explanation of what lies behind the symptom. It is most important not to rush things; repeated successes will consolidate improvement, but a failure will retard progress.

The technique can be varied considerably. However, it is probable that the vital component of all successful techniques is that somehow the patient is enabled to approach rather than avoid feared objects or situations.

Desensitization is particularly effective in single or specific phobias. In social phobias, and patients with the agoraphobia/claustrophobia syndrome, personality disorders are frequently associated and a combination of desensitization and drugs or interpretive psychotherapy may be required.

Systemization

The degree to which a single subject's delusions (q.v.) cohere and form a composite picture. Delusions may be expressed having no connection with each other, in which case they are unsystematized. On the other hand, delusions may show a reasonable and understandable connection. If the connection is loose the delusions are described as 'poorly systematized, if it is close and logical as 'well systematized'. Paranoid illnesses in intelligent, articular subjects who show little schizophrenic thought disorder and who are in good contact with their surroundings are most likely to produce well systematized delusions.

't' Test
SEE Students 't' test

Tantrums in childhood

Unrestrained motor outbursts of rage in situations of frustration are common in early childhood and often persist as troublesome behaviour at least into the early teens.
The causes and manifestations of the tantrums change as the child gets older, the rage reactions becoming more verbal, less physically violent, and more directed against the frustrating object or person. The outburst may be a temporary exhibition of fury in a well-adjusted child, or they may represent the expression of enduring hostility or unbearable inner tension in a depressed or anxious child. Knowledge of the rest of the child's emotional life and behaviour is essential to make the diagnosis.
In the toddler, in whom the tantrum represents a successful means of obtaining attention, consistently ignoring the child in the tantrum and giving him plenty of attention at other times is an effective way of reducing their frequency.

Tardive dyskinesia

A late onset and sometimes permanent oral dyskinesia with writhing, chewing, sucking movements of the tongue, mouth and jaws, frequently accompanied by akathisia (q.v.) and minor choreiform movements of the limbs.
Tardive dyskinesias begin insidiously and are usually first noticed after an average of two years neuroleptic therapy with either phenothiazines or butyrophenones. Their appearance seems to bear no relationship to the particular drug used or dosage, nor is there a correlation with the occurrence of reversible extrapyramidal disturbances earlier in the course of treatment. The dyskinesias are not alleviated but are often made worse by anti-Parkinsonian agents. Often they first appear when the neuroleptic drug is reduced in dosage or stopped and improves when the drug is reintroduced or the dosage increased. The incidence is small but many more cases might be masked by continuing neuroleptic therapy. The syndrome may be secondary to dopamine receptor sensitivity, secondary to prolonged blockade by neuroleptics.

Tay-Sachs disease
SEE Amaurotic family idiocy.

Temperament

Temperament refers to the characteristic features of an individual's emotional nature: the prevailing quality and lability of his mood, the readiness and intensity of his emotional reactions. The temperamental aspect of personality (q.v.) is usually regarded as constitutionally determined and genetically based.
Galen, in the second century AD, extended earlier notions of Hippocrates to propose four temperamental types – melancholic, choleric, sanguine, and phlegmatic – produced by a preponderance of the appropriate body 'humour'. Of more recent theories, the most influential in the field of psychiatry has been that of Kretschmer (q.v.) who described two contrasting types of body-build, the pyknic – stocky and well-rounded – and the leptosomatic (q.v.) or asthenic – small-boned, long and thin. He also refers to an athletic type in some ways intermediate between these two. Kretschmer claimed that the pyknic develops a cyclothymic (q.v.) personality with mood swings, is essentially sociable and good-natured, but is vulnerable to manic-depressive psychosis. The leptosome on the other hand is schizothymic – withdrawn, shy, and eccentric – and is liable to develop schizophrenia. There is some empirical support for weak correlations of this nature and a similar but more elaborate theory has been proposed by Sheldon (q.v.) who somatotypes (q.v.) individuals in terms of the relative strengths of their tendencies towards three basic bodily builds – ectomorphic (q.v.), mesomorphic (q.v.), and endomorphic (q.v.) – rather similar to Kretschmer's types and similarly considered to be reflected in characteristic temperaments.
SEE ALSO Constitution.

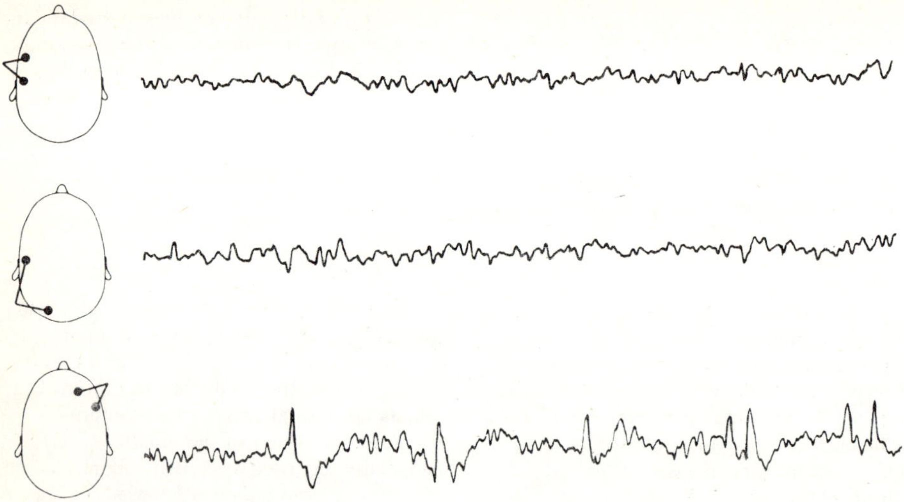

Typical EEG in temporal lobe epilepsy

Temporal lobe epilepsy

Epileptic seizures of any sort, of focal origin in the temporal lobe. The most characteristic seizures are psychomotor (q.v.), but are frequently accompanied by major convulsions. The focal origin of the attacks is associated with focal pathology in the majority of cases. Mesial temporal sclerosis (q.v.) accounts for half these lesions. Other lesions divide equally between post-natal trauma or infections, and indolent tumours. Mesial temporal sclerosis follows inadequately treated status epilepticus in early childhood. Many chronic epilepsies have psychomotor manifestations.

The EEG in adults classically reveals sharp spikes anti-phasing over the temporal lobe. In children obvious psychomotor seizures with clinically lateralizing features may show generalized abnormalities in their EEG. Only gradually does the spike focus become consistently located.

Management includes control of the psychomotor seizures by anti-convulsants, but also requires that the attendant behavioural disturbances are not thereby exacerbated. Barbiturates (and primidone) often cause severe disorders of mood and hyperkinesis (q.v.) in children. Hydantoin derivates are useful, but aberrant metabolism may lead to high serum levels. Carbamezepine may be useful as is succinamide, but in children may cause air hunger and weight loss. Behaviour disorders, rude and aggressive behaviour, neuroses and psychotic disorders are frequently associated. A chronic hallucinatory paranoid psychosis of onset in early adult life may follow a variable period after the onset of epilepsy. Depression is common and suicide rates are high.

SEE ALSO Epilepsy.

Tension

This denotes a state of strain evoked by stress experienced by the subject and manifests itself mainly in those muscle groups supplied by the voluntary nervous system. However, there are definite autonomic, biochemical and endocrinological correlates.

It is regarded as one component of an anxiety state and even used as a synonym for anxiety. Muscle tension is frequently associated with anxiety from any cause. There is increased muscle tonus, tremor of the extremities and strained and furrowed facial expression. Hands may be clenched so that knuckles appear white and the typical headache is described as aching or vice-like in character, affects the whole head and is usually worse at the end of the day. It is rapidly relieved by intravenous injection of short-acting barbiturates in subhypnotic doses, which have been used as a diagnostic test. Medication with chlordiazepoxide and diazepam is of value because of the muscle relaxant as well as anxiolytic properties of these drugs. Pre-menstrual tension is a syndrome which usually occurs some days before the menses in predisposed subjects and includes increased tendency to depression, irritability and anxiety as well as headache. Water retention, weight gain, swollen ankles, breasts and abdomen may be experienced. Polydipsia, hyperphagia, and hypersomnia have also been reported.

Teratogenic agents

Teratogenic agents are physical, chemical and biological agents acting upon the embryo or foetus. In general, the earlier the action of a teratogenic agent in gestation, the more severe the effects. The conceptus is most vulnerable during the embryonic period (i.e. from fertilization to the eighth week). Embryopathy caused by teratogenic agents often produces multiple defects because many organs are appearing simultaneously at the time of insult. Damage to the central nervous system by teratogenic agents may result in severe neurological damage and mental subnormality. Much that is known about teratogenesis depends upon experimental work with animals. Maternal diets deficient in vitamins have produced abnormalities in animals, especially with respect to the central nervous system. Excess of vitamin A has also been shown to be teratogenic in such experiments. Other examples of teratogenic agents are X-rays and other forms of hard irradiation; certain drugs, including thalidomide, and heavy metals.

Testamentary capacity

The capacity of an individual to make a will depends on his appreciation of his estate and of the claims which ties of family or friendship impose on him in the disposal of his property. 'A sound disposing mind' may be found in individuals suffering from both mental or physical disease, as long as judgement is preserved. The use by old people of promises to 'remember you in my will' is a common mode of manipulating their environment. Difficulties may arise when a succession of wills is made – some duly executed by a solicitor, some on post-office forms, and some on scraps of paper witnessed perhaps by a friend or casual acquaintance. The mental state of the legator at the time of making the different wills may be the source of a legal action by interested parties. It is important to remember that in the common arteriosclerotic dementia, lucid intervals may occur, and although the patient may be clearly demented, never-the-less his will may have been formulated entirely sensibly and properly. The doctor in attendance must never be witness to a will from which he may benefit, and in general is ill-advised to witness wills except in the most urgent circumstances. He should insist on the correct legal procedure being followed, and should confine his activities to keeping careful notes of his patient's mental and physical state over the period in question. Depressive and manic-depressive schizophrenic illnesses may all disturb an individual's judgement, as may organic cerebral disease, such as frontal lobe tumours, encephalitis, and other conditions.
SEE ALSO Court of protection and Dementia.

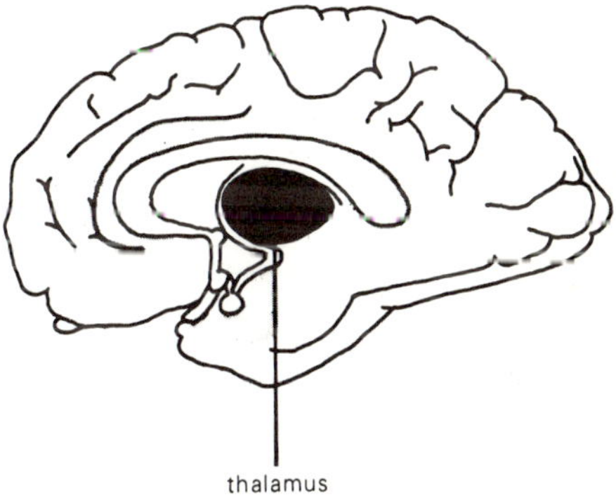

Thalamus

The thalamus is the final relay-station of the afferent fibre-systems to the cerebral cortex. It comprises three groups of nuclei, anterior, medial, and lateral, separated by the internal medullary lamina. Functionally, the thalamus can be divided into (a) specific regions receiving impulses from the somatic sensory systems, the cerebellum and the hypothalamus and projecting to well-defined cortical areas, and (b) nonspecific nuclei lying medially which evoke activity over wide cortical areas of both hemispheres. Lesions of the thalamus result in impairment of contralateral sensory functions, especially discriminatory and deep sensation, and are often accompanied by spontaneous pain of a widespread, severe and intractable nature.

Thematic apperception test (TAT)

The TAT is a popular projective technique for the assessment of personality (q.v.). It consists of a series of twenty cards displaying a variety of scenes involving human characters. The subject is asked to make up a story about each card, including an account of what is happening in the portrayed situation, what has led up to it, and what the outcome will be. Murray, the original designer of this test, assumed that the subject would project his own personality on to the main character or 'hero' of his stories and that recurring themes would reveal the main social needs of the subject and the main stresses or environmental pressures to which he is subject. Later workers have evolved other scoring and interpretative schemes. As with other projective tests of personality, attempts at objective validation have proved disappointing, but give some support to more restricted usages of the test. Thus the TAT has proved useful in research on achievement motivation and can be scored as an intelligence test. It may also provide diagnostic indications of some value, particularly in relation to schizophrenia (q.v.).
SEE ALSO Apperception and Psychological tests.

Therapeutic communities

This term, which was introduced by Maxwell Jones, refers to the deliberate structuring of relationships within hospital units, so that patients can benefit from the experience. In the past, much of the interpersonal atmosphere of psychiatric hospitals was actually harmful. The opening up of communications (both between staff and patients and between different levels of staff) and the fostering of informality and collective responsibility have proved to be valuable – especially for those with neurotic and personality disorders.
SEE ALSO Social psychiatry.

Therapy

The origins of almost all psychiatric disorders remain obscure and for the majority there is probably a multifactorial aetiology. With such a complicated causation and so many divergent views on the relative importance of each cause it is scarcely surprising that equally controversial views are held on the question of therapy. Most patients are likely to receive a composite therapy based on a number of differing types of therapy.
The individual types of therapy are described separately viz.: behaviour therapy, electroconvulsive therapy, occupational therapy, psychotherapy, psychopharmacology, physical therapy, play therapy, psychosurgery.

Theta rhythm

SEE EEG.

Thiamine deficiency

Thiamine (vitamin B_1) deficiency may arise naturally from a poor diet, from disproportionate carbohydrate intake, or in chronic alcoholism (q.v.). Gross thiamine deficiency is rare in Europe except in alcoholism, but minor deficiency disorders are common in the elderly and may explain some of their mental deterioration. Severe deficiency state is at times productive of Wernicke's encephalopathy (q.v.).

Thioxanthines

The thioxanthines are a series of compounds structurally similar to the phenothiazines (q.v.), but most have not achieved clinical use. Chloroprothixene, analogous to chlorpromazine, was the first used, while thiothixene has become available recently. Absorption, metabolism, and actions resemble the phenothiazines, but side effects are few. Extrapyramidal reactions may occur. They are mainly used in the treatment of schizophrenia, although

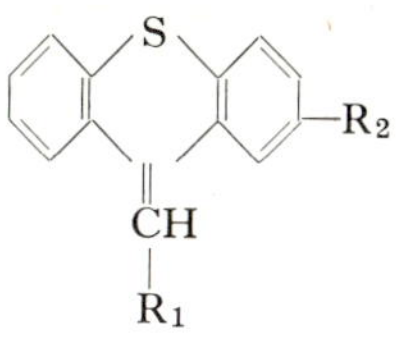

Thioxanthines

they potentially have the same clinical spectrum as phenothiazines. Chlorprothixene may be particularly useful when depressive features are present, while thiothixene with an alerting action has found a special place in the treatment of chronic schizophrenia.

Thought blocking

A sudden cessation of thought as though his mind has gone blank, alternatively called 'thought deprivation' as if an external force had suddenly taken his thoughts away (see 'passivity feelings'). The symptom is characteristic of schizophrenia but sometimes is difficult to diagnose as much reliance has to be put on the patient's description which is often vague. Behaviourally the effect is often very similar to the 'absences' of petit mal.

Thought, thinking

Idea is the most general term for a cognitive (q.v.) process not directly dependent upon perception (q.v.). It includes images, internal reconstructions of sensory experience, and thoughts which represent more conceptual and symbolic processes. The term thinking refers, in its most general sense, to any train of ideas or, in a more strict sense, to ideational activity initiated by and directed to the solution of a problem. The least-controlled form of thinking is the train of images referred to as fantasy (q.v.) which occurs in day-dreaming and similar states. Freud (q.v.) considered that fantasy is largely directed from the unconscious (q.v.) and represents vicarious wish-fulfilment. He also regarded dreams during sleep as a special type of fantasy in which repressed material gained expression in disguised and symbolic forms. Reality orientated thinking, by contrast, utilizes complex, hierarchically organized conceptual schemata, mediated by language (q.v.) or other symbolic codes such as those employed in mathematical reasoning. The course of child development in relation to thinking has been studied in detail, especially by the Swiss psychologist, Piaget. His studies have been particularly directed to the manner in which conceptual schemata are acquired and he lays great stress on two interelated processes described as assimilation and accommodation. Assimilation is the absorption and integration of new experience into pre-existing schemata, whereas accommodation implies the modification of old and the formation of new schemata. Piaget considers that intellectual development occurs in stages. During the early (0–2 years) sensorimotor period, the infant's behaviour is directly determined by innate or conditioned reflexes (q.v.) with little or no cognitive mediation. During this period the child learns to differentiate himself from his environment and the permanence of other objects. The second, pre-operational stage (2–7) includes an early phase (2–4) in which his thinking is egocentric and his concepts primitive. During the later (4–7) intuitive phase he can form classes of objects and deal with numbers but cannot describe the basis of his classifications. Next, from 7 to 11 years, comes the period of 'concrete operations' during which the child can handle a variety of logical operations but is largely dependent upon practical situations. Finally, during the period of formal operations (11–15), he achieves truly abstract thinking which extends to the hypothetical.
In mental illness, disorders of thinking are very common, affecting either the content or the form of thought or both. Numerous specific examples are described in other sections of this work. There is, however, a general tendency to more autistic or dereistic (q.v.) thinking governed by personal needs and fantasies. The similarity between some disorders of this nature and the primitive, magical and egocentric thinking of young children lends support to the concept of regression (q.v.), a reversion to an earlier or more primitive form of behaviour and expression.
SEE ALSO Conceptual thinking and Concrete thinking.

Thought stopping

A behavioural technique for the treatment of obsessional ruminations. The patient deliberately thinks his distressing ruminative thoughts which the therapist interrupts by shouting 'stop'. The patient is trained to do the same, eventually learning to control his thoughts by a subvocal 'stop' or even by introducing a neutral thought. The technique is probably a form of training in self-regulation.

Thumb sucking

An almost universal habit at some stage of life, the habit in itself is harmless. It is the anxieties engendered in the parents by overly-excessive thumb sucking which will bring the child to the doctor. It is only in rare cases when oral deformities are being produced that referral to a psychiatrist is necessary. Behaviour therapy (q.v.) is useful in these cases.

Thymeretics

SEE Monoamine oxidase inhibitors.

Thymoleptics

Drugs which exert their main clinical effect by elevating mood are known as antidepressants. The importance of their action in correcting disturbance of mood may be emphasized by using the alternative term thymoleptic. Although this is the strict use of the term it has recently been used as a synonym for the tricyclic anti-depressants to distinguish them from the monoamine oxidase inhibitors.
SEE ALSO Tricyclic anti-depressants.

Thyroid gland

The thyroid gland by its secretion of thyroxin affects the metabolism of all tissue, including the brain. Abnormalities of the thyroid gland can in consequence give rise to mental disorders. Hypothyroidism produces mental retardation, which in the congenital form (cretinism) can present as mental subnormality. In the adult form (myxoedema), delusions and hallucinations may occur.

Hyperthyroidism frequently produces a picture which is very difficult to distinguish from that of anxiety states.

Thyroid stimulating hormone (TSH-Thyrotrophin)

An anterior pituitary hormone which stimulates the thyroid gland.
SEE ALSO Thyrotrophin releasing hormone.

Thyrotrophin releasing hormone (TRH)

A tripeptide secreted by the hypothalamus which via the hypothalamic-hypophyseal portal blood system stimulates thyrotrophin (TSH) which activates the thyroid gland. Both TRH and TSH have been studied recently as antidepressants but the results so far are equivocal.

Tic

A tic is a repetitive co-ordinated movement involving a number of muscles in their normal synergistic relationship. It may be a simple habit spasm as seen in the states of intense concentration illustrated in close-up television, or it may be more complex – tossing the head, wriggling the shoulder, grimacing, skipping. While usually emotionally determined, tics may follow epidemic encephalitis and are associated with post-encephalitic Parkinsonism (q.v.). The motor element may be accompanied by a compulsive utterance – often blasphemous – the association forming the syndrome of Gilles de la Tourette (q.v.). Children usually 'grow out of' habits. Behaviour therapy and physical treatments of all kinds have been advocated. Haloperidol enjoys a current vogue.

Tics in childhood

Repetitive, involuntary jerky movements of the body are quite common in childhood, and usually take the form of blinking or sideways movements of the head. Occasionally they become more widespread. In the Gilles de la Tourette syndrome

(q.v.), widespread tics are accompanied by compulsive grunting and sometimes obscene utterances.
Tics are usually mild and monosymptomatic, and if the parents can be encouraged to ignore them they usually disappear over a few weeks. Tics accompanied by signs of emotional disturbance or becoming persistent require more active treatment.

Token economy
SEE Operant conditioning therapies.

Tone in muscle
SEE Muscle tone.

Torticollis

A distortion of the normal posture of the neck, torticollis may be tonic or spasmodic. Most commonly the neck is turned laterally, spasm of the sternocleidomastoid muscle is marked and the neck is held painfully rigid. Although often regarded as functional in nature, resistant spasmodic torticollis is, in fact, due to ill-defined cerebral disturbance.

Torts

A term used in English law, they are civil (as distinct from criminal) wrongs. The remedy for a tort is a common law action for damages. They are offences of one person on another (e.g. trespass, assault) whether or not an offence against the crown has been committed.
In general a person of unsound mind is liable for his torts. However, if such a person is incapable of forming intention or of notice he is not liable.
SEE ALSO Criminal responsibility and McNaughton Rules.

Toxic psychoses
(Synonym: Toxi-exhaustive psychoses)

The general signs of a toxic psychosis are disorientation for time, place, or person; impairment of recent memory; illusions resulting from misperception of sounds and of the enviroment; visual, aural, tactile, and olfactory hallucinations, and finally emotional changes with either apathy or anxiety, agitation and restlessness. One or other part of the syndrome may dominate the picture. For example, a psychosis following amphetamine (q.v.) overdose is most often marked by restlessness and hallucinosis, with little clouding or intellectual impairment. On the other hand, the psychosis following chronic barbiturate (q.v.) abuse usually shows marked clouding with confused, restless behaviour. The toxin implicated may be either exogenous or endogenous. Drug abuse has already been mentioned in the former category, and therapeutic substances must also be considered, for example isoniazid, steroids, and anaesthetics. Infections, the puerperium, and metabolic disturbances such as uraemia are precipitants in the second group. The elderly and the undernourished are particularly prone to toxic psychoses.
SEE ALSO Brain syndrome and Poisons affecting mental state.

Toxoplasmosis

Maternal infection in pregnancy by the protozoal organism Toxoplasma gondii may lead to embryopathy leading to early intrauterine death. If the pregnancy continues to term, the child may show severe signs in the neonatal period including choroidoretinitis, jaundice, hepatosplenomegaly, and encephalitis. Surviving children may be severely mentally subnormal with extensive neurological damage, blindness and epilepsy.

Training centres

Originally called 'occupation centres', these facilities are among the most important form of community service for the mentally subnormal. Recent years have seen an increase both in their numbers and in the quality of service they provide, with a recognition that the subnormal are capable of much greater response to appropriate training methods than had been thought. Some centres have special care units for those who are also physically handicapped.

Trance

A state of diminished consciousness resembling sleep. The EEG is characteristic of the waking state. Trance states may occur under hypnotic suggestion (q.v.), as an hysterical disturbance of consciousness, in catalepsy (q.v.); and may be the end result of states of ecstatic excitement. This last form is characteristically encouraged in certain rituals of the voodoo cult.

Tranquillizers

The concept of tranquillizing drugs was introduced with the advent of chlorpromazine, and comprises the ability to calm patients without impairment of consciousness. Thus a distinction is drawn between tranquillizing and sedative or hypnotic effects. In practice this distinction is by no means clear, and the majority of drugs classed as tranquillizers show a sedative component, and indeed the term tranquillosedative is now in common use.
The terms neuroleptic and ataractic were introduced as alternatives to the general term tranquillizer, but only neuroleptic has achieved any substantial use.
With the introduction of a large number of substances with varying tranquillizing properties, classification into major and minor tranquillizers is important, since these have differences in actions.
Major tranquillizers or neuroleptic drugs (q.v.) have a central anti-psychotic action and are used extensively to relieve the symptoms and behavioural disturbances of psychotic illness. Examples of this group are the phenothiazines (q.v.), rauwolfia alkaloids (q.v.), butyrophenones (q.v.), and thioxanthines (q.v.). In spite of their chemical diversity all are liable to produce extrapyramidal syndromes.
In contrast, the minor tranquillizers or anxiolytic drugs mainly relieve anxiety and have mild sedative effects. They are used widely in the treatment of psychoneurotic disorder and tension states. Examples of this category include the benzodiazepines (q.v.) and glycol derivatives (q.v.). These compounds do not produce extrapyramidal manifestations.

Trans-cultural psychiatry

SEE Culture.

Transexualism

Transexualism or eonism is the complete conviction by an individual that he or she is a member of the opposite sex. After adolescence there is an increasing desire to dress and to live as a member of the opposite sex and the patient presents to the doctor with a demand for a 'change of sex' operation. Cross gender identification dates back to childhood with a history often of imposed cross-dressing by parents due to effeminancy in the boy or tomboyishness in the girl. There is never any evidence of gonadal, chromosomal. or endocrinological abnormality. It is totally resistent to psychotherapy, hypnosis, behaviour therapy and drug therapy. There is an increasing pressure (commonly resisted in the United Kingdom) for cosmetic surgery. This consists of penotomy and castration in the male with oestrogen-provoked gynaecomastia or bilateral mastectomy with radium menopause and plastic operation on the genitals in the female.
Transexualism is to be distinguished from the true delusions of sex change which occur in schizophrenia and from cases of pseudo-hermaphroditism discovered at adolescence.

Transactional analysis

Associated with the work of Eric Berne (1910–70). Transactional analysis now has a large following, particularly in the USA. Berne believed that human behaviour could be seen in simpler terms than Freudian psychodynamics. The individual was a sort of automaton, with a script, a routine set of transactions, of games (predictable stereotyped inter-actions), and a repertoire of ego states, child, adult, and parent. All these activities had to be analysed in the simplest type of language – words that could be understood by the most and the least intellectual. Using certain novel techniques, notably the contract, Berne attempted to reduce human problems to their simplest terms. The contract between the therapist and the patient was an explicit statement regarding therapy agreed by therapist and patient – 'I will not treat you if this happens', 'What do you want from the treatment?', 'What is the end point or cure?' Intuition had its place and the therapist aimed to reactivate the child in the adult, and to cut through the verbiage and the tyranny of words. Ego states were conscious, the concept of the Freudian unconscious receiving little place in Berne's theories. Essentially transactional analysis deals with the here and now, the understanding of an individuals transactions with others and with the society in which he moves, a sort of psychological behaviourism. The method appeals to the educated layman and Berne's book *The Games People Play* (1964) was a best seller.

Transference

The transfer of previously experienced feelings for important figures in the patient's personal life onto the therapist. Thus the therapist, during the course of psychotherapy, may come to represent the father or the mother, rarely siblings or other family members. Eventually the patient-therapist interaction reduplicates the situation in which the neurosis itself began, and so a transference neurosis occurs. The original and repressed emotional problems are now totally transferred onto the therapist, the patient regresses and lives out, during and outside therapy, his earlier infantile and childhood hates, loves, fears and jealousies. The resolution of the transference neurosis is essential for the successful completion of the analysis.

Transmission in synapses of brain cells

Impulses within the nervous system pass from one nerve fibre to another at the synapses. These consist of fine clefts between the pre-synaptic membrane of the axon of one nerve cell and the post-synaptic membrane of the dendrites of the next. Transmission within the synapse depends upon the release of a neuro-transmitter (q.v.) substance from minute vesicles in the terminal portion of the axon. These neuro-transmitters diffuse across the synaptic cleft and affect the post-synaptic membrane. They may produce excitation, leading to an impulse in the next neurone or inhibition, reducing the chance of impulses in the next neurone. While the nature of the neuro-transmitters in the peripheral portions of both voluntary and autonomic nervous systems are well established, those in the brain are less well known.

For many years, there has been doubt as to whether cholinergic transmission occurred within the brain, but current evidence suggests that acetyl choline (q.v.) is a neuro-transmitter for certain areas of the cortex at least. Noradrenaline (q.v.) has been identified in the hypothalamus, mid brain, pons and medulla and its concentration alters with neuronal activity. Similarly, dopamine (q.v.) is found in the caudate nucleus and is believed to be one of the neuro-transmitters in the extra-pyramidal motor system. Serotonin (q.v.) (5-hydroxytryptamine) is also found in various mid brain sites and is probably also a neuro-transmitter. γ-aminobutyric acid (GABA (q.v.)) is localized exclusively in the central nervous system and the current evidence suggests that it is one of the many main inhibitory transmitters. Other possible central neuro-transmitters include a large number of amino acids such as glycine and glutamic acid, substance P, histamine and prostaglandins. SEE ALSO Synapse transmission.

Transvestism

Transvestism is the wearing of the clothing, commonly underclothing, of the opposite sex in order to induce sexual excitement. In some cases it is the fixed and exclusive stimulus for sexual orgasm. It occurs predominantly in males and is a form of 'fetishism'. Sexual arousal by female underclothing often dates back to childhood when the patient identified himself as the mother or sister by dressing in their clothes and masturbating to the incestuous fantasies provoked. Many transvestists are repressed homosexuals (q.v.). Transvestists may be brought before the courts after stealing articles of underwear for transvestist purposes. The condition is often transient and occurs under conditions of enforced heterosexual abstention, e.g. during a wife's pregnancy. The habitual transvestist can be effectively treated by electrical aversion therapy.

Trauma

For mental symptoms following trauma SEE Head injury. For symptoms from trauma during birth SEE Birth trauma and Mental subnormality.

Treatment, psychiatric

It is only from a proper assessment of the aetiology and diagnosis, that one can formulate a plan of treatment. This will be directed on three lines.
1. Removal of stress factors.
2. Assisting the patient to make more of his personality assets and cover his defects; in other words, helping him to adjust better by means of psychotherapy.
3. Physical treatment, which may be aimed at specific treatment of an endogenous factor, or simply at symptom relief until psychotherapy or enviromental adjustments are under way.

Treatment should be aimed at what is treatable, not necessarily at the most important aetiological factor. However, it is useful to make a note of the contribution each of the aetiological factors is thought to play, e.g. environmental 30%, personality 10%, endogenous (genetic, biochemical) 60%. In such a patient the therapeutic emphasis would be on physical measures and, if possible, on methods designed to alleviate the precipitating cause. On the other hand, in a patient where the aetiological factors were assessed as reactive 30%, personality 60%, endogenous 10%, it may be impracticable to modify either the defective personality or the environmental factors. In this case the small improvement to be gained by physical treatment may be the best means of enabling the patient, with support, to overcome his environmental difficulties.

With these ends in mind the doctor should use all methods of treatment available to him.

Occupational therapy is often the first stage in rehabilitation, diverting the patient from his symptoms, stimulating his interests and encouraging social intercourse. A social worker is often useful in helping with home problems and the Disablement Rehabilitation Officer (DRO) is specially trained to place disabled persons in suitable work.

Psychotherapy aims at removing, modifying, and retarding existing symptoms or disturbed patterns of behaviour, and promoting positive personality growth and development. Before embarking on treatment, it is most important to decide the objective for each individual case. Methods vary from supportive therapy and abreactive techniques to intensive psychoanalytic types of psychotherapy and may be individual or in groups.

Physical methods of treatment may be specific or non-specific. The former includes ECT (q.v.) or tricyclic anti-depressants (q.v.) in endogenous cases of depression, or the phenothiazines (q.v.) in cases of schizophrenia when an identifiable psychiatric illness has been diagnosed and the treatment is directed to its cure. Non-specific treatments, such as hypnotics (q.v.) and tranquillizers (q.v.), or specialized techniques, such as modified insulin therapy (q.v.), are aimed at providing relief from symptoms which are causing a vicious circle to be set up (e.g. anxiety and tension causing insomnia and loss of weight which themselves result in increased anxiety and tension), or are hindering the establishment of normal interests, social activity, or return to work which themselves could be therapeutic."

Tremor

Tremor may have an organic, a psychiatric, or an iatrogenic basis.

Among the organic tremors are intention tremor of a cerebellar lesion; coarse tremor at rest in Parkinsonism; senile tremor, most marked in the hands, is present at rest but made worse by movement. The flapping movement manifested by subjects with portal-systemic encephalopathy (rapid flexion-extension movement at the metacarpophalangeal and wrist joints) is associated with clouding of consciousness

(usually with associated jaundice and ascites).
Psychiatric tremors include hysterical – usually coarse which may disappear when the attention is redirected; anxiety – usually fine and resembling that of thyrotoxic subjects.
Psychotropic drugs frequently cause tremor and these include an extrapyramidal tremor with phenothiazines; a fine tremor similar to that of anxiety or thyrotoxicosis with the tricyclic anti-depressants and the amphetamines. Lithium frequently results in a fine tremor, though this is usually temporary. A coarse tremor, resulting in difficulty in picking up a cup, is a sign of lithium intoxication.

Trichotillomania

Hair plucking is seen in adolescent girls and, at times, in mentally subnormal patients. It is a form of self-mutilation, making the girl unattractive sexually, for it is sexual conflicts which most often trigger off the behaviour. Patches of alopecia make the girl unsightly, but this may be preferable to other self-mutilant behaviour, such as wrist slashing. Hair plucking is a sign of serious emotional problems, and the girl should be referred to a psychiatrist for treatment.

Tricyclic anti-depressants

The term tricyclic is derived from the three-ringed nucleus structure, and the term dibenzazepine (q.v.) is an alternative. They are structurally related to the phenothiazine tranquillizers. The prototype was imipramine and the last decade has seen several other tricyclic compounds introduced into clinical use. These drugs are widely used in the treatment of all types of depression. The majority are thought to exert their action by preventing the reabsorption of transmitter amines at synaptic junctions within the central nervous system, thereby increasing the availability of amines at receptor sites. However, one related compound iprindole may act by blocking 'marked inhibitory' monoamine receptors.
There are two main sub-groups of the tricyclic compounds, the iminodibenzyl (q.v.) compounds and the dibenzocycloheptadiene (q.v.) compounds, although there is now a miscellaneous group embracing some of the more recently introduced drugs which may be considered within the over-all category – iprindole, prothiadene, doxepin, dibenzepin, and opipramol.
In clinical terms the most useful distinction lies between drugs which have a well-marked sedative action for depressive states accompanied by agitation, and non-sedative compounds, best used when retardation and apathy are prominent (see table).
Absorption is rapid and the compounds pass freely into the tissues; relatively high levels are found in the brain. Tricyclic compounds are extensively and rapidly metabolized and little is excreted unchanged.
Their average success rate in depression is about 60% and relief occurs between three and twenty-one days on full dosage, but usually within a week. Like the related phenothiazines, tricyclic anti-depressants have other pharmacological actions; they include anti-cholinergic, adrenolytic, anti-serotonin and anti-histaminic effects.
These actions account for many of the side effects. The common side effects are mostly of nuisance value and tolerable, including drowsiness, dry mouth, black tongue, blurred vision, fine rapid tremor of the hands, sweating, tachycardia, constipation, and impotence. Recovery from depression is typically associated with some gain in body weight, but this may be excessive if tricyclic treatment is at all prolonged. Less common side effects include hypotension, skin rashes, hypomania, jaundice, and grand mal convulsions. Certain paradoxical reactions occur, particularly in the elderly; insomnia and agitation may appear, and on occasion a confusional state with delusions and hallucinations can be dramatic and disturbing. The more serious side effects require prompt withdrawal of the drug, but the minor adverse reaction can usually be tolerated or will respond to either reduction in dosage or change to an alternative compound.
A number of other compounds with actions broadly resembling the tricyclic groups have now been introduced. Prothiaden and dibenzepin are closely related

Activating	Neutral	Sedative
Desipramine	Nortriptyline	Amitriptyline
Imipramine	Dibenzepin	Trimipramine
Protriptyline	Iprindole	Doxepin
	Clomipramine	Opipramol
	Prothiaden	

The relative sedative effect of tricyclic anti-depressants. These compounds form a spectrum of varying sedative potency, but may conveniently be considered in three groups.

to the tricyclic compounds and have similar properties; iprindole is an indole derivative with an anti-depressant action like the tricyclic group; doxepin has well-marked tranquillizing properties as well as an anti-depressant action and is sedative; opipramol is a less-potent anti-depressant than the tricyclic compounds, is sedative, and has a limited use in neurotic depression.

Triple X syndrome
SEE Trisomy.

Trisomy

The ordinary human somatic cell contains forty-six chromosomes, consisting of twenty-three pairs (twenty-two pairs of autosomes; one pair of sex chromosomes). Trisomy is an abnormal condition in which an extra chromosome is present, so that one of the pairs of chromosomes of the normal complement is replaced by three chromosomes. The presence of these three chromosomes (which are apparently identical in the case of autosomal chromosomes) is known as trisomy for the chromosome concerned. Syndromes associated with trisomy of specific chromosomes include mongolism or Down's syndrome (q.v.) (trisomy of an autosomal chromosome of the G group), Edwards' syndrome (q.v.) (trisomy of an E group chromosome), and Patau's syndrome (q.v.) (trisomy of a D group chromosome). These are all associated with severe mental subnormality. Syndromes associated with trisomy of the sex chromosomes include Klinefelter's syndrome (XXY) and the XXX and XYY syndromes. These sex chromosome abnormalities appear to be associated not infrequently with personality deviations; mental subnormality may also be a feature, but in general it is of less severity than in the case of autosomal trisomies.
SEE ALSO Klinefelter's syndrome.

Truancy

Truancy involves absence from school where anxiety is absent, and an attempt is made to conceal the non-attendance. It must be sharply differentiated from school phobia (q.v.) where no attempt is made to conceal the symptoms which arise out of anxiety. The aetiology, treatment, and prognosis of the two conditions are quite different.
Truancy is particularly common in boys, especially in urban areas and during their last year of compulsory schooling. When the non-attendance is infrequent and in company with other boys, it is usually of no medical or psychiatric significance. When it is persistent it is often associated with other evidence of delinquent behaviour, especially stealing and offences against property. The isolated boy who repeatedly truants alone is often also unhappy and in difficulty over his relationships both at home and at school.

Tuberous sclerosis
SEE Epiloia.

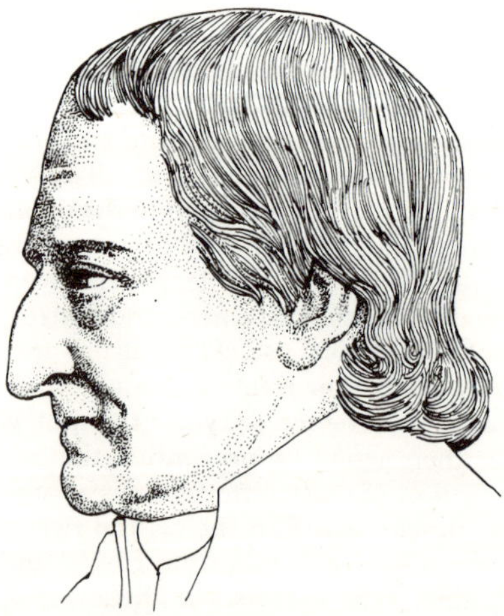

Tuke, William (1732–1822)

A Quaker tea merchant, Tuke founded the York Retreat, a hospital in which kindness and tolerance was to set the tone for the future care of the psychiatric patient and provide an administrative model for the mental hospitals which were to proliferate during the second half of the nineteenth century. His son Henry (1755–1814) and his grandson Samuel Tuke (1784–1857) continued his work, and Dr Daniel Hack Tuke (1827–1895), his great grandson, became one of the leading psychiatrists of the Victorian era.

Tumour, cerebral

SEE Brain tumour.

Turner's syndrome (Monosomy X)

Turner's syndrome is a manifestation of ovarian dysgenesis; the ovary being represented by a mere streak of non-functioning tissue. Primary amenorrhoea and sterility are constant findings and the physical features include lack of secondary sexual development and abnormalities of head, hands and viscera. The syndrome is associated with an XO chromosome complement. Personality traits include passivity, vagueness, abnormal social reactions from tomboyishness to exaggerated prissiness. In many cases intelligence is within the normal range; in some there is mild mental retardation.

Twilight states

States of partial consciousness, from a variety of causes, in which awareness seems limited, comprehension dulled, and in which abnormal behaviour may be associated with, and reflect, abnormal mental phenomena. Post ictal twilight states, which may last an hour or so after a seizure or series of seizures may be regarded as reflecting only a partial return to normal function. Some seizures likewise only disrupt, in Hughlings Jackson's terminology, the highest level of consciousness.

Thus a variety of circumstances, including intoxication with drugs (cannabis and cocaine especially), hysterical dissociative states (especially where triggered by minor cerebral trauma), may produce a similar effect. Physical and mental slowing, irritability and impulsive behaviour, hallucinations and paranoid ideas occur. Their separation from other states depends upon their relative brevity.

Tyramine

This sympathomimetic monoamine is found in large amounts in foods such as marmite, cheese, red wine and snails, and is responsible for the hypertensive reaction to such foods in patients on a monoamine oxidase inhibitor (MAOI (q.v.)). It is thought to act partly by releasing the pressor amines from their stores.

Ulcerative colitis

A severe inflammatory disease of the colon characterized by loose stools containing blood, pus, and mucus, and a generalized systemic disturbance with fever, weight loss, and anaemia. Allergic, infectious, and genetic factors have been implicated in the aetiology, as have psychological factors, since stress (q.v.) may produce vascular and secretory changes in the colon. Patients with a vulnerable personality may develop an exacerbation of symptoms at times of emotional conflict, and require psychiatric treatment.
SEE ALSO Psychosomatic disorders and Colitis.

Uncinate fit

A variety of epileptic attack characterized by auras of taste and smell and a dreamy state. The hallucinations are most commonly unpleasant in nature, and may precede or follow the dreamy state, which itself may defy description by the patient. The attack indicates a lesion of the temporal lobe.
SEE ALSO Psychomotor seizures.

Undinism

A perverse interest in urination and in urine – the individual getting pleasure from observing men or women urinate, from being urinated upon, from bathing in urine, or drinking urine.

Undoing

One of the methods of expiating or atoning for guilt-laden thoughts or actions, undoing is a defence mechanism developed at the stage when the child thinks in magical or animistic terms. Freud considered that many religious rituals were examples of undoing, and linked them with obsessional-compulsive behaviour. Simple acts, such as touching wood, or very complex ritualistic behaviour enable both the individual, and society, to guard against the retribution expected as a consequence of instinctually driven activities.

Unemployment

Loss of work, due to general economic conditions, advancing age or physical ill-health, may often cause reactive depression and emotional maladjustment. Then, shame and loss of a person's self-esteem may lead to actual suicide; 21% of a series of suicides in elderly people were associated with lack of employment. Schizophrenics tend to drift down the ladder of skill, as the illness progresses and those who are mentally handicapped in any way are likely to be the first to lose their jobs whenever employment is reduced. The loss of unskilled employment resulting from automation and other modern work processes may be causing permanent unemployment for these workers.

Unipolar psychosis

SEE Unipolar depression.

Unmarried mothers

Though recent changes in our society have greatly reduced the stigma of illegitimate pregnancy, it may still be the cause of much psychiatric disturbance. Even when the pregnancy is emotionally accepted and the woman does not suffer social rejection, there may be serious practical and financial problems. Emotional lability and vomiting during the pregnancy tend to be worse in these circumstances. Puerperal psychoses (schizophrenic and depressive) are more common in unmarried than in married mothers. If the pregnancy occurs in a woman of abnormal personality – which is not uncommon – the stress of childbirth and of responsibility for the infant may result in overt psychiatric disorder. The prognosis will depend on the degree of personality disturbance and on external circumstances.

Unreality – feelings of

Feelings of unreality may relate to the subject (the person himself feels unreal or changed: depersonalization) or to the world around (everything seems different, the streets, people etc., derealization). The disorder comes on rapidly or even suddenly, is always unpleasant and the feeling is so strange that, at first, the patient may worry in case it is a symptom of impending psychosis. It may last a few minutes or several days; rarely for months or years, but a recurrence is frequent. This symptom occurs in the context of an anxiety reaction, usually affecting a young adult and women are more often affected than men. The underlying personality is often obsessional; phobic symptoms are often found in association. Some patients with depressive reactions complain of a complete loss of feeling with the secondary complaint that the world around seems changed, unreal. An even more nihilistic variety of unreality feeling may be observed in some agitated depressions occurring in later life. In epilepsy (psychomotor seizures) feelings of unreality may occur, associated with clouding of consciousness, affective disturbance and visual or auditory hallucinations. Feelings of unreality can occur in normal people experiencing unusual fatigue or sleep deprivation. In schizophrenia unreality feelings seem to have a different quality; they are usually associated with passivity feelings and disturbances in the form of thought. LSD is alleged to induce unreality feelings, but these seem more akin to those reported by subjects with anxiety reactions.

Uraemia

Uraemia is the complex syndrome caused by severe impairment of kidney function. Biochemical changes include effects on water, electrolytes and the accumulation of nitrogenous compounds in the blood. Of the latter, creatinine levels indicate kidney function more accurately than urea, as they are dependent on constant endogenous factors rather than diet and catabolic rate. Symptoms include lassitude, depression, dullness, and a toxi-organic mental syndrome. Loss of appetite, vomiting, diarrhoea, hypertension, and anaemia in a grey-brown pigmented patient with a 'uraemic' breath odour, complete a picture progressing through muscle twitching and drowsiness to coma. Treatment is by control of dietary protein, short-acting sedatives, and symptomatic measures for the heart and blood pressure, or if a more radical approach is essential, by chronic intermittent haemodialysis or kidney transplant.

Urticaria

Urticaria or hives is an eruption of wheals which are sharply demarcated, red and itchy. The rash may occur alone, or as part of a more generalized systemic reaction. It may be due to a wide variety of allergens, foods such as shell fish, drugs such as penicillin, or materials such as silk, wool or fur. Stress and emotional factors often play a major part in the chronic form of the disease. Itching which is often severe, leads to scratching and the production of new lesions and this tends to occur at times when anxiety, hostility or frustration are increased and lead to further distress. An important aspect of treatment is the relief of the emotional factors.
SEE ALSO Skin disorders and Psychosomatic disorders.

Vaginismus

Vaginismus results in contraction of the pelvic musculature which may make sexual intercourse impossible. Spasm may spread to the thigh muscles and any attempt at penetration will lead to pain. Vaginismus is invariably of psychogenic origin, but dyspareunia (q.v.) may also arise from pelvic abnormality or disease. It may also be due to lack of sexual arousal leading to diminished or absent vaginal secretion. Frigidity (q.v.) may result from traumatic early experiences or phantasies where the sexual act is seen as harmful, distasteful or painful. For example menstruation may be regarded as unclean and masturbation, the first genital sexual act, may have been severely criticized or even ridiculed. Other aetiological factors may be fear of venereal disease or pregnancy, and uncongenial surroundings may also play a part. Conflict over the sexual partner may arise because of love for another, or latent homosexuality may be present. Psychotherapy (q.v.) should be the main form of treatment often beneficially combined with behaviour therapy.

Vasomotor rhinitis

Rhinitis is a reaction of the nasal mucosa characterized by increased secretion, oedema, sneezing, and itching which may be produced by an allergic or psychosomatic cause. Psychological factors may predominate, but more commonly they are contributory, with allergic, non-allergic irritants and infection all playing a part. The relationship between allergic and psychological precipitants is a close one because a patient with an allergy for primulas, for example, may start to sneeze at the sight of an artificial flower, because of the development of a conditioned reflex (q.v.). Allergic rhinitis which is perennial often results in chronic congestion of the nasal mucosa, and differs from hay fever (q.v.) which is characterized by seasonal recurrence during pollination.
SEE ALSO Psychosomatic disorders and Allergy.

Verbigeration

The senseless repetition of empty phrases, which occurs in association with other behavioural disorders in schizophrenia (q.v.) of long-standing. Speech seems separated from thought and almost accidental. Such manifestations are most common in under-occupied, institutionalized schizophrenics.

Vital depression
SEE Endogenous depression

Vitamin B_{12}
SEE Cobalamin

Vitamins

Brain metabolism (q.v.) is based essentially upon the oxidative breakdown of glucose. Thus co-factors utilized in glycolysis and the Krebs citric acid cycle will affect brain metabolism. Among such co-factors are vitamins of the B complex, and deficiency of these vitamins produces psychiatric disorders.
Although a mixed diet will provide an adequate intake of each of these vitamins, an inadequate intake of food, food fads and deficient absorption can all lead to a vitamin deficiency. Among the people in whom such a deficiency may be an important factor in the illness are those with gastro-intestinal disease, including post gastrectomy patients, in the elderly, in alcoholics, in association with chronic infections and in the severely depressed.
The vitamin deficiencies associated with mental symptoms are: thiamine, a major factor in Wernicke's encephalopathy (q.v.) and delirium tremens (q.v.); nicotinamide, in pellagra (q.v.); cobalamin (vitamin B_{12} (q.v.)); and folic acid.

Vogt-Speilmeyer disease
SEE Amaurotic family idiocy.

Voluntary movement

The voluntary muscles consist of numerous contractile cells arranged in parallel, attached either directly or through a tendon to the bone. Controlled contraction of the muscles gives rise to voluntary movement. This muscle contraction must be carefully co-ordinated if effective movement is to be achieved. The movement itself must be appropriate and antagonist, protagonist and synergist muscles must maintain the body posture. Movement is thus a carefully integrated process involving many muscle groups.

The idea of the movement is believed to be initiated in the 'premotor' area in the frontal cortex. The current concept is that the motor cortex, basal ganglia (q.v.), cerebellum (q.v.) and sensory cortex are involved in feedback circuits that initiate muscle contraction. According to this theory there are two possible planning pathways from the pre-motor area to area 4 of the motor cortex. Both involve the basal ganglia as an integral part.

One pathway is for unlearned movements. Its exact anatomical structure is unknown. In this type of movement concentration on the action is necessary, as for example in a child that is just walking. But there is a learned response through the lateral cerebellar cortex in which the movements are preprogrammed and thus need no concentration.

It appears that the basal ganglia are mainly concerned with muscle tone and slow movements, the cerebellum with rapid fine movements.

It is only after this process that the motor area 4 fires, probably mainly down the pyramidal tract to activate the 'final common path'. The stimulation of the 'final common path' takes place simultaneously through both the α pathway to the extrafusal fibres and the γ pathway to the intrafusal fibres – the so-called α/γ coactivation. This would mean that there is both a direct component of muscle contraction and a servo-assisted control.

There is an added recent complication to this theory. Local anaesthesia of the portion of the body surface related to the muscle depresses the servo response leading to the need for a greater conscious effort to initiate movement.

In this stage of movement somatosensory information from various parts including eyes and vestibular apparatus and proprioceptive impulses from the limbs feedback to both the cerebellum and motor cortex and enable those areas to mutually control the finesse of the movement. Thus, the picture emerges of muscle activity through the pyramidal tracts but under the control of three feedback loops – the γ motor path, the basal ganglia loop and the cerebellar-loop each with its own specific function.

Vomiting

Vomiting may arise from alimentary or central causes. In psychiatric practice it is a not uncommon hysterical symptom and in pregnancy is said to symbolize rejection. Persistent nausea and vomiting is a feature of lithium toxicity.

Von Hippel-Lindau's disease

Angiomatous lesions in the cerebellum associated with retinal angioma, and accompanied at times by cysts of liver, pancreas or kidney. The cerebellar lesion is often cystic, with a small angioma in the wall of the cyst.

Von Recklinghausen's disease

SEE Neurofibromatosis.

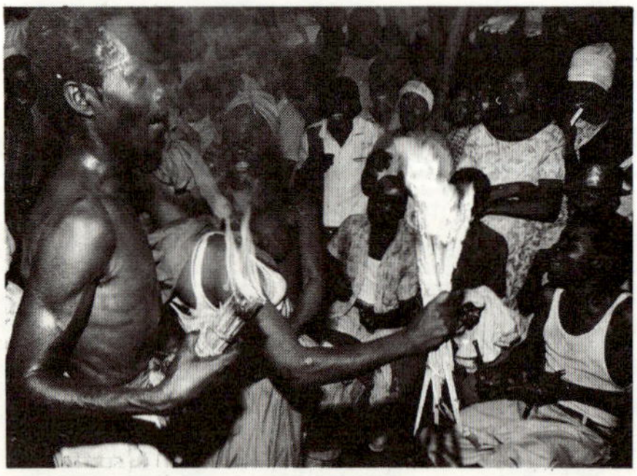

Voodoo cult

One of several forms of spirit worship, developed in the West Indies between about 1700 and 1900 and now most widespread in Haiti. It derives from a mixture of African religions (brought by slaves), local cults and elements of Christian liturgy. The cult involves homage to deities (called loa), the use of magic by sorcerers,

and powerful curses, which may actually cause death. Primitive peoples are very dependent on their immediate social group, rejection by whom may mean the loss of the will to live; another sorcerer may be found, possessing even stronger voodoo powers, who can practise counter-suggestion to the spell.
SEE Brainwashing.

Voyeurism

Voyeurism or scoptophilia is the exclusive attainment of sexual gratification through passive observation of sexual display in others. It is socially accommodated for in the striptease show, the 'blue film', or the enactment of coitus by prostitutes and their partners.
Secretive observation from the outside of a house after dark, of a young, attractive female in the act of undressing is the offence of the 'peeping Tom'. The excitement aroused through the possibility of being caught is contributory to the total sexual excitement necessary to induce orgasm in the observer. Voyeurs and 'peepers' are generally inoffensive, sexually inadequate men with strong fears of female rejection; only rarely is the act associated with sadistic fantasies and impulses.
Voyeuristic fantasies are said to date from early childhood sexual arousal, commonly related to seeing or imagining the parents having sexual intercourse. Most 'peepers' deny the habitual compulsive nature of their behaviour.
SEE ALSO Scoptophilia and Sexual disorders.

WAIS (Wechsler adult intelligence test)

A standard test of intelligence incorporating a wide range of tasks and which is administered individually by a person with special training. The tests are divided into two groups, verbal and performance, for which separate IQs can be determined in addition to the full-scale IQ. Since some of the tests, such as information, comprehension, object assembly, picture completion and vocabulary hold up well with ageing, whereas digit span, arithmetic, digit symbol, block design and similarities do not, a comparison between these groups can be used as an index of mental deterioration.
A special Wechsler intelligence scale for children (WISC) is a downward extension of the adult scale and is especially useful for children between the ages of 7 and 15 years.
SEE ALSO Intelligence, Mental deterioration, and Psychological tests.

Wandering in the elderly

Medical advice is often sought by the police when an elderly person is found wandering. This is usually due to an acute confusional state (q.v.) or dementia (q.v.). It is therefore necessary to test for recent memory, orientation in space and time, to look for perplexity and fluctuation of attention and concentration, and to exclude the possibility of any serious physical ill-health underlying a delirious state.

Wernicke's encephalopathy

Wernicke's encephalopathy is the result of thiamine deficiency, and is found in chronic alcoholics, and in patients suffering from conditions which lead to deficiency of thamine, such as gastric carcinoma, pernicious anaemia, hyperemesis gravidarum, and starvation. There is a sudden onset of delirium, or a change in consciousness; nystagmus, pupil abnormalities and ophthalmoplegia reflect the neuropathological changes which occur in the mid brain, and particularly in the corpora mammillaria. These neuropathological changes are characteristic of the condition. Prompt treatment by the administration of large doses of thiamine intravenously and intramuscularly is life saving (thiamine hydrochloride 100 mg. immediate slow i.v. injection followed by up to 1000 mg by intramuscular injection daily until recovery takes place).

Will

Operation of the will involves a conscious and deliberate decision to act in a particular way and the initiation of that action. Reference to decision-making implies choice between alternative lines of action and awareness of the ends to which these paths are directed. In important decisions of this nature, reference may be made to the dominant values of the self. Thus willed action may be contrasted with impulsive action: both are conative (q.v.) processes. Otto Rank introduced will therapy based on his theory of birth trauma. Self-control and self-assertion are seen as the equivalents of the separation of the baby from the mother's womb.
SEE ALSO Emotion and Impulse.

Wilson's disease
SEE Hepatolenticular degeneration

Withdrawal

This is a defence mechanism to protect the integrity of the ego (q.v.) (self) from real or imagined phantasied threat. It is an unconsciously and protectively motivated retreat from the reality of the external world. Through it, the subject withdraws to a greater or lesser extent from contacts, relationships, social situations and painful conflicts any or all of which may be experienced as a threat to personal integrity. Persistant use of this mechanism of defence is seen especially in shy, sensitive, schizoid personalities. It is basically a primitive mechanism and is seen in psychotic patients of the schizophrenia simplex type. Markedly obsessional personalities also display this defence.

Withdrawal symptoms

The manifestations of withdrawal of drugs of physical dependence. For details of the symptoms see both Abstinence syndrome and descriptions under the individual drugs. A list of the drugs of physical dependence is given under Addiction.

Word-association tests
SEE Free association.

Word blindness
SEE Dyslexia.

Word-salad

A mixture of words and/or phrases which have no logical meaning. Commonly associated with schizophrenia.

XXX syndrome
SEE Trisomy

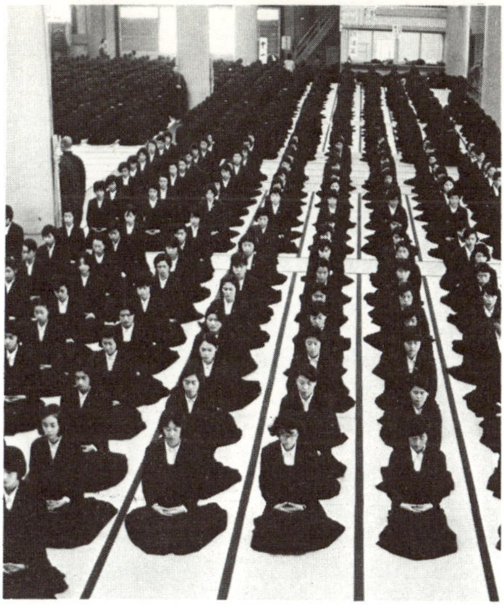

Zen psychotherapy

Based on a sect of Mahayana Buddhism, originated in China, Zen involves a variety of training techniques designed to guide the subject into a new mode of experiencing himself. The major turning point (termed 'satori') is attained after years of training in meditation, but it is considered impossible to express the experience in rational language which makes the concepts and effects difficult to assess scientifically. The individual with satori is described as living an increasingly effective and satisfying life, but the concepts and technique involved do not hold much value for therapy in the Western world – particularly because of the lack of clarity and scientific method of approach.

Appendix of Drugs*

** Editor's Note: This appendix includes some of the most widely used trade names but should in no way be regarded as fully comprehensive.*

Acepromazine maleate
(Available as Notensil[R], Plegizil[R])
Acepromazine is a phenothiazine derivative with anxiolytic and antipsychotic activity, having its greatest use in psychotic patients with excitement and aggressiveness. The dose is 10–25 mg tds for neuroses; 50–100 mg tds for psychoses. Side effects resemble those of chlorpromazine (q.v.) but occur less frequently and the contra-indications are as for chlorpromazine.

Acetylcarbromal
(Abasin[R])
Acetylcarbromal is a mild sedative with less hypnotic effect than carbromal (q.v.). It produces sleep of short duration and is also used as an ambulatory sedative. The normal dose is 250–500 mg tds. Few side effects occur at therapeutic doses but over longer periods symptoms resembling chronic bromide poisoning may occur.

Acetophenazine maleate
(Tindal[R])
A phenothiazine derivative with action and uses as chlorpromazine (q.v.) in anxiety and schizophrenia. The daily dose ranges from 40–80 mg. Its usefulness has not been fully established.

Amiphenazole hydrochloride
(Daptazole[R])
Amiphenazole is an analeptic with an action similar to leptazol (q.v.) but less potent. It is used in respiratory depression or failure and where large doses of morphine are necessary. Dosage is 15–20 mg with each dose of morphine, intramuscularly, and 100–200 mg tds or qds in respiratory insufficiency. Side effects include nausea, vomiting, skin rashes and insomnia. Amiphenazole may lead to bone marrow depression following long term usage.

Amitriptyline hydrochloride
(Laroxyl[R], Lentizol[R] and Saroten[R], Tryptizol[R]; also a constituent of combinations with various tranquillizers)
Amitriptyline is a dibenzocycloheptadiene derivative with potent anti-depressant activity and mild anxiolytic properties. It is used in all forms of depression. It has stronger anti-cholinergic and anti-histaminic actions than imipramine (q.v.), but causes less potentiation of noradrenaline. Dosage is normally 25 mg tds but this is often increased to 50 mg tds. The commonest side effects are drowsiness and dry mouth. Other anti-cholinergic effects are not uncommon. Amitriptyline should be used cautiously in patients with cardiovascular disorders, and it is contra-indicated in glaucoma, prostatic enlargement and urinary retention. Care should be taken when amitriptyline is given at the same time as anti-hypertensive drugs. Except in special circumstances it should not be combined with a monoamine oxidase inhibitor, and usually it is preferable to wait at least three weeks after discontinuing a monoamine oxidase inhibitor before starting treatment with amitriptyline.

Amphetamine sulphate
Amphetamine is a sympathomimetic amine with central nervous system stimulant and anorectic activity. It is used to treat mild depressive neuroses and as an adjuvant in the treatment of chronic alcoholism. The dose is 5 to 10 mg morning and midday. Side effects include dryness of the mouth, restlessness, headache, insomnia, irritability, dizziness, tremor and anorexia. Larger doses may give rise to fatigue, mental depression, an increase in BP, fever, cardiovascular reactions, cyanosis and respiratory failure, disorientation, hallucinations, convulsions, and coma. Continued use of amphetamine sulphate may cause addiction in some patients. It is contra-indicated in cardiovascular disease and thyrotoxicosis, and in those patients showing anxiety, hyper-excitability and restlessness.
The drug should be used with caution in patients with anorexia, insomnia and nephritis. Caution should be taken if amphetamine is used concurrently with monoamine oxidase inhibitors. Due to the liability of abuse the use of amphetamine is no longer recommended.

Amylobarbitone
(Amytal[R])
Amylobarbitone is an intermediate-acting barbiturate. It is used as a sedative and hypnotic. The sedative dose is 15–50 mg bd or tds and 100–300 mg as a hypnotic. Its action, side effects and contra-indications are as for barbiturates (q.v.) generally.

Amylobarbitone sodium
(Sodium Amytal[R])
Being more speedily absorbed, amylobarbitone sodium provides a quicker hypnotic action, otherwise its properties are the same as amylobarbitone (q.v.). Hypnotic dose 100 to 200 mg nocte. Its action, side effects and contra-indications are as for barbiturates (q.v.) generally.

Anisoperidone
Anisoperidone is a butyrophenone derivative used as a tranquillizer. It is less effective than haloperidol in schizophrenia, but greater anxiolytic activity than chlorpromazine (q.v.) has been reported. Dose: 5 to 20 mg daily. Side effects include lack of drive, mild catatonia, nausea, vomiting and Parkinsonism. The place of this substance in clinical therapeutics has not yet been established.

Apomorphine hydrochloride
Apomorphine at a dose of 2–8 mg subcutaneously is used as an emetic in the treatment of non-corrosive poisoning and for aversion therapy in alcoholism. At 2 mg it has sedative and hypnotic effects. Adverse reactions include hypotension, tachycardia and hypoventilation. It is contra-indicated in patients in shock or deep narcosis.

Azocyclonol hydrochloride
(Formerly available as Frenquel)
Azocyclonol is a neuroleptic found effective mainly in the treatment of acute schizophrenia. The dose of 20 to 100 mg tds produces few side effects, no sedation results but skin rashes may occur.

Barbitone
(Hypnogen[R], formerly Veronal[R])
Barbitone is one of the long-acting group of barbiturates, but is slow in producing hypnosis. Although one of the least toxic of the barbiturates, an intermediate or short-acting barbiturate is preferred as a hypnotic. Normal dose is 300 to 600 mg. As barbitone is excreted slowly its cumulation is a problem.

Barbitone sodium
(Previously available as Medinal[R])
Barbitone sodium produces hypnosis rather quicker than barbitone (q.v.), otherwise its properties are the same. Dose: 300 to 600 mg nocte.

Bemegride
(Megimide[R])
An analeptic drug with a similar, but longer, action to leptazol (q.v.) and nikethamide (q.v.), but less potent than picrotoxin (q.v.). In use 10 ml of injection solution (50 mg of bemegride) are injected every three to five minutes until the desired result is obtained, or until a total dose of 1 g is reached.
Toxic effects include retching, vomiting, muscular twitching and hypotension.

Benactyzine hydrochloride
(Formerly marketed as Cafron[R], Cevonol[R], Lucidil[R], Nutinal[R], Suavitil[R], and as an ingredient of Deprol[R], Procalm[R], Stoikon[R])
A diphenylmethane derivative with actions similar to meprobomate (q.v.). Used as a tranquillizer but now in disfavour owing to the number of side effects. Dosage 3–5 mg tds.

Benanserin
An indole derivative, benanserin has psychotropic properties. The place of this substance in clinical therapeutics has not yet been established.

Benzoctamine hydrochloride
(Tacitin[R])
Benzoctamine is an anthracene derivative with anxiolytic and muscle relaxant properties. It is used in anxiety and tension in dosages between 10 and 20 mg tds. Side effects include lassitude, hypotension, impaired vision, sweating, gastrointestinal upsets and tachycardia.

Benzperidol
(Synonym: benzperidol)
(Anquil[R], Frenactyl[R], Glianimon[R])
A butyrophenone derivative reputed to be particularly effective in schizophrenia in agitated geriatric patients and in the control of deviant and anti-social behaviour. The recommended daily dose is 0·25–1·5 mg. Side effects are typical of the butyrophenones.

Benzquinamide
(Quantril[R]; Quantril[R] in the UK is a brand of caffeine citrate)

Benzquinamide is a weak tranquillizer used in the treatment of anxiety and tension. The dose varies from 0·3 to 1 g daily and side effects include extrapyramidal effects, headache, vomiting, and dizziness.

Bromazepam
(Lexomil[R], Lexotan[R], Lexotane[R], Lexotanil[R])
Bromazepam is a new member of the benzodiazepine group. It resembles diazepam (q.v.) in clinical effects, particularly as an antianxiety agent at a daily dose of 4·5–9 mg. Its side effects are also similar to those of diazepam.

Bromocriptine
A dopamine agonist which increases the production of prolactin inhibitory factor in the hypothalamus. A recent study suggests that bromocriptine may have a part to play in the treatment of certain cases of mania.

Bromvaletone
(Bromural[R])
Bromvaletone is chemically related to carbromal. It is a mild, rapidly acting hypnotic with moderately short length of action. It has low toxicity but the habituation liability is similar to that of carbromal (q.v.). It is of no value in insomnia associated with pain. Dose: 300–600 mg. Chronic intoxication may produce bromism.

Buclizine hydrochloride
(Vibazine[R], Softran[R])
Buclizine is an anti-histamine also used for its anti-emetic properties, which are potent but not prolonged. Sedative effect is pronounced and buclizine has been used as an anxiolytic. Used for the symptomatic treatment of allergic conditions and of vertigo. The usual dose is 20–50 mg tds.

Butaperazine
(Synonym: butyrylperazine)
(Randolectil[R])
Butaperazine is an anti-psychotic related to phenothiazine with strong tranquillizing properties. It is used in treating chronic schizophrenia in doses ranging from 30 to 200 mg. daily. Side effects including extrapyramidal symptoms, hypotension, constipation and blurred vision are those associated with the phenothiazines.

Butobarbitone
(Soneryl[R])
Butobarbitone is a member of the intermediate acting barbiturates and used mainly as a hypnotic in insomnia, nervous or mental excitement and anxiety states. Dose: 100–200 mg. Side effects are those normally associated with barbiturates (q.v.).

Butriptyline hydrochloride
(Evadyne[R])
Butriptyline is a moderately sedative tricyclic antidepressant used in patients with depression associated with anxiety. The daily dosage is between 75 and 150 mg/day. Anticholinergic side effects are present.

Butyrylperazine
SEE Butaperazine.

Captodiame hydrochloride
(Formerly marketed in the United Kingdom as Covantin[R], Covatix[R])
(Marketed in USA as Suvren[R])
Captodiame hydrochloride has sedative and anti-spasmodic properties and has been used for the relief of tension, agitation and anxiety in minor neuroses and psychosomatic disorders. Dose: 50–100 mg tds. It is contra-indicated in coma due to central nervous depressants such as alcohol, barbiturates and opiates.

Carbromal
(Adalin[R])
Carbromal is a mild hypnotic of value in mild insomnia. The dose is 300–1000 mg. Side effects resemble those of chloral hydrate (q.v.). After long periods, symptoms of chronic toxicity resembling bromism may occur.

Carphenazine maleate
(Marketed in the USA as Proketazine[R] Maleate)
A phenothiazine derivative with tranquillizing properties similar to those of chlorpromazine (q.v.). It is used in the treatment of anxiey and schizophrenia, but in the latter maximum response is often slow. Its mild stimulating effect is valuable in the apathetic withdrawn schizophrenic. The dose is gradually increased at intervals of seven to fourteen days, being between 25 and 400 mg. Side effects and contra-indication are as for chlorpromazine (q.v.).

Centrophenoxine hydrochloride
(Lucidril[R])
SEE Meclofenoxate hydrochloride.

Chloral betaine
(Formerly marketed as Somilan[R])
A complex of chloral hydrate and betaine with similar actions and uses to chloral hydrate. It is claimed not to cause gastric irritation. Hypnotic dose 0·87–1·75 g half an hour before bedtime. Toxic effects and contra-indications as for chloral hydrate (q.v.).

Chloral hydrate
(Somnos[R], Noctec[R])
Chloral hydrate has been in use as a hypnotic for over 100 years. The dose is 300 mg–2g. Although considered a safe hypnotic, an adult death occurred with a 1·3 g dose. It should not be given as tablets as damage of the mucous membrane of the alimentary tract may occur.
Side effects include deep stupor, vasodilation, hypotension, hypothermia and respiratory depression. Gastric irritation may cause vomiting. Fatal dose averages about 10 g and doses over 2 g should be used with caution.
Chronic poisoning resembles chronic alcoholism. It is contra-indicated in patients with marked hepatic or renal impairment or severe cardiac disease and is best avoided in gastritis.

Chlordiazepoxide
(Librium[R], Calmoden[R])
(Also a constituent of Limbitrol[R])
Chlordiazepoxide is a minor tranquillizer and widely used prototype member of the benzodiazepines (q.v.). This compound has a strong anxiolytic effect, but less muscle relaxant properties than diazepam. It is valuable in all disorders in which anxiety is either causative, or a prominent symptom: these include the psychosomatic disorders. The normal dose is 10 mg tds. In chronic alcoholism up to 100 mg may be given. Excellent tolerance is reported and the side effects which are few and mild include ataxia and drowsiness. If psychological dependence does occur it is very weak. Although additive sedative effects may be encountered, chlordiazepoxide may be given safely with other psychotropic drugs.

Chlorhexadol
(Medodorm[R]; Dormax[R], Danish; Lova[R], USA)
Chlorhexadol, a chloral hydrate (q.v.) derivative, is a sedative and hypnotic. The dose is 200–800 mg tds as a sedative and 0·8–1·6 g as a hypnotic. Toxic effects and contra-indications are as for chloral hydrate (q.v.).

Chlorimipramine
SEE Clomipramine

Chlormethazanone
SEE Chlormezanone

Chlormethiazole edisylate
(Heminevrin[R])
Chlormethiazole is a hypnotic with muscle relaxant and anti-convulsant properties. It is used mainly in the treatment of delerium tremens, acute withdrawal symptoms in alcoholics and drug addicts, sleep disturbances and pre-eclamptic toxaemia. Dosage for insomnia is 1–2 g nocte. Side effects include gastrointestinal upsets and it is contra-indicated in depression. Due to additive or potentiating effects, chlormethiazole should be used with caution with other drugs.

Chlormezanone
(Synonym: Chlormethazanone)
(Trancopal[R])
Chlormezanone is a minor tranquillizer with actions similar to those of meprobamate (q.v.), and is used in the treatment of mild tension and anxiety states. It also relieves muscle spasm. Dose: 200 mg tds. Side effects are mild and relatively infrequent. Its use is contra-indicated with phenothiazines or monoamine oxidase inhibitors.

Chlorperphanazine
SEE Perphenazine.

Chlorproethazine
(Neuriplège[R])
A phenothiazine derivative chlorproethazine is a tranquillizer with actions and uses as chlorpromazine (q.v.).

Chlorproheptadiene
Chlorproheptadiene is a cycloheptene derivative which shows possible tranquillizing properties. The place of this

substance in clinical therapeutics has not yet been established.

Chlorpromazine hydrochloride
(Largactil[R], Megaphen[R], Propaphen[R] and in various combinations)
(Thorazine[R], Hydrochloride in the USA)
Chlorpromazine is a major tranquillizer (neuroleptic) and widely used prototype member of the phenothiazine (q.v.) group, having sedative and anxiolytic properties. It is used to alleviate anxiety, tension and agitation in neurotic and psychotic patients. It is especially valuable in schizophrenia. The dose varies from 25 to 100 mg tds. Side effects include drowsiness, dryness of the mouth, dizziness, headache, constipation, lassitude, Parkinsonism, hypotension, skin disorders, occasionally severe and rarely fatal blood dyscrasias and jaundice.
Chlorpromazine is contra-indicated in cases of coma due to direct central nervous system depression such as with alcohol, barbiturates; in patients with liver and cardiovascular disease.

Chlorprothixene
(Taractan[R], Truxal[R])
Chlorprothixene is a thioxanthene derivative with similar actions and uses as chlorpromazine (q.v.) and with some anti-depressant effect. It is used in the treatment of agitation, anxiety, hallucinations and delusions without the risk of exacerbating any underlying depression. Dose: 10–50 mg tds. Side effects include dryness of mouth, sweating, tachycardia, drowsiness and hypotension.

Citrated calcium carbimide
(Abstem[R])
Citrated calcium carbimide is used as an adjunct in alcoholism therapy. Like disulfiram (q.v.) it interferes with normal alcohol metabolism, an increase of acetaldehyde in the blood producing an unpleasant syndrome, flushing, headache, giddiness, and tachycardia. The dose is 1 tablet bd. It produces fewer and milder side effects than disulfiram, but mild or transitory leucocytosis has been reported. It is contra-indicated in patients with myocardial or coronary artery disease.

Clomacran
Clomacran is an acridan derivative used as a neuroleptic in schizophrenia in dosages between 100 to 600 mg daily. Side effects include drowsiness, akathisia (to an extent that anti-Parkinsonism treatment may be required) and insomnia. The place of this substance in clinical therapeutics has not yet been established.

Clomipramine hydrochloride
(Synonym: chlorimipramine)
(Anafranil[R])
Clomipramine is an iminodibenzyl derivative with anti-depressant properties. The dose is 25 mg tds for two to three days, increasing to 50 mg tds.
Side effects include dry mouth, difficulty with accommodation, disturbances of micturition, hypotension, and gastro-intestinal upsets, and are similar to those of the other iminodibenzyl derivatives (e.g. imipramine (q.v.)).
Contra-indications include liver damage, circulatory failure, glaucoma and urinary retention. It should not be used concurrently or within fourteen days of treatment with monoamine oxidase inhibitors.

Clonazepam
(Rivotril[R])
Clonazepam is one of the most recently introduced benzodiazepines with anti-epileptic properties. The adult daily dosage is 4–8 mg. Side effects are those of the benzodiazepines.

Clopenthixol
(Sordinol[R])
Clopenthixol is a thioxanthene derivative with anxiolytic activity and similar uses to the phenothiazines. It is used to produce sedation in the treatment of severe agitation acute schizophrenia and manic depression. Side effects include extrapyramidal symptoms, dyskinesia, hypotension and tachycardia. Dose: 30–150 mg tds.

Clorazepate (as potassium salt)
(Tranxene[R], Tranxilium[R])
An anxiolytic benzodiazepine used in anxiety states at a dosage of 15 mg at night. Side effects resemble those of other benzodiazepines.

Clorgyline
A non-hydrazine monoamine oxidase inhibitor, clorgyline has anti-depressant activity. The usual dose is 5 mg tds. Side effects reported include postural hypotension and fainting. The place of this substance in clinical therapeutics has not yet been established.

Clothiapine
(Etumin[R], Etomine[R], Etomina[R])
Clothiapine is a tranquillizer of the dibenzothiazepine group. Used in schizophrenia, the dose varies between 30 and 360 mg daily. The place of clothiapine in medical practice is not yet established.

Clozapine
(Leponex[R])
Clozapine is a dibenzodiazepine derivative with neuroleptic activity at a daily dose of 100–300 mg. The place of this substance in therapeutics is still not clear.

Codeine
Codeine, a narcotic analgesic (q.v.), is methylated morphine, much less toxic than morphine and death directly attributable to codeine is rare. Tolerance and addiction (q.v.) can occur. Orally its euphoric action is weak, but large doses subcutaneously can act as a morphine substitute for the addict. Codeine has a mild hypnotic action and less analgesic potency than morphine. It causes less respiratory depression and is less constipating than morphine. It is used as an analgesic and to relieve dry cough. Dose: 10–60 mg. The signs of codeine intoxication are narcosis, sometimes preceded by exhilaration and followed by convulsions; nausea and vomiting are prominent, the pupils are contracted and the pulse rate is increased. Codeine is also contained in many analgesic and antitussive combinations.

Cyclarbamate
(Calmalone[R])
A cyclopentane derivative with muscle relaxant and tranquillizer activity cyclarbamate has a dosage of 0·5 to 1·5 g daily, in divided doses.

Cyclobarbitone
(Phanodorm[R])
Cyclobarbitone is a member of the short-acting barbiturates (q.v.) with a comparatively mild action. It is used as a sedative and hypnotic in anxiety states and insomnia.
Dose: 200 to 400 mg.

Cyclobarbitone calcium
(Rapidal[R], Phanodorm[R])
Cyclobarbitone calcium has the same action and uses as cyclobarbitone, but since cyclobarbitone gradually decomposes the more stable cyclobarbitone calcium is preferred.

Cyprolidol
A pyridyl-cyclopropane derivative, cyprolidol has anti-depressant activity and is used in the treatment of depression. The daily dose is 500–600 mg. The place of cyprolidol in therapy is not yet established.

Deanol acetamidobenzoate
(Previously available as Deaner[R])
Deanol was claimed to stimulate the central nervous system including the reticular activating system so improving mood and behaviour, but its value was not proven. It was reputed to be of value in chronic fatigue states, mild depression and in chronic headaches and migraine. Dose: 50 mg initially, maintenance 25–75 mg daily. Side effects were typical of a parasympathomimetic agent.
Contra-indicated in grand mal.

Dehydrobenzperidol
(Droleptan[R])
SEE Droperidol.

Deserpidine
(Harmony[R])
Deserpidine is a Rauwolfia alkaloid with central depressant and sedative action and an antihypertensive effect. It is used for mild anxiety states and chronic psychoses. Dosage in mild mental disturbances is 0·1 mg od and in psychosis 0·5–1 mg tds. Although deserpidine produces less lethargy and depression than reserpine (q.v.), nasal congestion, drowsiness, gastro-intestinal upsets and depression may occur. It is specifically contra-indicated when there is any evidence of depression.

Desipramine hydrochloride
(Pertofran^R, Norpramin^R)
An iminodibenzyl derivative with antidepressant activity and side effects similar to imipramine (q.v.). The initial dose is 25 mg tds for three days, increasing as necessary to a maximum of 50 mg tds or qds; the usual maintenance dose is 50–100 mg daily. Contra-indications and special precautions as imipramine (q.v.). In severe depression and retardation, supervision is necessary because the suicidal risk is often temporarily enhanced.

Dexamphetamine sulphate
(Dephadren^R, Dexamed^R, Dexedrine^R)
SEE Amphetamines.

Dextromoramide acid tartrate
(Palfium^R)
Dextromoramide is a narcotic analgesic used in severe pain. The dose is 5 mg, increasing up to 20 mg if necessary. There is addiction liability (q.v.) and side effects include light-headedness, dizziness, nausea, vomiting and sleepiness. Respiratory depression may occur after intravenous administration. Contra-indications include patients with hepatic disease, hypotension and cerebral disease. The action of barbiturates, chlorpromazine and anaesthetics is enhanced.

Dextropropoxyphene hydrochloride
(Doloxene^R, Depronal; Darvon^R, in USA.) Also available in analgesic combinations
Dextropropoxyphene is a narcotic analgesic used in acute and chronic pain. Unlike levopropoxyphene, it has little antitussive activity. It has some addiction (q.v.) liability and side effects include nausea, vomiting and in high doses, drowsiness and dizziness. Dose: 30–65 mg tds or qds.

Dibenzepin hydrochloride
(Noveril^R, Neodalit^R)
Dibenzepin is a dibenzodiazin antidepressant with effectiveness intermediate between imipramine and amitriptyline. Side effects include dryness of mouth and precipitation of manic phases. Initial dose is 80 mg to 120 mg tds with maintenance doses of 80 mg tds.

Diacetylmorphine hydrochloride
SEE Diamorphine hydrochloride.

Diamorphine hydrochloride
(Synonym: heroin)
Diamorphine hydrochloride (heroin) is a derivative of the natural alkaloid morphine. It is a powerful analgesic and narcotic, having a more potent, but shorter analgesic action than morphine. Although it is a very effective cough suppressant, it should not be used for this purpose, because of its addictive properties. When administered subcutaneously or intramuscularly, it is used for the relief of severe pain in the terminal stages of cancer when morphine in safe dosage is no longer effective. It is also occasionally used in the immediate post-operative period. The oral, intramuscular or intravenous dose is 5 to 10 mg. Heroin produces intense euphoria and fewer side effects than morphine, such as constipation, nausea and vomiting, although it has a more powerful respiratory depressant action than morphine.
The treatment of the heroin addict is the same as for morphine addiction, but heroin addiction is considered to be much more difficult to break and the mental and moral deterioration of the addict is much worse than with morphine.

Diazepam
(Valium^R)
Diazepam is a benzodiazepine with stronger anxiolytic properties than chlordiazepoxide, is sedative and shows central muscle-relaxant action. It is used in anxiety and tension states, psychosomatic and organic illnesses with associated anxiety, in muscle spasm and as premedication. The dose varies from 2 mg tds in mild anxiety to 15–30 mg tds in severe anxiety and other psychiatric disorders. In muscle spasm the dose is 2–60 mg tds. 10–20 mg is given intravenously for minor operations. Side effects are similar to chlordiazepoxide.

Dichloralphenazone
(Welldorm^R, Bonadorm^R in Australia, and Dormwell^R, elsewhere)
(Fenzol^R)
Dichloralphenazone is a complex of chloral hydrate and phenazone used as a hypnotic and sedative. The hypnotic dose is 1·3 g and the sedative dose is 650 mg bd or tds. Side effects include hypersensitivity reaction, rashes and nausea. It is contra-indicated in acute intermittent porphyria,

marked hepatic or renal impairment and in severe cardiac disease.

Dihydrocodeine acid tartrate
(DF 118R)
Dihydrocodeine acid tartrate is a codeine derivative used as an analgesic and a cough suppressant. Side effects are less pronounced than with morphine (q.v.) and are similar to codeine (q.v.). Tolerance and addiction (q.v.) may occur. It is contra-indicated in liver disease and asthma. Dose: 10–60 mg.

Dimethacrine tartrate
(IstonilR)
Dimethacrine is an acridan derivative having antidepressant activity. The dose is 25 to 75 mg tds orally or 50 mg tds intravenously or intramuscularly.

Diphenhydramine
A sedative antihistamine which is used as a component of certain hypnotic combinations, typically with methaqualone (q.v.).

Diphenoxylate hydrochloride
(as a constituent in LomotilR)
Diphenoxylate is a narcotic analgesic used mainly in the treatment of acute and chronic diarrhoea. The usual dose is 5 mg tds or qds. Side effects include rash, pruritis, drowsiness, insomnia, dizziness, restlessness, euphoria, depression, abdominal distension and nausea. Diphenoxylate is contra-indicated in patients with impaired liver function. Long term administration of diphenoxylate carries the risk of addiction (q.v.)

Dipipanone
(PipadoneR. Also a constituent of DiconalR)
Dipipanone is a potent analgesic (25 mg ≡ 10 mg morphine sulphate) with a rapid onset of action. Its side effects include drowsiness, nausea and vomiting; and there is a risk of addiction (q.v.). Contra-indications are severe lung and kidney disease and in patients who have undergone thoracic operations. Administration is usually by subcutaneous or intramuscular injection, 25 mg bd or qds.

Dipiperon
(Synonyms: Pipamperon, Floropipamide), (DipiperonR, PiperonylR, PropitanR)
Dipiperon is a butyrophenone derivative used as a tranquilliser in chronic schizophrenia. The initial dose is 60 mg daily increasing to 200 to 600 mg daily. Side effects include extrapyramidal symptoms and hypotension.

Disulfiram
(Synonym: tenraethylthirum disulphide) (AntabuseR 200)
(Also available as: AbstinylR, Sweden; AlcophobinR, USA)
Disulfiram taken by itself rarely produces any pharmacological effects other than perhaps peripheral neuropathy, but when taken with alcohol unpleasant side effects occur, e.g. flushing, palpitations, dizziness. For this reason, it is used in the treatment of chronic alcoholism. It is not curative and requires concomitant psychotherapy. Because of the varying intensity of the side effects produced, initial treatment should be carried out in hospital. There are numerous contra-indications and doubt now exists about the merits of disulfiram therapy.

Dixyrazine
(EsucosR)
Dixyrazine is a phenothiazine derivative with actions and uses similar to chlorpromazine hydrochloride (q.v.). Side effects reported include fatigue, alopecia and other scalp and skin disorders. Dose: 15–75 mg bd.

Dothiepin
(ProthiadenR)
Dothiepin is a tricyclic anti-depressant compound used in the treatment of depression and anxiety. The dose is 25 mg tds, increasing to 50 mg tds or as necessary. Contra-indications include glaucoma, urinary retention, epilepsy. It should be given with caution with or within two or three weeks of cessation of treatment with a monoamine oxidase inhibitor.

Doxepin hydrochloride
(SinequanR, SinquanR, AponalR)
A tricyclic anti-depressant claimed to have associated anxiolytic properties, indicated in the treatment of depression and anxiety. Dose: 10 to 100 mg tds depending on

severity of condition. Contra-indications include glaucoma and urinary retention. Side effects include drowsiness, dryness of the mouth, tremor, blurring of vision, urinary retention, and constipation.

Droperidol
(Synonym dehydrobenzperidol)
(Droleptan[R], Thalamonal[R])
Droperidol is a butyrophenone derivative with actions similar to haloperidol. It produces a state of mental detachment and indifference to surroundings. It is used for the technique of neuroleptanalgesia and for premedication. Dose: 10–20 mg orally, 5 mg intravenously, 10 mg intramuscularly. Side effects include extrapyramidal effects. It is contra-indicated in depressive illness or in severe hepatic disease.

Ectylurea
(Levanil[R], Nostyn[R])
A mild sedative, ectylurea, is used in treating simple anxiety and tension. It appears to be of low toxicity, but it may cause skin rashes and occasionally, jaundice. It is contra-indicated in liver disease. Dose: 150–300 mg tds or qds.

Emetine hydrochloride
Emetine hydrochloride has been used in the past as a nauseant in aversion therapy of chronic alcoholism (q.v.).

Emylcamate
(Nuncital[R], Resteral[R])
(Formerly marketed as Striatran[R])
Emylcamate has tranquillizing and muscle-relaxant properties. It is used as an adjunct in the treatment of fractures, muscle pain, and inflammation. Dose: 20 mg tds before food and at night if necessary.
Side effects include various gastro-intestinal upsets, headache, palpitations, and skin rash. If used over long periods or in large doses periodic blood counts and liver function tests should be carried out especially if the patient already has hepatic disease.

Ephedrine
Ephedrine is a sympathomimetic amine. It has a more prolonged though less potent action than adrenaline, and is effective orally. It possesses a central stimulant action and is used in narcolepsy and catalepsy in doses of 8 to 60 mg tds by mouth. It is also a constituent of many combination preparations.

Ethamivan
(Vandid[R])
Ethamivan is an analeptic with quick action and short duration. It is used as a respiratory stimulant in barbiturate poisoning, in comatose states where respiration is depressed, and in neonatal asphyxia. Side effects include spontaneous motor activity, and in overdosage, convulsions. Ethamivan is contra-indicated in epileptic patients or in respiratory failure caused by a convulsive drug. It should not be given at the same time as a monoamine oxidase inhibitor.

Ethchlorvynol
(Arvynol[R], Serenesil[R])
Ethchlorvynol is a chlorinated carbinol with a mild hypnotic action and anticonvulsant activity approximately equivalent to that of phenobarbitone. It is used for the treatment of simple insomnia without pain, but the possibility of dependence should be borne in mind. Hypnotic dose: 500 mg nocte. Side effects include dizziness, bad taste in the mouth, vomiting, and ataxia which may be lessened by taking ethchlorvynol with milk. Hypotension, skin rashes, hangover effect and mental confusion may also occur.

Ethinamate
(Valmidate[R], formerly known as Valmid)
Ethinamate is an unsaturated carbinol with mild hypnotic properties, used in simple insomnia at a dose of 500–1,000 mg nocte. Side effects include vomiting and hangover. Dependence has been reported.

Ethoheptazine citrate
Ethoheptazine is a narcotic analgesic chemically allied to pethidine. It is used in the treatment of moderately severe pain, particularly associated with musculo-skeletal disorders. It is only available in combination with other analgesics such as aspirin or paracetamol (Equagesic[R], Zactipar[R], and Zactirin[R]. Side effects include nausea, dizziness, epigastric distress and pruritus. Dose: 75–150 mg tds or qds.

Ethotrimeprazine
(Synonym: Ethylisobutrazine, Etymenazine)
(Diquel^R, Sergetye^R)
Ethotrimeprozine is a phenothiozine derivative with sedative properties. It is an effective neuroleptic at a daily dose of 5–80 mg and the side effects are similar to those of chlorpromazine.

Fencamfamin hydrochloride
(Euvitol^R)
Fencamfamin hydrochloride is claimed to act as a central nervous stimulant and to be of value in the treatment of fatigue and depression following illness. Dose: 10–20 mg bd. It is contra-indicated in conditions of hyperexcitability and thyrotoxicosis. It should be used cautiously in patients with angina pectoris.

Fentanyl citrate
(Sublimaze^R)
Fentanyl citrate is a potent narcotic analgesic with actions similar to morphine (q.v.). It is used in conjunction with a neuroleptic drug such as droperidol, to produce anaesthesia. Side effects include depression of respiration and addiction may develop. Fentanyl should not be given with monoamine oxidase inhibitors (q.v.). Dose: 0·1 to 0·6 mg intravenously.

Flunitrazepam
(Rohypnol^R)
Flunitrazepam is one of the new benzodiazepine compounds with marked sedative effects. It is therefore used mainly as a hypnotic and a dose each night of 1–2 mg. The side effects are those of sedative benzodiazepines.

Floropipamide
(Synonyms: Dipiperon, Pipamperon)
SEE Dipiperon.

Fluanisone
(Sedalande^R, Haloanisone^R)
SEE Haloanisone.

Fluopromazine
(Psyquil^R, Siquil^R)
Fluopromazine hydrochloride has actions and side effects similar to those of chlorpromazine and has its main place in the treatment of schizophrenia. The daily dose is 20–150 mg daily.

Flupenthixol
(Fluanxol^R, Dapixol^R and Fluanxol^R Depot)
Flupenthixol is a thioxanthene derivative showing anti-anxiety properties. It has been used in chronic schizophrenia in doses of 1 to 6 mg daily. Side effects include extra-pyramidal symptoms. The depot form has several advantages for maintenance therapy.

Fluphenazine decanoate
(Modecate^R, Moditan^R enanthate, Darpotum^R D, Lyogen^R Depot)
Fluphenazine decanoate and enanthate are prolonged injectable forms of fluphenazine, with uses and properties similar to fluphenazine hydrochloride (q.v.).
Their chief advantage is the ease of administration for they can be given at intervals of one to four weeks. This is an important feature for it has been shown that 48% of schizophrenics do not take their tablets as prescribed and relapse is often due to stopping medication prematurely.
While the side effects are similar to those of oral fluphenazine, depressions may occur more commonly.

Fluphenazine enanthate
SEE Fluphenazine decanoate.

Fluphenazine hydrochloride
(Moditen^R, Lyogen^R, Omca^R, Sevenal^R)
(Prolixin^R and Permitil^R in USA)
Fluphenazine is a phenothiazine derivative with actions and uses similar to chlorpromazine (q.v.), but it has greater tranquillizing action and less sedative effect. It is used for the relief of anxiety and tension in manic-depressive states and schizophrenia. It has a powerful antiemetic action and is used to control postoperative vomiting. Dose: 1 to 5 mg od, although up to 15 mg od may be necessary in severe cases. Side effects see trifluoperazine hydrochloride.

Flurazepam
(Dalmane^R, Dalmadorm^R, USA)
Flurazepam is a benzodiazepine (q.v.) with potent hypnotic properties. It has greater hypnotic activity than nitrazepam (q.v.) but otherwise it has similar actions and uses. The usual dose is 15 to 30 mg nocte. In common with benzodiazepines the

safety of flurazepam is good and side effects are of a minor nature.

Fluspirilene
(Redeptin[R], Imap[R])
Fluspirilene is a diphenylbutylpiperidine derivative with antipsychotic activity used in the treatment of schizophrenia. It is long acting and initially a 2 mg dose is given im weekly. The dose is then increased in 2 mg increments weekly, up to 8 mg which is the maintenance dose. Side effects include extrapyramidal symptoms, nausea and vomiting.

Glutethimide
(Doriden[R])
Glutethimide is a piperidinedione derivative with hypnotic properties. Its action may be compared with the intermediate acting barbiturates, inducing sleep in about 20 minutes with some 6 hours duration. It is used for the treatment of insomnia but is not effective in the presence of pain or mental disturbance. The usual dose is 500 mg nocte. Side effects include nausea, excitement, and occasional skin rashes. It is contra-indicated in the first trimester of pregnancy.

Haloanisone
(Synonym fluanisone)
(Sedalande[R])
Haloanisone is a butyrophenone derivative having tranquillising activity. It is used in schizophrenia. Dosage varies between 75 and 300 mg. Side effects include extrapyramidal symptoms and hypotension.

Haloperidol
(Serenace[R])
(Haldol[R], in the USA)
A butyrophenone derivative, haloperidol is a tranquillizer with particular value in the treatment of mania and schizophrenic excitement. Delusions, hallucinations and paranoia are controlled and behaviour disorders in the mentally subnormal also respond. It is also used in the treatment of phobic anxiety. The dose is 0·5 mg bd in anxiety states, but in severe agitation up to 5 mg bd may be given. Side effects include extrapyramidal symptoms, motor restlessness and dystonic reactions. Other side effects include drowsiness, dizziness, and it should not be given alone where depression is prominent as this may be worsened.

Heptabarbitone
(Medomin[R])
A short acting barbiturate, heptabarbitone is used as a sedative and hypnotic. The sedative dose is 50 to 100 mg bd or tds and the usual hypnotic dose is 200 to 400 mg nocte. Side effects and contra-indications are as for barbiturates (q.v.) generally.

Heroin
(Synonyms: diamorphine hydrochloride; diacetylmorphine hydrochloride)
SEE Diamorphine hydrochloride.

Hexapropymate
(Mérinax[R])
Hexapropymate is a non-barbiturate hypnotic which promptly induces sleep of good duration. Dose: 200 to 600 mg nocte.

Hexobarbitone
Hexobarbitone is a short acting barbiturate (q.v.) used as a hypnotic, often in conjunction with other barbiturates (e.g. Evidorm[R]). Its sodium salt (q.v.) is a very short-acting barbiturate. The hypnotic dose of hexobarbitone is 250 to 500 mg. Side effects and contra-indications are as for the barbiturates (q.v.).

Hexobarbitone sodium
(Previously available as Cyclonal Sodium[R] and as combinations)
Hexobarbitone sodium is a very short-acting barbiturate used for inducing anaesthesia before the administration of gaseous anaesthetics and also as a general anaesthetic for short minor operations. Hexobarbitone has been largely superseded by thiopentone sodium.
Convulsions may be controlled by the intramuscular injection of hexobarbitone sodium, and up to 1 g has been used in status epilepticus. Dose: 0·2 to 1 g intravenously; 40 mg per kg bodyweight with a maximum dose of 2 g by rectal injection. It is contra-indicated in respiratory tract infections, in impaired liver function and low blood pressure.

Hydroxyphenamate
(Listica[R])
Hydroxyphenamate is a tranquillizer resembling meprobamate in its sedative properties. It is used in the treatment of anxiety and tension. Dose: 600 to 800 mg daily. Side effects include drowsiness,

dizziness, depression and occasionally hypotension and urticaria.

Hydroxyzine hydrochloride
(Atarax[R])
(Vistaril[R] in the USA)
Hydroxyzine, a diphenylmethane derivative, is a central nervous depressant with antihistaminic and antispasmodic actions. It is used in anxiety and tension states and as an adjuvant in the treatment of urticaria and dermatoses where emotional disturbances are prominent. Dose: 25 to 100 mg tds or qds. Side effects include slight hypotension, headache, drowsiness, and dry mouth. Hydroxyzine should be used cautiously with hypnotics, analgesics and dicoumarol type anticoagulants. Its use has been largely replaced by more effective anxiolytics.

Hyoscine hydrobromide
(Kwells[R] brand)
Hyoscine is a member of the Belladonna group of alkaloids having central and peripheral actions. Unlike atropine it depresses the motor areas of the cerebral cortex and acts as a hypnotic and does not have the stimulating effect of atropine on the brain. It is used to calm and induce sleep in delirium, acute mania, and in severe agitation. Hyoscine is a symptomatic treatment for Parkinson's syndrome, and is used to prevent motion sickness, and in pre-operative medication. Dose: 0·3 to 0·6 mg; larger doses are given in Parkinson's syndrome.
Side effects include dry mouth, blurring of vision, constipation, and drowsiness.

Imipramine hydrochloride
(Tofranil[R], Berkomine[R], Norpramine[R], Dimipressin[R], IA–Pram[R], Impamin[R], Praminal[R])
(Also a constituent of Tofranil[R] with Promazine)
Imipramine hydrochloride is the prototype iminodibenzyl derivative with antidepressant activity (thymoleptic). It is used mainly in the treatment of endogenous depression. It may be less effective than the monoamine oxidase inhibitors in the treatment of neurotic or reactive depression. Unfortunately it is difficult to recognise in advance which patient is best treated with which drug. Two or three weeks treatment may be necessary before the response is apparent at a dose of 25 to 50 mg tds. Side effects include atropine-like side effects, and imipramine is contra-indicated in glaucoma and epilepsy. Caution should be observed where pronounced circulatory or cardiac failure exists.

Iprindole
(Prondol[R], Galatur[R], Tertran[R])
Iprindole is a hexahydrocycloöcta [b] indole derivative with potent antidepressant activity. It is used in all forms of depression. The dose is usually 30 mg tds and 15 mg tds for elderly patients.
Side effects include dry-mouth, blurred vision, dizziness, unsteadiness on standing, tremors and hypotension. Iprindole should not be given concurrently or within two weeks of treatment with monoamine oxidase inhibitors. It is contra-indicated with a previous history of hepatic disorders and caution is necessary in patients with enlarged prostate or glaucoma.

Iproclozide
(Sursum[R])
Iproclozide is an antidepressant, of the hydrazine monoamine oxidase inhibitor group. In depression the dose is 10 mg three times daily. The side effects and contra-indications are as for other monoamine oxidase inhibitors (q.v.).

Iproniazid
(Marsilid[R])
The anti depressant iproniazid is the prototype monoamine oxidase inhibitor of the hydrazide group. It is used in the treatment of exogenous and reactive depression. The initial dose is 50 to 100 mg tds; maintenance, 25 to 50 mg tds. For general side effects and contra-indications see monoamine oxidase inhibitors. Iproniazid is one of the most effective monoamine oxidase inhibitors but its use should be limited to patients who have failed to respond to other drugs for the toxic and side effects (particularly jaundice and hypotension) are more common and serious than with some other amine oxidase inhibitors.

Isocarboxazid
(Marplan[R])
Isocarboxazid, a hydrazine derivative, is a monoamine oxidase inhibitor antidepressant drug used in the treatment of

depression. The initial dose is 10 mg tds, when the optimal effect may be seen between one and four weeks. A dose of 10 mg od or bd is then sufficient for maintenance. Isocarboxazide has the general side effects and contra-indications of the monoamine oxidase inhibitors (q.v.). The incidence of the side effects is however less than with most drugs in this class.

Laevopromazine
(Veractil[R])
SEE Methotrimeprazine maleate.

Leptazol
(Cardiazol[R])
(Metrazol[R], USA)
(Pentrazol[R], USA)
An analeptic, leptazol stimulates the respiratory and motor centres. Its action is more potent but shorter than picrotoxin. Leptazol is used to counteract respiratory depression caused by drugs. Electroconvulsive therapy has now superseded convulsive therapy in psychiatry induced by intravenous leptazol. Dose: 50–100 mg. Side effects on high doses include epileptiform convulsions.

Levallorphan tartrate
(Lorfan[R])
Levallorphan is a narcotic antagonist having greater potency and more prolonged action than nalorphine (q.v.). In small doses it is used to counteract the respiratory depression caused by morphine-like drugs with minimal alteration of the analgesic effect. Levallorphan can be given either before or with the analgesic. Dose: 0·5 to 1 mg intravenously to restore respiration. Half the initial dose may be repeated after 10 minutes if necessary.

Levomepromazine
(Veractil[R])
SEE Methotrimeprazine maleate.

Levorphanol tartrate
(Dromoran[R])
Levorphanol tartrate is a more potent, longer acting narcotic analgesic than morphine (q.v.). It is used in severe, acute and chronic pain. Dose: 1·5–3 mg orally bd, and 2–4 mg by injection in very severe pain. Levorphanol is well tolerated producing less hypnotic effect than morphine and less morphine-like side effects generally.

Lithium carbonate
(Priadel[R], Camcolit[R])
(Lithane[R], Eskalith[R], and Lithonate[R] in the USA)
Lithium carbonate is used in the treatment of manic phases of manic depressive psychoses, and as a prophylactic in recurrent affective disorders. To avoid tremor and nausea initial dosage should be small and gradually increased to between 600 and 1600 mg daily.
The drug is potentially toxic and treatment should be maintained under careful clinical and laboratory control. Early morning serum lithium levels should be between 0·8–1·2 mEq/litre.
Vomiting, ataxia, coarse tremor, fasciculation, marked drowsiness, slurred speech and confusion are signs of overdosage, and lithium poisoning results in coma with hyper-reflexia, muscle tremor. Contra-indications include cardiac or renal decompensation.

Lorazepam
(Ativan[R], Tavor[R], Temesta[R])
Lorazepam is a benzodiazepine with moderate anxiolytic activity and some sedation and muscle relaxant effects. It is used in anxiety and tension states. The dosage for mild anxiety is 1–9 mg daily and for severe cases up to 10 mg daily. Side effects resemble those found with all benzodiazepines.

Loxapine succinate
(Synonym: Oxilapine)
Loxapine is a dibenzoxazepin derivative used in the treatment of schizophrenia. Dose ranges from 20–140 mg with a mean daily dose of 50 mg. Side-effects include facial dystonia, extrapyramidal reactions, liver and haematological abnormalities.

L–tryptophan
(A constituent of Optimax[R])
L-tryptophan is a naturally occurring amino acid which when metabolised to 5-hydroxytryptamine exerts antidepressant properties. In the treatment of depression the daily dose of L-tryptophan is 2/6 g. Half the dose should be taken in the evening and the remaining half given in divided doses during the day. Side effects

include nausea, hypotension and drowsiness. Optimax also contains ascorbic acid and pyridoxine which is utilised in the metabolism of L-tryptophan to 5-hydroxytryptamine.

Lysergic Acid Diethylamide
SEE Lysergide

Lysergide
Synonyms: Lysergic Acid Diethylamide; LSD
Lysergide is a hallucinogen producing transient mental perceptional and behavioural changes resembling the symptoms of psychotic disease. Perceptional changes produced especially affect the visual system with alteration of colour perception, illusions and hallucinations. Personality changes occur and the sense of time and space is affected. Lysergide has been used to assist psychotherapy of neurotic patients, including obsessional neuroses, character disorders and psychopaths. Latent schizophrenia may develop and depressive states occasionally develop leading to suicidal intent. The greatest danger of treatment lies in the production of a drug-dependent sociopathic individual, and the therapeutic use of lysergide is now condemned by many psychiatrists.

Maprotiline hydrochloride
(Ludiomil[R])
Maprotiline is a novel antidepressant in the dibenzobicyclo-octadiene group. It is one of sedative antidepressants and is used in doses of 20–150 mg daily. Side effects resemble those of tricyclic antidepressants with sedative properties.

Mebanazine
(Actomol[R])
A hydrazine derivative, mebanazine is an anti-depressant with monoamine oxidase inhibitor activity. Used for depression the dose is 5 mg bd to qds with a maximum daily dose of 30 mg. The usual maintenance dose is 5 mg bd or tds. For side effects, contra-indications and precautions see monoamine oxidase inhibitors.

Mebutamate
(Formerly available as Capla[R])
Related to meprobamate, mebutamate is a central nervous system depressant which has been used as a tranquillizer. The dose is 0·6–1·2 g daily in divided doses. Side effects include dizziness, headache, nausea and constipation.

Meclofenoxate hydrochloride
(Synonym centrophenoxine hydrochloride)
(Lucidril[R])
Meclofenoxate hydrochloride is a central nervous stimulant used in the treatment of confusional states in the elderly, anoxia of newborn, intoxication by alcohol or carbon monoxide. It has also been used in delirium tremens and depression. The dose is 300–400 mg tds but the oral dose does not take effect for 4–6 days. Intravenously or intramuscularly the dose is 250–500 mg. Side effects include agitation and insomnia.

Medazepam
(Nobrium[R])
Medazepam is a minor tranquillizer of the benzodiazepine (q.v.) group. It has potent anxiolytic activity and is used in anxiety, tension and psychosomatic disorders affecting the skin, cardiovascular, respiratory, or gastrointestinal systems. The usual dose is 5 mg tds with a further 5 mg nocte if insomnia is a problem. Tolerance is good. Side effects are rare, dose related and include fatigue and drowsiness.

Melitracene
(Trausabun[R])
A dihydroanthracene derivative used in the treatment of depression with anxiety in daily doses of 50–250 mg. Side effects reported include dryness of the mouth, palpitation, sweating, and fatigue. The place of this substance in clinical therapeutics has not yet been established.

Mepazine
SEE Pecazine

Mephenesin
(Myanesin[R] and Tolseram[R], mephenesin carbamate)
Having muscle relaxant, sedative and anxiolytic activity mephenesin is used in the treatment of anxiety, tension and insomnia. However, its therapeutic efficacy has not been firmly established. The dose is 0·5 –1 g one to six times daily after meals. Orally mephenesin has low

toxicity but lassitude, anorexia, nausea and vomiting may occur.
The somewhat longer acting carbamate (Tolseram[R]) has a dose of 1–3 g, three to five times daily after meals.

Mephenoxalone
(Available in the USA as:
Lenetran[R], Tranpoise[R], Trepidone[R])
A mild tranquillizer, mephenoxalone resembles meprobamate in its pharmacological activity. Used for the treatment of anxiety and tension, but ineffective in psychoses. The usual dose is 400 mg qds. Side effects include drowsiness, headache, dizziness, nausea and skin reactions.

Meprobamate
(Equanil[R], Mepavlon[R], Miltown[R])
Meprobamate is a mild tranquillizer having slight muscle relaxant properties. It is used for anxiety, nervous tension and insomnia in doses of 200–400 mg tds. For insomnia 400 mg nocte. Some patients show idiosyncrasy to meprobamate when skin reactions may be produced. There is an addiction risk and patients should be warned of the effects of their lowered tolerance to alcohol.

Mesoridazine
(Synonym: mesuridazine)
(Available in the USA as Serentil[R], Lidanar[R], Lidanil[R], Lidanor[R])
A phenothiazine, mesoridazine is a metabolite of thioridazine (q.v.). It is used in the treatment of chronic schizophrenia and depression. Doses of 75 mg daily, increased over five weeks to a maximum of 300 mg daily have been used. Side effects include parkinsonism, orthostatic hypotension, dyskinesia, sedation and agranulocytosis.

Mesuridazine
SEE Mesoridazine.

Metaxalone
(Available in the USA as Skelaxin[R], and Zorane[R])
Metaxalone is a muscle relaxant with anxiolytic and sedative properties similar to mephenesin having additional analgesic properties. The dose is 2·4–3·2 g daily for not more than 10 consecutive days. Because of the reported side effects including gastro-intestinal upsets, drowsiness, dizziness, blood disorders and abnormal liver function tests the use of less toxic drugs has been recommended.

Methadone hydrochloride
(Physeptone[R])
Methadone hydrochloride is a narcotic analgesic having a longer duration of action than morphine but with less sedative effect. It is used for the relief of severe pain and to control non-productive coughing. The side effects are generally mild but the danger of addiction should be borne in mind. Dose: 5–10 mg orally or subcutaneously.

Methamphetamine
SEE Methylamphetamine hydrochloride.

Methaqualone hydrochloride
(Melsedin[R], Quaalude[R], Sedaquin[R], Mequelon[R], Tuazole[R], Paxidorm[R], Revonal[R])
(A constituent of Mandrax[R] and Matthodorm[R])
Melsed[R] contains methaqualone base.
Methaqualone is a hypnotic producing sleep of 6 to 10 hours duration. It is used in insomnia and as a daytime sedative. The usual hypnotic dose is 150 mg and for daytime sedation 75 mg bd or tds. Anticonvulsant action is also claimed. Side effects include gastric upsets, headache and hang-over effects. The drug has been liable to abuse.
SEE ALSO Mandrax[R] and Matthodorm[R].

Metharbitone
(Metharbital[R])
Metharbitone is a long-acting barbiturate with weak hypnotic activity but potent anticonvulsive properties. It is used in the treatment of grand and petit mal. The dose is 100 mg tds but due to tolerance up to 800 mg daily to control seizures may be required.
The side effects and contra-indications are as for barbiturates (q.v.).

Methiomeprazine
A phenothiazine derivative with anti-anxiety properties possibly useful in chronic alcoholism. The place of this substance in clinical therapeutics has not yet been established.

Methotrimeprazine maleate
(Synonyms: laevopromazine, levomepromazine)
(Veractil[R], Neurocil[R], Minozinan[R], Levoprome[R], Nozinan[R])
Methotrimeprazine is a phenothiazine used in the treatment of psychotic illnesses as an alternative to chlorpromazine (q.v.), but additionally it has been used in the treatment of moderate depression. It may be given alone or with analgesics or narcotics for the relief of pain and anxiety. The usual ambulatory dose is 10–15 mg tds or qds, increasing slowly to the most effective dose. The most common side effects are drowsiness and hypotension. Extrapyramidal symptoms and tachycardia occur less than with chlorpromazine, but a few cases, some fatal, of agranulocytosis have occurred.

Methoxypromazine maleate
(Tentone[R], USA)
A phenothiazine derivative, methoxypromazine has actions and uses similar to those of chlorpromazine hydrochloride (q.v.) Dose: 10–125 mg tds or qds.

Methperine sulphate
SEE Modaline sulphate.

Methylamphetamine hydrochloride
(Synonym: methamphetamine).
(Methedrine[R], Bophen[R] and Pervitin[R])
Methylamphetamine has the same actions and uses as amphetamine sulphate (q.v.), but it has a more rapid and prolonged action. Methedrine[R] is supplied only to hospitals, as a precaution against abuse, and is used to restore blood pressure during surgery and for abreaction in psychiatric diagnosis. Dose: 10–30 mg intravenously. For side effects and contra-indications see amphetamines (q.v.).

Methylpentynol
(Oblivon[R], Insomnol[R])
Methylpentynol has anxiolytic and hypnotic properties with a rapid but short action lasting about 3 hours. As a tranquillizer the dose is 250–500 mg, while the hypnotic dose is 0·5–1·0 g. Although methylpentynol seldom produces side effects, repeated use may induce toxic skin and liver reactions. Errors of judgement may be produced and the patient should be advised not to drive.

Methylpentynol Carbamate
Oblivon-C[R] has the same uses as methylpentynol but has a longer duration of action. As a sedative the dose is 200 mg tds and for hypnosis the dose is 200–600 mg.

Methylperidol
(Luvatren[R])
(Synonym: Moperon)
Methylperidol is a butyrophenone derivative with antipsychotic properties used mainly in the treatment of chronic schizophrenia. The usual daily dose is 15–30 mg and side effects include extrapyramidal symptoms.

Methylperone
(Buranil[R])
A butyrophenone derivative effective in severe agitation, mania and schizophrenia at a daily dose of 75–300 mg. The main side effects are drowsiness and the extrapyramidal syndrome.

Methylphenobarbitone
(Prominal[R])
Methylphenobarbitone has a more pronounced anti-convulsant action and less marked hypnotic action than phenobarbitone (q.v.). It is used in the treatment of epilepsy when the average dose is between 400–600 mg daily. Its side effects and contra-indications are as for barbiturates (q.v.) generally.

Methyl phenidate hydrochloride
(Ritalin[R])
Methyl phenidate hydrochloride is a central nervous stimulant resembling the activity of amphetamine (q.v.) but with little action on the appetite, blood pressure, heart rate, or respiration. It is used to improve mental activity, to relieve mild depression and fatigue, and is of value in treating lassitude and exhaustion following debilitating illness. The usual dose is 20 mg bd or tds. Side effects are as for amphetamines (q.v.), but are less pronounced and occur less frequently. Contra-indications include patients with agitation and hyperexcitability, and it should be used cautiously with pressor or hypertensive drugs.

Methyprylone
(Nodular[R])
A piperidinedione derivative, methyprylone is a central nervous depressant with sedative and hypnotic properties which last about 6 hours. It is used in mild or moderate insomnia and as a daytime sedative. Sedative dose: 50–100 mg tds or qds, hypnotic dose: 200–400 mg nocte. Methyprylone has about half the acute toxicity of phenobarbitone and is generally well tolerated. Minor side effects include dizziness, nausea, vomiting, headache and diarrhoea.

Methysergide
(Desiril[R], Sansert[R])
Methysergide is a serotonin antagonist and is used as a prophylactic in migraine. It is not recommended for treatment of acute attack. Dose: 1–2 mg bd or tds. Side effects resemble those of ergot (q.v.) and include nausea, gastric disorders, dizziness, lassitude and drowsiness. Inflammatory fibrosis in various areas, vascular reaction including arterial spasm may also occur. Contra-indications include peripheral vascular disease, phlebitis, impaired liver and kidney function and heart disease. Regular clinical supervision of patients under treatment is essential.

Modaline sulphate
(Synonym: methperine sulphate).
An antidepressant of the monoamine oxidase inhibitor group, modaline has actions, uses, and side effects as described for monoamine oxidase inhibitors (q.v.). It has been given in a dosage equivalent to 10–30 mg of modaline base tds.

Moperon
SEE Methylperidol

Morphine
(Duramorph[R])
The principal alkaloid of opium, morphine is a narcotic analgesic also having central stimulant action. It is used for the relief of severe pain, as a hypnotic where sleeplessness is due to pain, the arrest of haemorrhagic shock, the checking of peristalsis, the suppression of cough and the relief of anxiety and apprehension. Morphine produces euphoria and tolerance is rapidly acquired. There is a danger of addiction and it should therefore be used with discrimination. Dose: 8 to 20 mg. Toxic effects in large doses include coma, with slow respiration, cyanosis, hypotension. In smaller doses nausea, vomiting, tremors, constipation and miosis occur.

Nalorphine hydrobromide
(Lethidrone[R])
Nalorphine is a narcotic antagonist which in small doses counteracts most of the characteristic actions of morphine-like drugs, especially respiratory depression, without appreciably altering the analgesic effect. Nalorphine is used as an antidote in the treatment of overdosage produced by narcotic analgesics (q.v.). Dose: 5–10 mg intravenously, repeated according to patient's needs to a total dose not exceeding 40 mg. Side effects seldom occur but drowsiness, irritability, hypotension, and sweating may arise.

Nealbarbitone
(Censedal[R], Nevental[R])
Nealbarbitone is a member of the intermediate acting barbiturates and has slight anti-convulsant properties similar to phenobarbitone. It is used as a daytime sedative for anxiety and tension, in phobic and psychotic states, and it is claimed to rarely produce drowsiness. Dose: 60 to 200 mg tds, adjusting to the patient's needs. Toxic effects and contra-indications are those of the barbiturates (q.v.).

Nialamide
(Niamid[R])
Nialamide is an anti-depressant of the monoamine oxidase inhibitor group. It is used in treating reactive, mixed and psychotic depressive states. Dose: 25 mg. – 100 mg tds. Side effects and contra-indications are as for the monoamine oxidase inhibitors (q.v.).

Nitrazepam
(Mogadon[R], Mogadan[R])
Nitrazepam is a benzodiazepine derivative with hypnotic properties. It is used for insomnia and sleep disturbance due to anxiety, tension, depression, overwork or conflict. The dose is 5–10 mg prn. Unlike other hypnotics nitrazepam does not enforce sleep by generalised depression of the brain, but induces sleep lasting six to eight hours by blocking some inflow areas.

The safety of nitrazepam is good; over-dosage up to 70 times the normal dose has produced no harmful effects. Side effects or hang-over occur only very rarely.

Nortriptyline hydrochloride
(Allegron[R], Aventyl[R], Altilev[R], Acetexa[R], Noritren[R], Nortrilen[R], Sensival[R])
Nortriptyline is a dibenzocycloheptadiene derivative chemically very similar to amitriptyline (q.v.). It has anti-depressant properties, and uses, side effects and contra-indications similar to those of amitriptyline. Dose: 25 mg tds or qds, to 50 mg tds.

Noxiptyline
(Agedal[R])
A dibenzocycloheptadiene derivative, noxiptyline is used in simple depression or in mixed anxiety with depression. Efficacy is reported to be similar to amitriptyline (q.v.). The average daily dose is 120–200 mg. Side effects include dryness of the mouth, tremor of fingers, vertigo, disturbed binocular vision, sweating, and disturbance of micturition.

Opipramol hydrochloride
(Insidon[R])
An iminostilbene derivative, opipramol possesses sedative and mild anti-depressant properties. It is used in the treatment of mild depression and emotional fatigue resulting from anxiety and tension. Dose: initial, 50 mg tds; maintenance, 50 mg bd. Side effects include nausea, giddiness, and dryness of the mouth. It should not be given concurrently with or within two to three weeks of cessation of therapy with monamine oxidase inhibitors.

Orphenadrine
(as the hydrochloride – Disipal[R],
(as the citrate – Norflex[R])
Orphenadrine has an inhibitory effect on the cerebral motor areas and also produces a euphoriant effect. It is used in the symptomatic treatment of paralysis agitans relieving rigidity but having little effect on tremors. An initial 50 mg tds dose is adjusted according to the response and side effects. Up to 100 mg qds may be used. The side effects are mild atropine-like effects which tend to disappear as tolerance develops.
It may be given in conjunction with phenothiazines, butyrophenones, or thioxanthenes to control the extrapyramidal side effects produced by these drugs in higher doses.

Oxanamide
(Quiactin[R])
Oxanamide has anxiolytic properties with actions similar to meprobamate (q.v.) with some additional muscle relaxant properties. It is used in the treatment of anxiety and tension. Dose: 400 mg qds.

Oxazepam
(Serenid[R]-D., Adumbran[R], Anxiolit[R], Praxiten[R], Serox[R], Serepax[R], Seresta[R])
A benzodiazepine, oxazepam is chemically closely related to chlordiazepoxide (q.v.). It has anxiolytic properties and is used in the treatment of anxiety, tension and agitation. Dose: 15–30 mg tds. Side effects and contra-indications are as for chlor-diazepoxide.

Oxilapine
Oxilapine is a dibenzthiazepine derivative having anxiolytic activity. It is not yet established in clinical practice.

Oxycodone pectinate
(Proladone[R])
Oxycodone is a narcotic analgesic used for the control of post-operative pain and inoperable cancer. It is effective intra-muscularly for about 10 hours. Dose: 5–15 mg every eight to twelve hours. Side effects and contra-indications are as for morphine (q.v.).

Oxypendyl
(Pervetral[R])
A substituted phenothiazine with anti-psychotic activity. The place of this substance in clinical therapeutics has not yet been established.

Oxypertine hydrochloride
(Integrin[R])
Oxypertine, a butyrophenone derivative, is a tranquillizer used in the treatment of schizophrenia, particularly in withdrawn or apathetic patients. Dose: 40 mg bd or tds. Used in anxiety neuroses the dose is 10 mg tds or qds. Side effects include drowsiness, dry mouth and dizziness. It should not be given concurrently with or within two or three weeks of cessation of

treatment with a monoamine oxidase inhibitor. Blood counts and liver function tests are desirable for patients on long term dosage.

Papaverine hydrochloride
(Available as a component of: Hypersin[R], Monotrean[R], Placadol[R])
An opium alkaloid, papaverine has no analgesic or hypnotic actions. It is used as an anti-spasmodic to produce relaxation of involuntary muscle in peripheral vascular disease, coronary spasm, intestinal, ureteric and biliary colic, and dysmenorrhoea. Dose: 60–300 mg orally. Side effects include cardiac arrhythmias. It should be used cautiously intravenously owing to its action on cardiac muscle.

Paraldehyde
Paraldehyde has a depressant effect on the nervous system similar to that produced by chloral hydrate (q.v.). It acts as a sedative and hypnotic. It induces sleep of about eight hours duration and is useful as a sedative in the treatment of status epilepticus and in the control of delirium tremens. The dose is 5–10 ml by mouth or by intramuscular injection, and 15–30 ml by rectal injection. Side effects include erythematous rash and gastric irritation. It is contra-indicated in gastro-enteritis, broncho-pulmonary disease, and hepatic insufficiency. Paraldehyde decomposes on storage and deaths have occurred from the use of such material. It must not be used if it has a brownish colour or an odour of acetic acid.

Pargyline
(Eutonyl[R])
Pargyline is a monoamine oxidase inhibitor with a pronounced orthostatic hypotensive action and negligible anti-depressant effect. It is used mainly in the treatment of benign hypertension. Dose: 10–50 mg od increasing according to the patient's needs. Side effects and contra-indications are as for monamine oxidase inhibitors (q.v.). Additionally pargyline is contra-indicated in severe myocardial ischaemia, uraemia, renal failure, pyloric stenosis, glaucoma, and shock or severe haemorrhage.

Pecazine hydrochloride
(Pacatal[R], Laevmin[R])
A phenothiazine derivative, pecazine is a tranquillizer with actions and uses similar to chlorpromazine (q.v.).
Being less potent than chlorpromazine it produces less side-effects. The concomitant use of chlorpromazine and pecazine produces fewer side-effects than an equal use of either drug alone. Dose: 50–400 mg daily, in divided doses.

Pemoline
(Kethamed[R], Ronyl[R], Volital[R], Deltamine[R], Hyton[R], Pioxol[R], Stimul[R])
A central nervous stimulant, pemoline is used in the treatment of fatigue, epilepsy complicated by lethargy, drowsiness, and reactive depression. It is claimed to stimulate respiration depressed by morphine and to shorten barbiturate anaesthesia. Dose: 10–20 mg tds. Side effects in large doses include nervousness and tachycardia. If given in the evening insomnia is likely.

Pentazocine
(Fortral[R])
Pentazocine is a benzmorphan with narcotic analgesic properties, having a potency between that of morphine and codeine. The usual oral dose is 25 mg to 100 mg. every 3 to 4 hours after meals or im 30 mg tds. Side effects include nausea, vomiting, dizziness and drowsiness. Sweating, vertigo, tachycardia and hypertension may also occur. In larger doses hallucinations and delusions may result together with feelings of depersonalization. However a low addiction potential is likely.
Contra-indications include respiratory disease, raised intracranial pressure, head injury, convulsive states, hypertension, hepatic and renal disease. It is not recommended for children under 12.

Penthrichloral
(Clorased[R], Danuctene[R])
Penthrichloral has sedative and hypnotic properties similar to those of chloral hydrate but it is more palatable and causes less gastric irritation. Side effects and contra-indications are as for chloral hydrate (q.v). Dose: 0·5–1 g.

Pentobarbitone sodium
(Nembutal[R], and in combinations)
Pentobarbitone sodium is a short-acting barbiturate having hypnotic and anticonvulsant activity. It is used in insomnia, as a basal hypnotic prior to anaesthesia, and as an obstetric amnesiant. As an anticonvulsant it is used to control seizures due to chorea, eclampsia, tetanus, and strychnine or picrotoxin poisoning. Relaxation and hypnosis occur in about a minute. Dose: 100–200 mg. Side effects and contra-indications are as for barbiturates.

Perazine
(Taxilan[R])
Perazine is a phenothiazine tranquillizer with actions and uses similar to those of chlorpromazine (q.v.), but with a more pronounced anti-emetic effect. It is used in the treatment of schizophrenia in doses varying from 75 to 600 mg daily. Side effects include extra-pyramidal symptoms.

Pericyazine
(Synonym propericiazine).
(Neulactil[R], Aolept[R])
Pericyazine is a phenothiazine derivative with actions and uses similar to chlorpromazine (q.v.). It is used in the treatment of schizophrenia and behaviour disorders in severe psychiatric illness. It is also effective in the treatment of severe anxiety and tension states. Dose: 5–90 mg according to the condition under treatment. Side effects include extra-pyramidal effects, drowsiness, postural hypotension, and tachycardia. Other side effects and contra-indications are as chlorpromazine.

Perphenazine
(Synonym: chlorperphenazine)
(Fentazin[R], Decentan[R], Trilafon[R])
(Also a constituent of Triptafen[R])
A phenothiazine derivative, perphenazine has actions and uses similar to those of chlorpromazine (q.v.), but is effective in smaller doses. It produces sedation without hypnosis and has little effect on the blood pressure. It is an effective anti-emetic. Perphenazine is used chiefly in the treatment of anxiety, tension, psychomotor activity, nausea, and vomiting. In anxiety and tension the dose is 2 mg tds. In psychotic states, 8–16 mg tds or qds. Side effects are as for chlorpromazine and include extra-pyramidal dysfunction, drowsiness, dryness of the mouth. Contra-indications are as for chlorpromazine.
SEE ALSO Triptafen[R]–DA.

Pethidine hydrochloride
Pethidine hydrochloride is a narcotic analgesic which relieves most types of pain. Pethidine analgesia lasts two to five hours. Usually 100 mg intramuscularly is effective, but 200 mg may be given. It is used for obstetric analgesia and as an adjunct in nitrous oxide/oxygen anaesthesia. Side effects include dizziness, perspiration, dry mouth, nausea, and vomiting, but are less frequent than with morphine (q.v.). Pethidine is contra-indicated in severe liver disease, head injuries, and should not be used with some monoamine oxidase inhibitors.
Its use is accompanied by euphoria and addiction may occur, which in severe cases is as difficult to break as morphine addiction. As tolerance develops doses as large as 3–4 g daily may be taken by addicts, at which doses muscle twitching, tremor, mental confusion, hallucination and sometimes convulsions may be present, and occasionally death has occurred. The abstinence syndrome (q.v.) is similar to that of morphine abstinence but appears more readily. Addiction is treated as for morphine addiction (q.v.).

Petrichloral
(Periclor[R])
Petrichloral is a chloral hydrate derivative. It has similar sedative and hypnotic properties to chloral hydrate (q.v.) but is more palatable and causes less gastric irritation. Dose: as a daytime sedative, 300 mg, qds, as a hypnotic, 0·5 –1 g nocte.

Phenaglycodol
(Ultran[R], Sinforil[R], Acalo[R])
Phenaglycodol is a weak central nervous system depressant which has tranquillizing properties. It is used for the relief of anxiety and depression. Dose 0·8–1·2 g daily, in four to six divided doses. Side effects include drowsiness and dizziness.

Phenazocine hydrobromide
(Narphen[R])
Phenazocine is a narcotic analgesic with similar actions and uses to morphine (q.v.) but it is effective in smaller doses, acts quicker and its effects last longer. It is used

pre-operatively as an adjunct to anaesthesia or post-operatively. The usual dose is 1–3 mg intramuscularly, or 5 mg orally. Its effects last about six hours. Side effects resemble those of morphine although phenazocine has less sedative effect and causes less constipation. Contra-indications are as for morphine.

Phencyclidine hydrochloride
(Available in the USA as Sernyl[R] and Sernylan[R])
Phencyclidine is a potent analgesic and anaesthetic which is said not to cause depression of cardio-vascular and respiratory functions. When given intravenously in doses of 0·2 mg per Kg an amnesic trance-like state with analgesia is produced. The chief disadvantage of phencyclidine is the small difference between the effective and toxic dose. The toxic effects include hallucinations, agitation, and catatonic rigidity and inco-ordination. It has also been used in the treatment of psycho-neuroses and to assist psychtherapy in obsessional illness.

Phendimetrazine tartrate
(Available in the USA as Plegine[R] and in Canada as Dietrol)
Phendimetrazine is a central nervous stimulant used as an anorectic in the treatment of obesity in doses of 17·5 – 70 mg bd or tds, one hour before meals. Side-effects as for amphetamine sulphate. Other side effects include glossitis, stomatitis, constipation and abdominal cramps. Contra-indications as for amphetamine sulphate (q.v.).

Phenelzine sulphate
(Nardil[R])
Phenelzine sulphate is a monoamine oxidase inhibitor with anti-depressant activity. The usual dose is the equivalent of 15 mg of the base, tds or qds. Side effects and contra-indications are as for monoamine oxidase inhibitors (q.v.).

Phenmetrazine hydrochloride
(Preludin[R])
A sympathomimetic, phenmetrazine has less stimulant action on the central nervous system than amphetamine (q.v.). It has a potent anorectic action and is used in the treatment of obesity. Dose: 25 mg bd or tds, half an hour before meals. Side-effects are slight, but similar to those of amphetamine sulphate. Because large doses and prolonged treatment may lead to addiction treatment should be limited to one month. Contra-indications include severe hypotension, thyrotoxicosis and acute coronary disease.

Phenobarbitone
(Gardenal[R], Luminal[R], Phenobarbitone Spansule[R])
Phenobarbitone is a long-acting barbiturate, used as a sedative, hypnotic and anti-convulsant. In the treatment of anxiety and psychosomatic conditions the dose ranges from 30–120 mg daily with a maximum of 600 mg in 24 hrs.
Drowsiness and sedation accompany daytime use and following hypnotic use hangover effects are commonly reported.
The chief danger lies in a cumulative action on regular administration which may result in chronic poisoning.
The action, side effects and contra-indications are as for barbiturates (q.v.) generally.

Phenoperidine hydrochloride
(Operidine[R])
Phenoperidine is a narcotic analgesic with similar actions to morphine (q.v.). It provides analgesic supplement in conjunction with the neuroleptic droperidol in anaesthesia. It is also used in cases of prolonged assisted ventilation where it acts as a respiratory depressant and analgesic.

Phenoxypropazine maleate
(Drazine[R]) Now discontinued.
Phenoxypropazine is a monoamine oxidase inhibitor with antidepressant activity. It is a potent antidepressant, but serious side-effects including hepatotoxicity outweighed the advantages of effectiveness and the drug is no longer available. The usual dose was 10 mg bd. For general toxic-effects and contra-indications see monoamine oxidase inhibitors.

Phenprobamate
(Gamaquil[R])
Phenprobamate is a carbinol derivative showing muscle relaxant, anti-convulsant and tranquillizer properties. Dose: 400–800 mg tds. It is used in the treatment of

anxiety and tension and side effects include disturbances of coordination.

Phenylmethylbarbituric acid
(Rutonal[R])
Phenylmethylbarbituric acid is used as an anti-convulsant and in epilepsy like phenobarbitone, but has half the potency of phenobarbitone as an hypnotic. Dose: up to 200 mg five times daily.

Pimozide
(Orap[R])
Pimozide is a diphenylbutylpiperidine with antipsychotic activity used in the treatment of schizophrenia with the exception of the manic phase. Pimozide's long action enables a single daily dose, initially 2–4 mg increasing to 10 mg as necessary. The usual dose is 6 mg daily. Side effects include extrapyramidal effects, rashes and occasionally glycosuria. Pimozide is contra-indicated in endogenous depression, pre-existing Parkinsonism or epilepsy.

Pipamazine
(Mornidine[R])
Pipamazine is a phenothiazine derivative with actions similar to those of chlorpromazine (q.v.), but having less potent tranquillizing activity than chlorpromazine it is no longer used for this purpose. Side effects and contra-indications as for chlorpromazine. Dose: 5 mg every four hours.

Pipethanate hydrochloride
(Sycotrol[R])
Pipethanate hydrochloride is a minor tranquillizer. Since it also has peripheral anticholinergic activity it is used in the treatment of anxiety and tension associated with psychosomatic conditions and senile paraesthesia. Dose: 3–6 mg tds. Side effects include drowsiness.

Pipradol hydrochloride
(Available in the USA as Meratran[R])
Pipradol is a central nervous stimulant which increases mental activity without causing after depression. It produces less anorexia, insomnia and euphoria than amphetamine (q.v.) and has little effect on blood pressure, heart rate and respiration. It is used in the treatment of depression without anxiety and in narcolepsy. Dose: 2 mg tds. Overdoses may cause nausea, anorexia, anxiety and insomnia. It should be avoided when tension and agitation are present.

Piritamide
(Dipidolor[R])
Piritamide is a parenteral narcotic analgesic effective in severe pain. The maximum daily dose is 80 mg. It is metabolized in the liver and care should be exercised in patients with hepatic disorders. Although not yet recorded, dependence may be anticipated.

Pizotifan maleate
A thienobenzocycloheptene, pizotifan is a serotonin, tryptamine, histamine and acetylcholine antagonist used in the treatment of migraine and which has reported to show antidepressant activity. The dose ranges between 0·5–3 mg daily. Side effects include drowsiness, venous thrombosis, peripheral paraesthesia. Disturbances of reality have also been reported.
The place of pizotifan in therapeutics is not yet established.

Prazepam
Prazepam is a benzodiazepine derivative having tranquillizing, anti-convulsant and muscle relaxant actions. It has been used as an anxiolytic and particular effectiveness is claimed in somatised anxiety. The usual dose is 20 mg tds and side effects include drowsiness, dizziness and mild nausea. The exact value of prazepam in therapy is yet to be established.

Prochlorperazine
(Stemetil[R], Compazine[R], Tementil[R])
Prochlorperazine is a phenothiazine derivative having a more potent tranquillizing activity than chlorpromazine (q.v.) It is used in mild to moderate anxiety, tension and agitation in doses of 5–10 mg tds or qds. For psychotic disorders 5–25 mg tds or qds is given. Prochlorperazine is effective in Ménière's syndrome and labyrinthitis when 5–10 mg tds or qds is given. It has less sedative effect than chlorpromazine but it gives rise to extrapyramidal symptoms more frequently and in greater intensity. Contra-indications as chlorpromazine (q.v.).

Proheptatriene
A dibenzocycloheptatriene derivative which is reputed to have anti-depressant activity equivalent to or better than that of other trycyclic compounds. Further assessment is required and the preparation is not yet commercially available.

Promazine
(Sparine[R], Prazine[R], Verophen[R])
(Also a constituent of Tofranil[R] with Promazine)
A phenothiazine closely related to chlorpromazine (q.v.) promazine is less potent and less liable to produce toxic side effects such as jaundice and severe hypotension. It is used as a tranquillizer in psychotic conditions, in senile agitation, alcoholism, and as an anti-emetic. Dose: 50 mg tds. Side effects include dizziness and drowsiness. Epileptic fits are provoked more often than with other phenothiazines. Contra-indications as for chlorpromazine.
SEE ALSO Tofranil[R] with Promazine

Promethazine hydrochloride
(Phenergan[R], Atosil[R], Prothazin[R])
(Also a constituent of Protamyl[R])
Promethazine is an antihistamine, particularly effective in the treatment of urticaria and motion sickness. It has pronounced sedative effects and is used as a short acting hypnotic in psychiatric practice, and as an anxiolytic in anxiety and tension. It also possesses anticholinergic properties and is used in the treatment of parkinsonism. Dose: 25 mg, od, bd or tds. Side effects include those of the antihistamines generally. Jaundice and agranulocytosis have been reported. Contra-indications include patients with hepatic disease.
SEE ALSO Protamyl[R].

Propanolol hydrochloride
(Inderal[R])
Propanolol is a beta-adrenergic receptor blocking drug which is effective in reducing the somatic manifestations of anxiety. It has its greatest value in those patients showing maximum somatic symptomatology at a dosage of 80–160 mg/day. Side effects are uncommon but in patients at special risk, cardiac failure and bronchospasm may occur.

Propericiazine
SEE Pericyazine.

Propiomazine
(Indorm[R])
Propiomazine, a phenothiazine derivative, is a central nervous depressant. It is used as a sedative or hypnotic. Dose: 10–20 mg. Side effects include dry mouth, gastro-intestinal upset, allergic rash, occasional mild mental confusion, and nightmares. Care should be exercised when used with other central nervous depressants.

Prothipendyl hydrochloride
(Tolnate[R], Dominal[R])
Prothipendyl is an azaphenothiazine derivative with anxiolytic, sedative and anti-emetic properties. It is used to treat anxiety and agitation in psychoneuroses and psychoses. It is also used as a hypnotic in insomnia and as a sedative in surgical premedication. Dose: 20 mg bd–qds. Side effects may include dry mouth, abdominal discomfort, and drowsiness. More serious side effects include photosensitivity and epilepsy. Tachycardia and hypotension may occur at higher dosages.

Protriptyline
(Concordin[R], Maximed[R], Triptil[R])
A dibenzocycloheptatriene derivative, protriptyline is chemically closely related to amitriptyline, having similar anti-depressant activity. It is used in psychotic and reactive depression, the dose range being 5–15 mg tds or qds. For maintenance the dosage should be reduced to the smallest necessary. Common side effects include restlessness, tachycardia, excitement, and anticholinergic effects. It is contra-indicated in predisposition to urinary retention and glaucoma. Caution is necessary when used with adrenergic blocking agents, and it should not be administered with or within 2–3 weeks of cessation of treatment with monoamine oxidase inhibitors (q.v.).

Pyrovalerone
Pyrovalerone is an anti-depressant compound. The place of this substance in clinical therapeutics has not yet been established.

Quinalbarbitone
(Seconal Sodium[R], Quinalspan[R])
Quinalbarbitone is a short-acting barbiturate used in simple insomnia and anxiety states in doses of up to 100 mg

tds. Side effects and contra-indications are as for barbiturates (q.v.).

Reserpine
(Serpasil[R], Rausedan[R], Reserpin[R], Sedaraupin[R])
Reserpine is a Rauwolfia alkaloid (q.v.) with central depressant and sedative action and an anti-hypertensive effect. It is used for its sedative action in mild anxiety states and chronic psychoses. Dose in mild anxiety states, 0·5 to 2 mg. and in severe psychoses, 2 –3 mg od or bd. Side effects include nasal congestion, lethargy, drowsiness and gastro-intestinal upset. Higher doses may cause insomnia, bradycardia, parkinsonian-like syndrome and severe depression which may lead to suicide.
It is contra-indicated in anxiety depressive states, in gastric ulcer, and in cardiac damage.

Spiroperidol
Spiroperidol is a butyrophenone derivative with anti-psychotic activity particularly useful in schizophrenia. The usual daily dose is 0·3 mg to 0·9 mg. Side effects include extra-pyramidal symptoms, perspiration, dry mouth, hypotension, and urinary retention.

Sulphonal
Sulphonal is now seldom prescribed, but it was formerly used as a hypnotic for producing prolonged sleep in psychiatric cases and in nervous insomnia. Sulphonal is slowly excreted and has a cumulative effect which makes it one of the most dangerous hypnotics. Side effects include gastric disturbances, liver damage and the formation of methaemoglobin. Dose: 0·3 to 1·2 g. Contra-indicated in heart disease.

Temazepam
Temazepam is a benzodiazepine with anxiolytic properties. It has been used as a tranquillizer but its place in therapeutics is not yet established.

Tetrabenazine
(Nitoman[R])
Tetrabenazine has central effects similar to those of reserpine (q.v.), but its action is more rapid and of shorter duration. It causes depletion of serotonin (q.v.), dopamine (q.v.) and noradrenaline (q.v.) in brain tissue, but not peripherally. It has been used in the treatment of acute and chronic mental disorders. More recently it has found successful use in hyperkinesia and Huntingdon's chorea (q.v.). Toxic effects include Parkinsonism, agitation and suicidal depression. Dose: 25–50 mg bd or tds. Contra-indicated with or immediately after a course of monoamine oxidase inhibitors.

Tetraethylthiuram disulphide
SEE Disulfiram.

Thalidomide
Preparations previously marketed in the UK or abroad included:
Algosedir, Asmaval, Calmorex, Contergan, Countergan Forte, Distaval, Distaval Forte, Enterosedir, Gastrimide, Grippex, Imida-Lab, Imidan, Imidene, Kevadon, Lulamin, Neosedyn, Pentosedir, Peracon-Expectorans, Polygripan, Predni-Sedir, Profarmil, Quetimiol, Quietoplex, Sedalis, Sedi-Lab, Sedimide, Sedoval K–17, Softenon, Softenon Forte, Talimol, Tensival, Theophyl-choline, Ulcerfen, Valgis, and Valgraine.
A piperidinedione derivative, Thalidomide was an effective hypnotic available in the United Kingdom in 1958. In November 1961 the first report of teratogenic effects appeared and in December 1961 it was withdrawn from the British market.
When given during the first trimester of pregnancy, inhibition of limb bud development in the foetus was likely.
Thalidomide has been shown to have immunosuppressive activity and it has therefore also been used in the treatment of cancer and of lepra reactions.

Thialbarbitone sodium
(Kemithal[R], Sodium)
Thialbarbitone sodium is a very short-acting barbiturate about half as potent as thiopentone sodium, but with a similar duration of action. It is used as a basal narcotic producing anaesthesia of short or long duration intravenously. Respiratory depression is said to be less than with other intravenous barbiturates and laryngeal spasm occurs less. General side effects and contra-indications are as for barbiturates (q.v.).

Thiopropazate hydrochloride
(Dartalan[R], Dartal[R] and in combinations Tonoquil[R] and Vesitan[R])
A phenothiazine derivative, thiopropazate has actions and uses similar to those of chlorpromazine (q.v.), but it is effective in smaller doses. It is used in the treatment of psychoses where agitation and aggressiveness predominate. It is used for psychoneuroses in anxiety states and as an anti-emetic and anti-nauseant. The dose is 5–10 mg tds. Side effects include blurring of vision, dryness of the mouth, hypotension, nasal congestion, and extrapyramidal symptoms. Contra-indications as for chlorpromazine.

Thioproperazine
(Majeptil[R], Vontil[R])
Thioproperazine is a phenothiazine derivative with tranquillizing activity similar to chlorpromazine (q.v.). Its sedative, hypotensive and hypothermic properties are less than those of chlorpromazine, but it has a much more potent anti-emetic action. It is used in the treatment of acute and chronic schizophrenia, mania, and delirium, and to control excitement and aggression. The dose is 10–30 mg tds. Side effects frequently include extrapyramidal disturbances, respiratory depression may occur and sweating, salivation and seborrhoea are severe. Contra-indications as for chlorpromazine.

Thioridazine hydrochloride
(Melleril[R], Mellerettes)
A phenothiazine derivative, thioridazine has anxiolytic activity and is used as a tranquillizer in anxiety tension, psychoneuroses, senile agitation and confusion, and behavioural disorders in children. The dose is 10–30 mg tds initially, increasing to 200 mg tds as required. It is less effective in schizophrenia than some other phenothiazines. Side effects are less than with most other phenothiazines. Extra-pyramidal effects are rare, and jaundice, agranulocytosis or severe dermititis are also rare. Drowsiness, dizziness and dry mouth may occur. It is contra-indicated in severely depressed or comatose states.

Thiothixene
(Navane[R], Orbinamon[R])
A thioxanthene derivative, thiothixene is an anti-psychotic agent which has been used in the treatment of schizophrenia. Dose: 10–30 mg daily. Contra-indications are circulatory collapse, coma, C.N.S. depression due to any cause and blood dyscrasias. It is not recommended for children under 12 years.

Tofenacin hydrochloride
(Elamol[R])
Tofenacin is a tricyclic antidepressant with mild sedative properties. It is administered in dosages up to 240 mg daily. Side effects are those of anticholinergic drugs.

Tolboxane
(Clarmil[R], Clarphoril[R])
A propanediol derivative showing muscle relaxant and anxiolytic properties. The place of this substance in clinical therapeutics has not yet been established.

Tranylcypromine
(Parnate[R])
Tranylcypromine is a monoamine oxidase inhibitor with anti-depressant properties. It is used in the treatment of severe mental depression. The initial dose is 10 mg bd. If there is no response after 2 to 3 weeks, the dose is increased to 10 mg tds. Hypertensive crisis is an occasional side effect, which may lead to intracranial haemorrhage. Other side effects and contra-indications are as for monoamine oxidase inhibitors (q.v.).

Triclofos sodium
(Tricloryl[R])
A chloral derivative, triclofos has similar sedative and hypnotic actions to chloral hydrate but it is more palatable and relatively free from the tendency to cause gastric irritation. The dose for daytime sedation is 500 mg od or bd the hypnotic dose is 1 g (2 g in some cases) nocte. Some gastric irritation and headache have been reported. Contra-indications as for chloral hydrate (q.v.).

Trifluperidol
(Triperidol[R], Psicoperidol[R])
A butyrophenone derivative, trifluperidol is a tranquillizer with properties similar to those of haloperidol (q.v.). It has been used in the treatment of schizophrenia and manic-depressive psychoses. The dose is, initially, 0·5 mg od, increasing by 0·5 mg

at three day intervals until the desired effect is achieved. Maintenance: 1·5–2·5 mg od. Side effects include hypotension, hyper-salivation, and effects similar to haloperidol. Contra-indications include pregnancy, neurological disorders exhibiting pyramidal or extra-pyramidal symptoms.

Trifluoperazine hydrochloride
(Stelazine[R], Amylozine Spansule[R], Eskazinyl[R], Jatronevral[R])
Trifluoperazine hydrochloride is a tranquillizer of the phenothiazine group. In low doses, 2–4 mg bd, it is used to treat anxiety states, nervous and emotional stress, senile agitation and confusion. At higher dosages, 5–10 mg bd or tds it is used to treat acute mania, delirium tremens and schizophrenia. Side effects include agitation, dizziness, drowsiness, insomnia and nasal congestion. Above 10 mg tds reversible extra-pyramidal symptoms are frequently produced. Blood dyscrasias have occasionally been reported. Contra-indications include existing blood dyscrasias, bone marrow depression, and liver damage.

Triflupromazine hydrochloride
(Formerly available in Great Britain as Vespral[R] Available in the USA as Vesprin[R])
Triflupromazine is a member of the phenothiazine group of tranquillizers, having actions and uses similar to those of chlorpromazine (q.v.). It has been used in the management of acute and chronic psychoses when hallucinations and delusions are prominent. Uses also include treatment of anxiety and tension. The dose is 10 to 50 mg depending on the severity of the condition. Side effects and contra-indications are as for chlorpromazine.

Trimetozine
(Trioxazine[R])
Trimetozine is a morpholine derivative used as a sedative and tranquillizer. Usual dose 300 mg. three to six times daily. Although few side effects are reported its weak anxiolytic activity has probably precluded widespread use.

Trimipramine
(Surmontil[R])
An iminodibenzyl derivative, trimipramine has anti-depressant properties resembling those of imipramine (q.v.). It is used in the treatment of all types of depression, particularly if associated with anxiety or agitation. The initial dose is 25 mg tds increased by 25 mg daily to 50 –100 mg tds. The usual maintenance dose is 25 mg bd to 50 mg tds. Side effects and contra-indications are as for imipramine.

Tybamate
(Benvil[R])
Chemically related to meprobamate (q.v.), tybamate is a minor tranquillizer used in the treatment of anxiety and tension. Dose: 1 tablet tds or qds. The sedative effects are less than those of meprobamate otherwise the side effects and contra-indications are as for meprobamate.

Valnoctamide
(Axiquel[R], Nirvanil[R])
Valnoctamide is a valeramide derivative having tranquillizing action reported to be of value in anxiety and tension. Dose: 400–800 mg daily in divided doses.

Viloxazine hydrochloride
(Vivalan[R])
Viloxazine is a novel antidepressant without sedative or anticholinergic side effects. It also possesses anti-epileptic properties. It is used at a daily dosage of 150–300 mg. Its place in therapy has not yet been thoroughly assessed.

The Concise Encyclopaedia of Psychiatry is based upon a series of publications sponsored under the Roche Continuing Medical Education campaign.
The contributors to the original series were:

K. Bergmann, MD, FRCPSYCH, DPM, Department of Psychological Medicine, Newcastle General Hospital, Newcastle upon Tyne

J. A. Bonn, MB, MRCP, MRCPSYCH, DPM, Department of Psychological Medicine, St Bartholomew's Hospital, London EC1

Valerie Cowie, MD, PHD, FRCPSYCH, DPM, Queen Mary's Hospital for Children, Carshalton, Surrey

A. D. Forrest, MD, MRCP, FRCPE, FRCPSYCH, DPM, Department of Psychiatry, University of Edinburgh

H. L. Freeman, MA, BM, FRCPSYCH, DPM, Psychiatry Department, Hope Hospital, Salford

Professor J. L. Gibbons, MD, FRCP, FRCPSYCH, DPM, Department of Psychiatry, The Medical School, Southampton University

P. J. Graham, MB, FRCP, FRCPSYCH, DPM, Department of Psychological Medicine, The Hospital for Sick Children, Great Ormond Street, London WC1

J. C. Gunn, MD, MRCPSYCH, DPM, Director of the Special Hospital Research Unit, Institute of Psychiatry, London SE5

Professor H. Gwynne Jones, BSC, FBPSS, Department of Psychology, University of Leeds

Professor R. A. Hinde, FRS, SCD, DPHIL, M.R.C. Unit on the Development and Integration of Behaviour, Sub-Department of Animal Behaviour, Madingley, University of Cambridge

J. Johnson, MD, FRCPE, FRCPSYCH, University Department of Psychiatry, Manchester Royal Infirmary

D. W. Kay, DM, FRCP, FRCPSYCH, DPM, Department of Psychiatry, University of Tasmania, Hobart, Tasmania

D. H. W. Kelly, MD, MRCP, FRCPSYCH, DPM, St George's Hospital, London SW1

Professor R. E. Kendell, MD, FRCP, MRCPSYCH, DPM, Department of Psychiatry, University of Edinburgh

M. H. Lader, MD, PHD, MRCPSYCH, CPM, Institute of Psychiatry, The Maudsley Hospital, London SE5

Denis Leigh, MD, BSC, FRCP, FRCPSYCH, The Maudsley Hospital, London SE5

C. McDonald, MD, MRCPSYCH, MANZCP, DPM, Warlingham Park Hospital, Surrey

J. Marks, MA, MD, FRCP, FRCPATH, MRCPSYCH, Downing College, University of Cambridge

C. M. B. Pare, MD, FRCP, FRCPSYCH, DPM, Department of Psychological Medicine, St Bartholomew's Hospital, London EC1

I. B. Pearson, MD, MRCPSYCH, DPM, University Department of Psychiatry, Mapperley Hospital, Nottingham

A. A. Robin, MD, FRCPSYCH, DPM, Runwell Hospital, Wickford, Essex

Professor J. R. Smythies, MA, MSC, MD, FRCP, FRCPSYCH, FAPA, DPM, School of Medicine, Birmingham, Alabama, USA

J. Stevenson, PHD, M.R.C. Unit on the Development and Integration of Behaviour, Madingley, University of Cambridge

D. C. Taylor, MD, MRCP, FRCPSYCH, DPM, Human Development Research Unit, The Park Hospital for Children, Headington, Oxford

J. M. Taylor, BPHARM, MPS, Bishop's Stortford, Hertfordshire

Professor J. P. Watson, MD, MRCP, MRCPSYCH, DPM, DCH, Guy's Hospital, London, SE1

D. Watt, BSC, MD, FRCPSYCH, DPM, St John's Hospital, Stone, Bucks

J. H. P. Willis, MB, FRCPE, FRCPSYCH, DPM, Department of Psychological Medicine, Guy's Hospital, London SE1

The editors wish to express their appreciation for the help provided by the original contributors. For the new book the editors have tried to bring the entries up to date and in consequence, take full responsibility for the opinions expressed.